Vestibular Rehabilitation
Second Edition

Contemporary Perspectives in Rehabilitation

Steven L. Wolf, PhD, FAPTA, Editor-in-Chief

Vestibular Rehabilitation
Second Edition

Susan J. Herdman, PT, PhD
Professor, Division of Physical Therapy,
   Dizziness and Balance Center
Department of Orthopaedics and Rehabilitation
University of Miami School of Medicine
Coral Gables, Florida

F. A. DAVIS COMPANY • **Philadelphia**

F. A. Davis Company
1915 Arch Street
Philadelphia, PA 19103

Printed in the United States of America

Last digit indicates print number: 10 9 8 7 6 5 4 3 2 1

Publisher, Health Professions: Jean-François Vilain
Developmental Editor: Christa Fratantoro
Production Editor: Stephen D. Johnson
Cover Designer: Louis J. Forgione

Library of Congress Cataloging-in-Publication Data
Vestibular rehabilitation / [edited by] Susan J. Herdman, — 2nd ed.
    p.   cm.
    Includes bibliographical references and index.
    ISBN 0-8036-0444-0 (alk. paper)
    1. Vestibular apparatus—Diseases. 2. Vestibular apparatus—Diseases—Treatment. 3. Vestibular apparatus—Diseases—Exercises therapy. 4. Vestibular apparatus—Diseases—Patients—Rehabilitation.
I. Herdman, Susan.
    [DNLM: 1.   Vestibular Diseases—rehabilitation.   WV 255 V5836
2000]
RF260.V4725   2000
617.8'82—dc21
DNLM/DLC
for Library of Congress   99-39686
                                                                                CIP

Foreword to the Second Edition

When we asked Susan Herdman to take on this project in the earlier part of this decade, I must admit that I had little concern about her expertise as a clinician/scientist and even less about her passion for rehabilitation of patients with vestibular disease. What concerned me was the uncertainty with which the rehabilitation community would embrace a text on this subject. After all, *vestibular rehabilitation* was something that many clinicians knew a little about but have scarcely studied. At the time, Susan was adamant about the emerging role of rehabilitation therapists in the treatment of patients with dizziness and accompanying sequelae because of vestibular impairments. Her enthusiasm was contagious and her premonitions accurate.

The first edition of *Vestibular Rehabilitation* is now seen by some as a guidebook and by others as the definitive text on the rehabilitation of vestibular disorders. In the 5 years since the first edition was published, Dr. Herdman's courses and certification procedures for competence in treating patients with the diagnoses embodied in this book have become legendary. In fact, many of the contributors to this new edition assist in teaching that course. Even more remarkable than the skill and reputation that Dr. Herdman brings to her work is her ability to anticipate those topics that still might be needed for students and clinicians to become more knowledgeable and better skilled in this specialty area.

The respect shown to Susan by her colleagues is manifest in this second edition. Most of the contributors from the first edition have been retained. They have done an admirable job in updating their references and concepts. This fact is not surprising. Drs. Hain, Horak, Shupert, Keshner, Zee, Fetter, Honrubia, Erskine, Tusa, Leigh, Maddox, Whitney, and Shumway-Cook are well respected in the fields of vestibular rehabilitation or otolaryngology, and one would expect nothing less than a comprehensive contemporization of their previous work. Dr. Herdman has overseen the updating of their materials and has found other outstanding contributors to address those topics not covered in the first edition. Consequently, an 18-chapter text has now been expanded to 25 contributions.

The seven new contributions include the following: one in the Medical Assessment section (Chapter 8, Assessment of Otolith Dysfunction by Drs. Halmagyi and Curthoys); one in the Medical Management section (Chapter 14, Psychological Problems and the Dizzy Patient by Dr. Tusa); and five in the Rehabilitation Assessment and Management section (Chapter 16, Disability in Vestibular Disorders by Dr. Cohen; Chapter 21, Cervical Vertigo by Dr. Clendaniel; Chapter 22, Management of the Elderly Person with Vestibular Dysfunction, Dr. Whitney; Chapter 23, Treatment of Patients with Nonvestibular Dizziness and Disequilibrium, by Dr. Shepard and Annamarie Asher, PT; and Chapter 25, Physical Therapy Diagnosis for Vestibular Disorders, by Dr. Herdman). Dr. Rine has rewritten Chapter 24 on assessment of children with vestibular disorders and postural dysregulation.

The contribution from G. M. Halmagyi and I. S. Curthoys provides insight into tests for otolith integrity including subjective visual-horizontal and vestibular-evoked myogenic potential measures. Ron Tusa reminds us that with persistent dizziness comes concurrent behavioral problems that must be identified and treated, and Helen Cohen provides a comprehensive review of existing enablement models and how we can objectively measure changes in task-directed vestibular patient abilities. Richard Clendaniel reviews the often-overlooked relationship between cervical spinal pathology and its interface to balance problems.

The second edition addresses the needs for vestibular system analyses and treatment for older adults. Sue Whitney reviews factors that contribute to imbalance in senior citizens and how such factors may be remediated. Specific checklists and assessment tools are also included. Neil Shepard and Annamarie Asher address the fact that people of all ages may acquire dizziness symptoms that are not of vestibular origin. They offer an interesting framework in which to screen patients for nonvestibular imbalance and provide treatment options and measures.

This edition closes with Dr. Herdman taking to heart the calling of her professional physical therapy colleagues. She has developed a chapter on physical therapy diagnosis for vestibular problems and guides the reader through a logical progression of deductive reasoning, including historical notation and application of clinical tests. A treatment plan can be derived from this approach. The exercise, appropriately referred to by Dr. Herdman as a "work in progress," is totally compatible with the *Guidelines to Physical Therapy Practice* (*Physical Therapy*, **77,** November 1997). In this regard, *Vestibular Rehabilitation* now becomes a forerunner for future clinical specialty texts that seek to inform within the context of professional practice.

As recently as 15 years ago we were advocating for inclusion of case studies and problem-solving approaches as the benchmark for defining clinical relevance in textbooks. We now seek to relate our emerging guidelines for practice to the thought processes that make us unique and essential to the rehabilitation process, including seeking and documenting evidence for our actions. We concluded the Foreword to the First Edition (1994) with the metaphor of a labor of love to foster the delivery of this book. We can now proudly say that the child has learned to walk unassisted and unencumbered by anyone's expectations but our own.

Stephen L. Wolf, PhD, FAPTA
Series Editor

Foreword to the First Edition

As scientists and clinicians we sometime marvel at how an apparently small and innocuous system of ossicles and semicircular canals, deeply embedded within the petrous portions of temporal cortical bone, can have such an intricate and profound influence on our ability to exist in an ever-changing environment. Yet as students and users of rehabilitation procedures, we spend little time learning about the complexities of the vestibular system. We know that intimate ties exist between the vestibular apparatus, our sense of "dizziness," and postural stability. Despite this knowledge, the use of exercise within a rehabilitative context is relatively new, and many health-related professionals are naive about both the rationales inherent in exercise protocols and their potential benefit as an adjunct to surgical or pharmacologic interventions. With these realities in mind, Susan Herdman, an experienced physical therapist with extensive clinical and research experience in vestibular system pathology, has assembled an expert team of researchers and clinicians to help fill the gaps in our knowledge of vestibular system pathophysiology and rehabilitative treatment options.

All the contributors are sensitive to the fact that few texts addressing this topic have been geared to the varied needs of rehabilitation personnel. Accordingly, this book is written with both student and clinician in mind. Dr. Herdman has carefully grouped the chapters into four sections covering, respectively: fundamentals, medical assessment, medical management, and rehabilitation. In this manner all readers can follow a logical progression from fundamental physiology to pathophysiologic occurrences following deafferentation, inflammatory disease, or trauma. Medical assessment issues are presented to acquaint (or reacquaint) the reader with typical methods for quantifying vestibular function and addressing concurrent auditory problems. The section on medical management offers rehabilitation providers insight into how physicians decide on pharmacologic or surgical interventions and medical treatments (including treatment of disorders related to migraine). Most important, and in keeping with the underlying philosophy of the Contemporary Perspectives in Rehabilitation series, several of these contributions contain case studies presented in a decision-making format so that the reader can "think along" with the clinician/author. This approach is most obvious in the remarkably comprehensive yet diversified section on rehabilitation assessment and management. The six chapters in this section, while filled with valuable clinical information, also challenge the clinician or student to think logically and deductively as master clinicians write about their treatment approaches to vestibular hypofunction, bilateral vestibular loss, benign paroxysmal positional vertigo, and vestibular pathology among traumatic brain-injured patients and in children with vestibular disorders. These contributions are heavily documented and offer many opportunities for applying the clinical experience bestowed in each chapter with case-study formats.

At the risk of flaunting the excellence embodied in this text, I can say unequivocally that this text is unparalleled in its breadth of content and sensitivity to the needs of its diversified readership. If the process of absorbing the context and fresh ideas in this very special but important area of rehabilitation spawns new ideas or yields treatment insights, this labor of love will have been well worth the many hours spent in its delivery.

Stephen L. Wolf, PhD, FAPTA
Series Editor

Preface to the Second Edition

During the 5 years since the publication of the First Edition of *Vestibular Rehabilitation*, we realized that we needed to extend the material presented to cover a wider range of problems than those associated with only clearly defined vestibular deficits. To address this awareness, the Second Edition includes seven new chapters. Four of these chapters address the management of migraine-related dizziness and vertigo, the psychological management of patients with vestibular disfunction, cervical vertigo, and the management of patients with complaints of dizziness who have normal vestibular function. The fifth new chapter addresses the special management problems of the elderly person with a vestibular deficit, and the sixth specifically deals with assessment of otolith dysfunction.

In addition to these new chapters, the Second Edition contains significant revisions that reflect new information about rehabilitation of patients with vestibular deficits. For example, in the past 5 years, there have been tremendous changes in the treatment of BPPV with the development of specific exercises for the canalithiasis and cupulolithiasis forms involving each canal. Specific sections of the chapters on treatment of BPPV, of unilateral and of bilateral vestibular loss, have been included that provide support for evidence-based practice.

Finally, a new chapter has been added that offers a paradigm for arriving at a physical therapy diagnosis through history and clinical examination. A physical therapy diagnosis enables the therapist to identify a constellation of symptoms and signs toward which therapy will be directed. Once the diagnosis has been reached, the general exercise approach can be identified. Other elements of the examination identify problems that will modify the exercise program for each patient, such as disorders affecting other systems and subjective complaints. Finally, there are specific assessments that must be performed to establish the patient's baseline performance so that changes in status can be assessed following treatment.

Susan J. Herdman

Preface to the First Edition

Management of patients with vestibular disorders is a formidable problem. Dizziness and balance problems account for 5 to 10 percent of all physician visits and affect 40 percent of people over the age of 40. Dizziness is the number one reason for physician visits by people over the age of 65. One of the difficulties in managing these patients is that the term "dizzy" is used to mean a variety of sensations, from vertigo to disequilibrium to lightheadedness. Dizziness, therefore, can be due to any of a myriad of problems including vestibular pathology, drug interactions, orthostatic hypotension, anxiety, and somatosensory loss in the lower extremities.

Identifying dizziness due to vestibular pathology is not always easy. Although vertigo is sometimes considered to be a marker for a vestibular deficit, patients can have severe vestibular dysfunction without vertigo. Furthermore, although we assess the health of the vestibular system by measuring the vestibulo-ocular reflex, this measurement gauges only the function of the horizontal canals and not that of the vertical canals or otoliths. This means that patients may have vestibular problems that cannot be measured. Attempts to isolate the function of the vestibulospinal system also have had limited success. Although patients with vestibular deficits may have difficulty maintaining their balance when both visual and somatosensory cues are altered, patients with nonvestibular balance disorders have similar difficulties.

Treatment of patients with vestibular problems also has been difficult. Sixty years ago, Dandy treated vertigo by performing bilateral vestibular nerve sections. He knew that vestibular deficits resulted in vertigo and believed that the loss of vestibular inputs would have no effect on a person's function. Fifteen years ago, patients with vertigo were given drugs, placed on bedrest, and often told they would have to "learn to live with it."

Today, management of the patient with a vestibular problem is more sophisticated. Although surgical management is still primarily ablative, care is taken to limit the surgical destruction of the inner ear, and the results of these procedures are carefully studied. Medical management recognizes that the use of vestibular suppressant medications may not be appropriate in all patients and that prolonged use in certain patients may actually delay recovery. New medical treatments have been developed for a variety of vestibular disorders.

The use of exercises as a treatment modality is the third approach that is now used extensively for patients with vestibular deficits. Although Cawthorne and Cooksey introduced the use of exercises as a treatment for patients with vestibular disorders in the 1940s, it is only in the last few years that physical therapists have become interested in treating this common and complicated patient population. Originally, this interest was due to an increased awareness of the importance of the vestibular system in balance control; now, it reflects the added awareness that many patients with vestibular deficits can be treated for the vestibular problem itself.

This text provides a thorough introduction of vestibular disorders to rehabilitation students and is a comprehensive resource for clinicians treating patients with vestibular dysfunction. Chapters on vestibular anatomy and physiology, vestibular adaptation, and the role of the vestibular system in postural control provide the basis for understanding how the normal vestibular system functions. The main concern in this book, however, is the assessment of patients with vestibular disorders and the development of different treatments. Because a diagnosis often is not available in patients with complaints of vertigo and disequilibrium, the assessment and identification of problems and goals become even more critical. The intent of the book is to provide the information necessary to enable the student to understand and the clinician to make appropriate decisions about the use of exercises for patients with vestibular lesions. The book is suitable for the therapist who has extensive experience with the dizzy patient, those therapists who are just beginning to work with these patients, and students who are contemplating working with such patients. Physical therapists who may find this book of interest include those in general hospital settings, private practice, or rehabilitation centers. Because vestibular disorders can be due to a variety of problems including viral infection, head trauma, motor vehicle accidents, stroke and aging, all physical therapists should find this book useful. In addition, this book should be a useful resource to occupational therapists, audiologists, otolaryngology nurses, and otolaryngologists.

Susan J. Herdman

Acknowledgments

In addition to those who actually set words to paper, many people contributed to this book. First are the patients with vestibular and other balance disorders, whose experiences with vertigo and with the process of diagnosis and treatment are the basis for this book. Second, I would like to thank all my colleagues who wrote individual chapters. I have enjoyed working with them very much.

Contributors

Annamarie Asher, PT
Vestibular Clinic
University of Michigan
Ann Arbor, Michigan

Thomas Brandt, MD, FRCP
Director and Professor of Neurology
Klinikum Grohadern
University of Munich
Munich, Germany

Richard A. Clendaniel, PT, PhD
Department of Otolaryngology—Head
  and Neck Surgery
The Johns Hopkins Hospital
Baltimore, Maryland

Helen S. Cohen, EdD, OTR, FAOTA
Associate Director, Center for Balance
  Disorders
  and Assistant Professor
Bobby R. Alford Department of
  Otorhinolaryngology and
  Communicative Sciences
Baylor College of Medicine
Houston, Texas

Ian S. Curthoys, PhD
Department of Psychology
University of Sydney
Sydney, Australia

Marianne Dietrich, MD
Department of Neurology
Klinikum Grohadern
University of Munich
Munich, Germany

M. Cara Erskine, MEd, CCC, SLP/A
Department of Rehabilitation Medicine
University of Maryland Medical System
  and
The Johns Hopkins University School of
  Medicine
Baltimore, Maryland

Michael Fetter, MD
Eberhard-Karl University
Department of Neurology
Tubingen, Germany

Timothy C. Hain, MD
Associate Professor of Neurology and
  Otolaryngology
Northwestern University School of
  Medicine
Chicago, Illinois

G. Michael Halmagyi, MD
Institute of Clinical Neurosciences
Royal Prince Albert Hospital and the
  University of Sydney
Sydney, Australia

Susan J. Herdman, PT, PhD
Professor
Division of Physical Therapy
Dizziness and Balance Center
Department of Orthopaedics and
  Rehabilitation
University of Miami School of Medicine
Coral Gables, Florida

Michael A. Hillman, MD
Director of the Vestibular Testing
    Center
Marshfield Clinic
Marshfield, Wisconsin

Vicente Honrubia, MD
Professor
Division of Head and Neck Surgery
Victor Goodhill Ear Center
UCLA School of Medicine
Los Angeles, California

Fay B. Horak, PT, PhD
Senior Scientist
R. S. Dow Neurological Sciences
    Institute
Good Samaritan Hospital and Medical
    Center
Portland, Oregon

Emily A. Keshner, PT, EdD
Sensory Motor Performance Program
Rehabilitation Institute of Chicago
Chicago, Illinois

R. John Leigh, MD
Departments of Neurology,
    Neuroscience, Otolaryngology, and
    Biomedical Engineering
Department of Veterans Medical Affairs
    Medical Center and Case Western
    Reserve University
Cleveland, Ohio

Douglas E. Mattox, MD
Professor and Chair
Department of Otolaryngology—Head
    and Neck Surgery
The Emory Clinic
Atlanta, Georgia

Tanya S. Ramaswamy, MD
Former Instructor of Otolaryngology
Northwestern University School of
    Medicine
Chicago, Illinois

Rosemary Rine, PT, PhD
Assistant Professor
Division of Physical Therapy
Department of Orthopaedics and
    Rehabilitation
University of Miami
Coral Gables, Florida

Neil Shepard, PhD
Speech Pathology Department
Hospital of the University of
    Pennsylvania
Philadelphia, Pennsylvania

Hiroshi Shimizu, MD
Department of Otolaryngology—Head
    and Neck Surgery
University of Maryland Medical System
    and
The Johns Hopkins University School of
    Medicine
Baltimore, Maryland

Anne Shumway-Cook, PT, PhD
Research Coordinator
Division of Physical Therapy
University of Washington
Seattle, Washington

Charlotte L. Shupert, PhD
Assistant Scientist
R. S. Dow Neurological Sciences
    Institute
Good Samaritan Hospital and Medical
    Center
Portland, Oregon

Ronald J. Tusa, MD, PhD
Professor of Neurology,
    Ophthalmology, and Otolaryngology
Bascom Palmer Eye Institute
University of Miami
Miami, Florida

Susan L. Whitney, PT, ATC, PhD
Director of Vestibular Rehabilitation
  Program
Centers for Rehabilitation Services
Assistant Professor
Departments of Physical Therapy and
  Otolaryngology
School of Health and Rehabilitation
  Sciences
University of Pittsburgh
Pittsburgh, Pennsylvania

David S. Zee, MD
Professor of Neurology and
  Otolaryngology—Head and Neck
  Surgery
Johns Hopkins Hospital
Baltimore, Maryland

Contents

SECTION III: Medical Management 235

SECTION I

Fundamentals

CHAPTER 1

Anatomy and Physiology of the Normal Vestibular System

Timothy C. Hain, MD
Tanya S. Ramaswamy, MD
Michael A. Hillman, MD

PURPOSE OF THE VESTIBULAR SYSTEM

The human vestibular system is made up of three components: a peripheral sensory apparatus, a central processor, and a mechanism for motor output (Fig. 1–1). The peripheral apparatus consists of a set of motion sensors, which send information to the central nervous system, specifically the vestibular nucleus complex and the cerebellum, about head angular velocity, linear acceleration, and orientation of the head with respect to the gravitational axis. The central nervous system processes these signals and combines them with other sensory information to estimate head orientation. The output of the central vestibular system goes to the ocular muscles and spinal cord to serve two important reflexes, the *vestibulo-ocular reflex* (VOR) and the *vestibulospinal reflex* (VSR). The VOR generates eye movements, which enable clear vision while the head is in motion. The VSR generates compensatory body movement in order to maintain head and postural stability, thereby preventing falls. The performance of the VOR and VSR are monitored by the central nervous system, and are readjusted as necessary by an adaptive processor. From a rehabilitation perspective, it is crucially important to realize that there are multiple fail-safe mechanisms closely integrated into these reflexes. The capability for repair and adaptation is so remarkable that after removal of half of the peripheral vestibular system, such as by a unilateral vestibular nerve section, finding clinical evidence of vestibular dysfunction is often quite difficult. The ability of central mechanisms to use vision, proprioception, auditory input, tactile input, or cognitive knowledge regarding an impending movement allows vestibular responses to be based on a richly textured, multimodal sensory array. With these general philosophical considerations in mind, the purpose of this chapter is to describe the anatomy and the physiologic responses of the vestibular system, paying particular at-

Sensory Input   **Central Processing**   **Motor Output**

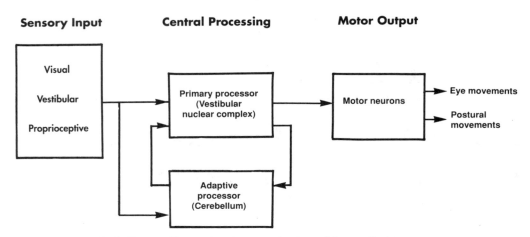

FIGURE 1–1. Block diagram illustrating the organization of the vestibular system.

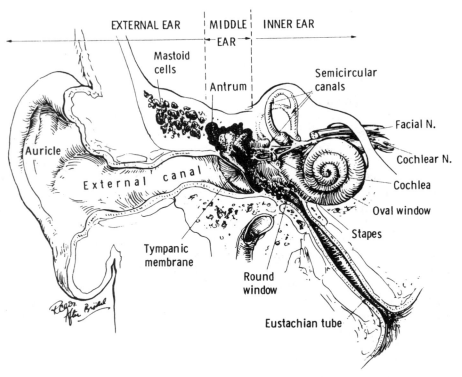

FIGURE 1–2. Anatomy of the peripheral vestibular system. Illustration by Brodal, from Templer, 1987 with permission from Ishiyaku EuroAmerica.[1]

tention to aspects relevant to rehabilitation. We will proceed from the peripheral to central structures, and conclude with a discussion of "higher-level" problems in vestibular physiology, which are relevant to rehabilitation.

THE PERIPHERAL SENSORY APPARATUS

Figure 1–2 illustrates the peripheral vestibular system in relation to the ear. The peripheral vestibular system includes the membranous and bony labyrinths, and the motion sensors of the vestibular system, the hair cells. The peripheral vestibular system lies within the inner ear, which is bordered laterally by the air-filled middle ear, and medially by temporal bone.

Bony Labyrinth

The *bony labyrinth* consists of three semicircular canals (SCC), the cochlea, and a central chamber, called the *vestibule* (see Fig. 1–3). The bony labyrinth is filled with perilymphatic fluid, which has a chemistry similar to cerebrospinal fluid (high Na:K

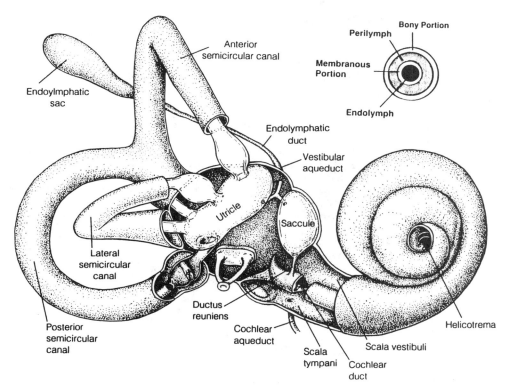

FIGURE 1–3. The membranous and bony labyrinths. The inset illustrates the perilymphatic and endolymphatic fluid compartments. Majority of the illustration by Mary Dersch from Pender, 1992, with permission from Lippincott-Raven.[2]

ratio). Perilymphatic fluid communicates via the cochlear aqueduct (not shown) with cerebrospinal fluid in the subarachnoid space.

Membranous Labyrinth

The membranous labyrinth is suspended within the bony labyrinth by fluid and supportive connective tissue. It contains five sensory organs, the membranous portions of the three semicircular canals and the two otolith organs, the utricle and saccule. One end of each semicircular canal is widened in diameter to form an ampulla.

The membranous labyrinth is filled with endolymphatic fluid (Fig. 1–3). In contrast to perilymph, the electrolyte composition of endolymph resembles intracellular fluid (high K:Na ratio). Under normal circumstances, no direct communication exists between the endolymph and perilymph compartments.

Hair Cells

Specialized hair cells contained in each ampulla and otolith organ are biological sensors that convert displacement due to head motion into neural firing (Fig. 1–4). The hair cells of the ampullae rest on a tuft of blood vessels, nerve fibers, and supporting tissue, called the *crista ampullaris*. The hair cells of the saccule and utricle, the maculae,

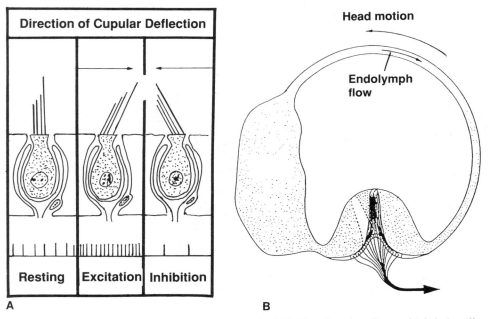

FIGURE 1–4. Effects of head rotation on the canals. (*A*) The direction from which hair cells are deflected determines whether or not hair-cell discharge frequency increases or decreases. (*B*) Cross-section of the membranous labyrinth illustrating endolymph flow and cupular deflection in response to head motion. Reprinted from Bach-Y-Rita, et al, 1971 (© 1965, IEEE) with permission from Academic Press.[3]

are located on the medial wall of the saccule and the floor of the utricle. Each hair cell is innervated by an afferent neuron located in Scarpa's ganglion, which is located close to the ampulae. When hairs are bent toward or away from the longest process of the hair cell, firing rate increases or decreases in the vestibular nerve (see Fig. 1–4A). A gelatinous membrane called the cupula overlies each crista. The cupula causes endolymphatic pressure differentials across the cupula, associated with head motion, to be coupled to the hair cells (Fig. 1–4B).

These otolithic membranes are structures similar to the cupulae, but as they contain calcium carbonate crystals called *otoconia*, they have substantially more mass than the cupulae (Fig. 1–5). The mass of the otolithic membrane causes the maculae to be sensitive to gravity. In contrast, the cupulae normally have the same density as the surrounding endolymphatic fluid and are insensitive to gravity.

Vascular Supply

The labyrinthine artery supplies the peripheral vestibular system (Fig. 1–6; see also Fig. 1–11). The labyrinthine artery has a variable origin. Most often it is a branch of the anterior-inferior cerebellar artery (AICA), but occasionally it is a direct branch of the basilar artery. Upon entering the inner ear, the labyrinthine artery divides into the anterior vestibular artery and the common cochlear artery. The anterior vestibular artery supplies the vestibular nerve, most of the utricle, and the ampullae of the lateral and anterior semicircular canals. The common cochlear artery divides into a main branch, the main cochlear artery, and the vestibulocochlear artery. The main cochlear artery supplies the cochlea. The vestibulocochlear artery supplies part of the cochlea, the ampulla of the posterior semicircular canal, and the inferior part of the saccule.

The labyrinth has no collateral anastomotic network and is highly susceptible to ischemia. Only 15 seconds of selective blood flow cessation is needed to abolish auditory nerve excitability.[5,6]

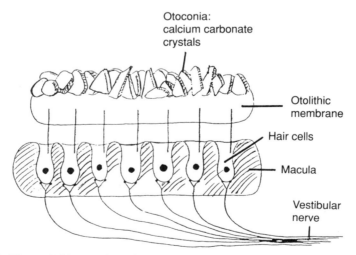

FIGURE 1–5. The otolithic macula and its overlying membrane. Reprinted from Baloh RW, Honrubia V, 1990, with permission of the publisher, F. A. Davis.[4]

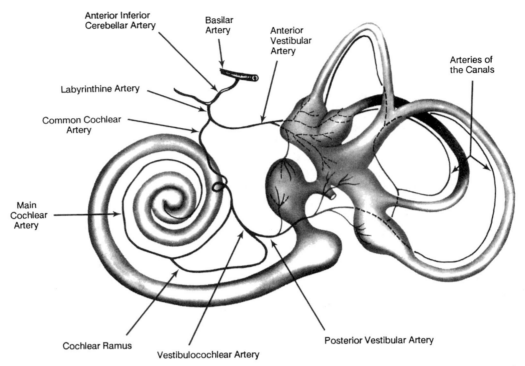

FIGURE 1–6. The arterial supply of the labyrinth. Reprinted from Schuknecht, HF, 1974, with permission of the publisher, Harvard University Press.[7]

PHYSIOLOGY OF THE PERIPHERY

The hair cells of the canals and otoliths convert the mechanical energy generated by head motion into neural discharges directed to specific areas of the brainstem and the cerebellum. By virtue of their orientation, the canals and otolith organs are able to respond selectively to head motion in particular directions. By virtue of differences in the mechanics, the canals are able to respond to velocity, and the otoliths to acceleration.

Semicircular Canals

The semicircular canals provide sensory input about head velocity, which enables the VOR to generate an eye movement that matches the velocity of the head movement. The desired result is that the eye remains still in space during head motion, enabling clear vision. Neural firing in the vestibular nerve is proportional to head velocity over the range of frequencies in which the head commonly moves (0.5 to 7 Hz). In engineering terms, the canals are *rate sensors*.

This fact poses a significant problem: How do the hair cells of the semicircular canals, which are activated by displacement, produce sensory input proportional to velocity? The labyrinth must have a method of converting head velocity into displacement. Certain biophysical properties of the semicircular canals loops accomplish the conversion.[8] The membranous canal loops have very thin walls and a small lumen diameter relative to the radius of the loop curvature. These characteristics make viscous drag on the endolymph very powerful. Viscosity is essentially fluidic friction and causes endolymph motion to be slowed down in a way similar to how honey slowly runs down the side of a jar. In a frictionless system, for a step of constant rotational velocity, endolymph displacement would be proportional to velocity times time. The viscosity creates resistance to endolymph displacement, causing rapid damping of displacement. In approximate mathematical terms, the viscosity puts a differential operator into the displacement equation, so that displacement becomes proportional to head velocity. Because of these considerations, over the usual frequencies of head movement, endolymph displacement is proportional to angular head velocity, and the canals function as rate sensors.

A second important dynamic characteristic of the canals has to do with their response to prolonged rotation at constant velocity. Instead of producing a signal proportional to velocity, as a perfect rate sensor should, the canals respond reasonably well only in the first second or so, because output decays exponentially with a time constant of about 7 seconds. This behavior is due to a springlike action of the cupula which tends to restore it to its resting position.[6]

There are three important spatial arrangements that characterize the alignment of the semicircular canals loops. First, each canal plane within each labyrinth is perpendicular to the other canal planes, analogous to the spatial relationship between two walls and the floor of a rectangular room (Fig. 1–7). Second, the planes of the semicircular canals between the labyrinths conform very closely to each other. The six individual semicircular canals become three coplanar pairs: (1) right and left lateral, (2) left anterior and right posterior, and (3) left posterior and right anterior. Third, the planes of the canals are close to the planes of the extraocular muscles, thus allowing relatively simple connections between sensory neurons related to individual canals, and motor output neurons, related to individual ocular muscles.

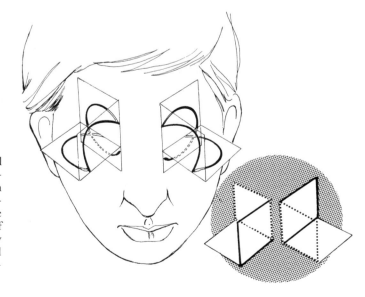

FIGURE 1–7. The spatial arrangement of the semicircular canals. The canals on each side are mutually perpendicular, are paired with conjugate canals on the opposite side of the head, and also are closely aligned with the optimal pulling directions of the extraocular muscles.

The coplanar pairing of canals is associated with a push-pull change in the quantity of semicircular canals output. When angular head motion occurs within their shared plane, the endolymph of the coplanar pair is displaced in opposite directions with respect to their ampullae, and neural firing increases in one vestibular nerve and decreases on the opposite side. For the lateral canals, displacement of the cupula towards the ampulla (ampullopetal flow) is excitatory, whereas for the vertical canals, displacement of the cupula away from the ampulla (ampullofugal flow) is excitatory.

There are three advantages to the push-pull arrangement of coplanar pairing. First, pairing provides *sensory redundancy.* If disease affects the semicircular canals input from one member of a pair (e.g., as in vestibular neuritis), the central nervous system will still receive vestibular information about head velocity within that plane from the contralateral member of the coplanar pair.

Second, such a pairing allows the brain to ignore changes in neural firing that occur on both sides simultaneously, such as might occur due to changes in body temperature or chemistry. These changes are not related to head motion and are *common-mode noise.* The engineering term for this desirable characteristic is *common-mode rejection.* Third, as will be discussed in a later section, a push-pull configuration assists in compensation for sensor overload.

Otoliths

The otoliths register forces related to linear acceleration (Fig. 1–8). They respond to both linear head motion and static tilt with respect to the gravitational axis. The function of the otoliths is illustrated by the situation of a passenger in a commercial jet. During flight at a constant velocity, we have no sense that we are travelling at 300 miles per hour. However, in the process of taking off and ascending to cruising altitude, we sense the change in velocity (acceleration) as well as the tilt of the plane on ascent. The otoliths therefore differ from the semicircular canals in two basic ways: they respond to linear motion instead of angular motion and they respond to acceleration rather than to velocity.[8]

The otoliths have a simpler task to perform than the canals. Unlike the canals, which must convert head velocity into displacement to properly activate the hair cells of the cristae, the otoliths need no special hydrodynamic system. Exquisite sensitivity to gravity and linear acceleration is obtained by incorporating the mass of the otoconia into the otolithic membrane (see Fig. 1–5). As force is equal to mass times acceleration, by incorporating a large mass, a given acceleration produces enough shearing force to make the otoliths extremely sensitive (*shearing force* refers to force that is directed perpendicularly to the processes of the hair cells).

Like the canals, the otoliths are arranged to enable them to respond to motion in all three dimensions (Fig. 1–9). However, unlike the canals, which have one sensory organ per axis of angular motion, there are only two sensory organs for three axes of linear motion. In an upright individual, the saccule is vertical (parasagittal), while the utricle is horizontally oriented (near the plane of the lateral semicircular canals). In this posture, the saccule can sense linear acceleration in its plane, which includes the acceleration oriented along the occipitocaudal axis and also linear motion along the anterior-posterior axis. The utricle senses acceleration in its plane, which includes lateral accelerations along the interaural axis, as well as again, anterior-posterior motion.

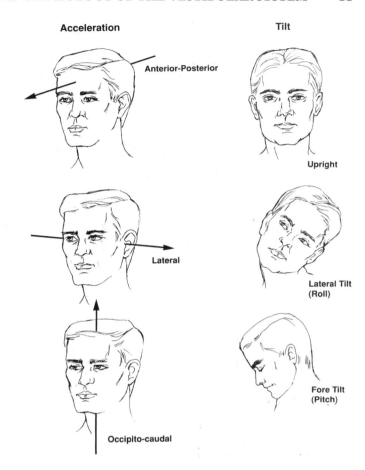

FIGURE 1–8. The otoliths register linear acceleration and static tilt.

Because earth's gravitational field is a linear acceleration field, on earth, the otoliths register tilt. For example, as the head is tilted laterally (which is also called *roll*; see Fig. 1–8), shear force is exerted upon the utricle, causing excitation, while shear force is lessened upon the saccule. Similar changes occur when the head is tilted forwards or backwards (called *pitch*). Because linear acceleration can come from two sources—earth's gravitational field as well as from linear motion—there is a sensor ambiguity problem. We will discuss strategies that the central nervous system might use to solve this problem in our section on higher-level vestibular processing.

In the otoliths, as in the canals, there is a push-pull arrangement of sensors, but in addition to splitting the sensors across sides of the head, the push-pull processing arrangement for the otoliths is also incorporated into the geometry of the otolithic membranes. Within each otolithic macula, a curving zone, the striola, separates the direction of hair cell polarization on each side. Consequently, head tilt results in increased afferent discharge from one part of a macula, while reducing the afferent discharge from another portion of the same macula.

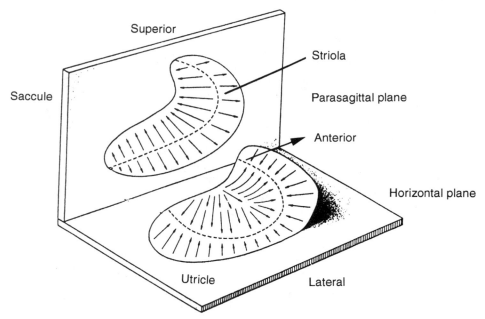

FIGURE 1–9. Geometry of the otoliths. This diagram is a schematic showing orientation only, as the saccule is actually inferior to the utricle. Reprinted from Barber HO, Stockwell CW, 1976, with permission of the publisher, C. V. Mosby.[9]

The Vestibular Nerve

Vestibular nerve fibers are the afferent projections from the bipolar neurons of Scarpa's (vestibular) ganglion. The vestibular nerve transmits afferent signals from the labyrinths along its course through the internal auditory canal (IAC). In addition to the vestibular nerve, the IAC also contains the cochlear nerve (hearing), the facial nerve, the nervus intermedius (a branch of the facial nerve, which carries sensation), and the labyrinthine artery. The IAC travels through the petrous portion of the temporal bone to open into the posterior fossa at the level of the pons. The vestibular nerve enters the brainstem at the pontomedullary junction. Because the vestibular nerve is interposed between the labyrinth and the brainstem, some authors consider this nerve a peripheral structure, whereas others consider it a central structure.

There are two patterns of firing in vestibular afferent neurons. Regular afferents usually have a tonic rate and little variability in interspike intervals. Irregular afferents often show no firing at rest, and when stimulated by head motion develop highly variable interspike intervals.[10] Regular afferents appear to be the most important type for the VOR, because irregular afferents can be ablated without much change in the VOR of experimental animals. However, irregular afferents may be important for the VSR.

Regular afferents of the monkey have tonic firing rates of about 90 spikes per second, and sensitivity to head velocity of about 0.5 spikes per degree per second.[11,12] We can speculate about what happens immediately after a sudden change in head velocity. Humans can easily move their heads at velocities exceeding 300° per second. As noted previously, the semicircular canals are connected in push-pull, so that one side is always being inhibited while the other is being excited. Given the sensitivity and tonic rate noted above, the vestibular nerve, which is being inhibited, should be driven to a firing rate of 0 spikes per second, for head velocities of only 180° per second! In other words, head velocities greater than 180° per second may be unquantifiable by half of the vestibular system. This cutoff behavior has been advanced as the explanation for Ewald's second law, which says that responses to rotations that excite a canal are greater than for rotation that inhibits a canal.[13,14] Cutoff behavior may explain why patients with unilateral vestibular loss avoid head motion towards the side of their lesion. More will be said about this when we discuss how the central nervous system may compensate for overload.

CENTRAL PROCESSING OF VESTIBULAR INPUT

There are two main targets for vestibular input from primary afferents: the vestibular nuclear complex and the cerebellum (see Fig. 1–1). The vestibular nuclear complex is the primary processor of vestibular input, and implements direct, fast connections between incoming afferent information and motor output neurons. The cerebellum is the adaptive processor—it monitors vestibular performance and readjusts central vestibular processing if necessary. At both locations vestibular sensory input is processed in association with somatosensory and visual sensory input.

Vestibular Nucleus

The vestibular nuclear complex consists of 4 "major" nuclei (superior, medial, lateral, and descending) and at least 7 "minor" nuclei (Fig. 1–10). This large structure, located primarily within the pons, also extends caudally into the medulla. The superior and medial vestibular nuclei are relays for the VOR. The medial vestibular nucleus is also involved in vestibulospinal reflexes, and coordinates head and eye movements that occur together. The lateral vestibular nucleus is the principal nucleus for the vestibulospinal reflex. The descending nucleus is connected to all of the other nuclei and the cerebellum, but has no primary outflow of its own. The vestibular nuclei are laced together via a system of commissures, which for the most part, are mutually inhibitory. The commissures allow information to be shared between the two sides of the brainstem and implements the push-pull pairing of canals discussed earlier.

In the vestibular nuclear complex, processing of the vestibular sensory input occurs concurrently with the processing of extravestibular sensory information (proprioceptive, visual, tactile, and auditory). Extensive connections between the vestibular nuclear complex, cerebellum, ocular motor nuclei, and brainstem reticular activating systems are required to formulate appropriate efferent signals to the VOR and VSR effector organs, the extraocular and skeletal muscles.

Vascular Supply

The vertebral-basilar arterial system provides the vascular supply for both the peripheral and central vestibular system (Fig. 1–11). The posterior-inferior cerebellar arteries (PICA) branch off the vertebral arteries. They supply the surface of the inferior portions of the cerebellar hemispheres, as well as the dorsolateral medulla, which in-

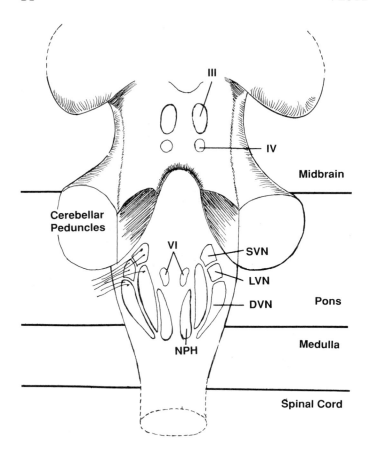

FIGURE 1–10. The vestibular nuclear complex. This section shows the brainstem with the cerebellum removed. DVN = descending vestibular nucleus; LVN = lateral; MVN = medial; NPH = nucleus prepositus hypoglossi; III = oculomotor nucleus (inferior oblique muscle and medial, superior, and inferior rectus muscles); IV = trochlear nucleus (superior oblique muscle); VI = abducens nucleus (lateral rectus). The MVN (not labeled) lies between NPH and DVN.

cludes the inferior aspects of the vestibular nuclear complex. The basilar artery is the principal artery of the pons. The basilar artery supplies central vestibular structures via perforator branches, which penetrate the medial pons, short circumferential branches, which supply the anterolateral aspect of the pons, and long circumferential branches, which supply the dorsolateral pons. The AICA supplies both the peripheral vestibular system, via the labyrinthine artery, as well as the ventrolateral cerebellum and the lateral tegmentum of the lower two-thirds of the pons. Recognizable clinical syndromes with vestibular components may appear after occlusions of the basilar artery, the labyrinthine artery, the AICA, and the PICA.

Cerebellum

The cerebellum is a major recipient of outflow from the vestibular nucleus complex, and is also a major source of input itself. Although not required for vestibular reflexes, vestibular reflexes become uncalibrated and ineffective when the cerebellum is removed. Originally, the vestibulocerebellum was defined as the portions of the cerebellum receiving direct input from the primary vestibular afferents. We now understand that most parts of the cerebellar vermis (midline) respond to vestibular stimula-

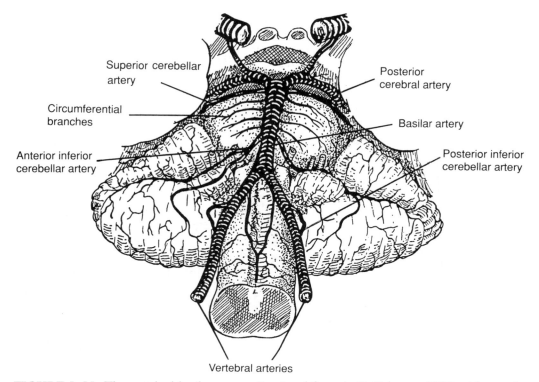

Superior cerebellar artery

Posterior cerebral artery

Circumferential branches

Basilar artery

Anterior inferior cerebellar artery

Posterior inferior cerebellar artery

Vertebral arteries

FIGURE 1–11. The vertebral-basilar system. Reprinted from A. G. Osborne, 1980, with permission of the publisher, Harper & Row.[15]

tion. The cerebellar projections to the vestibular nuclear complex have an inhibitory influence on the vestibular nuclear complex.

The cerebellar flocculus adjusts and maintains the gain of the VOR.[16] Lesions of the flocculus reduce the ability of experimental animals to adapt to disorders, which reduce or increase the gain of the VOR. Patients with cerebellar degenerations or the Arnold-Chiari malformation typically have floccular disorders.

The cerebellar nodulus adjusts the duration of VOR responses, and is also involved with processing of otolith input. Patients with lesions of the cerebellar nodulus, such as patients with medulloblastoma, show gait ataxia and often have nystagmus, which is strongly affected by the position of the head with respect to the gravitational axis.

Lesions of the anterior-superior vermis of the cerebellum affect the VSR, and cause a profound gait ataxia with truncal instability. These patients are unable to use sensory input from their lower extremities to stabilize their posture. These lesions are commonly related to excessive alcohol intake and thiamine deficiency.

Neural Integrator

Thus far we have discussed processing of velocity signals from the canals or acceleration signals from the otoliths. These signals are not suitable for driving the ocular motor neurons, which need a neural signal encoding eye position. The transformation of velocity to position is accomplished by a brainstem structure called the *neural integrator*. The location of the neural integrator has been identified only recently. The nucleus prepositus hypoglossi, located just below the medial vestibular nucleus, appears to provide this function for the horizontal oculomotor system.[17] Although a similar structure must exist for the vestibulospinal system, the location of the VSR neural integrator is presently unknown.

MOTOR OUTPUT OF THE VESTIBULAR SYSTEM NEURONS

Output for the Vestibulo-Ocular Reflex

The output neurons of the VOR are the motor neurons of the ocular motor nuclei, which drive the extraocular muscles. The extraocular muscles are arranged in pairs, which are oriented in planes very close to those of the canals. This geometrical arrangement enables a single pair of canals to be connected predominantly to a single pair of extraocular muscles. The result is conjugate movements of the eyes in same plane as head motion.

There are two white matter tracts that carry output from the vestibular nuclear complex to the ocular motor nuclei. The ascending tract of Deiters carries output from the vestibular nucleus to the ipsilateral abducens nucleus (lateral rectus) during the horizontal VOR. All other VOR-related output to the ocular motor nuclei is transmitted by the medial longitudinal fasciculus (Fig. 1–12).

Output for the Vestibulospinal Reflex

The output neurons of the VSR are the anterior horn cells of the spinal cord gray matter, which drive skeletal muscle. However, the connection between the vestibular nuclear complex and the motor neurons is more complicated than for the VOR. The VSR has a much more difficult task than the VOR, because there are multiple strategies that can be used to prevent falls, which involve entirely different motor synergies. For example, when shoved from behind, one's center of gravity might become displaced anteriorly. In order to restore "balance," one might (1) plantar-flex at the ankles; (2) take a step; (3) grab for support; or (4) use some combination of all three activities. The VSR also has to adjust limb motion appropriately for the position of the head on the body (see the frame of reference problem discussed in the section on higher-level problems in vestibular processing), and must also use otolith input to a greater extent than does the VOR.

There are three major white matter pathways that connect the vestibular nucleus to the anterior horn cells of the spinal cord. The lateral vestibulospinal tract originates from the ipsilateral lateral vestibular nucleus, which receives the majority of its input from the otoliths and the cerebellum (see Fig. 1–12). This pathway generates antigravity postural motor activity, primarily in the lower extremities, in response to the head position changes which occur with respect to gravity. The medial vestibulospinal tract originates from the contralateral medial, superior, and descending vestibular nuclei (see Fig. 1–12) and mediates ongoing postural changes in response to semicircular canal sensory input (angular head motion). The medial vestibulospinal tract descends

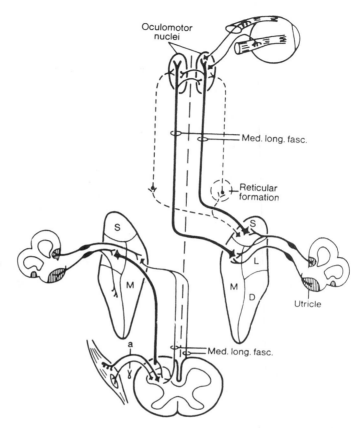

FIGURE 1–12. The VOR and VSR arcs. S, L, M, and D indicate the superior, lateral, medial, and descending vestibular nuclei, respectively. The lateral vestibulospinal and medial vestibulospinal tracts are shown as heavy and light lines, beginning in the lateral vestibular nucleus, respectively. From Brodal A, 1981, with permission of the publisher, Oxford University Press.[18]

only through the cervical spinal cord in the medial longitudinal fasciculus and activates cervical axial musculature.

The reticulospinal tract receives sensory input from all of the vestibular nuclei, as well as all of the other sensory and motor systems involved with maintaining balance. This projection has both crossed and uncrossed components, and is very highly collateralized. As a result, the reticulospinal tract through the entire extent of the spinal cord is poorly defined, but is probably involved in most balance reflex motor actions, including postural adjustments made to extravestibular sensory input (auditory, visual, and tactile stimuli).

VESTIBULAR REFLEXES

The sensory, central, and motor output components of the vestibular system have been described. We will now discuss their integration into reflexes called the VOR, VSR, and VCR. Additionally, we include brief descriptions of cervical, visual, and somatosensory reflexes. Although not directly mediated by the vestibular apparatus, these reflexes have a close interaction with vestibular reflexes.

The Vestibulo-Ocular Reflex

The VOR normally acts to maintain stable vision during head motion. The VOR has two components. The angular VOR, mediated by the semicircular canals, compensates for rotation. The linear VOR, mediated by the otoliths, compensates for translation. The angular VOR is primarily responsible for gaze stabilization. The linear VOR is most important in situations where near targets are being viewed and the head is being moved at relatively high frequencies. An example of how the horizontal canal VOR is orchestrated is given below:

1. When the head turns to the right, endolymphatic flow deflects the cupulae to the left (see Fig. 1–4B).
2. The discharge rate from hair cells in the right crista increases in proportion to the velocity of the head motion, while the discharge rate from hair cells in the left lateral crista decreases (see Fig. 1–4A).
3. These changes in firing rate are transmitted along the vestibular nerve and influence the discharge of the neurons of the medial and superior vestibular nucleii.
4. Excitatory impulses are transmitted via white matter tracts in the brainstem to the oculomotor nuclei which activate the right (ipsilateral) medial rectus and the left (contralateral) lateral rectus. Inhibitory impulses are also transmitted to their antagonists.
5. Simultaneous contraction of the left lateral rectus and right medial rectus muscles, and relaxation of the left medial rectus and right lateral rectus occurs, resulting in lateral compensatory eye movements toward the left.

The Vestibulospinal Reflex

The purpose of the VSR is to stabilize the body. The VSR actually consists of an assemblage of several reflexes named according to the timing (dynamic vs. static or tonic) and sensory input (canal vs. otolith). These reflexes are discussed in more detail in Chapter 2. As an example of a vestibulospinal reflex, let us examine the sequence of events involved in generating a labyrinthine reflex.

1. When the head is tilted to one side, both the canals and otoliths are stimulated.
2. The vestibular nerve and vestibular nucleus are activated.
3. Impulses are transmitted via the lateral and medial vestibulospinal tracts to the spinal cord.
4. Extensor activity is induced on the side to which the head is inclined, and flexor activity is induced on the opposite side.

The Vestibulocollic Reflex

The vestibulocollic reflex (VCR) acts on the neck musculature in order to stabilize the head. The reflex head movement produced counters the movement sensed by the otolithic or semicircular canal organs. The precise pathways mediating this reflex have yet to be detailed.

CERVICAL REFLEXES

The Cervico-Ocular Reflex

The cervico-ocular reflex (COR) interacts with the VOR and becomes relevant when considering recovery from vestibular lesions. The COR consists of eye movements driven by neck proprioceptors that can supplement the VOR under certain circumstances. Normally, the gain of the COR is very low.[19] However, the COR is facilitated when the vestibular apparatus is injured,[20,21] and may become important in subjects with labyrinthine injury.

The Cervicospinal Reflex

The cervicospinal reflex (CSR) is defined as changes in limb position driven by neck afferent activity. Analogous to the COR, which supplements the VOR under certain circumstances, the CSR can supplement the VSR by altering motor tone in the body. Like the VSR, the CSR consists of an assemblage of several reflexes. Two pathways are thought to mediate these reflex signals—an excitatory pathway from the lateral vestibular nucleus and an inhibitory pathway from the medial part of the medullary reticular formation. When the body is rotated with head stable, neurons of the excitatory vestibulospinal system increase their rate of firing on the side to which the chin is pointed. At the same time, neurons thought to be in the inhibitory reticulospinal system show a reduced rate of firing. This activity leads to extension of the limb on the side to which the chain is pointed and flexion of the limb on the contralateral side. Vestibular receptors influence both of these systems by modulating the firing of medullary neurons in a pattern opposite to that elicited by neck receptors. The interaction between the effects on the body of vestibular and neck inputs tend to cancel one another when the head moves freely on the body so that posture remains stable.[22]

The Cervicocollic Reflex

The cervicocollic reflex (CCR) is a cervical reflex that stabilizes the head on the body. The afferent sensory changes caused by changes in neck position create opposition to that stretch by way of reflexive contractions of appropriate neck muscles. The reflex was thought to be primarily a monosynaptic one; however, long-loop influences are being investigated.[19] The degree to which the CCR contributes to head stabilization in normal humans is presently uncertain, but it seems likely that it is useful primarily to stabilize head movement in the vertical plane, and it may also be facilitated after labyrinthine loss.

VISUAL REFLEXES

The visual system is a capable and sophisticated sensory system that influences vestibular central circuitry and drive visual following responses (i.e., smooth pursuit) and postural reactions. Because of intrinsic delays in multisynaptic visual mechanisms, visual responses occur at a substantially longer latency and are much less suited to tracking at frequencies above about 0.5 Hz than vestibular responses. Visual tracking responses may be facilitated after vestibular loss.

SOMATOSENSORY REFLEXES

Somatosensory mechanisms appear to be involved in postural stability as well. Bles and associates documented somatosensory induced nystagmus ("stepping around nystagmus").[23] Interestingly, the subjects with bilateral vestibular loss developed a more pronounced nystagmus than did normal subjects. This group implies that subjects with bilateral vestibular loss use somatosensory information to a greater level than controls.

HIGHER-LEVEL PROBLEMS IN VESTIBULAR PROCESSING

In this section we will identify some of the more sophisticated aspects of central vestibular processing, which are especially apt to be disrupted by disease and, for this reason, are especially relevant to rehabilitation. The underlying theme repeated throughout is the multimodal nature of the vestibular system. Over and over we will see a need to resolve multiple, partially redundant sensory inputs and to produce a motor signal distributed to multiple, highly redundant motor output mechanisms.

Velocity Storage

How good does the VOR have to be? In order to keep the eye still in space while the head is moving, the velocity of eyes should be exactly opposite to head movement. When this happens, the ratio of eye movement to head movement amplitude, called the *gain*, equals −1.0. In order to maintain normal vision, retinal image motion must be less than 2° per second. In other words, for a head velocity of 100° per second, which is easily produced by an ordinary head movement, the gain of the VOR must be 98 percent accurate, as any greater error would cause vision to be obscured.

The normal VOR can deliver this high standard of performance only for brief head movements. In other words, the VOR is compensatory for high-frequency head motion, but is not compensatory for low-frequency head motion. This fact can be most easily seen by considering the response of the semicircular canals to a sustained head movement, which has a constant velocity. The canals respond by producing an exponentially decaying change in neural firing in the vestibular nerve. The *time constant* of the exponential is about 7 seconds, or in other words, the firing rate decays to 32 percent of the initial amount in 7 seconds. Ideally, the time constant should be infinite, which would be associated with no response decline. Apparently, a time constant of 7 seconds is not long enough, because the central nervous system goes to the trouble to perseverate the response, and replace the peripheral time constant of 7 seconds with a central time constant of about 20 seconds. The perseveration is provided via a brainstem structure called the *velocity storage mechanism*.[24]

The velocity storage mechanism is used as a repository for information about head velocity derived from several kinds of motion sensors. During rotation in the light, the vestibular nucleus is supplied with *retinal slip* information. Retinal slip is the difference between eye velocity and head velocity. Retinal slip can drive the velocity storage mechanism, and keep vestibular-related responses going even after vestibular afferent information decays. The vestibular system also uses somatosensory and otolithic information to drive the velocity storage mechanism.[25] This example shows how the vestibular system resolves multiple, partially redundant sensory inputs.

Compensation for Overload

A second problem related to an imperfection in sensors is the response to high-velocity head movement. Humans can easily move their heads at velocities exceeding 300° per second. For example, while driving in the car, when one hears a horn to the side, the head may rapidly rotate to visualize the problem and potentially to avoid an impending collision. Similarly, during certain sports (e.g., racquet ball), head velocity and acceleration reach high levels. One must be able to see during these sorts of activities, but the vestibular nerve is not well suited to transmission of high velocity signals. The reason is the cutoff behavior discussed in the section regarding the motor output of the vestibular system. High-velocity head movement may cause the nerve on the inhibited side to be driven to a firing rate of 0.

In this instance, the vestibular system must depend on the excited side, which is wired in "push-pull" with the inhibited side. Whereas the inhibited side can only be driven to 0 spikes per second, the side being excited can be driven to much higher levels. Thus, the push-pull arrangement takes care of part of the overload problem. Note, however, that patients with unilateral vestibular loss do not have this mechanism available to deal with the overload problem, and are commonly disturbed by rapid head motion toward the side of their lesion.

Sensor Ambiguity

Sensory input from the otoliths is intrinsically ambiguous, as the same pattern of otolith activation can be produced by either a linear acceleration or a tilt. In other words, in the absence of other information, we have no method of deciding whether we are being whisked off along an axis, or if the whole room just tilted. Canal information may not be that useful in resolving the ambiguity, because one might be rotating *and* tilting at the same time. These sorts of problems are graphically demonstrated in subway cars and airplanes, which can both tilt and/or translate briskly.

Outside of moving vehicles, vision and tactile sensation can be used to decide what is happening. As long as one does not have to make a quick decision, these senses may be perfectly adequate. However, remember that visual input takes 80 ms to get to the vestibular nucleus, and that tactile input must be considered in the context of joint position, and intrinsic neural transmission delays between the point of contact and the vestibular nuclear complex.

Another strategy that the brain can use to separate tilt from linear acceleration is *filtering*. In most instances, tilts are prolonged, while linear accelerations are brief. Neural filters that pass low and high frequencies can be used to tell one from the other. Nevertheless, in humans, evolution apparently has decided that the ambiguity problem is not worth solving. Otolith-ocular reflexes appropriate to compensate for linear acceleration or tilt do exist in darkness, but are extremely weak in normal humans.[26] Stronger otolith-ocular reflexes are generally only seen in the light when vision is available to solve the ambiguity problem. Sensory ambiguity becomes most problematic for patients who have multiple sensory deficits because they cannot use other senses to formulate appropriate vestibulospinal responses.

Motion Sickness

An instructive illustration of how the brain routinely processes multiple channels of sensory information simultaneously is found in the motion sickness syndrome. The motion sickness syndrome consists of dizziness, nausea or emesis, and malaise following motion. It is thought to be caused by a conflict between movement information in related sensory channels, such as visual-vestibular conflicts or conflict between an actual and an anticipated sensory input. For example, motion sickness is often triggered by reading a book while riding in a car. In this instance, the vestibular and proprioceptive systems signal movement but the visual system signals relative stability.

The vestibular apparatus provides partially redundant information, and this allows for the possibility of intralabyrinthine conflict. Space motion sickness is thought to be caused by intralabyrinthine conflict. About 50 percent of space shuttle astronauts experience motion sickness during the initial 24 to 72 hours of orbital flight. It is currently thought that space motion sickness is due to a disturbance in "otolith-tilt translation."[27] The otoliths normally function in the context of a gravitational field, so that, at any moment, the total force acting on the otoliths is the vector sum of that due to gravity and that due to linear acceleration of the head. The central nervous system expects linear acceleration to be mainly related to tilt because linear acceleration due to gravity is usually much greater than that due to acceleration of the head. When outside of earth's gravitational field, such as is the situation for astronauts in outer space, the only source of otolith stimulation is linear acceleration of the head. In susceptible individuals, the central nervous system continues to interpret linear acceleration as being primarily related to tilt, which is now untrue, causing the motion sickness syndrome.[27,28]

Structures that appear to be essential for the production of motion sickness include: (1) intact labyrinth and central vestibular connections, (2) cerebellar nodulus and uvula that coordinate labyrinthine stimuli, (3) the chemoreceptive trigger zone located in the area postrema, and (4) the medullary vomiting center.[29] Why certain subjects are more prone to motion sickness than others is not completely understood.

Repair

Thus far, we have described some of the problems posed by the limitations of the vestibular sensor apparatus and the constraints of physics. In normal individuals, these problems can be satisfactorily resolved by relying on redundancy of sensory input and central signal processing. In addition to these intrinsic problems, there are also extrinsic problems that are related to ongoing changes in sensory apparatus, central processing capabilities, and motor output channels. Because being able to see while one's head is moving and avoiding falls is so important to survival, the *repair facility* of the vestibular system must be considered as an integral part of its physiology, and for this reason, it is our final topic.

Adaptive plasticity for peripheral vestibular lesions is dealt with elsewhere in this volume. Suffice it to say that repair is amazingly competent, even enabling the vestibular system to adapt to peculiar sensory situations requiring a reversal of the VOR.[30] However, one should consider the high degree of *context dependency* to the repair of peripheral vestibular lesions. In other words, adaptations learned within one sensory context may not work within another. For example, a patient who can stabilize gaze on a target with the head upright may not be able to do so when making the same head movements from a supine posture. Experimentally, in the cat, VOR gain adaptations can be produced that depend on the orientation of the head.[31] Similarly, when the VOR of cats is trained using head movements of low frequency, no training effect is seen at high frequencies.[32]

Another type of context dependency relates to the vestibulospinal reflexes and has to do with the difference in reference frames between the head and body. Because the head can move on the body, information about how the head is moving may be rotated with respect to the body. For example, consider the situation when the head is turned 90° to the right. In this situation, the coronal plane of the head is aligned with the sagittal plane of the body and motor synergies intended to prevent a fall for a given vestibular input must also be rotated by 90°. For example, patients with vestibular impairment who undergo gait training in which all procedures are performed only in a particular head posture (such as upright) may show little improvement in natural situations where the head assumes other postures, such as looking down at one's feet. Little is understood about the physiology of context dependency.

Repair of central lesions is much more limited than that available for peripheral lesions; this is the "Achilles' heel" of the vestibular apparatus. Symptoms due to central lesions last much longer than symptoms due to peripheral vestibular problems. The reason for this vulnerability is not difficult to understand. To use a commonplace analogy, if your television breaks down you can take it to the repair shop and get it fixed. If, however, both your television and the repair shop are broken, you have a much bigger problem. The cerebellum fulfills the role of the repair shop for the vestibular system. When there are cerebellar lesions, or lesions in the pathways to and from the cerebellum, symptoms of vestibular dysfunction can be profound and permanent. Clinicians use this reasoning when they attempt to separate peripheral from central vestibular lesions. A spontaneous nystagmus, which persists over several weeks, is generally due to a central lesion; a peripheral nystagmus can be repaired by an intact brainstem and cerebellum.

SUMMARY

The vestibular system is an old and sophisticated human control system. Accurate processing of sensory input about rapid head and postural motion is difficult, as well as critical to survival. Not surprisingly, the body uses multiple, partially redundant sensory inputs and motor outputs, combined with a competent central repair capability. The system as a whole can withstand and adapt to major amounts of peripheral vestibular dysfunction. The Achilles' heel of the vestibular system is a relative inability to repair central vestibular dysfunction.

REFERENCES

1. Templer, JW, et al: Otolaryngology—Head and Neck Surgery: Principles and Concepts. Ishiyaku EuroAmerica, St. Louis, 1987.
2. Pender, DJ: Practical Otology. JB Lippincott Company, Philadelphia, 1992, p. 7.
3. Bach-Y-Rita, P, et al (eds): The control of eye movements. Academic Press, New York, 1971.
4. Baloh, RW, and Honrubia, V. Clinical Neurophysiology of the Vestibular System. F. A. Davis, Philadelphia, 1990.
5. Ledoux, A: Les canaux semi-circulaires etude electrophysiologique. Contribution a l'effort d'uniformisation des epreuves vestibulaires. Essai d'interpretation de la semiologie vestibulaire. Acta Oto-Rhino-Laryngol, Belgica. 12:109, 1958.
6. Perlman, HB, et al: Experiments on temporary obstruction of the internal auditory artery. Laryngoscope 69:591, 1959.
7. Schuknecht, HF: Pathology of the Ear. Harvard Univ. Pr., Cambridge, 1974.
8. Wilson, VJ, and Jones, MJ: Mammalian Vestibular Physiology. Plenum, New York, 1979.
9. Barber, HO, and Stockwell, CW: Manual of Electronystagmography. C.V. Mosby, St. Louis, 1976.
10. Goldberg, JM, and Fernandez, C: Physiology of peripheral neurons innervating semicircular canals of the squirrel monkey. I. Resting discharge and response to constant angular acceleration. J Neurophysiol 34:634, 1971.
11. Fernandez, C, and Goldberg, JM: Physiology of peripheral neurons innervating semicircular canals of the squirrel monkey. II. Response to sinusoidal stimulation and dynamics of the peripheral vestibular system. J Neurophysiol 34:661, 1971.
12. Miles, FA, and Braitman, DJ: Long term adaptive changes in primate vestibulo-ocular reflex. II. Electrophysiological observations and semicircular canal primary afferents. J Neurophysiol 43:1426, 1980.
13. Baloh, RW, et al: Ewald's second law re-evaluated. Acta Otolaryngol 83:474, 1977.
14. Ewald, R: Physiologische Untersuchungen ueber das Endorgan des Nervus Octavus. Bergmann, Wiesbaden, 1892.
15. Osborne, AG: Introduction to Cerebral Angiography. Harper & Row, New York, 1980.
16. Robinson, DA: Adaptive gain control of the vestibulo-ocular reflex by the cerebellum. J Neurophysiol 39:995, 1976.
17. Cannon, SC, and Robinson, DA: Loss of the neural integrator of the oculomotor system from brain stem lesions in the monkey. J Neurophysiol 57:1383, 1987.
18. Brodal, A: Neurological Anatomy in Relation to Clinical Medicine, ed 3. Oxford Univ. Pr., New York, 1981.
19. Peterson, BW: Cervicocollic and cervicoocular reflexes. In Peterson, BW, and Richmond, FJ (eds): Control of Head Movement. Oxford Univ. Pr., New York, 1988, pp 90–99.
20. Kasai, T, and Zee, DS: Eye-head coordination in labyrinthine-defective human beings. Brain Res 144:123, 1978.
21. Botros, G: The tonic oculomotor function of the cervical joint and muscle receptors. Adv Otorhinolaryngol 25:214, 1979.
22. Pompeiano, O: The tonic neck reflex: Supraspinal control. In Peterson, BW, and Richmond, FJ (eds): Control of Head Movement. Oxford Univ. Pr., New York, 1988, pp 108–119
23. Bles, W, et al: Somatosensory compensation for loss of labyrinthine function. Acta Otolaryngol (Stockh) 97:213, 1984.
24. Raphan, T, et al: Velocity storage in the vestibulo-ocular reflex arc (VOR). Exp Brain Res 35:229, 1979.
25. Hain TC: A model of the nystagmus induced by off-vertical axis rotation. Biological Cybernetics 54:337, 1986.
26. Israel, I, and Berthoz, A: Contribution of the otoliths to the calculation of linear displacement. J Neurophysiol 62:247, 1989.
27. Parker, DE, et al: Otolith tilt-translation reinterpretation following prolonged weightlessness: Implications for preflight training. Aviat Space Environ Med 56:601, 1985.
28. Oman, CM, et al: MIT/Canadian vestibular experiments on the spacelab-1 mission: 4. Space motion sickness: Symptoms, stimuli and predictability. Exp Brain Res 64:316, 1986.
29. Harm, DL: Physiology of motion sickness symptoms. In Crampton, GH (ed): Motion and Space Sickness. CRC Press, Boca Raton, 1990, pp 153–170.
30. Gonshor, A, and Melvill, JG: Extreme vestibulo-ocular adaptation induced by prolonged optical reversal of vision. J Physiol (Lond) 256:381, 1976.
31. Baker, J, et al: Dependence of cat vestibulo-ocular reflex direction adaptation on animal orientation during adaptation and rotation in darkness. Brain Res 408:339, 1987.
32. Godeaux, E, et al: Adaptive change of the vestibulo-ocular reflex in the cat: The effects of a long-term frequency selective procedure. Exp Brain Res 49:28, 1983.

CHAPTER 2

Role of the Vestibular System in Postural Control

Fay B. Horak, PT, PhD
Charlotte Shupert, PhD

One of the most important tasks of the human postural control system is that of balancing the body over the small base of support provided by the feet. As a sensor of gravity, the vestibular system is one of the nervous system's most important tools in controlling posture. The vestibular system is *both a sensory and a motor system*. As a sensory system, the vestibular system provides the central nervous system (CNS) with information about the position and motion of the head and the direction of gravity. The CNS uses this information, together with information from other sensory systems, to construct a picture (sometimes called a "model" or "schema" or an "internal representation" or "map") of the position and movement of the entire body and the surrounding environment. In addition to providing sensory information, the vestibular system also contributes directly to motor control. The CNS uses descending motor pathways, which receive vestibular and other types of information to control static head and body positions and to coordinate postural movements.

Because the vestibular system is both a sensory and a motor system, it plays many different roles in postural control. In this chapter we explore the four most important roles (Fig. 2–1). First, we discuss the role of the vestibular system in the sensation and perception of position and motion. Second, we discuss its role in orienting the head and body to vertical, including the static alignment of the head and body and the selection of appropriate sensory cues for postural orientation in different sensory environments. These two roles are primarily sensory in nature; the vestibular system provides the sensory information about head motion and position and the direction of gravity which the CNS needs to carry out these functions. Third, we discuss the role of the vestibular system in controlling the position of the body's center of mass, both for static positions and dynamic movements, and fourth, we discuss its role in stabilizing the head during postural movements. These two roles involve motor aspects of the vestibular system.

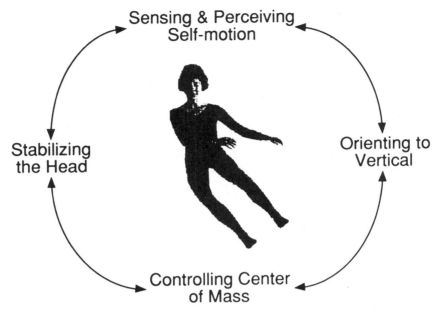

FIGURE 2–1. Four important roles of the vestibular system in postural control interact with other sensory and motor systems to accomplish tasks like maintaining equilibrium and body alignment on an unstable surface.

SENSING AND PERCEIVING POSITION AND MOTION

The vestibular system provides information about the movement of the head and its position with respect to gravity and other inertial forces (like those generated by moving vehicles). Therefore, this system contributes important information to the sensation and perception of the motion and position of the body as a whole. The vestibular system consists of two types of motion sensors, the semicircular canals and the otoliths. The canals sense rotational movement of the head. Rotational movements in the sagittal and frontal plane are detected by the vertical (anterior and posterior) canals. The horizontal canals are sensitive to motions in the horizontal plane. The largest head motions during quiet stance and walking or running occur in the sagittal (anterior-posterior) plane. Frontal plane (side to side) and horizontal plane (as if to shake the head "no") movements also occur, but they are smaller.[1] Information from all three sets of canals contributes directly to the perception of self-motion.

In contrast to the canals, which sense rotational motion, the *otoliths* sense linear accelerations. Vertical linear accelerations of the head, like the head translations generated during deep knee bends, are sensed by the *saccular otoliths*. Horizontal linear accelerations, like the translations of the head generated during walking forward, are sensed by the *utricular otoliths*. The otolith organs also provide information about the direction of gravity. Gravity, which is also a linear acceleration, produces an otolith signal that changes systematically as the head is tilted. The CNS uses this signal to determine head alignment with respect to gravitational vertical.

As important as good vestibular function is for determining the position and motion of the body, vestibular information by itself is not enough. First, the vestibular system can only provide information about head movements and not the position or movement of any of the other body segments. Second, vestibular information about head movements can be ambiguous. A signal from the vertical canals indicating anterior head rotation can be produced by the head flexing on the neck or by the body flexing at the waist, but the vestibular system alone cannot distinguish between the two. In addition to these problems, the vestibular system is not equally sensitive to the entire range of possible head movements. The semicircular canals are most sensitive to faster head movements, such as those that occur at heel strike during gait or as a result of a sudden trip or slip.[2-5] The canals respond poorly to slower head movements, such as the slow drifting movements that occur during quiet stance. The otolith organs can signal tilts with respect to gravity and slow, drifting movements, but only when these movements are linear, rather than rotational.[6-9]

In order to clarify the ambiguities inherent in vestibular information and to get good sensory information about the entire range of possible head and body movements, the CNS relies on information from all available sensory systems. Each sensory system contributes a different important kind of information about body position and motion to the CNS, and each sensory system is most sensitive to particular types of motion.[10-15] The *visual system* signals the position and movement of the head with respect to surrounding objects. The visual system can provide the CNS with the information necessary to determine whether a signal from the otoliths corresponds to a tilt with respect to gravity or a linear translation of the head. The visual system also provides information about the direction of vertical, because walls and door frames are typically aligned vertically, parallel to gravity. The visual system provides good information about slow movements or static tilts of the head with respect to the visual environment.[12,16,17]

In contrast to vision, the *somatosensory system* provides information about the position and motion of the body with respect to its support surface and about the position and motion of body segments with respect to each other. For example, somatosensory information can help the CNS distinguish whether a head rotation signal from the vertical canals is due to motion of the head on the neck or due to flexion of the body at the waist. The somatosensory system can also provide information about how body segments are aligned with respect to each other and the support surface by providing information about muscle stretch and joint position at the ankle or more proximal joints. The somatosensory system is particularly sensitive to fast movements, like those generated by sudden perturbations of joint positions.[18]

The contribution of each sensory system to the sensation of self-motion has been demonstrated experimentally by stimulating the individual sensory systems. Electrical stimulation of the vestibular nerve by means of current passed through electrodes placed on the skin over the mastoid bone produces sensations of self-motion or tilt in humans by mimicking the vestibular signals that would be generated by an actual head movement.[19,20] Similar results can be achieved by presenting subjects with large moving visual scenes (Fig. 2–2).[12,17,21-23] When the head is moved, the image of the entire visual scene moves in the opposite direction. When subjects watch a large moving visual scene, the CNS often misinterprets the visual stimulus and the observers feel self-motion in the opposite direction. Vibrating tendons in the neck and legs, which stimulate somatosensory motion detectors, can also give rise to sensations of body motion.[10,24,25]

The perception of self-motion and orientation depends on more than sensory cues alone, however. What the subject predicts and knows about the sensory environment or what the subject has experienced in the past (sometimes called the subject's "central

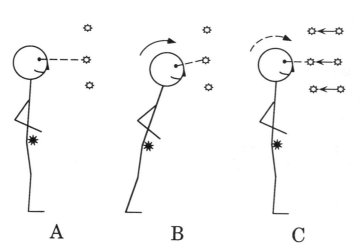

FIGURE 2–2. Visual information can be used to determine how the body is moving. In this and all subsequent stick figures, the asterisk corresponds to the position of the body's center of mass, which is located about 2 cm in front of the spinal column at the level of the pelvis. As the body sways forward (*B*) visual objects placed in front of the subject loom toward the observer. If visual objects are moved toward a stationary observer (*C*), the observer can experience an illusion of forward sway (*dotted arrow*), especially in cases of vestibular loss.

set") can contribute powerfully to how sensory signals are interpreted.[26] For example, imagine two cars stopped next to each other at a traffic light. If one car moves forward slightly, the driver of the second car may step on the brake, mistakenly believing that his car has rolled backward. This illusion is very powerful, because cars often do roll backward when stopped as most drivers know. The "central set" of the driver is to expect the car to move, and so the driver accepts the visual motion cue, despite the fact that both the driver's vestibular and somatosensory systems indicate that the driver has not moved. This phenomenon has also been demonstrated in the laboratory. Subjects seated in a stationary chair who observe a large moving visual scene may perceive either chair motion or visual scene motion depending on whether they are asked to concentrate on visual or somatosensory cues.[27] This observation is particularly interesting because these illusions of motion occur despite the fact that the vestibular system is signaling no motion in either case.

Given the vestibular system's important role in the sensation of self-motion, it is not surprising that patients with vestibular disorders often have abnormal perceptions of self-motion. Patients may report that they feel themselves spinning or rocking or that the room appears to spin around them. These sensations may be associated with particular head positions depending on the disorder. Patients may adopt leaning postures while insisting that they feel themselves aligned vertically, indicating that self-motion perception and automatic postural responses may be independent of each other to some degree. Patients with profound losses of vestibular function have difficulty determining how they are moving in environments lacking good visual and somatosensory orientation cues, such as walking at night on a sandy beach or swimming in muddy water.

In summary, the vestibular system, along with other sensory systems, provides the CNS with the information about body motion and position with respect to vertical, which is critical for sensing and perceiving self-motion. No sensory system alone provides all of the necessary information for sensing motion of the whole body; each sensory system contributes different and necessary information. In the next section, we explore how sensory information is used by the CNS to align the body to vertical, and how the CNS selects sensory information for body orientation in different environments.

ORIENTING THE BODY TO VERTICAL

Keeping the body properly aligned parallel to gravity and directly over the feet is one of the most important goals of the postural control system. The vestibular system, which can detect the direction of gravity, plays a very important role in maintaining the orientation of the whole body to vertical. Because the term "orientation" also includes the alignment of body segments other than the head with respect to each other and with respect to vertical, other sensory systems contribute to body orientation as well. In this section, we discuss the role of the vestibular system in the orientation of the head and body to vertical, and how the nervous system selects appropriate sensory information for orientation in different sensory environments.

Postural Alignment

Spinal x-rays and fluoroscopy have revealed that most vertebrates hold the vertical spine parallel to gravitational vertical.[28] The vestibular system, which signals the direction of gravity, plays an important, but not exclusive, role in the head and trunk alignment in animals. Unilateral vestibular lesions in animals result in head and body tilts toward the lesioned side.[28–30] The amount of asymmetrical posturing gradually diminishes over time, and the return to normal postural alignment has been considered a sign of vestibular compensation.[31] In humans, the vestibular system also plays an important role in the alignment of the head and body with respect to gravity, although the effect of unilateral vestibular lesions on postural alignment is more variable and more short-lived than in lower species.[29,30,32] Humans with sudden loss of vestibular function on one side can also show lateral flexion of the head to the side of the loss during the acute phase of the lesion.[31,32] However, within 6 months to 1 year following total unilateral vestibular loss in humans, postural alignment and control can be indistinguishable from that of normals.[33] Bilateral loss of vestibular function may be associated with a forward head position.[34] Altered postural alignment, sometimes associated with excessive muscle tension and pain, especially in the neck, is a familiar problem for patients with vestibular dysfunction.[35]

In addition to head tilts, the entire body seems to shift, temporarily, to the side of vestibular loss. Patients with unilateral vestibular lesions shift their weight to the side of their lesions and then regain normal weight distribution over the course of several weeks.[36] Fukuda[37] developed a stepping-in-place test to document the asymmetry and gradual compensation which follow unilateral vestibular loss. In this test, subjects attempt to step in place with eyes closed, and patients with unilateral losses typically rotate slowly toward the side of the lesion. Patients with bilateral vestibular loss have also been reported to shift their weight forward or backward.[38]

Another way to investigate the role of the vestibular system in aligning the body to gravity is to stimulate the vestibular system electrically by delivering low-level (<2 mA) direct currents through electrodes on the mastoid processes, with an anode placed on one mastoid and a cathode placed on the other.[19,20,39–46] Cathodal currents increase the tonic firing in the vestibular nerve, and anodal currents decrease the firing rate.[47] With the head facing forward, sway induced by galvanic current is lateral and toward the anode, because the galvanic current simulates the vestibular nerve signal, which would result if the body was tilted toward the side of the cathode. Subjects sway toward the anode to correct the apparent tilt induced by the galvanic stimulation. Although galvanic stimulation reliably results in tonic head tilts and weight shifts in normal humans,[19,20,39–46] these responses are typically absent or abnormal in patients with vestibular nerve sections, but can be normal in patients with loss of peripheral hair cell receptors, which confirms that the galvanic current directly stimulates the vestibular nerve.[48,49] Postural responses to electrical stimulation can be enhanced when subjects stand on a sway-referenced surface that provides poor somatosensory feedback for orientation or when galvanic current is delivered during responses to a platform movement.[46,48] These findings suggest that the role of the vestibular system in automatic postural alignment is increased when somatosensory information for postural control is unreliable.[19]

Studies of postural responses to electrical stimulation of the vestibular system also show that the nervous system takes both vestibular and somatosensory information into account when organizing these responses. The direction of body sway and the corresponding muscle activations induced by galvanic stimulation are modulated by the position of the head on the trunk. With the head facing forward, galvanically induced sway is lateral and toward the anode. If the head is turned on the trunk so that the ear with the anode is turned forward, the galvanically induced sway is forward.[19] This observation suggests that information about head position from neck receptors is combined with vestibular information to trigger an appropriate postural response regardless of head position with respect to the body.[19] When the head and lower limbs are aligned forward, but the trunk is aligned differently, postural responses to galvanic stimulation are appropriate to alignment of the head and feet, regardless of trunk alignment.[50] Thus, equilibrium control centers use information about body position and motion derived from proprioceptive afferents from many body segments, not just the neck, in combination with vestibular information to produce an accurate picture of body sway and appropriate postural responses.[51]

One hypothetical explanation for the altered postural alignment of patients with vestibular deficits is that the vestibular lesion has resulted in an altered internal map of body orientation in space. Gurfinkel and colleagues[13] have suggested that the CNS constructs a model or internal map of the direction of gravity based on vestibular and other sensory information, and that the CNS aligns the body according to this map. This hypothetical explanation could also account for the body realignments that result from galvanic stimulation. The galvanic current, which simulates the pattern of vestibular nerve firing that results when the body is tilted toward the cathode, may result in a change of the central nervous system's estimate of the position of gravity; that is, that it has shifted toward the anode. Subjects sway toward the anode to realign their bodies to the new estimate of the position of gravity. The tonic body and/or head misalignment in patients with vestibular disorders may also result from a faulty internal map based on abnormal information from their malfunctioning vestibular systems.

Vestibular information also contributes to another important internal map, the map of "stability limits," and vestibular pathology may lead to defects in this internal map as well. A human standing with feet planted on the ground may sway forward or backward a small amount (about 4° backward and about 8° forward) without losing balance and taking a step. The boundaries of the area over which an individual may

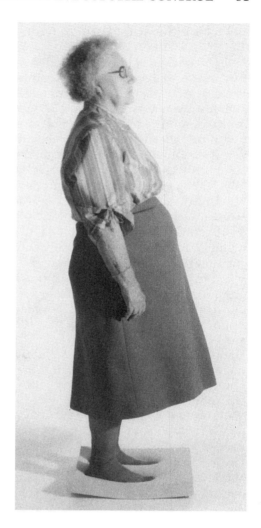

FIGURE 2–3. Elderly woman with loss of vestibular function, peripheral neuropathy, and cataracts who aligns herself near her backward limits of stability. In this photograph, she is standing on a compliant foam pad, which decreases her ability to use somatosensory cues for orientation.

safely sway are called the stability limits.[52] The actual stability limits for any individual in any situation are determined by biomechanical constraints, such as the firmness and size of the base of support, and by neuromuscular constraints, such as strength and swiftness of muscle responses.[53] Vestibular pathology might result in a poor match between a patient's actual stability limits and the internal map of those limits. The internal map could be smaller or larger than the actual stability limits, or the map could be poorly aligned with respect to gravity. As a result, patients may align themselves near the edges of their actual stability limits. Because visual and somatosensory information may substitute for vestibular information, alignment may be normal in patients with well-compensated vestibular losses, but may be very abnormal in patients with deficits in multiple sensory systems. Figure 2–3 shows a patient with bilateral loss of vestibular function, peripheral neuropathy, and cataracts, who aligns herself near her backwards limits of stability in stance.

Selecting Sensory Information

The studies of abnormal body alignment resulting from vestibular lesions show that the vestibular system plays an important role in the orientation of the body in space. The fact that normal alignment can be recovered with time even following bilateral vestibular loss, however, also argues that vestibular information is not the only source of sensory information that can be used for orientation. Visual and proprioceptive information also contribute to body alignment, as experiments with large, moving visual surrounds and tendon vibrations have shown.[17,21–24] Whether and how vestibular or other sensory information is used for orientation depends, in part, on the sensory information available in the environment.

Under normal conditions (i.e., a stable support surface and a well-lit visual environment), orientation information from all three sensory modalities is available and is congruent; that is, all three modalities yield similar estimates of body position and motion. There are, however, many environmental conditions in which the sensory orientation references are not congruent. For example, when the support surface is compliant (like mud, sand, or a raft floating on water) or uneven (like a ramp or rocky ground), the position of the ankle joint and other somatosensory and proprioceptive information from the feet and legs may bear little relationship to the orientation of the rest of the body; that is, the body could be aligned parallel to the direction of gravity and well within the stability limits despite large amounts of ankle motion (Fig. 2–4). Under such circumstances, it is critical that the nervous system be able to extract from the available sensory information the actual orientation of the body with respect to gravity and the base of support, because failure to align the body properly in a gravity environment will almost certainly lead to a fall.

The way in which the nervous system selects the appropriate sensory information for body orientation in different environments has been investigated experimentally using a paradigm developed by Nashner and his colleagues.[54–56] A similar protocol for testing the role of sensory interaction in balance was developed by Shumway-Cook and Horak.[57] In this paradigm, subjects are asked to stand quietly in each of six different sensory environments and the subject's postural sway is measured. In the first en-

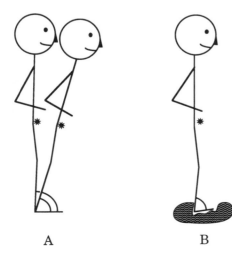

A   B

FIGURE 2–4. When subjects stand on a flat, firm support surface (*A*), ankle flexion corresponds to a forward body position. When the support surface is compliant or tilted (*B*), however, ankle flexion can correspond to an upright or even backward body position. Thus, vestibular information is more important for postural control in *B* than in *A*.

FIGURE 2–5. This figure shows how "sway-referencing" the subject's support surface and visual surround interferes with the ability to use somatosensory and visual information to orient the body to vertical. In *A*, the subject stands aligned to vertical and the center of mass projects directly over the foot. In *B*, the subject has swayed forward, resulting in a toe-down rotation of the platform and a forward rotation of the visual surround. Although the ankle angle and the position of the head with respect to the visual surround have not changed, the center of mass is now in front of the foot and the subject is in imminent danger of a fall. Normal subjects can detect this forward sway using vestibular information and avoid a fall, but patients with vestibular losses have difficulty doing so.

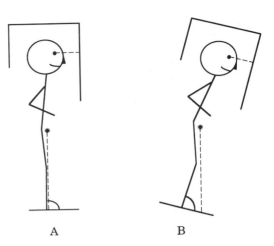

A   B

vironment, the subject's support surface and visual surround are fixed to the earth and the subject stands with eyes open; the second is the same, but subject stands with eyes closed. This part of the test is equivalent to the standard Romberg test used in clinical evaluations of standing balance.

In the remaining four environments, either the support surface, the visual surround, or both are moved in proportion to the subject's postural sway. This type of stimulation is referred to as "sway-referencing" (Fig. 2–5). By sway-referencing the support surface and/or the visual surround, the normal sensory feedback relationships between the different sensory systems can be disrupted. For example, when the support surface is sway-referenced, somatosensory information from the ankle joints correlates poorly with the position of the body. Support surface sway-referencing can be mimicked by placing the subject on compliant foam, and visual sway-referencing can be mimicked by placing a striped dome over the subject's head.[57] Vestibular information gives a more accurate estimate of body position and motion under these circumstances, and the CNS should rely more heavily on vestibular information for orientation.

Figure 2–6 shows how normal subjects react when exposed to such altered sensory environments. Normal subjects sway a small amount even under normal circumstances (condition 1), and this sway increases slightly when visual information is removed by eye closure (condition 2). Although sway increases slightly more when either the visual surround alone (condition 3) or the support surface (condition 4) alone is sway-referenced, subjects are still able to select useful sensory information from the sources available and maintain body orientation with respect to gravity. Even when the support surface is sway-referenced and visual information is eliminated by eye closure (condition 5) or altered by sway-referencing (condition 6), normal subjects are able to use vestibular cues to orient the body, albeit somewhat less efficiently. This is not surprising; conditions 5 and 6 are similar to walking on uneven surfaces in poorly lit environments (Fig. 2–7), swimming in murky water, or standing in the cabin of a ship, which are all tasks that normals can do without great difficulty.

Patients with clinically diagnosed vestibular disorders have also been tested using the same paradigm.[54–57] One of the most important findings from these studies is that not all patients with vestibular disorders respond in the same way. Patients identified

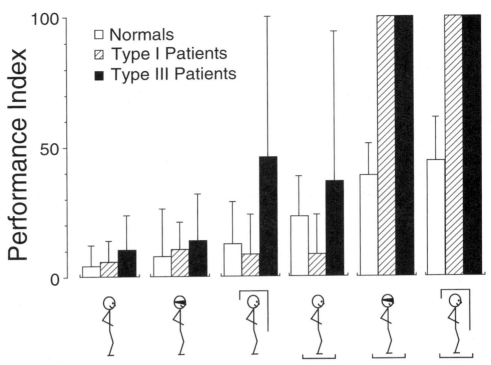

FIGURE 2–6. Median postural sway (as a percentage of the maximum sway possible without a fall) and 95th percentile limits for normal subjects and two groups of vestibular patients in six different sensory conditions. Stick figures along the abscissa show the sensory information available in each condition. Blindfold indicates eyes closed; a box around the feet indicates that the platform was sway-referenced. A box around the head indicates a sway-referenced visual surround.

in Figure 2–6 as type I lost all sense of orientation and fell in conditions 5 and 6, in which orientation information from both the surface and vision have been altered and the subject is forced to rely more heavily on vestibular information. One should note, however, that these patients performed as well as normals in conditions 1 to 4, in which at least one unaltered source of sensory information was available to them. In conditions 5 and 6, however, these patients lose balance when forced to rely on vestibular information, as though that information is missing or abnormal. This pattern of results is typical of patients with long-standing, well-compensated bilateral losses of peripheral vestibular function (although this pattern can also be seen in patients with other vestibular abnormalities). The fact that patients with well-compensated vestibular losses can use either visual or somatosensory information to orient the body limits the sensitivity and specificity of the standard Romberg test (equivalent to conditions 1 and 2) as a test of vestibular function.[58]

In contrast to the type I patients, type III patients, who had uncompensated vestibular disorders, showed increased sway in conditions 3 to 6 (see Fig. 2–6). That is, they had difficulty with orientation whenever somatosensory or visual information was altered or not available. Why type III patients have difficulty orienting in conditions 3 and 4, which have normal somatosensory and visual information (respectively), is not clear. They probably have chosen to orient their bodies to visual or support surface references which correspond poorly to gravity. Some investigators have hypothesized

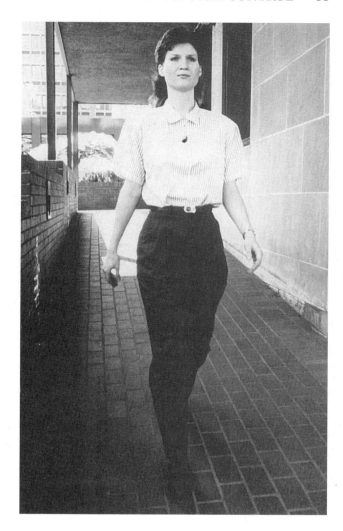

FIGURE 2–7. Walking in a poorly lighted environment on an uneven surface like a ramp puts demands on vestibular information for postural control.

that some humans are predisposed to "weight" (rely more heavily on) sensory information from a particular source, like vision or somatosensation,[15,27] particularly when vestibular cues to orientation are unreliable. Incomplete CNS adaptation to a vestibular lesion may also be a factor. This pattern of results is typical of patients in the acute stages of vestibular lesions. Patients who undergo postural testing shortly after surgery to destroy vestibular function on one side perform similarly to patients in type 1.[33] However, as these patients recover and the CNS adapts to the vestibular loss, their results come to resemble those of type 1 patients, and many patients with total unilateral loss eventually return to normal sensory orientation for postural control.[33]

In summary, these studies show that vestibular information for body orientation is most important in environments that lack good somatosensory or visual cues for orientation. Patients attempting to rely on faulty or missing vestibular information in these environments may align themselves poorly and fall. However, they may also choose another source of orientation information, regardless of its usefulness, when

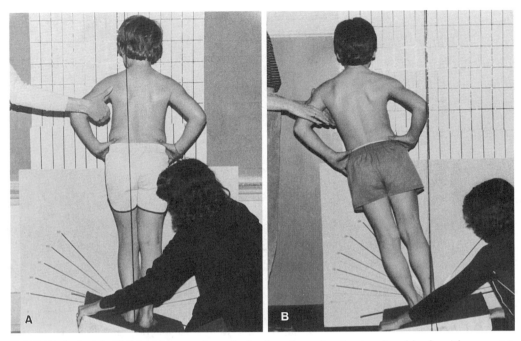

FIGURE 2–8. (*A*) Child with normal vestibular function orienting head and body with respect to gravity while surface is tipped and eyes are closed. (*B*) Child with absent vestibular function orienting head and body with respect to the tipped surface while eyes are closed.

vestibular information is bad or missing. Figure 2–8*A* shows a healthy child who maintains a normal orientation with respect to gravitational vertical despite standing on a tilted surface. Figure 2–8*B* shows a child with abnormal vestibular function who appears to rely most heavily on surface information for orientation; he maintains a perpendicular orientation to his tilted support surface. If the support surface is orthogonal with respect to gravity, this strategy may work fairly well. However, when the support surface is tilted, as it is in Figure 2–8, this strategy works poorly.

Although the subject shown in Figure 2–8*B* chooses somatosensory information for orientation, other vestibular patients behave as if they rely most heavily on vision for orientation and sway or fall when attempting to stand near large moving objects (like buses or cars). These patients appear to misinterpret the movement of external objects as self-motion in the opposite direction. As a result, they may throw themselves into disequilibrium as they attempt to maintain a constant orientation with reference to the moving visual object. Thus, vestibular patients may either align themselves with a faulty vestibular estimate of the direction of gravity or may align themselves with an estimate of the direction of gravity from another sensory system.

CONTROLLING CENTER OF BODY MASS

The previous sections described how the vestibular system detects the position and motion of the head, and how this sensory information is used for postural orientation. This section will describe how motor output from the vestibular system contributes to static body positions and dynamic postural movements, which help subserve the postural goal of maintaining equilibrium or controlling the center of body mass within its limits of stability. We know from anatomic studies that motor output pathways leave the central vestibular nuclei and descend in the spinal cord, where they terminate on the neurons which activate neck, trunk, and limb muscles. However, the functional significance of the descending vestibular system for the control of orientation and equilibrium in alert, intact humans and animals is still poorly understood. Nevertheless, there is evidence that vestibular signals probably play a variety of roles, including tonically activating antigravity (extensor) muscles, triggering postural responses, contributing to the selection of appropriate postural strategies for the environmental conditions, and coordinating head and trunk movements.

Orientation and equilibrium represent two distinct postural goals. In order to accomplish some tasks, greater priority must be placed on achieving a specific postural orientation, at the cost of postural equilibrium. For example, an experienced soccer or volleyball player may make contact with a ball even though making contact requires falling to the ground. Other tasks require equilibrium at the cost of postural orientation. For example, balancing across a wire may require rapid hip flexions and extensions to maintain equilibrium. In this task, trunk orientation with respect to vertical is sacrificed to achieve the goal of equilibrium. The way in which the CNS achieves the trade-off between control of orientation and control of equilibrium in postural tasks is not well understood. Both static positions and dynamic movements require a system that prioritizes behavioral goals and uses all the sensory information available to effectively and efficiently control the limbs and trunk to achieve both orientation and equilibrium.

Role in Static Positions

Magnus[59] was the first to investigate the role of descending vestibulospinal pathways in the control of static body position, and he used decerebrate animals to isolate the vestibulospinal system from other higher motor centers. He described reflexive movements of the limbs elicited by different head positions in decerebrate cats, and these descriptions were later refined and modified by Roberts.[60,61] Placing the head in different positions with respect to gravity and with respect to the body modifies activity in both the vestibular end organs and neck afferents (muscle spindles, joint receptors, etc.), which in turn affect limb muscle activity through the vestibulospinal and cervicospinal reflex pathways (see Chapter 1). To determine the role of the vestibular system alone, decerebrate animals are tilted in the dark with the head fixed to the trunk. To determine the role of neck afferents alone, the heads of decerebrate animals are held in a fixed position with reference to gravity and the body is tilted with respect to the head. The combined effect of cervicospinal and vestibulospinal reflexes can be examined by tilting both the head with respect to gravity and the neck with respect to the trunk.

In these experiments, Roberts found that vestibulospinal reflexes (VSR) and cervicospinal reflexes (CSR) seem to oppose each other in their effect on limb musculature. These effects are illustrated in Figure 2–9, which shows the nine different head and neck postures used in his experiment and their resulting effects on limb position. Normal neutral stance is shown in the center panel of Figure 2–9. When the cat's head and body were tilted nose-up (stimulating the vestibular system alone) forelimb flexion

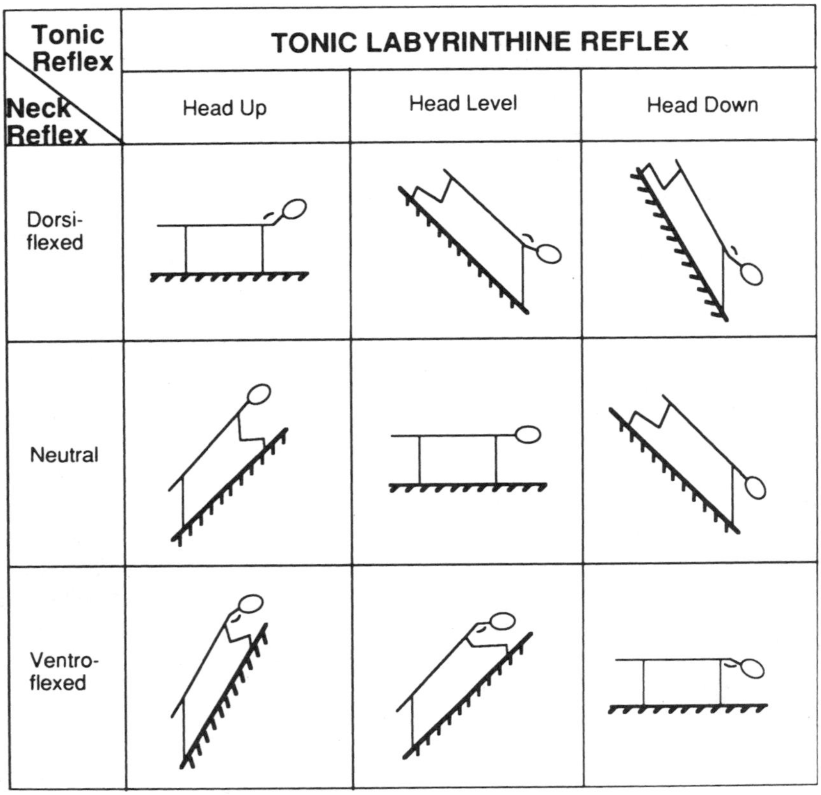

Tonic Reflex / Neck Reflex	TONIC LABYRINTHINE REFLEX		
	Head Up	Head Level	Head Down
Dorsi-flexed			
Neutral			
Ventro-flexed			

FIGURE 2–9. Effects of tonic neck and labyrinthine reflexes, in the forelimbs and hindlimbs of decerebrate cats. Adapted from Roberts.[61]

was observed (see Fig. 2–9, column 1, middle panel). When the cat's hindquarters were elevated above its fixed head to produce nose-up cervical stimulation alone, forelimb extension was observed (see Fig. 2–9, column 2, top panel). When the two reflexes were evoked simultaneously, limb position did not change (see Fig. 2–9, column 1, top panel), presumably because the two reflexes canceled each other.

Magnus hypothesized that the functional effect of this observed reflex cancellation is to permit the head to move independently with respect to the body without altering limb muscle activity. Roberts later proposed a second hypothesis: Simultaneous head and neck tilts would probably occur during stance on uneven or inclined surfaces, and the interaction of the CSR and VSR in these cases would produce the appropriate pattern of tonic limb muscle activity for stabilizing the trunk in a constant horizontal position with respect to gravity.[60] In other words, no matter what the orientation of the head and body, the combined action of the vestibular and cervical reflexes would always evoke extension of the downhill limbs and flexion of the uphill limbs.

Subsequent studies attempting to quantify the effects of VSRs and CSRs by recording electromyographic activity in triceps and biceps in decerebrate cats do not all confirm Roberts' findings, however. Some experimenters find little modulation of triceps with head movements in the pitch plane[62] and others[63–65] find limb activation in the opposite direction to that predicted by Roberts. Studies in intact, behaving animals, although quite limited, also fail to confirm Roberts' hypothesis. Recently, intact cats trained to stand freely on a tilted platform have been found to show a stereotypical postural strategy in which projection of the center of mass on the support surface and limb orientation with respect to vertical varied minimally with surface tilt angle.[66] Rather than stabilizing the trunk in space as suggested by Roberts, intact cats seem to maintain the orientation of their trunks parallel to the tilted surface and stabilize center of body mass and limb orientation with respect to gravity.

Thus, although static VSRs and CSRs may be seen in decerebrate animals, they may not play a dominant role in static body postures in intact animals. Also, although the effects of tonic labyrinthine or neck reflexes may be observed very early in development or in cases of brain injury, they have not been conclusively demonstrated in intact human subjects. In healthy adults, the stretch reflex of the soleus muscle becomes more excitable when the head is placed in different positions with respect to gravity. However, unlike Roberts' decerebrate cats, who increased forelimb or hindlimb extension when the head was tilted with respect to gravity, human ankle extensors are *less* excitable when the head is out of normal position with respect to gravity; that is, when the subject is supine or prone.[67] Also, the excitability of ankle extensors is suppressed by foot support in standing subjects. Thus, static postures in intact animals and humans are probably dominated by proprioceptive inputs from the limbs and/or movement patterns programmed at a higher level of the nervous system, rather than vestibular and neck reflexes.[68–70]

Role in Automatic Postural Responses

TRIGGERING AUTOMATIC POSTURAL RESPONSES

If balance is disturbed in a standing human, limb muscles are activated at short latencies to restore equilibrium. Because the latencies of these muscle activations are shorter than a voluntary reaction time, and because they act to restore equilibrium, they are called "automatic postural responses." Substantial research has been devoted to determining the role of the vestibular system in automatic postural responses. As noted above, direct vestibulospinal pathways from both the canals and the otoliths, which could convey automatic postural responses to perturbations in stance, have been identified anatomically. Both cats and humans respond to sudden drops with short latency ankle extensor activations (50 to 100 ms in cat; 80 to 200 ms in humans). These muscle responses are present with eyes closed, so they are not likely to be a result of visual stimulation. These responses are missing in patients with absent vestibular function, but survive procedures in animals that eliminate the canals but spare the otoliths. The magnitude of the responses is also proportional to head acceleration, all of which suggests a vestibular and, more specifically, an otolith origin.[71–74]

Quick displacements directly to the head during stance also result in muscle activations in the neck (45 ms), trunk (85 ms), thigh (90 ms), and ankle (70 ms).[75–77] These responses are absent in patients with adult-onset vestibular loss, suggesting a vestibular origin. However, adults who lost vestibular function as infants may show normal patterns of response to these head perturbations, suggesting that cervicospinal responses may adaptively compensate for the loss of vestibular input early in life.[76,77]

Because limb muscles are activated in response to sudden drops, perturbations in head position, and galvanic stimulation,[44–46] investigators have hypothesized that

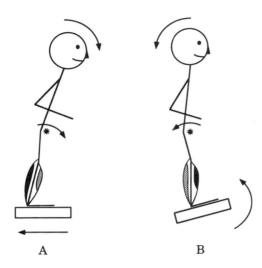

FIGURE 2–10. Platform translations and rotations. In (*A*), backward horizontal translation of the platform results in stretch of ankle plantarflexors (*shaded*) and forward sway of the body. Medium latency activation of ankle plantarflexors and other muscles restores equilibrium in response to backward platform translations. In (*B*), however, toe-up rotation of the platform, which also results in stretch of ankle plantarflexors, results in backward sway of the body. For toe-up platform rotations, medium latency activation of the shortened ankle dorsiflexors (*shaded*) restores equilibrium. The CNS relies more heavily on vestibular information for postural control for platform rotations.

A   B

vestibulospinal mechanisms may also play a role in automatic postural responses to stance perturbations induced at the feet by movable platforms.[78,79] Two types of platform perturbations have been used to test this hypothesis: backward or forward translations, which induce forward or backward sway respectively, and platform rotations, which induce ankle dorsiflexion or plantar flexion (Fig. 2–10). Platform translations result in activation of the stretched ankle muscles which occur at 80 to 100 ms following the onset of platform movement and act to restore the body to initial position. It does not appear, however, that vestibular inputs contribute a great deal to these responses. Human subjects and cats with complete absence of vestibular function can respond to surface translations using automatic postural responses with normal latencies and patterns, even when vision is not present.[34,54,80–82] Proprioceptive information from stretched muscles appears to be sufficient for recovery from platform translations. This conclusion is supported by the finding that automatic postural responses to surface translations are delayed when proprioceptive inputs are disrupted by sway-referencing of the surface or eliminated with pressure cuffs at the thigh or in peripheral neuropathy.[83–85] Finally, relatively large head accelerations are required to produce relatively weak responses in the limbs, and the head accelerations that occur in response to platform translations are quite small.[75–77] Therefore VSRs probably do not play a large role in the recovery of equilibrium following platform translations.

In contrast to responses to translations, responses to platform rotations may rely much more heavily on vestibular mechanisms. Platform rotations produce ankle dorsiflexion or plantar flexion, stretching muscles in the lower leg, but do not produce corresponding forward or backward body sway. Responses to platform rotations consist of two parts. First to occur is a response in the stretched ankle muscle at 70 to 100 ms, which is probably triggered by proprioceptive inputs[75,78,79,85–87] and which could, if unopposed, actually destabilize the body. Slightly later, a stabilizing response occurs in the shortened ankle muscle (at 100 to 120 ms), and this response is probably more dependent on vestibular and visual inputs. Patients with bilateral and unilateral loss of vestibular system have reduced magnitudes and delayed latencies of this stabilizing response.[79] The ability to adaptively reduce the magnitude of the destabilizing response to repeated surface tilts is impaired in some patients with loss of vestibular function.[54] The cause of this failure to adapt could either be that vestibular information is required to trigger the adaptive process or because patients with absent vestibular function become hypersensitive to proprioceptive information.[88]

These studies, as do many others, suggest that the role of the vestibular system automatic postural responses increases when proprioceptive information about body sway is lacking or inaccurate, and they also suggest that accurate, efficient recovery of equilibrium following stance perturbation requires a close interaction of vestibular and somatosensory information. This hypothesis is supported by studies that show that the magnitude of responses to head perturbations increases when subjects stand on compliant or moving surfaces.[76,86] Further, responses to peripheral vestibular stimuli are stronger in cats suspended by hammocks than in cats who support themselves on their legs. Cats suspended in hammocks have no access to proprioceptive information about body position, and are thus more dependent on vestibular stimulation.[89]

SELECTION OF POSTURAL STRATEGIES

Not all postural tasks require the same type of movement for the recovery of equilibrium, and different automatic postural responses are triggered in different situations. These different responses have different muscle activation patterns, different body movements, and different joint forces, and are called "postural control synergies" or "strategies."[87] Two very different strategies for moving the body's center of mass without moving the feet have been identified in previous studies: "ankle strategy" and "hip strategy" (Fig. 2–11).[90] An ankle strategy is used by most subjects recovering from a postural disturbance like a horizontal translation of the support surface when standing on a firm, flat support surface. The body sways roughly as an inverted pendulum by exerting force around the ankle joints. A hip strategy, which consists of rapid body motions about the hip joints is typically used on narrow support surfaces (beams), compliant or tilting support surfaces (foam, tiltboards), when stance is narrow (one-foot standing or tandem stance), or when center of mass position must be corrected quickly (i.e., when the perturbation velocity is high). There is evidence that these postural control strategies are centrally programmed and can be combined depending on biomechanical conditions, subject expectations, and prior experience. For example, normal subjects typically show a mixed ankle and hip strategy when responding to a translation of a 10-cm beam for the first time, or when responding to translations of a flat surface for the first time after responding to a series of beam trials, or when responding to intermediate or fast translations of a flat support surface.[91–93]

Vestibular information does not seem to be essential for initiation or execution of a normal ankle strategy, because subjects with complete absence of vestibular function show normal kinematic and EMG patterns associated with an ankle strategy.[34,82,92,93] This suggests that proprioceptive information from the body is sufficient to produce normal ankle strategy responses. In contrast, some evidence suggests that patients with vestibular loss have difficulty using hip strategy. Patients with bilateral vestibular loss show poor performance in tasks such as one-foot standing, heel-toe walking, and beam balancing, all tasks requiring hip strategy for good balance control.[34,80,82,94–96] There is also experimental evidence that signals from the vestibular system could act as a trigger for some postural responses. Subjects undergoing support surface translations show horizontal and vertical head acceleration peaks that are above threshold for the vestibular system at 40 to 60 ms following the onset of a platform translation.[92,93] Also, subjects with loss of somatosensory information from the feet due to ankle isch-

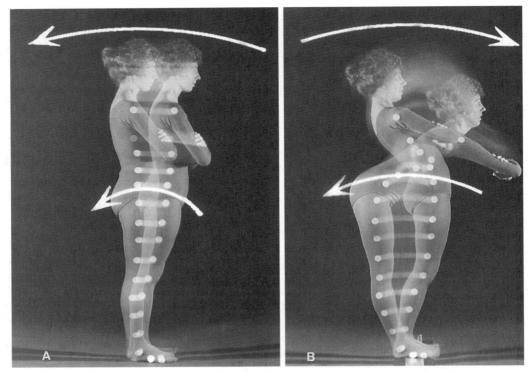

FIGURE 2–11. Normal subject using an ankle strategy (*A*) and a hip strategy (*B*) to control postural sway. Arrows at the hips show direction of corrective center of mass movement. Arrows at the heads show direction of corrective head movement. The relationship between vestibular and somatosensory information is different for ankle (*A*) and hip (*B*) strategy. In (*A*), a subject recovers from forward sway using ankle strategy, and ankle extension corresponds to backward movement of the center of mass and backward pitch of the head. In (*B*), the subject recovers using hip strategy. Ankle extension and backward movement of the center of mass now correspond to forward movement of the head and trunk. (Reprinted from Phys Ther 67:1881, 1987 with permission of the American Physical Therapy Association.)

emia, who presumably must increase their reliance on the vestibular system, use a hip strategy when an ankle strategy would be more efficient.[80] All of these findings suggest a critical link between the vestibular system and the use of hip strategy to control posture.

However, evidence also suggests that the relationship between vestibular information and the use of hip strategy is not simple. In a recent study, patients with bilateral vestibular loss were tested using fast platform translations and many of them showed bursts of abdominal muscle activity and early hip flexion torques similar to normals, indicating that normal vestibular function is not necessary to trigger hip strategy responses.[93] Why does vestibular information seem to be critical for a hip strategy in some circumstances, but not others? The answers to this question may lie both in the way sensory information from the vestibular and somatosensory systems is interpreted and in the way motor activity produces body movements in the different postural tasks. The tasks requiring hip strategy in which vestibular loss subjects perform poorly all involve changes in the support surface; that is, in its compliance (for foam or tiltboards), or in its size (beams), or in the way the body contacts the surface (beams, tandem stance, or stance on one foot). Further, these situations involve changes in the way forces generated at the ankle result in body movements; torques generated at the ankle cannot be used effectively to move the center of mass on short or compliant support surfaces. In these situations, body movements (either self-generated or due to a perturbation) do not result in the same somatosensory feedback as they do during normal bipedal stance on a firm surface, nor will an ankle strategy, which relies on generation of torque at the ankle joints, be very effective in correcting balance following a perturbation. It may be that normal subjects use vestibular information to interpret the changes in somatosensory information to produce an appropriately changed postural response in these special situations. Bilateral vestibular loss patients, who lack vestibular information, may not be able to accomplish the reinterpretation in time to prevent losses of balance when standing on compliant or short support surfaces. Responses to fast translations on a large, firm support surface, however, may not require reinterpretations of somatosensory information or changes in the way ankle torque can be used, and this may account for why patients with bilateral vestibular loss do not show obvious abnormalities in this task.

Although vestibular loss patients appear to be able to initiate hip strategy responses to fast platform translations, they take compensatory steps to maintain balance in response to these faster translations more frequently than normal subjects.[93] This suggests that they do have some difficulty with fast translations despite their ability to initiate a hip strategy. The fact that bilateral vestibular loss patients tend to step more often to correct balance when responding to fast platform perturbations also suggests a further connection between a failure of hip strategy and vestibular loss. Although they may be able to initiate hip torques, vestibular loss patients may be unable to execute hip strategy efficiently, and may resort to stepping because hip strategy may require efficient control of the trunk and good stabilization of the head with respect to gravity, which is likely to be faulty in patients lacking vestibular information.

Whereas vestibular loss is associated with a failure to use hip strategy in some conditions, some patients with pathology of the vestibular system habitually use hip movements to control center of mass position.[34,55,97] These patients typically report vertigo and ataxia consistent with vestibular dysfunction, and have histories consistent with vestibular pathology, but often show normal horizontal vestibulo-ocular reflex (VOR) function during rotation testing; these findings suggest that these patients have sustained damage to their vestibular systems, but have not lost a significant amount of vestibular function.[34,35,55,97,98] Preliminary results suggest that some vestibular patients who show hip sway use a coordinated pattern of active hip motions similar to hip strategy in normals. Others appear to generate large ankle forces which result in hip sway because the patients exert no control over their trunks. Coordination of head and trunk motions are abnormal in both types of patients.

There are several possible explanations for an overreliance on hip sway in some patients with vestibular disorders.

1. As a result of disease or damage, the vestibular system in these patients may become hyperresponsive. The hyperresponsive vestibular system may overestimate the velocity of head motion signals during body sway, and the CNS may respond to small perturbations as though they were much bigger.
2. The vestibular dysfunction may impair the patients' ability to interpret somatosensory input from feet, so they may perform similarly to normal subjects with acute somatosensory loss due to ankle ischemia and use hip strategy.

3. The abnormal vestibular information may contribute to abnormal internal representation of stability limits, so patients may behave as if small disturbances in stance push them beyond their stability limits.

Patients who perceive themselves to be in a different relation to their stability limits than they actually are may show inappropriate postural movement strategies in response to destabilization.[35,98] For example, some patients may not take a step necessary to recover equilibrium in response to a displacement of center of body mass outside their limits of stability because they perceive themselves to be well within their stability limits. In contrast, other patients may make exaggerated postural responses to small perturbations well within their limits of stability because they perceive themselves to be at their limits of stability and therefore at risk for a fall. The type of response may depend both on the type of vestibular dysfunction and the requirements of the task.

In summary, vestibular information is used, with information from other senses, to construct internal maps of the limits of stability, which in turn affect body alignment and recovery from postural disturbances. The information provided by the vestibular system and its relationship to information from the other senses changes depending on the movement strategy used in controlling equilibrium. We have hypothesized that postural strategies are specific prescriptions for mapping interactions among sensory and motor elements of postural system; these maps are, in essence, a method for solving a sensorimotor problem. Individuals need a variety of different movement strategies to choose from depending on current, past, and expected environmental conditions and task constraints. Although the vestibular system may not be prescribing the details of the coordinated motor pattern for postural movements, it seems to be intimately involved in the appropriate selection of movement strategies.

DEVELOPMENT OF MOTOR COORDINATION

Consistent with the concept that the vestibular system does not shape the details of coordinated postural patterns, intact vestibular function does not appear to be crucial for the normal development of many aspects of motor coordination. Deaf children who sustain complete or partial loss of vestibular function within the first year of life score within or above normal limits in tests of interlimb coordination such as kicking, walking, running, skipping, hopping, and fine coordination of the hands.[95,99,100] Clinical measures of balance function, such as duration of one foot standing and ability to walk on a balance beam, however, are affected by loss of vestibular function. These tasks are difficult because one-foot stance and balance beams compromise the patient's ability to use somatosensory information to control posture. However, these tasks also require hip strategy for center of mass control, which is usually abnormal in patients with absent vestibular function.[34,80,82] Preliminary results from patients with vestibular loss in infancy suggest that although they are capable of responding to very fast translations of a flat support surface without resorting to stepping, they do not generate torques at the hip (i.e., they do not adopt hip strategy) in the same way as either normal subjects or patients who have lost vestibular function as adults.[93] This suggests that children who lose vestibular function early in life are capable of developing highly efficient postural control responses, but that, due to their vestibular loss, they may avoid the hip strategy because of the increased trunk and head control required. Thus, these children may perform nearly normally in situations with normal support conditions, but show abnormalities in situations where hip strategy is unavoidable.

STABILIZING THE HEAD

The use of visual and vestibular information for the control of posture is complicated by the fact that these sense organs are located in the inertially unstable head. Because the center of gravity of the head is located above its axis of rotation, any movement of the body will result in head motion. Uncontrolled head motion complicates the use of vestibular information to make estimates of body motion and position. Also, if the range of head motions exceeds that which can be compensated for by the VOR, blurred vision could result. For these reasons, investigators have suggested that the nervous system might stabilize the head with respect to gravity during postural control, either to simplify the interpretation of vestibular information or facilitate gaze stabilization (Fig. 2–12A).[101,102] In the absence of good information about gravity from the vestibular system, or in an attempt to simplify the coordination of head and trunk movements, it has also been suggested that the nervous system might stabilize the head with respect to the trunk (Fig. 2–12B).[101]

Although there is some movement of the head in space during most locomotor tasks, the position of the head with respect to gravity is held relatively constant, despite the large movements of the body which can occur during tasks like hopping or running.[102–104] In these studies, neck muscle activity was not recorded, so it is difficult to know whether head position was being actively stabilized by the CNS. Head position does appear to be controlled actively during recovery from some types of postural disturbances. Normal subjects respond to fast translations and rotations of a large, rigid surface with neck muscle activations.[79,92,105] Neck muscle activations are also observed in normal subjects using hip strategy.[34,82,92,93] In these studies, the neck muscle activations occurred prior to any large change in head position, and so the activations appear to be a result of an anticipatory control strategy. In other words, these muscle activations serve to prevent the large tilts of the head with respect to gravity that could occur during the large trunk movements, characteristic of a hip strategy.

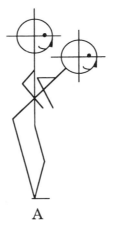
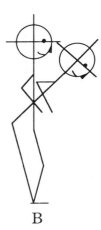

FIGURE 2–12. Alternative strategies for control of head position during postural movements. Example is given for a subject using hip strategy to control center of mass. Head is stabilized with respect to gravity in (*A*) and head is stabilized with respect to trunk in (*B*).

A   B

To determine the role of the vestibular system in maintaining head position with respect to gravity, the control of head position has also been studied in patients with vestibular loss.[34,82,106,107] During tasks like walking and running, patients with profound vestibular loss show variability in head position with respect to gravity. Profound loss of vestibular function has little effect on the control of head position in patients using ankle strategy to respond to platform translations, but both the control of the position of the center of mass and the control of head position are abnormal in vestibular loss patients in situations which require hip strategy.[34,82] As discussed, some vestibular patients with ataxia and vertigo, who have not lost vestibular function, tend to rely on hip sway to control posture. The control of head position is also abnormal in these patients. They fail to activate neck muscles in anticipation of their hip movements and, as a result, they control head position with respect to gravity poorly.[34,97]

The findings of these studies are fairly clear. The head appears to be approximately stabilized, with respect to gravity, for a wide range of movement tasks. The vestibular system plays an important role in this head stabilization. In contrast, the vestibular system appears to be less important for the control of the position of the center of mass, especially when good somatosensory cues about body position are available. These observations are consistent with the hypothesis that the distal-to-proximal muscle activations which control the center of mass are triggered by somatosensory information from the feet and legs, and that the neck and trunk muscle activations which control of head position are triggered by vestibular mechanisms.[3,4,5]

SUMMARY

The vestibular system plays many potential roles in postural control. The role it plays in any given postural task will depend both on the nature of the task and on the environmental conditions. When the stabilization of the head is critical for good performance, the vestibular system assumes a very important role. Likewise, when somatosensory (and, to a lesser degree, visual) information is not available, vestibular information for postural control assumes a dominant role. Table 2–1 suggests some tasks and conditions in which vestibular information for postural control is important, and some balance abnormalities that suggest a vestibular disorder. It is also important to

TABLE 2–1 Roles of the Vestibular System in Postural Control

Role of the Vestibular System	Clinical Assessment	Findings Suggestive of Vestibular Disorder
Sensing and perceiving self-motion	Patient performs head motions and/or positions in different planes	Patient reports abnormal sensations of motion and/or vertigo
Orienting to vertical	Patient stands on inclined surface	Trunk oriented to support surface instead of gravity
	Patient stands on foam with eyes closed	Patient falls or sway increases markedly
Controlling center of mass	Patient stands or walks on a beam	Patient is not able to use hip strategy to control center of mass and falls
Stabilizing the head	Patient leans or is tilted	Head not stabilized with respect to vertical

note that although this table and this chapter have been devoted to the role of the vestibular system in the control of standing balance, the vestibular system is equally important during locomotion, and problems with sensing movement, orienting to vertical, controlling the position of the center of mass, and stabilizing the head result in impairments in gait as well as standing balance.

Consider, for example, a task and a set of environmental conditions that occur frequently in clinical examinations of postural control: the patient sits, with eyes closed, on a board, which is tilted (see Fig. 2–1). This task is appropriate to test the ability of the patient to use vestibular information for the control of posture because visual and somatosensory cues for orientation are poor, and normal subjects typically stabilize their heads with respect to gravity while executing such tasks. When asked to perform this task, patients who have recently lost vestibular function will demonstrate abnormalities in the use of vestibular information in each of its four roles. First, they will have difficulty perceiving and reporting when their bodies or heads are properly oriented to gravity; that is, they will have difficulty identifying when they are upright. Second, they will orient head and body position poorly to gravity, showing tilts rather than upright orientations when asked to right themselves. Third, if the board is tipped suddenly, they may not be able to recover balance, and fourth, head position with respect to gravity will vary a great deal as they attempt to recover from the perturbation.

Unfortunately, the assessment of vestibular function in a clinical setting is not so straightforward with patients whose vestibular losses are well compensated. What one observes in these patients is often not the primary action of the vestibular system, but the result of the body's attempt to compensate for the loss. For example, vestibular patients often have difficulty with stiffness in the neck and shoulders. Assuming, however, that this neck stiffness is a primary result of vestibular activation of tonic neck reflexes would be a mistake. The stiffness may be the result of an increase in gain in the cervicocollic system, or a change in strategy; if the head can no longer be aligned to gravity because the direction of gravity cannot be detected, the CNS may choose to stabilize the head to the trunk. Alternatively, the neck stiffness could be a result of voluntary attempts to stabilize head position to limit vertigo or oscillopsia.

Whereas we once assumed that the abnormal balance of patients with vestibular disorders was the simple and necessary consequence of the loss of vestibular reflexes, we now know that the role of the vestibular system in the control of posture is much more complex. In addition to providing (together with vision and somatosensation) the sensory information necessary for orientation and balance, the vestibular system also interacts with the parts of the CNS responsible for expectation and learning. Although automatic and rapid, postural control is also flexible, capable of adaptation to many different sensory environments and musculoskeletal constraints. The role of the vestibular system in postural control will not be fully appreciated until we better understand the complex and multifaceted nature of postural control itself.

REFERENCES

1. Grossman, GE, et al: Frequency and velocity of rotational head perturbations during locomotion. Exp Brain Res 70:470, 1988.
2. Winters, JM, and Peles, JD: Neck muscle activity and 3-D head kinematics during quasi-static and dynamic tracking movements. In Winters, JM, and Woo, SLY (eds): Multiple Muscle Systems: Biomechanics and Movement Organization. Springer-Verlag, New York, 1990, p 461.

3. Keshner, EA, and Peterson, BW: Mechanisms controlling human head stability: I. Head-neck dynamics during random rotations in the vertical plane. J Neurophys 73:2293, 1995.
4. Keshner, EA, et al: Mechanisms controlling human head stability: II. Head-neck dynamics during random rotations in the horizontal plane. J Neurophys 73:2302, 1995.
5. Keshner, EA, and Peterson, BW: Neural and mechanical contributions to voluntary control of the head and neck. In Berthoz, A, et al (eds): The Head-Neck Sensory-Motor System. Oxford Univ. Pr., New York, 1992, p 381.
6. Barmack, NH: A comparison of the horizontal and vertical vestibulo-ocular reflexes of the rabbit. J Physiol (Lond) 314:547, 1981.
7. Van der Steen, J, and Collewijn, H: Ocular stability in the horizontal, frontal, and sagittal planes in the rabbit. Exp Brain Res 56:263, 1984.
8. Pettorossi, V, et al: Contribution of the maculo-ocular reflex to gaze stability in the rabbit. Exp Brain Res 83:366, 1991.
9. Nashner, L, et al: Organization of posture controls: An analysis of sensory and mechanical constraints. In Allum, JHJ, and Hulliger, M (eds): Progress in Brain Research, Vol 80, Afferent Control of Posture and Locomotion. Elsevier, Amsterdam, 1989, p 411.
10. Lackner, JR: Some mechanisms underlying sensory and postural stability in man. In Held, R, et al (eds): Handbook of Sensory Physiology. Springer-Verlag, New York, 1978, p 806.
11. Stoffregen, TA, and Riccio, GE: An ecological theory of orientation and the vestibular system. Psychol Rev 95:3, 1988.
12. Lestienne, F, et al: Postural readjustments induced by linear motion of visual scenes. Exp Brain Res 28:363, 1977.
13. Gurfinkel, VS, et al: Body scheme in the control of postural activity. In Gurfinkel, VS, et al (eds): Stance and Motion: Facts and Theories. Plenum, New York, 1988, p 185.
14. Xerri, C, et al: Synergistic interactions and functional working range of the visual and vestibular systems in postural control: Neural correlates. In Pompeiano, O, and Allum, JHJ (eds): Progress in Brain Research, Vol 76, Vestibulospinal Control of Posture and Locomotion. Elsevier, Amsterdam, 1988, p 193.
15. Zacharias, G, and Young, L: Influence of combined visual and vestibular cues on human perception and control of horizontal rotation. Exp Brain Res 41:159, 1981.
16. Mauritz, KH, et al: Frequency characteristics of postural sway in response to self-induced and conflicting visual stimulation. Pfluegers Arch Ges Physiol 335:37, 1975.
17. van Asten, W, et al. Postural adjustments induced by simulated motion of differently structured environments. Exp Brain Res 73:371, 1988.
18. Matthews, PBC: Mammalian Muscle Receptors and their Central Actions. Arnold, London, 1972.
19. Nashner, L, and Wolfson, P: Influence of head position and proprioceptive cues on short latency postural reflexes evoked by galvanic stimulation of the human labyrinth. Brain Res 67:255, 1974.
20. Magnusson, M, et al: Galvanically induced body sway in the anterior-posterior plane. Acta Otolaryngol (Stockh) 110:11, 1990.
21. Dichgans, J, and Brandt, T: Visual-vestibular interaction: Effects on self-motion perception and postural control. In Held, R, et al (eds): Handbook of Sensory Physiology, Vol VIII, Perception. Springer-Verlag, Berlin, 1978, p 755.
22. Howard, I: Human Visual Orientation. Wiley, Chichester, 1982.
23. Stoffregen, T: Flow structure versus retinal location in the optical control of stance. J Exp Psych: Hum Perc Perf 11:554, 1985.
24. Pyykko, I, et al: Vibration-induced body sway. In Claussen, C, and Kirtane, M (eds): Computers in Neurootologic Diagnosis. Werner Rudat, 1983, p 139.
25. Johansson, R, et al: Identification of human postural dynamics. IEEE Trans Biomed Eng 35:858, 1988.
26. von Holst, E, and Mittelstaedt, H: Das Raefferenzprinzip. Naturwissenschaften 37:464, 1957.
27. Mergner, Y, and Becker, W: Perception of horizontal self-rotation: Multisensory and cognitive aspects. In Warren, R, and Wertheim, A (eds): Perception and Control of Self-Motion. Lawrence Erlbaum, New Jersey, 1990, p 219.
28. de Waele, C, et al: Vestibular control of skeletal geometry. In Amblard, B, et al (eds): Posture and Gait: Development, Adaptation and Modulation. Elsevier, Amsterdam, 1988, p 423.
29. Dow, RS: The effects of unilateral and bilateral labyrinthectomy in monkey, baboon, and chimpanzee. Am J Physiol 121:392, 1938.
30. Schaefer, K, and Meyer, D: Compensation of vestibular lesions. In Kornhuber, H (ed): Handbook of Sensory Physiology, Vol VI, The Vestibular System, Part 2: Psychophysics, Applied Aspects, and General Interpretation. Springer-Verlag, Berlin, 1978, p 463.
31. Precht, W: Recovery of some vestibuloocular and vestibulospinal functions following unilateral labyrinthectomy. In Freund, HJ, et al (eds): Progress in Brain Research, Vol 64, The Oculomotor and Skeletomotor Systems: Differences and Similarities. Elsevier, Amsterdam, 1986, p. 381.
32. Curthoys, IS, and Halmagyi, GM: Vestibular compensation: A review of the oculomotor, neural, and clinical consequences of unilateral vestibular loss. J Vestib Res 5:67, 1995.
33. Black, FO, et al: Effects of unilateral loss of vestibular function on the vestibulo-ocular reflex and postural control. Ann Otol Rhinol Laryngol 98:884, 1989.

34. Shupert, C, et al: The effect of peripheral vestibular disorders on head-trunk coordination during postural sway in humans. In Berthoz, A, et al (eds): The Head-Neck Sensory Motor System: Evolution, Development, Neuronal Mechanisms and Disorders. Oxford Univ. Pr., New York, 1991, p 607.

35. Shumway-Cook, A, and Horak, FB: Rehabilitation strategies for patients with vestibular deficits. In Arenberg, IK, and Smith, DB (eds): Neurologic Clinics, Vol 8, Diagnostic Neurotology. WB Saunders Co, Philadelphia, 1990, p 441.

36. Takemori, S, et al: Vestibular training after sudden loss of vestibular functions. Otorhinolaryngology 47:76, 1985.

37. Fukuda, T: The stepping test: Two phases of the labyrinthine reflex. Acta Otolaryngol (Stockh) 50:95, 1959.

38. Norre, M: Treatment of unilateral vestibular hypofunction. In Oosterveld, W (ed): Otoneurology. Wiley, Chichester, 1984, p 24.

39. Njiokiktjien, C, and Folkerts, JF: Displacement of the body's centre of gravity at galvanic stimulation of the labyrinth. Confin Neurol 33:46, 1971.

40. Coats, AC: The sinusoidal galvanic body-sway response. Acta Otolaryngol (Stockh) 74:155, 1972.

41. Kots, YM: Descending reflex influences during the organization of voluntary movement. In Evarts, EV (ed): The Organization of Voluntary Mechanisms: Neurophysiological Mechanisms. Plenum, New York, 1977, p 181.

42. Iles, JF, and Pisini, JV: Vestibular-evoked postural reactions in man and modulation of transmission in spinal reflex pathways. J Physiol 455:407, 1992.

43. Storper, I, and Honrubia, V: Is human galvanically induced triceps surae electromyogram a vestibulospinal reflex response? Otolaryngol Head Neck Surg 107:527, 1992.

44. Britton, TC, et al: Postural electromyographic responses in the arm and leg following galvanic vestibular stimulation in man. Exp Brain Res 94:143, 1993.

45. Fitzpatrick, R, et al: Task-dependent reflex responses and movement illusions evoked by galvanic vestibular stimulation in standing humans. J Physiol 478:363, 1994.

46. Inglis, JT, et al: The effect of galvanic vestibular stimulation on human postural responses during support surface translations. J Neurophysiol 73:896, 1995.

47. Goldberg, JM, et al: Responses of vestibular-nerve afferents in the squirrel monkey to externally applied galvanic currents. Brain Res 252:156, 1982.

48. Tokita, T, et al: Diagnosis of otolith and semicircular-canal lesions by galvanic nystagmus and spinal reflexes. In Graham, M, and Kemink, J, (eds): The Vestibular System: Neurophysiologic and Clinical Research. Raven, New York, 1987, p 305.

49. Watanabe, Y, et al: Clinical evaluation of vestibular-somatosensory interactions using galvanic body sway test. In Graham, M, and Kemink, J, (eds): The Vestibular System: Neurophysiologic and Clinical Research. Raven, New York, 1987, p 393.

50. Lund, S, and Broberg, C: Effects of different head positions on postural sway in man induced by a reproducible vestibular error signal. Acta Physiol Scand 117:307, 1983.

51. Gurfinkel, VS, et al: Is the stretch reflex the main mechanism in the system of regulation of the vertical posture of man? Biofizika 19:744, 1974.

52. McCollum, G, and Leen, TK: Form and exploration of mechanical stability limits in erect stance. J Motor Behav 21:225, 1989.

53. Shumway-Cook, A, and McCollum, G: Assessment and treatment of balance deficits in the neurologic patient. In Montgomery, P, and Connolly, B (eds): Theoretical Framework and Practical Application to Physical Therapy. Chattanooga Corporation, Chattanooga, 1991.

54. Nashner, L, et al: Adaptation to altered support and visual conditions during stance: Patients with vestibular deficits. J Neurosci 5:536, 1982.

55. Black, F, and Nashner, L: Vestibulospinal control differs in patients with reduced and distorted vestibular function. Acta Otolaryngol 406:110, 1984.

56. Black, FO, et al: Abnormal postural control associated with peripheral vestibular disorders. In Pompeiano, O, and Allum, JHJ (eds): Progress in Brain Research, Vol 76, Vestibulospinal Control of Posture and Locomotion. Elsevier, Amsterdam, 1988, p 263.

57. Shumway-Cook, A, and Horak, FB: Assessing the influence of sensory interaction on balance. Phys Ther 66:1548, 1986.

58. Black, FO, et al: Computerized screening of the human vestibulospinal system. Ann Otol Rhinol Laryngol 87:853, 1978.

59. Magnus, R: Body Posture. In Van Harreveld, A (ed): New Delhi, Amerind, 1989.

60. Roberts, TDM: Reflex balance. Nature 244:56, 1973.

61. Roberts, TDM: Neurophysiology of Postural Mechanisms. Butterworth-Heinemann, London, 1967.

62. Wilson, VJ, et al: Spatial organization of neck and vestibular reflexes acting on the forelimbs of the decerebrate cat. J Neurophys 55:514, 1986.

63. Anderson, JH, et al: Dynamic relations between natural vestibular inputs and activity of forelimb extensor muscles in the decerebrate cat: I. Motor output during sinusoidal linear accelerations. Brain Res 120:1, 1977.

64. Anderson, JH, et al: Dynamic relations between natural vestibular inputs and activity of forelimb ex-

tensor muscles in the decerebrate cat: II. Motor output during rotations in the horizontal plane. Brain Res 120:17, 1977.

65. Soechting, JF, et al: Dynamic relations between natural vestibular inputs and activity of forelimb extensor muscles in the decerebrate cat: III. Motor output during rotations in the vertical plane. Brain Res 120:35, 1977.
66. Lacquaniti, F, et al: The control of limb geometry in cat posture. J Physiol 426:177, 1990.
67. Chan, CWY, and Kearney, RE: Influence of static tilts on soleus motorneuron excitability in man. Neurosci Lett 33:333, 1982.
68. Macpherson, JM, et al: Stance dependence of automatic postural adjustments in humans. Exp Brain Res 78:557, 1989.
69. Massion, J, et al: Axial synergies under microgravity conditions. J Vestib Res 3:275, 1993.
70. Bernstein, N: The Coordination and Regulation of Movement. Pergamon, London, 1967.
71. Melvill-Jones, G, and Watt, DGD: Muscular control of landing from unexpected falls in man. J Physiol (Lond) 219:729, 1971.
72. Greenwood, R, and Hopkins, A: Landing from an unexpected fall and a voluntary step. Brain 99:375, 1976.
73. Watt, DGD: Effect of vertical linear acceleration on H-reflex in decerebrate cat: I. Transient stimuli. J Neurophys 45:644, 1981.
74. Lacour, M, et al: Muscle responses and monosynaptic reflexes in falling monkey: Role of the vestibular system. J Physiol Paris 74:427, 1978.
75. Dietz, V, et al: Interlimb coordination of leg-muscle activation during perturbation of stance in humans. J Neurophysiol 62:680, 1989.
76. Horak, FB, et al: Vestibular and somatosensory contributions to responses to head and body displacements in stance. Exp Brain Res 100:93, 1994.
77. Shupert, CL, and Horak, FB: Effects of vestibular loss on head stabilization in response to head and body perturbations. J Vestib Res 6:1, 1996.
78. Allum, JHJ, and Honegger, F: A postural model of balance-correcting movement strategies. J Vestib Res 2:323, 1992.
79. Allum, JHJ, et al: The influence of bilateral peripheral vestibular deficit on postural synergies. J Vestib Res 4:49, 1994.
80. Horak, F, et al: Postural strategies associated with somatosensory and vestibular loss. Exp Brain Res 82:167, 1991.
81. Thomson, DB, et al: Bilateral labyrinthectomy in the cat: Motor behavior and quiet stance parameters. Exp Brain Res 85:364, 1991.
82. Shupert, C, et al: Coordination of the head and body in response to support surface translations in normals and patients with bilaterally reduced vestibular function. In Amblard, B, et al (eds): Posture and Gait: Development, Adaptation, and Modulation. Elsevier, Amsterdam, 1988 p. 281.
83. Diener, HC, et al: The significance of proprioception on postural stabilization as assessed by ischemia. Brain Res 296:103, 1984.
84. Mauritz, KH, et al: Balancing as a clinical test in the differential diagnosis of sensory-motor disorders. J Neurol Neurosurg Psychiatr 43:407, 1980.
85. Nashner, L: Fixed patterns of rapid postural responses among leg muscles during stance. Exp Brain Res 30:59, 1977.
86. Diener, HC, et al: Stabilization of human posture during induced oscillations of the body. Exp Brain Res 45:126, 1982.
87. Nashner, L, and McCollum, G: The organization of human postural movements: A formal basis and experimental synthesis. Behav Brain Sci, 8:135, 1985.
88. Horak, FB: Comparison of cerebellar and vestibular loss on scaling of postural responses. In Brandt, T, et al (eds): Disorders of Posture and Gait. George Thieme Verlag, Stuttgart, 1990, p 370.
89. Kasper, J, et al: Influence of standing on vestibular neuronal activity in awake cats. Exp Neurol 92:37, 1986.
90. Horak, FB, and Nashner, L: Central programming of postural movements: Adaptation to altered support surface configurations. J Neurophysiol 55:1369, 1986.
91. McCollum, G, et al: Parsimony in neural calculations for postural movements. In Bloedel, J, et al (eds): Cerebellar Functions. Springer-Verlag, Berlin, 1984, p 52.
92. Runge, CF, et al: Postural strategies defined by joint torques. Gait & Posture (accepted).
93. Runge, CF, et al: Role of vestibular information in initiation of rapid postural responses. Exp Brain Res 122:403, 1998.
94. Horak, FB, et al: Vestibular function and motor proficiency in children with hearing impairments and in learning disabled children with motor impairments. Dev Med Child Neurol 30:64, 1988.
95. Kaga, K, et al: Influence of labyrinthine hypoactivity on gross motor development of infants. Ann NY Acad Sci 374:412, 1981.
96. Fregly, A: Vestibular ataxia and its measurement in man. In Kornhuber, H (ed): Handbook of Sensory Physiology, Vol VI, The Vestibular System, Part 2: Psychophysics, Applied Aspects, and General Interpretation. Springer-Verlag, Berlin, 1974, p 321.

97. Shupert, CL, et al: Hip sway associated with vestibulopathy. J Vestibular Res 4:231, 1994.
98. Shumway-Cook, A, and Horak, FB: Vestibular rehabilitation: An exercise approach to managing symptoms of vestibular dysfunction. Semin Hearing 10:196, 1989.
99. Shumway-Cook, A, et al: Critical examination of vestibular function in motor-impaired learning disabled children. Int J Ped Otorhinolaryngol 14:21, 1988.
100. Crowe, TK, and Horak, FB: Motor proficiency associated with vestibular deficits in children with hearing impairments. Phys Ther 68:1493, 1988.
101. Nashner, L: Strategies for organization of human posture. In Igarashi, M, and Black, FO (eds): Vestibular and Visual Control on Posture and Locomotor Equilibrium. Karger, Basel, 1985, p 1.
102. Pozzo, T, et al: Head stabilization during various locomotor tasks in humans: I. Normal subjects. Exp Brain Res 82:97, 1990.
103. Grossman, G, et al: Performance of the human vestibuloocular reflex during locomotion. J Neurophys 62:264, 1989.
104. Assaiante, C, and Amblard, B: Head-trunk coordination and locomotor equilibrium in 3- to 8-year old children. In Berthoz, A, et al (eds): The Head-Neck Sensory Motor System. Oxford Univ. Pr., New York, 1991, p 121.
105. Keshner, E, et al: Neck, trunk and limb muscle responses during postural perturbations in humans. Exp Brain Res 75:455, 1988.
106. Grossman, G, and Leigh, RJ: Instability of gaze during locomotion in patients with deficient vestibular function. Ann Neurol 27:528, 1990.
107. Pozzo, T, et al: Head stabilization during various locomotor tasks in humans: II. Patients with bilateral peripheral vestibular deficits. Exp Brain Res 85:208, 1991.

CHAPTER 3

Postural Abnormalities in Vestibular Disorders

Emily A. Keshner, PT, EdD

The vestibular system is considered to play an integral role in the control of posture and balance. Much of the evidence for this conclusion has, in fact, relied on findings of postural and orientation disorders in patients and animals with vestibular abnormalities.[1-5] Both clinical and experimental observations have shown that along with symptoms of vertigo, past pointing, and nystagmus, equilibrium disturbances are one of the major complaints of patients with partial or total destruction of the vestibular labyrinths.[6] Despite these fairly consistent symptoms, examination of any one patient with postural abnormalities arising from damage to the vestibular system could yield an uncertain diagnosis.[6,7] Most diagnoses are based on subjective complaints, and patient descriptions of a symptom may differ. One patient might experience a perception of the world spinning about, while another complains of imbalance and falling, yet both could have the same vestibular pathology.[7] Because the process of central nervous compensation proceeds over a lengthy period of time, patients can also have different symptoms when they finally arrive at a clinic, although suffering a similar deficit.

The question for the clinician and the clinical investigator is whether any one compensatory strategy is more efficient or effective for the population of patients with a vestibular deficit. If one strategy is better, then a systematic approach to treatment could be followed. But to determine the effectiveness of the compensation, we must first determine how to reliably detect whether the patient is suffering from postural dyscontrol, and whether vestibular dysfunction is responsible for the symptoms. In this chapter, some of the methods available for testing postural disorders associated with vestibular pathology are briefly discussed. Then, postural behaviors that have been quantified and associated with specific vestibular pathologies will be described. Finally, the issue of how the postural system compensates for loss or damage to vestibular signals will be discussed.

EXAMINING THE VESTIBULOSPINAL SYSTEM

Advantages and Limitations of Clinical Tests

Although vestibular disorders continue to be diagnosed through measures of the vestibulo-ocular system such as electronystagmography and rotational testing, these cannot fully describe all disorders of the vestibular system. One problem is that tests of vestibulo-ocular integrity and vestibulospinal function may not be correlated.[7] First, the well-defined loop of the vestibulo-ocular reflex (VOR) does not, in any way, reveal the integrity of the more complex vestibulospinal pathways, which are intimately involved in the control of posture and balance. Second, tests of the VOR are commonly performed in the plane of the horizontal semicircular canals, whereas vestibulospinal reflexes (VSR) are dependent on inputs from the vertical semicircular canals and the otoliths.

There is increasing evidence that dynamic posturography is a useful tool for identifying disorders of the vestibulospinal system.[8–10] Dynamic posturography is not a direct assessment of peripheral or central vestibular function: it assesses balance rather than specific vestibular function. But response patterns specific to individuals with vestibular dysfunction are elicited with dynamic posturography; thus it is a useful adjunct to more traditional methods of testing vestibular function. Diagnostic tests of the vestibulospinal system that are more easily available to the clinician, and less expensive, than dynamic posturography are discussed in this chapter, as well as some of the problems inherent in each method of testing. Table 3–1 presents a summary of the advantages and disadvantages of the tests discussed here.

TABLE 3–1 Advantages and Disadvantages of Clinical Tests of Postural Instability

Static Tests		
	Advantages	**Disadvantages**
Romberg	Easily performed in clinic	Qualitative
		Does not test adaptive responses
Stabilometry	Quantitative	Requires a force platform
	Can manipulate sensory inputs	Intersegmental shifts confound results
		Does not test adaptive responses
Dynamic Tests		
Stepping tests	Easily performed in clinic	Does not test adaptive responses
	Can be quantified	Has not been shown to be reliable
Tiltboards	Easily performed in clinic	Qualitative
	Requires adaptation to external forces	Amplitude and application of force are not controlled
Posturography	Quantitative	Requires a posture platform
	Requires adaptation to external forces	
	Can manipulate sensory signals	

Dynamic Posturography

AUTOMATIC POSTURAL RESPONSES

In the 1970s, Nashner reported stereotypical, automatic responses to postural disturbances initiated at the base of support, introducing the measurement of postural reactions on a moving platform as a powerful experimental approach.[11,12] Since that time, the majority of studies of postural kinematics have concentrated on the elec-

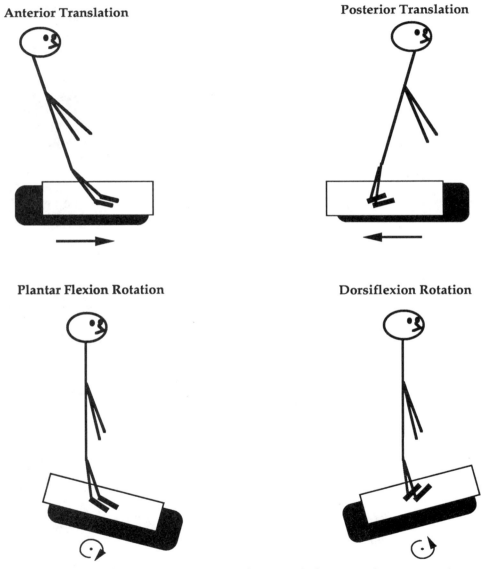

FIGURE 3–1. The four standard directions of posture platform perturbation. Note that in anterior translations and plantar flexion rotations, ankle angles increase. In posterior translations and dorsiflexion rotations, ankle angles decrease.

tromyographic (EMG) responses from muscles in the lower limb, from which most descriptions about restabilizing actions have been drawn.[11–16] Subjects stand on a platform that could be translated in an anterior and posterior direction, or rotated so that the ankles are moved into plantar flexion or dorsiflexion (Fig. 3–1). The expected response to anterior motion of the platform is backwards sway (base of support moved in front of the center of mass), producing a decreased angle at the ankle and a stretch of the ankle muscles on the anterior surface of the body (i.e., tibialis anterior). If the platform moves posteriorly, the subject sways forward (base of support moved behind the center of mass), thereby decreasing the ankle angle and stretching the gastrocnemius and soleus muscles. Rotating the platform into plantar flexion or dorsiflexion would produce equivalent changes at the ankle (see Fig. 3–1), but the center of mass remains in line with the base of support.

Although the monosynaptic stretch reflex does not act functionally to replace the center of mass over the base of support, EMG analysis of the lower limb muscles revealed that the muscles being stretched also responded at latencies longer than the stretch reflex but shorter than voluntary reactions in order to bring the body back over the base of support. These restabilizing ankle muscle responses (at latencies of 90 to 120 ms) were followed within 10 to 20 ms by the muscle in the upper leg on the same side of the body (i.e., soleus followed by the hamstrings; tibialis anterior followed by the quadriceps). Thus, from these early studies, patterns of muscle activation initiated by ankle proprioceptive inputs, and arising from distal to proximal lower limb muscles, were identified as ascending muscle synergies responsible for restabilization after platform movement.[11,12]

Nashner's original conclusion that the body acts as a rigid, inverted pendulum, relying primarily on ankle proprioceptive inputs to initiate the restabilizing actions, does not accurately describe the complex, multisegmental actions that occur during postural restabilization.[14,16–19] The "ankle strategy" is most effective when sway is slow and the support surface is firm. When it is impossible to exert adequate torque around the ankle joint, as when the base of support is narrow or pliant, balance is recovered with flexion at the hip or a "hip strategy."[20] Allum et al[21] concluded that all balance corrections result from one of two basic synergies defined by the timing between segmental responses, and that the selected synergy was amplitude modulated according to the initial movement velocities at all joint segments, thereby producing a continuous repertoire of movement strategies for balance. With more realistic stimuli (i.e., rapid perturbations and a center of mass moving far beyond the base of support), the ability to take a step has been found to be the relevant criteria for recovery of balance.[22,23] Other studies have demonstrated that the initiation of the balance reactions is highly dependent both on the ability to predict the occurrence of the perturbation,[24–27] and on the location of the disturbance on the body.[28–31]

IDENTIFYING VESTIBULAR CONTRIBUTIONS TO AUTOMATIC POSTURAL RESPONSES

Since the earliest presentation of Nashner's findings, investigators have been attempting to define the contribution of the vestibular system to the automatic postural responses.[32–36] Studies in which the labyrinthine receptors were directly stimulated by vertically dropping human and animal subjects, thereby producing linear acceleratory stimuli,[33–36] demonstrated that direct labyrinthine stimulation can produce automatic or "triggered" postural reactions in the lower limb. Nashner[13] hypothesized, however, that the vestibular system only contributes to the control of lower-limb balance reactions when proprioceptive signals are absent or unreliable. Using a servomechanism, the posture platform was made to match the sway at the hip, thereby maintaining a neutral position at the ankle and, assumably, eliminating any change in the proprioceptive feedback from the ankle during normal quiet standing.[13] In these subjects, automatic postural responses were significantly delayed when the subjects had to rely on vestibular signals in the absence of proprioceptive feedback from the ankles.

Quite possibly the servomechanism did not fully remove the ankle proprioceptor feedback, but rather produced distorted or modified signals that altered the automatic postural reactions, or responses to vestibular inputs during quiet stance may not be transferable to those responses observed during dynamic gait and a loss of balance. In an attempt to resolve the issue of labyrinthine involvement in the generation of postural reactions to support surface displacements, Allum et al.[37] devised a novel experiment. Angular displacement of the ankle was kept equal for both platform translations and rotations, thereby producing equivalent proprioceptive signals from the ankle, although the labyrinthine inputs differed. When head acceleration and neck and lower-limb muscle EMG responses recorded during both perturbations did not exhibit the same response patterns, these investigators concluded that labyrinthine signals must be directly involved in the generation of lower-limb postural reactions. The differences between the subject groups were greatest and most consistent during platform rotations,[38] leading these researchers to believe that vestibular loss is best diagnosed using a rotation of the support surface. Using a range of platform translation velocities (5 to 35 cm/sec) others[39] found that equivalent head accelerations produced very different torques at the hip and knee in healthy subjects and patients with bilateral vestibular deficit, suggesting that the magnitude and force pattern of the muscles depend on vestibular inputs from early head movements.

ALTERING SENSORY CUES

Manipulating the visual and somatosensory inputs that are available during dynamic posturography is another method employed to isolate a person's ability to use vestibular signals. As mentioned previously, protocols to alter somatosensory inputs currently include using a servoed platform that matches the normal sway at the ankle during quiet standing, or adding a layer of dense foam to the base of support to make somatosensory inputs less effective.[40] Visual conditions have been controlled by either stabilizing or rotating the visual field in an anterior-posterior plane.[40–42] When the visual field is rotated in phase with the anterior-posterior sway of the subject, the subject experiences a distortion of visual signals by way of the unexpected and inappropriate visual feedback.

Although normal subjects, elderly individuals, and those with vestibular deficit exhibit an increased tendency to fall under conditions of altered sensory input,[40,41,44,45] concluding that the cause is a vestibulospinal system unable to compensate for the loss of other sensory signals may be premature. Modification of somatosensory and visual inputs is not necessarily equivalent to a loss of those signals, and the central nervous system may well compensate for distorted or minimized inputs by altering the sensorimotor transformation algorithm. For example, the system may select a compensatory strategy that relies on enhancing the gains of somatosensory and visual responsiveness to the distorted inputs rather than shifting responsibility for the response on to the vestibulospinal system.

In summary, postural responses to support surface displacements have been tested by: (1) translating a standing subject along the earth's horizontal plane on a moving platform; (2) rotating the foot about the horizontal axis of the ankle into dorsi-flexion or plantar flexion; and (3) keeping the platform fixed to the earth horizontal or servoing the angle of the platform to match the angle at the ankle during quiet sway. Experiments using the posture platform have been performed with a wide range of ve-locities and amplitudes of displacement that alter the transmission of forces from the lower limb to the head and make the comparison of vestibular influences on balance difficult across laboratory settings. Instructions to the subjects and monitoring of past experiences with the paradigm are not regulated. A further restriction on the interpre-tation of results is that measurement of postural responses should incorporate the mechanics of body sway with the threshold properties and dynamic characteristics of the labyrinthine receptors,[16,39,46–48] because knowing the mechanics of the head and motions of the center of mass is necessary for predicting the role of canal and otolith feedback in restabilization. Despite its limitations, and the multitude of variables that should be controlled, the posture platform continues to be employed as a method for obtaining quantitative measures of postural reactions in clinical populations. Many of the results reported in this chapter have, in fact, depended on the posture platform methodology to examine disturbances in postural control as a result of vestibular dysfunction.

Tests of Quiet Stance

Traditional clinical examinations of vestibulospinal function include tests of self-localization, such as the Romberg test.[49] Initially, Romberg's test of instability was based on a population of patients with proprioceptive loss from tabes dorsalis who were unable to stand with feet together and eyes closed. But the Romberg test is insen-sitive for detection of chronic unilateral labyrinthine impairment, and is highly vari-able, even within a subject.[50] Modifying the test by having the patient stand in a tan-dem heel-to-toe position (sharpened or tandem Romberg) has made the test more sensitive,[6] probably because of the narrowed base of support. Even so, tests of quiet stance fail to measure the adaptive components of the postural response that are essen-tial to dynamic balance during most daily activities.[51]

Tests of quiet stance may indicate the severity of a balance problem because pa-tients with vestibular system damage will demonstrate increased sway and falling when the base of support is constrained during quiet standing. Conclusions about the neural processes contributing to postural imbalance are severely limited, however. The effect of altered proprioceptive and cutaneous information on low-frequency sway sta-bilization cannot be determined by tests of quiet standing. Changing velocity of the vi-sual field is a significant parameter controlling body sway during quiet standing,[51] but simple removal of vision does not alter the temporal or spatial organization of the au-tomatic postural reactions.[32] Furthermore, behavioral measures as to how often a sub-ject falls, or to which direction he deviates, do not convey information about the motor and sensory mechanisms that may be involved in postural control.[52,53] Thus, attempt-ing to assess the integrity of the vestibular system through a test of quiet standing opens the door to many confounding variables, and is far from specific to the vestibu-lospinal disorders that may produce a postural deficit.[54,55] Despite these limitations, the concept of deviation from the vertical during quiet standing continues to underlie most clinical testing of vestibular dysfunction.

Stabilometry

Stabilometry is a clinical tool that measures anterior-posterior and lateral excursions of the body in subjects standing quietly on a force platform, usually over time.[56-58] During that time, the subject stands quietly on a force plate, and the excursion of the center of gravity is measured across several conditions that can include eyes open, eyes closed, and eyes closed with head extension. Attempts to stress the vestibulospinal system have been incorporated into this system of measurement by altering signals from other sensory pathways. For example, adding a layer of foam rubber to the base of support to make somatosensory inputs less effective,[40] or placing the subjects within a visually controlled environment to modify visual feedback.[41] This attempt to quantify the classical Romberg test has made the measurement of postural sway during quiet standing more objective, but the mechanisms contributing to the observation of increased sway still cannot be identified. One problem is that changing the position of the body parts (either randomly or through experimenter directive) could shift the center of pressure without affecting the stability of the subject.[56] In general, because the sensory apparatus of the vestibular system is most responsive to changes in acceleration and orientation in space,[59] and because patients with vestibular deficits tend to have normal Romberg signs, tests of quiet standing on a stabilometer are not compelling measures of vestibulospinal function.

Tiltboards

Tilt reactions, or reflexes opposing bodily displacement, traditionally were evoked through a lateral tilt or anterior-posterior tilt of the supporting surface about a horizontal axis.[1-3] On tilting the base of support, the reaction to regain a stable equilibrium occurred by moving the body against the angular momentum and repositioning the center of gravity within the vertical projection of its base of support.[1-5] These reactions have also been elicited in the clinic by simply pushing the patient at the shoulder girdle. Problems with the accuracy of this test are threefold. First, because the tilt reactions are measured by observational techniques, later voluntary responses (greater than 150 ms) rather than automatic postural reactions are being evaluated. Second, the response pattern alters if the force is applied directly to the trunk rather than to the support surface. Third, tilt responses will be organized differently depending on whether the patient is pushed or trips over an obstacle in the environment, whether the application of perturbation is predictable, and whether it is self-induced or elicited.

Stepping Tests

The Unterberger[60] or stepping test of Fukuda[61] examines the ability of patients to turn about a vertical axis when marching or stepping in place. Marked variability in the amount of rotation produced by even the same subject, however, makes these tests unreliable.[6] Patients with severe disruption of the vestibular system may stagger so uncontrollably that the stepping tests cannot reliably indicate the side of the lesion.[62] A battery of tests developed by Graybiel and Fregly[63] (Ataxia Test Battery) examine subjects standing upright, on one leg, and with feet aligned in tandem position with eyes open or closed, as well as tandem walking in a straight line on the floor or on a narrow rail. This test is useful for patients that have compensated for a labyrinthine deficit because, when a narrowed base of support is required, even those patients score more poorly than normal subjects on measures of deviation from the straight line or of the number of steps made prior to falling from the rail.

POSTURAL REACTIONS IN PERIPHERAL VESTIBULAR DISORDERS

A discussion of etiology and diagnostic testing of vestibular system disease is beyond the scope of this chapter, but can be found in other sources.[6,64,65] The focus here will be on those vestibular disturbances that have been found to produce a postural disturbance, and those that have been tested for changes in vestibulospinal function. Dysfunction in the vestibulospinal system can be divided into two categories: distortion and deficiency.[66,67] A *deficiency* in the system usually implies that the sensory (i.e., labyrinthine) inputs have been reduced or abolished, resulting mostly in complaints of unsteadiness and instability. *Distortion* means that the signal is present but disturbed, and does not correspond with expectations about the sensory feedback. The result would be inappropriate or false motor responses to the existing situation (e.g., vertigo and ataxia). A summary of postural disturbances is presented in Table 3–2 for the disorders discussed in this chapter.

Deficient Labyrinthine Inputs

Damage along the eighth nerve or within the vestibular labyrinth produces lost or diminished signals from the peripheral vestibular apparatus.[59] Central disturbances originate at the vestibular nuclei or in the higher central pathways that communicate with the vestibular nuclei. In both cases, patients can experience disequilibrium, im-

TABLE 3–2 Postural Disturbances Observed with Vestibular Disorders

Peripheral Vestibular Disorders	
Deficient Inputs	Need more energy to maintain the upright position
	Instability increases in the presence of inappropriate sensory signals
	Amplitudes of EMG and torque are inversely related to severity of deficit
Distorted Inputs	Still able to process vestibular inputs
	Falls increase in the presence of inappropriate sensory signals
Central Vestibular Disorders	
	Impaired perception and location of the gravitational vertical
	Direction-specific ataxia
	Falling tends to occur in the direction of quick phase nystagmus
Aging	
	Longer response latencies and delayed reaction times
	Diminished sensory acuity and impaired signal detection
	Postural response patterns are temporally disordered

balance, and ataxia. With unilateral lesions of the peripheral system, the normal symmetry of inputs from the right and left labyrinths become disordered, resulting in a decreased firing rate of the vestibular nuclei on one side. A unilateral lesion affects the system as if the intact side were being stimulated, thus generating an illusion of change in head orientation and movement. The inherent disequilibrium then activates the vestibulospinal system to respond inappropriately, resulting in vertigo, nystagmus, and postural instability.

Another effect of vestibular system stimulation, maintaining tone of the muscles against gravity, appears to be directly correlated with labyrinthine inputs; the activation of extensor muscles in the extremities of both monkeys[68] and humans[69] with unilateral deficit were found to be enhanced contralateral to the side of the lesion. But postural reactions are more complex than single-pathway vestibular reflexes, and cannot be traced and localized as easily as these direct-line responses. For example, when both labyrinths are lesioned, an artificial sense of motion does not occur, and neither do the symptoms of nystagmus and vertigo. Yet equilibrium is still disturbed, suggesting that the balance function of the vestibular system is not a simple response to stimulation of the labyrinthine receptors.

Indicators of Vestibulospinal Deficiency

UNILATERAL AND BILATERAL LABYRINTHINE DEFICIT

Variability of the responses measured from the many methods of posturography confirms the complexity of control of these disordered postural responses. After repeated attempts to quantify the results of the Romberg test, the most reliable effort seems to be measuring energy of the power spectral densities of the center of force trajectories when maintaining an upright position.[70] Both in this study and in others using force plates to record sway during quiet stance,[7,58] intersubject variability and overlap between normal and clinical populations reduced the strength of the findings. Results suggest, however, that more energy needs be expended to maintain an upright position when visual inputs are removed (eyes closed) from patients with a labyrinthine deficit.

In a series of papers presented by Black and Nashner,[44,66,70] postural sway was recorded through a potentiometer placed at the level of the hips. Patients stood on a platform that could be either earth fixed, or moved proportional to body sway (servoed). The visual environment was then manipulated so that patients experienced a visual field that was either (1) earth fixed, (2) proportional to body sway, or (3) removed by eye closure. Patients with reduced or absent labyrinthine inputs were more unstable than normal controls only when ankle proprioceptive references were proportional to body sway and visual references were either removed or inappropriate (conditions 2 and 3 above). When the only reliable source of feedback was the vestibular inputs, it was believed that patients with vestibular deficiencies would fall because they were dependent on the somatosensory and visual reference to correctly organize their postural responses. From these studies, Black and colleagues suggested that vestibular deficits could be quantified by systematically altering the sensory information provided by the support surface and the visual surround.

Several problems limit our reliance on these results for clinical diagnosis and measurement, however. First, patients with unilateral or partial bilateral deficits at times were as unstable as patients with total loss of vestibular function,[52] thus rendering this a poor test of graduated function in the vestibular system. Second, the authors tested only well-compensated patients. As will be discussed later, compensation could occur as a central reorganization in the system. Thus, these experiments may not be testing a vestibular deficit, but rather a compensatory subsystem that responds inadequately to the presented stimuli. Third, patients with postural instability from other, nonvestibular disorders may have test results similar to those of patients with vestibular deficits (Hain and Herdman, personal communication).

Allum and colleagues examined both the latencies and amplitudes of muscle EMG responses on a platform that dorsiflexed the ankle.[14,32,37,53,71,72] Areas under the EMG bursts in the ankle muscles, soleus and tibialis anterior, and ankle torque recordings of patients with complete bilateral labyrinthine deficit were significantly diminished when compared with normal subjects with eyes both open and closed. Using these data, the presence of a linear correlation between EMG amplitudes and the extent of the peripheral vestibular deficit was explored.[54] The population measured included those with intact labyrinths (normal subjects), acute unilateral labyrinthine deficit patients, chronic unilateral labyrinthine deficit patients, and bilateral labyrinthine deficit patients, thus covering a graduated range of labyrinthine function.

A stepwise discriminant analysis technique performed on the data suggested that muscle response amplitudes in the soleus and tibialis anterior muscles, as well as amplitude of torque exerted on the platform, were inversely related to the severity of the labyrinthine deficit. Muscle and torque responses diminished in amplitude as the reception of labyrinthine inputs decreased. Because lower-limb EMG activity was still present in the patients with complete loss of labyrinthine inputs, a linear correlation of the amount of EMG activity with extent of peripheral vestibular deficit suggests that lower-limb postural reflexes could be triggered by proprioceptive stretch reflexes, but that amplitude modulation is under the control of, or requires the presence of, vestibulospinal signals. EMG activity in the neck muscles was not obviously altered in these patients, implying local control of neck muscle responses. Thus the effectiveness of the ankle muscle responses to produce a functional forward torque in patients rotated backward on a platform was diminished, and these patients tended to fall backward.

EMG responses of patients with vestibular deficit during horizontal translations of a platform were also examined.[38,73] Although latencies of the postural reactions were produced without significant time delays, segmental organization of the postural response were disordered. Allum et al[72] found that angular velocity measures of rotation of the trunk about the hip were not significantly altered in patients with a bilateral peripheral vestibular deficit, and that a hip strategy was a common component in the postural response to platform rotations. These investigators suggested that the movement strategy selected depended on the initial direction of trunk and head acceleration (which is oppositely directed in platform rotations and translations), and was executed as if preprogrammed from the beginning. Although Horak et al[73] previously stated that hip strategies were not seen in patients with vestibular disorders, new measures of hip torques emphasize the importance of identifying the proper response variables when using dynamic posturography as a diagnostic tool. Runge et al[39] have found that the joint torques at the hip and knee were abnormal over a range of velocities during rearward translations for patients with bilateral deficit. Because head accelerations were the same in the patients and healthy subjects, these investigators agreed with other findings[14,32] that the magnitude and force pattern of the muscles depends on vestibular inputs from early head movements.

We can conclude that patients with partial or total loss of labyrinthine input exhibit diminished amplitudes of EMG response and thus require greater energy expenditure to maintain balance, particularly when another source of stimulation to the system (e.g., visual inputs) has been removed. These patients also exhibit greater sway in sensory conflict situations, and variability between patients is a common clinical occurrence because of the dynamic central compensatory processes. With unilateral deficit, the initial perception of apparent body motion is directed away from the side of the lesion. Postural reactions are usually in a direction opposite to the direction of vertigo, causing a tendency to fall and deviate toward the affected side. Severe postural disturbances occur when these individuals have to rely on vestibular inputs, but the deficit is compensated within 2 weeks after the lesion.[74] Individuals with bilateral deficit exhibit normal postural sway in quiet stance.[73] Removal of vision with eye closure increases this sway by only a small amount.[66] These patients tend to fall backward when their eyes are closed during dorsiflexion tilts of a platform. Their diminished amplitudes of muscle activity presumably result in the reduced restabilizing torques recorded at the ankle, knee, and hip.[75]

MÉNIÈRE'S SYNDROME

Ménière's syndrome, or endolymphatic hydrops, is considered to be a vestibular deficiency, although it presents as fluctuating vestibular function. Symptoms of acute Ménière's syndrome include a fluctuating low-frequency hearing loss, tinnitus, and a sensation of fullness or pressure in the ear.[6] Patients with this syndrome exhibit a negative Romberg sign during remission,[76] but symptoms of dizziness and instability can occur for several days following intermittent episodes of vertigo. These episodes appear at irregular intervals for years, and about one-third of the patients eventually develop bilateral involvement.[6]

Objective diagnosis of Ménière's syndrome has been dependent on long-term documentation of the fluctuating hearing loss. More recently, quantitative posturography measures have been able to identify consistent changes in the postural response of these patients, even during periods of remission. The movement pattern of the center of gravity was measured during a stepping test after observing that patients deviated toward the affected side even during the remission period.[76] Stepping was performed in the dark with eyes open and closed, and patients were required to perform at a frequency that was both optimal for normal walking and that elicited a smooth rhythmical pattern (i.e., 1.2 Hz). When eyes were closed, the patients exhibited angular deviations of 30° or more toward the affected side after 8 to 12 seconds of stepping. Time to deviation indicated a degrading central motor program that was initiated by visual inputs, but which required vestibular inputs (in the absence of vision) to be maintained over time.

Measures of sway during quiet standing have included analyses of the pattern of motion, displacement, and power spectrum of the center of gravity. With all of these measures, position of the center of gravity changed in an irregular fashion, and deviated primarily toward the affected side.[77,78] High-frequency components of standing sway were observed during acute phases of Ménière's syndrome, but not during remission periods.[78] Patients with Ménière's syndrome who had not developed vestibular hypofunction, as determined from VOR gains, were also tested under conditions of sensory conflict during quiet standing (see earlier description in section on "Indicators of Vestibulospinal Dysfunction").[70] These patients responded very much like well-compensated patients with unilateral or bilateral loss of labyrinthine inputs. The group had nearly normal responses on all trials with the platform fixed to earth horizontal. Responses fell outside the normal range when either the platform or the visual field was perceptually stabilized, again suggesting dependence on reliable inputs from the vestibular labyrinths during these test conditions.

Indications of Vestibulospinal Distortion

BENIGN PAROXYSMAL PERIPHERAL POSITIONAL VERTIGO

To study the effects of distorted labyrinthine inputs on posture, patients with benign paroxysmal peripheral positional vertigo (BPPV) have been examined.[70] The key to this syndrome is that brief episodes of vertigo (usually less than 1 minute) are generated with position change. Paroxysmal positional nystagmus can be observed with rapid changes of position. After a period of several attacks, symptoms can become more prolonged, and include dizziness and nausea lasting for hours or days.[6] Degeneration of the utricular macula releasing otoconia that settle on the cupula of the posterior semicircular canal is strongly implicated as the cause of BPPV, and could result from a variety of etiologies (i.e., trauma, infection, ischemia). The intensity of BPPV depends on the velocity of the positional changes, and attacks can be avoided if positions are assumed very slowly.[79]

Because of the positional component of this syndrome, postural changes are easily recorded during quiet standing by having patients alter the position of their head in space. After tilting the head, large amplitudes of anterior-posterior sway and sway ipsilateral to the direction of head tilt were observed.[79] Instability gradually decreased as the vertigo diminished, but with eyes closed, the sway could not be compensated by other inputs, and falling occurred.

Unlike patients with a loss of vestibular inputs, patients with distorted inputs from BPPV reacted normally on a moving platform when forced to rely only on vestibular inputs. More disturbing to this group of patients were inappropriate (perceptually stabilized) visual circumstances whether the platform was earth fixed or moving proportional to body sway.[52,66,70] Patients with BPPV probably rely primarily on visual information to organize their postural reactions, and have suppressed their response to the potentially unreliable vestibular inputs.

POSTURAL REACTIONS IN CENTRAL VESTIBULAR LESIONS

One could erroneously assume that function of the vestibular labyrinths is directly representative of the functional integrity of the vestibular system. Although receiving direct inputs from the peripheral labyrinths, the vestibular nuclear complex also receives visual and somatosensory inputs.[59] Convergence of vestibular and somatosensory input onto the vestibulospinal and reticulospinal[80] neurons can take place at the level of the vestibular nuclear complex, at the adjacent reticular formation, and upon spinal interneurons[81,82] and motoneurons.[80] Inputs from either of these modalities are not necessarily redundant because each represents different parameters and is effective within a particular frequency domain.[83–85] In fact, the frequency of stimulation is important to control with compensated patients because motor output of the visual system as well as the vestibular system has been found to be frequency dependent.[48,86–89] Thus it is unlikely that normal postural responses are reflective of the isolated labyrinthine and neck reflexes observed in the decerebrate animal.[90–92] Instead, postural reactions probably emerge from a dynamic coupling of all available sensory signals.

Several clinical findings have been suggested to differentiate between a peripheral and central disturbance in the vestibular system. Gradually increasing disturbances of standing, walking, and falling in the direction of the quick phase of spontaneous nystagmus have been identified as indications of a central vestibular lesion.[93] Balance disorders as a result of abnormalities of the vestibular nuclear complex have been observed,[94,95] but are poorly documented. The majority of the literature about central vestibular brain stem lesions reports only oculomotor abnormalities, but Brandt et al[95] have attempted to relate well-defined central vertigo syndromes to characteristics of postural imbalance. Briefly, these investigators reported five conditions for which postural imbalance has been consistently reported: downbeat nystagmus vertigo syndrome, ocular tilt reaction, Wallenberg's syndrome, paroxysmal and familial ataxia, and brain stem lesions that mimic labyrinthine dysfunction. One should recognize, however, that structures other than the vestibular system may be damaged and affect balance.

Downbeat nystagmus is specific for a lesion of the paramedian craniocervical junction (30 percent of cases due to Arnold-Chiari malformation), inducing a direction-specific vestibulospinal ataxia. Static head tilts modulate the intensity of the nystagmus and the postural sway, suggesting involvement of otolith function. The typical postural imbalance in this condition is an anterior-posterior sway with a tendency to fall backward, but many of these patients do not complain of vertigo or balance problems. Brandt et al[95] suggest that the backward sway is a vestibulospinal compensation to the forward vertigo resulting from the downbeat nystagmus. **Ocular tilt reaction** is actually a triad of responses, including ipsilateral head-trunk tilt, ocular torsion, and ocular deviation. This condition has been observed in patients with brain stem abscess, multiple sclerosis, and acute Wallenberg's syndrome. Patients seem to have a readjustment in their perception of the vertical that matches tilt deviation of the eye, head, and trunk. **Wallenberg's syndrome** is an infarction of the dorsolateral medulla resulting in ipsilateral dysmetria of the extremities, pain and temperature loss, and a lateropulsion of the eyes and head causing the body to deviate toward the side of the lesion and, consequently, fall. **Paroxysmal and familial ataxia** share the broad-based, unsteady gait that defines ataxia. Finally, pontomedullary lesions near the vestibular nuclei at the entry of the eighth nerve can mimic a peripheral labyrinthine disorder, and **drop attacks** (a sudden, unpredictable forward falling) can occur with basilar insufficiency. Thus, the evidence from clinical reports suggests that a central vestibular dysfunction results in impaired perception and location of the gravitational vertical exhibited throughout the body postural system. But with all of these syndromes, other motor structures are affected as well, and may contribute to the impairment.

POSTURAL DYSFUNCTION WITH PATHOLOGY OF OTHER SENSORY-MOTOR CENTERS

The vestibular nuclear complex communicates with motor as well as sensory centers.[93] In fact, extensive reciprocal connections between the vestibular nuclei and the cerebellum[96] argue for a prominent role of the cerebellum in regulating the output of the

vestibulospinal system, and lesions of the cerebellum result in severe postural disturbances. Three kinds of cerebellar ataxia have been identified, suggesting different
pathophysiological mechanisms that are dependent on the site of the lesion.[97] A test of
the sway stabilizing responses on a posture platform of patients with late cortical atrophy of the anterior lobe of the cerebellum revealed that response latencies were within
normal limits following dorsiflexion rotations and backward translations on a platform,
but amplitudes and durations of response were two to three times greater than normal,[98,99] and habituation to the stimulus was absent.[100] Postural response magnitudes of
the patients with anterior lobe damage were scaled correctly when relying on current
somatosensory feedback, but patients were unable to scale their responses when relying
on prior experience. Thus, the major effect of anterior lobe cerebellar damage on postural responses may be an impairment of responses based on predictive central set.[99]

A characteristic sway frequency of 3 Hz has been recorded in this population.[101]
Intersegmental counterbalancing actions were enhanced in these patients, so that
falling was not commonly observed, but they tend to exhibit a stiff-legged gait. Stance
ataxia was found to improve with visual feedback, unlike that appearing with vestibulospinal lesions.[102] Thus, in these patients, stabilizing responses occurred, but they
lacked the balance between opposing muscle forces and grading of response over time.

The postural system of patients with lesions of the vestibulocerebellum (flocculus,
nodulus, and uvula) may be so severely impaired that these patients cannot walk.
Ataxia of the head and trunk is observed while sitting, standing, and walking. These
patients exhibit unusually large sway in all directions with predominantly low frequencies of less than 1 Hz, and visual stabilization appears to be reduced when
Romberg tests with eyes open and closed are compared. These patients tend to fall
even when sitting down, which may be due to diminished intersegmental movement
for counterbalancing or to truncal ataxia.[97,103] Neocerebellum lesions produce little
postural instability or disturbance of stance, even with eyes closed. Control of position
of the body's center of mass seems to be disturbed, because these patients exhibit
ataxia during a limb and trunk pursuit task.[97] Reports of head and trunk deviation to
the side of the lesion have also appeared.[103]

With basal ganglia disorders, such as Parkinson's disease, equilibrium reactions are
often delayed or absent.[1] An anticipatory postural response in the soleus muscle, normally seen in response to a perturbation of the forearm, is absent or reduced in these patients,[104] although long latency responses to direct stretch of a muscle have been observed to be enhanced in the Parkinson population in both the upper arm[105] and lower
limb.[106] Response latencies to sudden platform displacements were found to be within
the normal range,[107,108] although the ability to suppress long latency muscle reactions to
a perturbation was impaired in these patients even under supported conditions.[109]
When required to scale the magnitude of their responses to amplitude and velocity of
backward platform translations, patients with Parkinson's disease produced smaller
than normal extensor bursts, larger than normal flexor bursts, and smaller torque responses.[110] On a sinusoidally moving treadmill, patients with Parkinson's disease were
able to maintain their balance with eyes open by using their leg flexor muscles, whereas
healthy subjects activated their extensor muscles. Timing and amplitude of this muscle
activity were also impaired.[111] The inability to generate adequate force in the stabilizing
muscles appears, therefore, to be hampering successful postural reactions in these patients. Inferring the contribution of the basal ganglia or the impairment of vestibular information during dynamic postural reactions in this patient population is difficult,
however, because the motor impairments could be as much an effect of akinesia, rigidity, or aging as of disruptions in the postural control system.

Lesions in the motor cortex have also resulted in disturbances to the automatic postural reactions. Patients with spastic paresis rarely exhibit disturbances of posture during quiet standing as in the Romberg test, but reactions to rapid displacements of the support surface indicate deficits in the dynamic postural reactions.[112] Hemiplegic adults demonstrate delayed onsets, a failure to respond, and disparate responses of agonist and antagonist muscles in the paretic lower limb during postural perturbations on a platform.[113] With augmented feedback, such as a warning tone and knowledge of perturbation direction, however, timing of the postural responses improved.[114] When balancing on a seesaw apparatus, patients with spastic hemiparesis minimized the high-frequency, anteroposterior sway on the affected side with a corresponding reduction of the EMG response in tibialis anterior.[115,116] Electrical stimulation of the tibial nerve in patients on the seesaw revealed a delayed and diminished EMG response of tibialis anterior in the affected leg, thereby interfering with the normal compensatory response to displacement of the support surface. Spastic paraparetic patients were observed to produce qualitatively similar results.[115,116]

Children with cerebral palsy were also studied on a posture platform.[117] Their instability seemed to correlate with the clinical diagnosis; children with spastic hemiplegia exhibited reversals in the expected order of muscular activation, whereas children with ataxia demonstrated normal muscle sequencing yet fell frequently. The timing, direction, and amplitude of their postural reactions were disturbed, particularly when the expected sensory inputs had been altered (see paradigm described in section on "Indicators of Vestibulospinal Dysfunction"). Thus, postural abnormalities of children with cerebral palsy were due either to muscle incoordination or instability as a result of an inability to deal with sensory conflict.

Results of these clinical studies suggest that the long latency, polysynaptic postural adjustments can be elicited at the spinal level, but require modulation by supraspinal structures to develop a sufficient response threshold and gain. Possibly there are an inappropriate number of nerve fibers within the damaged motor pathway to excite the motoneuron pool, or perhaps the damaged pathway sends a reduced drive to the interneurons at segmental levels that would normally facilitate the polysynaptic reflex response.[112]

MECHANISMS FOR RECOVERY OF POSTURAL STABILITY

Identification of compensatory mechanisms will improve therapeutic interventions that teach compensation for, or adaptation to, destabilizing conditions. These mechanisms are studied through clinical research, but we must be cautious about conclusions drawn about the function of an anatomic site that are based strictly on the absence of motor control in the presence of specific deficits or damage. We must remember that responses generated in the absence of a sensory or motor signal do not reveal the function of that input. Rather, these responses demonstrate how the system operates in the absence of certain inputs.

Sensory Substitution

Vestibular, visual, and somatosensory signals influence the organization of a normal postural response. When any one of these signals is lost or distorted, a central

reweighting occurs so that the remaining sensory inputs are used to elicit postural reactions, albeit in some altered fashion (Box 3–1). Changes in the postural response organization with loss of labyrinthine inputs have been described in detail in other sections of this chapter. Two modifications in particular should be noted. First, in the
absence of labyrinthine signals, the normal postural reactions to dorsiflexion of the ankle are elicited, but with significantly diminished amplitudes.[71] Thus, the response
does not reach an appropriate gain to maintain stability, and restabilizing torques at
the ankle are inadequate to prevent falls.

Second, peripheral vestibular deficit patients tend to hold the neck stiff so that little free head movement occurs. An analysis of the temporal relationship between
angular acceleration of the head and trunk in the flexor and extensor directions
demonstrates that patients move the head in the same direction as the body (head
locked to trunk) associated with absent neck torques,[118] whereas normal subjects exhibit a counter-rotation of the head and body in the sagittal plane.[46,72] This finding correlates with clinical observations that vestibular deficit patients increase gain of neck
muscles to hold the head stiff in relation to the body. A fast fourier transform performed on the head and trunk angular acceleration recordings revealed a loss of the
normal 2- to 3-Hz peak in the power spectrum of patients with bilateral labyrinthine
deficit.[32] This frequency has been cited as the operating frequency for the vestibulocollic reflexes in studies of normal subjects attempting to stabilize the head during
vertical and horizontal rotations in the seated position,[48,87] and is typical of natural
head movements during locomotion.[119,120] Stiffening of the muscles may, therefore, be
one compensatory strategy that actually works against successful restabilization by interfering with the normal balance of movement-dependent torques at the different
body segments, and with the reception of stimuli necessary to produce vestibular
adaptation.

Somatosensory inputs provide powerful feedback about motion of the limbs, and
stabilize body sway at the lower frequencies (less than 1 Hz). Studies have shown that
sensory input to the hand and arm through contact cues at the fingertip or through a
cane can reduce postural sway in individuals who have no impairments and in patients without a functioning vestibular system, even when contact force levels are inadequate to provide physical support of the body.[109,121] When proprioceptive feedback

---

**BOX 3–1 Modifications to Postural Stability Following Loss of Specific Sensory
Inputs**

Labyrinthine Deficits
>   Stiffening between body segments
>   Increased sway at high frequencies

Somatosensory Deficits
>   Low-frequency sway during quiet stance
>   Delayed restabilization
>   Increased lateral sway

Visual Deficits
>   Increased sway at low frequencies
>   Increased sway at high frequencies when labyrinthine inputs are also absent

from the ankle was excluded or suppressed in normal subjects during perturbations on a posture platform,[11,122] a characteristic low-frequency (1 Hz) sway emerged. Postural abnormalities have been observed with impairment of spinal pathways such as occurs with Friedreich's ataxia, a hereditary disorder affecting the spinocerebellar pathways and posterior columns.[123] In the absence of feedback from these pathways to the cerebellum, a significant delay of the restabilizing response of the tibialis anterior muscle following dorsiflexing ankle rotations on a posture platform has been observed.[98] These patients exhibit large lateral sway deviations in the low-frequency range (less than 1 Hz) with eyes closed, as do patients with tabes dorsalis.[122] Patients with sensory polyneuropathy of the lower extremities demonstrate ataxia and instability during quiet stance. Falls tended to occur when the eyes were closed,[123] suggesting that visual inputs are necessary along with vestibular inputs in the absence of lower limb proprioceptor signals.

Finally, cervical proprioceptors have been the focus of investigations related to the diagnosis of dizziness and ataxia.[124,125] The neck proprioceptors have intimate connections with the vestibular system and are probably used both as feedforward and feedback to the vestibulocolic reflexes.[126] Cervical ataxia has been a controversial diagnosis, however, because there are no hard signs to identify the neck as the source of the dizziness.[125] Recently, Karlberg et al[127–129] have engaged in a series of studies to verify ataxia or vertigo of cervical origin. Using posturography in which stance was perturbed by a vibratory stimulus applied toward the calf muscles, they studied patients with recent onset of neck pain and vertigo but normal otoneurological findings. Results demonstrated disturbed postural control in the patients with cervical vertigo that differed from patients with vestibular neuritis and suggest that disorders of the neck should be considered when assessing patients complaining of dizziness, vertigo, and balance disturbances.

Visual signals are used to accurately detect and reduce motion relative to the surroundings.[130,131] In normal subjects, vision is very influential, but does not appear to be an essential input for the recovery of balance. Many studies have shown that simply removing vision will not produce significant changes in the postural response organization, although greater sway amplitudes may appear.[32,42,43] Instead, visual information is thought to be redundant unless both vestibular and somatosensory inputs are lost.[131] To test the importance of visual inputs in the absence of labyrinthine inputs, sway was measured in subjects standing on a stabilometer placed within a laterally tilting room.[41] At low frequencies of sinusoidal tilt (0.0025 to 0.1 Hz), patients with unilateral and bilateral labyrinthine deficits exhibited sway similar to that of normals. At higher frequencies (0.2 Hz), the patients' sway increased beyond normal limits, indicating that patients with vestibular deficit could rely on visual inputs at lower frequencies, but suffered for the loss of vestibular signals at higher frequencies.[51,132] Labyrinthine deficit patients on a stabilometer were better able to stabilize sway when fixating on a stationary light.[133] When an optokinetic stimulus was introduced the patients became unstable, suggesting that velocity information received through peripheral vision is the cause of the increased sway.

In summary, patients lacking labyrinthine inputs become more dependent on accurate ankle proprioceptive and visual references to correctly organize their postural responses. Inappropriate or distorted signals along either of these sensory pathways will produce increased sway and falls in these patients. Although the sensory signals often provide congruent information, inputs from any of these modalities are not necessarily redundant because each represents different parameters and is affective within a particular frequency domain.[51,83,84] Thus, the falls observed in vestibular deficit patients, particularly following a platform perturbation or in the absence of other sensory signals, may be due to uncontrolled or poorly compensated oscillations of intersegmental structures at particular frequencies of sway.

Compensatory Processes

Compensation for vestibular pathology is a gradual process of functional recovery that is probably of central origin.[134,135] Numerous structures have been identified as participating in vestibular compensation including the vestibular nuclei, spinal cord, visual system, cerebellum, inferior olive, and more.[135] Thus, focusing specifically on a single site for functional recovery of postural control would be difficult. In fact, studies have shown that in both humans and animals, methods of compensation for vestibular dysfunction are not comparable either across subjects or within a subject for different functions.[135,136] The only consistency seems to be that the goal of postural compensation is to reorganize the neural circuitry so that bilateral stimulation of the vestibular system is kept in balance.

Central control over postural responses can be measured in studies examining predictive processes. For example, Guitton et al[86] assessed the influence of mental set on the relative importance of visual and vestibular cues for head stabilization in humans. Normal subjects and patients with bilateral vestibular deficit were tested on their ability to stabilize their heads voluntarily with visual feedback, in the dark, and while distracted with a mental arithmetic task while being rotated horizontally using a random (white noise) stimulus with a bandwidth of 0 to 1 Hz. Normal subjects stabilized their heads best when voluntarily attempting to keep the head coincident with a stationary visual target. Vestibular deficit patients had comparable response amplitudes with vision present, but much lower amplitudes when vision was removed. The apparent lack of head stabilization when all subjects performed mental arithmetic suggested that the short latency (approximately 50 ms) head stabilizing reflexes provided little effective head stabilization in humans at these frequencies of rotation. An analysis of response latencies revealed that long latency or voluntary mechanisms (occurring at greater than 150 ms) were primarily responsible for the observed head stabilization.

Anticipatory presetting of the static and dynamic sensitivity of the postural control system also assists in stabilization of the head at high frequencies.[137,138] Practice or prior experience with a postural task influences EMG output. With practice, decreasing size of the EMG response to a plateau level has commonly been observed during stabilizing reactions,[11,32,71] suggesting central habituation of these responses at the cortical or spinal levels. Selection of postural strategies on a translating platform is influenced by prior experience as well as current feedback information.[20] When the task is well practiced, subjects are able to combine complex movement strategies and respond quickly under a variety of different posture platform paradigms. Even chronic patients with labyrinthine deficits eventually demonstrate normal sway,[58] indicating that a central regulatory mechanism is compensating for the peripheral dysfunction.

A study of head stabilizing responses with random frequencies of sinusoidal rotation may have revealed the method by which the central nervous system (CNS) is regulating postural compensation.[139,140] When tested in the dark at high frequencies (up to 4 Hz), compensation for bilateral peripheral labyrinthine deficit manifested as a shift in system mechanics. In the horizontal plane, patients were able to compensate for trunk rotation by increasing stiffness of the head and neck. In the vertical plane, patients maintained a stable head over a broader frequency range than healthy adults, possibly by changing stiffness or increasing the gain of the cervicocollic reflex to compensate for instability at higher frequencies. The inability of the patients to stabilize at low frequencies (below 1 Hz) in the sagittal plane suggests that the system requires otolith inputs for quiet standing. The ability to maintain a stable head at more functional higher frequencies, however, suggests that individuals with a labyrinthine deficit have acquired an adaptive strategy, which reveals the complex integration of CNS control over the mechanical properties of the system.

AGING AND VESTIBULAR DYSFUNCTION

Falls among the elderly are a major public health concern because they are the leading cause of injury-related death and nonfatal injury in the United States.[141,142] The dynamic process of maintaining an upright posture is compromised in the elderly as evidenced by this increased incidence of falling. Lengthened response latencies, increased static sway, and muscle weakness have been cited as contributing to falls in the elderly,[143,144] but none of these have been identified as causal factors. Attentional demands and disorganized postural strategies are more global parameters that have been targeted as potentially generative causes of falls.[75,145–147]

An impaired vestibular system is believed to be involved in the increased instability of the elderly because anatomic studies have revealed a gradually decreasing density of labyrinthine hair cell receptors beginning at age 30, and a steeper decline in the number of vestibular receptor ganglion cells beginning around 55 to 60 years of age.[148–150] Although caloric measures of the peripheral vestibular system have demonstrated declining function with age,[149] these changes are not present in the central vestibular neurons. The gradual loss of labyrinthine acuity with age prompts viewing the elderly population as a model for compensation to vestibular dysfunction. But in the elderly, sensory loss occurs as a slow process along several feedback pathways, not just the vestibular pathways.[148–152] Thus, their compensatory approach to postural instability may not be the same as in those patients that have experienced an acute but sustained loss of a single input (see Table 3–2).

Age-related trends in the VOR and optokinetic reflexes have been shown to correlate well with anatomic changes found in the peripheral vestibular system.[150,151] Declining gains and increased time delays have been seen in the optokinetic response (OKR), and decreased VOR gains with larger phase leads appeared at frequencies below 1.5 Hz. This would suggest that elderly subjects have an increased reliance on the visual tracking reflexes, and that increased visuomotor processing time could contribute to feedback delays and poor performance.[151] Thus, elderly individuals will have more difficulty detecting sensory signals indicating a loss of stability, and when they do, longer response latencies may well interfere with their ability to produce timely stabilizing reactions.

A longitudinal study of elderly fallers[153] has found significant changes in the mean frequency of postural sway in the medial-lateral direction. A low frequency component that was identified in this plane suggests a slow postural drift during quiet standing.[154] On a posture platform, the stabilizing muscle synergies found to appear in a temporally consistent fashion in young normals exhibit a disorganized order of onset in the elderly.[45,155] Latencies of EMG responses and reaction times are increased in the elderly population.[145,155,156] Quiet sway tends to increase in the elderly.[157,158,159] Although both sway induced by platform perturbation and quiet sway measures demonstrated significant aging-related decreases in stability,[160] the differences between the young and the elderly were more pronounced for the perturbed sway data. Some of the quiet sway measures, however, were more successful in distinguishing elderly fallers from nonfallers. A study of elderly individuals on a rotating posture platform[75] has explored whether delayed latencies of lower-limb muscle responses are responsible for the failure to produce torque outputs necessary to compensate for unexpected falling. Results indicate that a disordered temporal relationship between tibialis anterior and soleus muscles, which are concurrently activated in younger individuals,[32] resulted in decreased stabilizing ankle torques. Weakness of the tibialis anterior muscle has also been described in the elderly,[144] and could be a major contributor to the diminished torque response. Because there is no significant difference in the trunk angular acceleration responses, we can infer that the elderly compensate for diminished ankle torque by increasing hip torque. Thus, impaired balance in the elderly may be produced by altered response synergies that are generated by delayed vestibulospinal and propriospinal reflex responses as a result of increased sensory thresholds and an aging musculoskeletal system.

SUMMARY

We can draw the following conclusions about mechanisms that contribute to postural stability from the existing data. First, central neural processes influence stability in the form of automatic, long latency reactions, voluntary movements, and changes in both the passive mechanical properties (e.g., stiffness) and active force outputs (e.g., joint torques) of the system. Second, the presence or absence of specific sensory inputs (e.g., vestibular or proprioceptive) alters the magnitude or temporal onset of the muscle response pattern, whereas distortion of sensory inputs seems to rearrange the directional organization of the muscle response patterns. Third, learning, attention, and predictive processes influence the performance of postural reactions, as does the motor activity in which the individual is currently engaged when the postural behavior is required. Finally, a particular compensatory strategy adopted by a patient may interfere with, rather than assist, postural stability. Thus, clinicians and researchers should identify the preplanned and automatic components of a postural response to determine how best to influence the postural response organization. Recognizing the multiple factors that contribute to the outcome of a postural response should assist clinicians in determining the approach and effectiveness of their intervention strategies for retraining and restoration of postural function.

REFERENCES

1. Brock, S, and Wechsler, IS: Loss of the righting reflex in man. Arch Neurol Psychiatr 17:12, 1927.
2. Martin, JP: Tilting reactions and disorders of the basal ganglia. Brain 88:855, 1965.
3. McNally, WJ: Labyrinthine reactions and their relation to the clinical tests. Proc Royal Soc Med 30:905, 1937.
4. Radmark, K: On the tipping reaction. Acta Otolaryngol 28:467, 1940.
5. Weisz, S: Studies in equilibrium reactions. J Nervous Ment Dis 88:150, 1938.
6. Baloh, RW, and Honrubia, V: Clinical Neurophysiology of the Vestibular System. FA Davis, Philadelphia, 1979.

7. Norre, ME, et al: Functional recovery of posture in peripheral vestibular disorders. In Amblard, B, et al (eds): Posture and Gait: Development, Adaptation and Modulation. Elsevier, Amsterdam, 1988, p 291.

8. Furman, JM: Role of posturography in the management of vestibular patients. Otolaryngol Head Neck Surg 112:8, 1995.

9. DiFabio, RP: Sensitivity and specificity of platform posturography for identifying patients with vestibular dysfunction. Phys Ther 75:290, 1995.

10. Norre, ME: Posturography: Head stabilisation compared with platform recording. Application in vestibular disorders. Acta Otolaryngol Suppl (Stockh) 520:434, 1995.

11. Nashner, LM: Adapting reflexes controlling human posture. Exp Brain Res 26:59, 1976.

12. Nashner, LM: Fixed patterns of rapid postural responses among leg muscles during stance. Exp Brain Res 30:13, 1977.

13. Nashner, LM: Vestibular and reflex control of normal standing. In Stein, RB, et al (eds): Control of Posture and Locomotion. Plenum, New York, 1973, p 2918.

14. Allum, JHJ, and Pfaltz, CR: Visual and vestibular contributions to pitch sway stabilization in the ankle muscles of normals and patients with bilateral peripheral vestibular deficits. Exp Brain Res 58:82, 1985.

15. Black, FO, et al: Abnormal postural control associated with peripheral vestibular disorders. In Pompeiano, O, and Allum, JHJ (eds): Vestibulospinal Control of Posture and Movement. Progress in Brain Research. Elsevier, Amsterdam, 1988, p 263.

16. Nashner, LM, et al: Organization of posture controls: An analysis of sensory and mechanical constraints. In Allum, JHJ, and Hulliger, M (eds): Afferent Control of Posture and Locomotion. Progress in Brain Research. Elsevier, Amsterdam, 1989, p 411.

17. Keshner, EA, et al: Neck and trunk muscle responses during postural perturbations in humans. Exp Brain Res 71:455, 1988.

18. Stockwell, CW, et al: A physical model of human postural dynamics. In Cohen, B (ed): Vestibular and Oculomotor Physiology. Ann NY Acad Sci 374:722, 1981.

19. Nashner, LM, and McCollum, G: The organization of human postural movements: A formal basis and experimental synthesis. Brain Behav 8:135, 1985.

20. Horak, FB, and Nashner, LM: Central programming of postural movements: Adaptation to altered support-surface configurations. J Neurophysiol 55:1369, 1986.

21. Allum, JHJ, et al: Vestibular and proprioceptive modulation of postural synergies in normal subjects. J Vestib Res 3:59, 1993.

22. Maki, BE, and McIlroy, WE: The role of limb movements in maintaining upright stance: The "change-in-support" strategy. Phys Ther 77:488, 1997.

23. Pai, YC, and Patton, J: Center of mass velocity-position predictions for balance control. J Biomech 30:347, 1997.

24. Bouisset, S, and Zattara, M: Segmental movement as a perturbation to balance? Facts and concepts. In Winters, JM, and Woo, SLY (eds): Multiple Muscle Systems: Biomechanics and Movement Organization. Springer-Verlag, New York, 1990, p 498.

25. Burleigh, A, and Horak, FB: Influence of instruction, prediction, and afferent sensory information on the postural organization of step initiation. J Neurophysiol 75:1619, 1996.

26. Horak, FB, et al: Influence of central set on human postural responses. J Neurophysiol 62:841, 1989.

27. Maki, BE, and Whitelaw, RS: Influence of expectation and arousal on center-of-pressure responses to transient postural perturbations. J Vestib Res 3:25, 1993.

28. Horak, FB, et al: Vestibular and somatosensory contributions to responses to head and body displacements in stance. Exp Brain Res 100:93, 1994.

29. Gu, MJ, et al: Postural control in young and elderly adults when stance is perturbed: Dynamics. J Biomech 29:319, 1996.

30. Massion, J, and Gahery, Y: Diagonal stance in quadrupeds: A postural support for movement. Prog Brain Res 50:2196, 1979.

31. Roberts, TDM, and Stenhouse, G: Reactions to overbalancing. Prog Brain Res 50:397, 1979.

32. Keshner, EA, et al: Postural coactivation and adaptation in the sway stabilizing responses of normals and patients with bilateral peripheral vestibular deficit. Exp Brain Res 69:66, 1987.

33. Greenwood, R, and Hopkins, AL: Muscle responses during sudden falls in man. J Physiol (Lond) 254:507, 1976.

34. Lacour, M, and Xerri, C: Compensation of postural reactions to free-fall in the vestibular neurectomized monkey. Exp Brain Res 40:103, 1980.

35. Melvill Jones, G, and Watt, DGD: Observations on the control of stepping and hopping movements in man. J Physiol 219:709, 1971.

36. Wicke, RW, and Oman, CM: Visual and graviceptive influences on lower leg EMG activity in humans during brief falls. Exp Brain Res 46:324, 1982.

37. Allum, JHJ, et al: The role of stretch and vestibulo-spinal reflexes in the generation of human equilibrating reactions. In Allum, JHJ, and Hulliger, M (eds): Afferent Control of Posture and Locomotion. Progress in Brain Research. Elsevier, Amsterdam, 1989, p 399.

38. Allum, JHJ, et al: The influence of a bilateral peripheral vestibular deficit in postural synergies. J Vestib Res 4:49, 1994.

39. Runge, C, et al: Vestibular loss patients show abnormal joint torque responses to fast perturbations. Soc Neurosci Abstr 22:1633, 1996.
40. Bles, W, et al: The mechanism of physiological height vertigo. II. Posturography. Acta Otolaryngol (Stockh) 89:534, 1980.
41. Bles, W, et al: Compensation for labyrinthine deficits examined by use of a tilting room. Acta Otolaryngol (Stockh) 95:576, 1983.
42. Nashner, LM, and Berthoz, A: Visual contributions to rapid motor responses during postural control. Brain Res 150:403, 1978.
43. Vidal, PP, et al: Difference between eye closure and visual stabilization in the control of posture in man. Aviat Space Environ Med 53:166, 1982.
44. Black, FO, et al: Effects of visual and support surface orientation references upon postural control in vestibular deficient subjects. Acta Otolaryngol 95:199, 1983.
45. Woollacott, MH, et al: Postural reflexes and aging. In: Mortimer JA (ed): The Aging Motor System. Praeger, New York, 1982, p 98.
46. Allum, JH, et al: The control of head movements during human balance corrections. J Vestib Res 7:189, 1997.
47. Gresty, M: Stability of the head: Studies in normal subjects and in patients with labyrinthine disease, head tremor, and dystonia. Movement Disorders 2:165, 1987.
48. Keshner, EA, and Peterson, BW: Mechanisms controlling human head stability: I. Head-neck dynamics during random rotations in the vertical plane. J Neurophysiol 73:2293, 1995.
49. Romberg, MH: Manual of nervous diseases of man. Sydenham Society, London, 1853, p 395.
50. Wall, C III, and Black, FO: Postural stability and rotational tests: Their effectiveness for screening dizzy patients. Acta Otolaryngol 95:235, 1983.
51. Xerri, C, et al: Synergistic interactions and functional working range of the visual and vestibular systems in postural control: Neuronal correlates. In Pompeiano, O, and Allum, JHJ (eds): Vestibulospinal Control of Posture and Movement. Progress in Brain Research. Elsevier, Amsterdam, 1988, p 193.
52. Black, FO: Vestibulospinal function assessment by moving platform posturography. Am J Otology (suppl)39, 1985.
53. Allum, JHJ, and Keshner, EA: Vestibular and proprioceptive control of sway stabilization. In Bles, W, and Brandt, T (eds): Disorders of Posture and Gait. Elsevier, Amsterdam, 1986, p 19.
54. Allum, JHJ, et al: Indicators of the influence a peripheral vestibular deficit has on vestibulo-spinal reflex responses controlling postural stability. Acta Otolaryngol (Stockh) 106:252, 1988.
55. Cohen, H, and Keshner, EA: Current concepts of the vestibular system reviewed: II. Visual/vestibular interaction and spatial orientation. Am J Occup Ther 43:331, 1989.
56. Bles, W, and de Jong, JMBV: Uni- and bilateral loss of vestibular function. In Bles, W, and Brandt, T (eds): Disorders of Posture and Gait. Elsevier, Amsterdam, 1986, p 127.
57. Kapteyn, TS, et al: Standardization in platform stabilometry being a part of posturography. Agressologie 24:321, 1983.
58. Norre, ME, and Forrez, G: Posture testing (posturography) in the diagnosis of peripheral vestibular pathology. Arch Otorhinolaryngol 243:186, 1986.
59. Hain, T: In Herdman, SJ (ed): Vestibular Rehabilitation. FA Davis, Philadelphia, 1999.
60. Unterberger, S: Neue objektive registrierbare vestibulariskorperdrehungen, erhalten durch treten auf der stelle. Der 'Tretversuch.' Arch Ohren Nasen Kehlkopfheilkd 145:478, 1938.
61. Fukuda, T: Statokinetic reflexes in equilibrium and movement. Tokyo Univ. Pr., Tokyo, 1983.
62. Bles, W, et al: Somatosensory compensation for loss of labyrinthine function. Acta Otolaryngol (Stockh) 95:576, 1984.
63. Graybiel, A, and Fregly, AR: A new quantitative ataxia test battery. Acta Otolaryngol (Stockh) 61:292, 1966.
64. Peitersen, E: Measurement of vestibulospinal responses in man. In Kornhuber, HH (ed): Handbook of Sensory Physiology, Vol VI, Vestibular System. Springer-Verlag, Berlin, 1974, p 267.
65. Baloh, RW, and Halmagyi, GM: Disorders of the Vestibular System. Oxford Univ. Pr., New York, 1996.
66. Black, FO, and Nashner, LM: Vestibulo-spinal control differs in patients with reduced versus distorted vestibular function. Acta Otolaryngol (Stockh) 406:110, 1984.
67. Norre, ME: Posture in otoneurology. Acta Oto-Rhino-Laryngol Belgica 44:55, 1990.
68. Dow, RS: The effects of bilateral and unilateral labyrinthectomy in monkey, baboon, and chimpanzee. Am J Physiol 121:392, 1938.
69. Allum, JHJ, and Pfaltz, CR: Postural control in man following acute unilateral peripheral vestibular deficit. In Igarashi, M, and Black, FO (eds): Vestibular and Visual Control of Posture and Locomotor Equilibrium. Karger, Basel, 1985, p 315.
70. Black, FO, et al: Computerized screening of the human vestibulospinal system. Ann Otol Rhinol Laryngol 87:853, 1978.
71. Keshner, EA, and Allum, JHJ: Plasticity in pitch sway stabilization: Normal habituation and compensation for peripheral vestibular deficits. In Bles, W, and Brandt, T (eds): Disorders of Posture and Gait. Elsevier, Amsterdam, 1986, p 289.
72. Allum, JHJ, et al: Organization of leg-trunk-head coordination in normals and patients with peripheral

vestibular deficits. In Pompeiano, O, and Allum, JHJ (eds): Vestibulospinal Control of Posture and Movement. Progress in Brain Research. Elsevier, Amsterdam, 1988, p 277.

73. Horak, FB, et al: Postural strategies associated with somatosensory and vestibular loss. Exp Brain Res 82:167, 1990.

74. Fetter, M, and Dichgans, J: Vestibular tests in evolution. II. Posturography. In: Baloh, RW, and Halmagyi, GM (eds): Disorders of the Vestibular System. Oxford Univ. Pr., New York, 1996, p 256.

75. Keshner, EA, et al: Predictors of less stable postural responses to support surface rotations in healthy human elderly. J Vestib Res 3:419, 1993.

76. Okubo, J, et al: Posture and gait in Meniere's disease. In Bles, W, and Brandt, T (eds): Disorders of Posture and Gait. Elsevier, Amsterdam, 1986, p 113.

77. Dichgans, J, et al: Postural sway in normals and atactic patients: Analysis of the stabilizing and destabilizing effects of vision. Agressologie 17C:15, 1976.

78. Kapteyn, TS, and De Wit, G: Posturography as an auxiliary in vestibular investigation. Acta Otolaryngol 73:104, 1972.

79. Buchele, W, and Brandt, T: Benign paroxysmal positional vertigo and posture. In Bles, W, and Brandt, T (eds): Disorders of Posture and Gait. Elsevier, Amsterdam, 1986, pp 101–111.

80. Brink, EE, et al: Influence of neck afferents on vestibulospinal neurons. Exp Brain Res 38:285, 1980.

81. Peterson, BW: The reticulospinal system and its role in the control of movement. In Barnes, CD (ed): Brainstem Control of Spinal Cord Function. Academic Press, New York, 1984, p 27.

82. Wilson, VJ, et al: Tonic neck reflex of the decerebrate cat: Response of spinal interneurons to natural stimulation of neck and vestibular receptors. J Neurophysiol 51:567, 1984.

83. Bilotto, G, et al: Dynamic properties of vestibular reflexes in the decerebrate cat. Exp Brain Res 47:343, 1982.

84. Peterson, BW, et al: The cervicocollic reflex: Its dynamic properties and interaction with vestibular reflexes. J Neurophysiol 54:90, 1985.

85. Keshner, EA, et al: Patterns of neck muscle activation in cats during reflex and voluntary head movements. Exp Brain Res 88:361, 1992.

86. Guitton, D, et al: Visual, vestibular and voluntary contributions to human head stabilization. Exp Brain Res 64:59, 1986.

87. Keshner, EA, et al: Mechanisms controlling human head stability: II. Head-neck dynamics during random rotations in the horizontal plane. J Neurophysiol 73:2302, 1995.

88. Masson, G, et al: Effects of the spatio-temporal structure of optical flow on postural readjustments in man. Exp Brain Res 103:137, 1995.

89. Dijkstra, TMH, et al: Temporal stability of the action-perception cycle of postural control in a moving visual environment. Exp Brain Res 97:477, 1994.

90. Roberts, TDM: Reflex balance. Nature 244:156, 1973.

91. Suzuki, J, and Cohen, B: Head, eye, body and limb movements from semicircular canal nerves. Exp Neurol 10:393, 1964.

92. Magnus, R: Physiology of posture. Lancet 2:531, 585, 1926.

93. Uemura, T, et al: Neuro-otological examination. University Park Press, Baltimore, 1977.

94. Rudge, P: Clinical neurootology. Churchill Livingstone, London, 1983.

95. Brandt, T, et al: Postural abnormalities in central vestibular brain stem lesions. In Bles, W, and Brandt, T (eds): Disorders of Posture and Gait. Elsevier, Amsterdam, 1986, p 141.

96. Shimazu, H, and Smith, CM: Cerebellar and labyrinthine influences on single vestibular neurons identified by natural stimuli. J Neurophysiol 34:493, 1971.

97. Mauritz, KH, et al: Quantitative analysis of stance in late cortical cerebellar atrophy of the anterior lobe and other forms of cerebellar ataxia. Brain 102:461, 1979.

98. Diener, HC, et al: Characteristic alterations of long-loop "reflexes" in patients with Friedreich's disease and late atrophy of the cerebellar anterior lobe. J Neurol Neurosurg Psychiatr 47:679, 1984.

99. Horak, FB, and Diener, HC: Cerebellar control of postural scaling and central set in stance. J Neurophysiol 72:479, 1994.

100. Nashner, LM, and Grimm, RJ: Analysis of multiloop dyscontrols in standing cerebellar patients. In Desmedt, JE (ed): Cerebellar Motor Control in Man: Long Loop Mechanisms. Karger, Basel, 1978, p 300.

101. Dichgans, J, and Mauritz, KH: Patterns and mechanisms of postural instability in patients with cerebellar lesions. In Desmedt, JE (ed): Motor Control Mechanisms in Health and Disease. Raven, New York, 1983, p 633.

102. Diener, HC, and Dichgans, J: Pathophysiology of cerebellar ataxia. Movement Disorders 7:95, 1992.

103. Dichgans, J, and Diener, HC: Different forms of postural ataxia in patients with cerebellar diseases. In Bles, W, and Brandt, T (eds): Disorders of Posture and Gait. Elsevier, Amsterdam, 1986, p 207.

104. Traub, MM, et al: Anticipatory postural reflexes in Parkinson's disease and other akinetic-rigid syndromes and cerebellar ataxia. Brain 103:393, 1980.

105. Berardelli, A, et al: Physiological mechanisms of rigidity in Parkinson's disease. J Neurol Neurosurg Psychiatr 46:45, 1983.

106. Allum, JHJ, et al: Disturbance of posture in patients with Parkinson's disease. In Amblard, B, et al (eds): Posture and Gait: Development, Adaptation and Modulation. Elsevier, Amsterdam, 1988, p 245.

107. Horak, FB, et al: Postural inflexibility in parkinsonian subjects. J Neurol Sci 111:46, 1992.
108. Dick, JP, et al: Associated postural adjustments in Parkinson's disease. J Neurol Neurosurg Psychiatr 49:1378, 1986.
109. Schieppati, M, and Nardone, A: Free and supported stance in Parkinson's disease: The effect of posture and 'postural set' on leg muscle responses to perturbation, and its relation to the severity of the disease. Brain 114:1227, 1991.
110. Horak, FB, et al: Effects of dopamine on postural control in parkinsonian subjects: Scaling, set, and tone. J Neurophysiol 75:2380, 1996.
111. Dietz, V, et al: Balance control in Parkinson's disease. Gait Posture 1:77, 1993.
112. Benecke, R, and Conrad, B: Disturbance of posture and gait in spastic syndromes. In Bles, W, and Brandt, T (eds): Disorders of Posture and Gait. Elsevier, Amsterdam, 1986, p 231.
113. DiFabio, RP, and Badke, MB: Influence of cerebrovascular accident on elongated and passively shortened muscle responses after forward sway. Phys Ther 68:1215, 1988.
114. Badke, MB, et al: Influence of prior knowledge on automatic and voluntary postural adjustments in healthy and hemiplegic subjects. Phys Ther 67:1495, 1987.
115. Dietz, V, et al: Body oscillations in balancing due to segmental stretch reflex activity. Exp Brain Res 40:89, 1980.
116. Dietz, V, and Berger, W: Interlimb coordination of posture in patients with spastic paresis. Brain 107:965, 1984.
117. Nashner, LM, et al: Stance posture control in select groups of children with cerebral palsy: Deficits in sensory organization and muscular coordination. Exp Brain Res 49:393, 1983.
118. Allum, JHJ, and Honegger, F: A postural model of balance-correcting responses. J Vestib Res 2:323, 1992.
119. Keshner, EA, and Peterson, BW: Frequency and velocity characteristics of head, neck, and trunk during normal locomotion. Soc Neurosci Abstr 15:1200, 1989.
120. Grossman, GE, et al: Frequency and velocity of rotational head perturbations during locomotion. Exp Brain Res 70:470, 1988.
121. Jeka, JJ: Light touch contact as a balance aid. Phys Ther 77:476, 1997.
122. Mauritz, KH, and Dietz, V: Characteristics of postural instability induced by ischaemic blocking of leg afferents. Exp Brain Res 38:117, 1980.
123. Kotaka, S, et al: Somatosensory ataxia. In Bles, W, and Brandt, T (eds): Disorders of Posture and Gait. Elsevier, Amsterdam, 1986, p 178.
124. Cohen, LA: Role of eye and neck proprioceptive mechanisms in body orientation and motor coordination. J Neurophysiol 24:1, 1961.
125. de Jong, JMBV, and Bles, W: Cervical dizziness and ataxia. In Bles, W, and Brandt, T (eds): Disorders of Posture and Gait. Elsevier, Amsterdam, 1986, p 185.
126. Wilson, VJ, and Melvill Jones, G: Mammalian vestibular physiology. Plenum, New York, 1979.
127. Karlberg, M, et al: Dizziness of suspected cervical origin distinguished by posturographic assessment of human postural dynamics. J Vestib Res 6:37, 1996.
128. Karlberg, M, et al: Postural and symptomatic improvement after physiotherapy in patients with dizziness of suspected cervical origin. Arch Phys Med Rehabil 77:874, 1996.
129. Karlberg, M, et al: Impaired postural control in patients with cervico-brachial pain. Acta Otolaryngol Suppl (Stockh) 520:440, 1995.
130. Gantchev, GN, et al: Influence of the stabilogram and statokinesigram visual feedback upon the body oscillations. In Igarashi, M, and Black, FO (eds): Vestibular and Visual Control of Posture and Locomotor Equilibrium. Karger, Basel, 1985, p 135.
131. Paulus, W, et al: Visual postural performance after loss of somatosensory and vestibular function. J Neurol Neurosurg Psychiatr 50:1542, 1987.
132. Waespe, W, and Henn, V: Neuronal activity in the vestibular nuclei of the alert monkey during vestibular and optokinetic stimulation. Exp Brain Res 27:523, 1977.
133. Kotaka, S, et al: The influence of eye movements and tactile information on postural sway in patients with peripheral vestibular lesions. Auris-Nasus-Larynx, Tokyo, 13(suppl II):S153, 1986.
134. Pfaltz, CR: Vestibular habituation and central compensation. Adv Oto-Rhino-Laryngol 22:136, 1977.
135. Igarashi, M: Vestibular compensation. Acta Otolaryngol (Stockh) (suppl)406:78, 1984.
136. Hart, CW, et al: Compensation following acute unilateral total loss of peripheral vestibular function. In Graham, MD, and Kemink, JL (eds): The Vestibular System. Neurophysiologic and Clinical Research. Raven, New York, 1987, p 187.
137. Viviani, P, and Berthoz, A: Dynamics of the head-neck system in response to small perturbations: Analysis and modelling in the frequency domain. Biol Cybern 19:19, 1985.
138. Jeannerod, M: The contribution of open-loop and closed-loop control modes in prehension movements. In Kornblum, S, and Requin, J (eds): Preparatory States and Processes. Lawrence Erlbaum Assoc, Hillsdale, NJ, 1984, p 323.
139. Keshner, EA, and Chen, KJ: Mechanisms controlling head stabilization in the elderly during random rotations in the vertical plane. J Motor Behav 28:324, 1996.
140. Chen, KJ, et al: Head stabilization in labyrinthine deficit patients during horizontal and vertical plane rotations. Soc Neurosci Abstr 22:1633, 1996.

141. Gryfe, CI, et al: A longitudinal study of falls in an elderly population. I. Incidence and morbidity. Age Aging 6:201, 1977.
142. Sattin, RW, et al: The incidence of fall injury events among elderly in a defined population. Am J Epidemiol 131:1028, 1990.
143. Manchester, D, et al: Visual, vestibular and somatosensory contributions to balance control in the older adult. J Gerontol 44:M118, 1989.
144. Whipple, RH, et al: The relationship of knee and ankle weakness to falls in nursing home residents: An isokinetic study. J Am Geriatr Soc 35:13, 1987.
145. Stelmach, GE, et al: Age related decline in postural control mechanisms. Int J Aging Hum Develop 29:205, 1989.
146. Woollacott, MH: Age-related changes in posture and movement. J Gerontol 48:56, 1993.
147. Woollacott, MH, et al: Are there varying attentional demands for different postural strategies? Soc Neurosci Abstr 21:1202, 1995.
148. Bergstrom, B: Morphology of the vestibular nerve. II. The number of myelinated vestibular nerve fibers in man at various ages. Acta Otolaryngol 76:173, 1973.
149. Richter, E: Quantitative study of human Scarpa's ganglion and vestibular sensory epithelia. Acta Otolaryngol 90:199, 1980.
150. Rosenhall, U: Degenerative patterns in the aging human vestibular neuro-epithelia. Acta Otolaryngol 76:208, 1973.
151. Peterka, RJ, and Black, FO: Age-related changes in human vestibulo-ocular reflexes: Pseudorandom rotation tests. J Vestib Res 1:61, 1990.
152. Peterka, RJ, et al: Age-related changes in human vestibulo-ocular reflexes: Sinusoidal rotation and caloric tests. J Vestib Res 1:49, 1990.
153. Skinner, HB, et al: Age-related declines in proprioception. Clin Orthop 184:208, 1984.
154. Maki, BE, et al: A prospective study of postural balance and risk of falling in an ambulatory and independent elderly population. J Gerontol Med Sci, 49:M72, 1994.
155. McClenaghan, BA, et al: Spectral characteristics of ageing postural control. Gait Posture 3:123, 1995.
156. Woollacott, MH: Gait and postural control in the aging adult. In Bles, W, and Brandt, T (eds): Disorders of Posture and Gait. Elsevier, New York, 1986, p 325.
157. Studenski, S, et al: The role of instability in falls among older persons. In Duncan, PW (ed): Balance. American Physical Therapy Association, Alexandria, VA, 1990, p 57.
158. Hasselkus, BR, and Shambes, GM: Aging and postural sway in women. J Gerontol 30:661, 1975.
159. Overstall, PW, et al: Falls in the elderly related to postural imbalance. Brit Med J 1:261, 1977.
160. Maki, BE, et al: Aging and postural control. A comparison of spontaneous- and induced-sway balance tests. J Am Geriatr Soc 38:1, 1990.

CHAPTER 4

Vestibular Adaptation

David S. Zee, M.D.

A robust and versatile capability for adaptive control of vestibular motor behavior is essential if an organism is to maintain optimal visual function and stable balance throughout life. Changes associated with normal development and aging, as well as with disease and trauma, demand mechanisms both to detect errors in performance and to correct them. An understanding of such mechanisms is crucial in the design and evaluation of programs of physical therapy that are used to rehabilitate patients with vestibular disorders.[1] The purpose of this chapter is to review new information about adaptive mechanisms that bears on the management of patients with disorders of their vestibular systems. By necessity, we will emphasize studies of the vestibulo-ocular reflex (VOR), because most is known about its adaptive control. When possible, however, we will also refer to vestibulospinal (VSR), vestibulocollic (VCR) and cervico-ocular (COR) reflexes.

RECALIBRATION, SUBSTITUTION, AND ALTERNATIVE STRATEGIES

Adaptive control of vestibular reflexes must be looked at in the larger context of overall compensation for vestibular deficits.* Restoring adequate motor behavior by readjusting the input-output relationships (e.g., gain, timing, or direction) of the VOR or VSR may be impossible, especially when deficits are large. Other mechanisms of compensation must then be invoked (Box 4–1). Examples include substitution of another sensory input to drive the same motor response (e.g., substitution of the COR for the VOR); substitution of an alternative motor response in lieu of the usual compensa-

---

*We will not make a rigid distinction here between the terms adaptation and compensation though, in general, the former is used in a more restricted sense, to imply adjustment in the basic VORs and VOSs, whereas the latter is used, in a larger sense, to include the entire repertoire of ways, including substitution, prediction, and other cognitive strategies, by which patients recover from, and learn to live with, vestibular disorders.

BOX 4–1   Compensatory Mechanisms

Adaptation
   Changing the gain, phase, or direction of the vestibular response

Substitution of
   Other sensory inputs mechanisms (e.g., COR)
   Alternative motor responses (e.g., saccades)
   Strategies based on prediction or anticipation

---

tory motor response (e.g., use of saccades instead of slow phases to help stabilize gaze during head rotation); and the use of strategies based on prediction or anticipation of intended motor behavior (e.g., preprogramming compensatory slow phases in anticipation of a combined eye-head movement towards a new target). Furthermore, there is considerable variability among subjects about which particular mechanisms are primarily used for compensation.[2] This heterogeneity dictates a need for quantitative testing of vestibular function in patients before and during rehabilitation. Any plan of therapy must focus on what is likely to work best, and what is working best. The promotion of different goals may require a different therapeutic emphasis, and different therapeutic programs may potentially work at cross purposes. Therefore, planning the program of therapy based on what is most likely to succeed in the context of the type and the degree of deficit, and the patient's inherent potential for compensation, is essential. To illustrate these points, we will first discuss two archetypal paradigms requiring vestibular compensation: unilateral and bilateral loss of labyrinthine function.

Loss of Unilateral Labyrinthine Function

Unilateral labyrinthectomy (UL) has been used as an experimental model to study motor learning and compensation for more than 100 years. Yet, until recently, little has been known about the error signals that drive the compensatory process, the precise mechanisms that underlie recovery from both the static and the dynamic disturbances that are created by the loss of labyrinthine input from one side, and the additional strategies that are available to assist in the overall goal of gaze and postural stability during movement.

THE DEFICIT TO BE CORRECTED AFTER UNILATERAL LABYRINTHECTOMY

Using the VOR as an example, UL creates two general types of deficits for which a correction is required: *static imbalance*, related to the differences in the levels of tonic discharge within the vestibular nuclei; and *dynamic disturbances*, related to the loss of one-half of the afferent input that normally contributes, in a push-pull fashion, to the generation of compensatory responses during head movement. Spontaneous nystagmus with the head still, and sustained torsion (ocular counter-roll) are examples of the static type of disturbance from an imbalance in semicircular canal and otolith inputs, respectively. Decreased amplitude (gain) and asymmetry of eye rotation during head rotation are examples of the dynamic type of disturbance.

THE ERROR SIGNALS THAT DRIVE VESTIBULO-OCULAR REFLEX ADAPTATION

What might be the error signals that drive VOR adaptation? Image motion or "slip" on the retina, when associated with head movements, is the obvious candidate; the raison d'être of the VOR is to keep images stable on the retina during head movements. We investigated the role of vision, and especially of visual information mediated by geniculostriate pathways, on both the acquisition and the maintenance of adaptation to UL in monkeys.[3] We recorded VOR function in three groups of animals. One group had undergone a prior bilateral occipital lobectomy many months before the labyrinthectomy. These "cortically blind" animals were allowed normal light exposure after UL. The other animals had undergone no prior lesions, and were divided into two groups: those that were kept in complete darkness for 4 days following UL, and those that were allowed normal exposure to light after the UL.

RESTORATION OF STATIC VESTIBULO-OCULAR REFLEX BALANCE AFTER UNILATERAL LABYRINTHECTOMY

The results from this experiment were clear cut. Restoration of static balance, as reflected in the disappearance of spontaneous nystagmus, proceeded independently of whether or not the animals had undergone a prior occipital lobectomy, or whether or not they were kept in the dark after UL. Furthermore, a bilateral occipital lobectomy performed nearly 1 year after the labyrinthectomy, when compensation to UL had taken place, did not result in the reappearance of spontaneous nystagmus. Thus, both the acquisition and the maintenance of static balance in canal-ocular reflexes after UL are independent of visual inputs. (Another example of restoration of static imbalance after UL is the elimination of cyclotorsion [ocular counter-roll] that follows UL.[4] This bias arises from imbalance in otolith-ocular reflexes. It is not known if this readjustment also requires visual inputs.)

RESTORATION OF DYNAMIC VESTIBULO-OCULAR REFLEX FUNCTION AFTER UNILATERAL LABYRINTHECTOMY

On the other hand, the restoration of dynamic performance after UL depended critically on visual experience. There was no increase in the amplitude (gain) of the VOR until exposure to light. Similar results occur in monkeys after unilateral plugging of a lateral semicircular canal, which causes a nearly 50 percent decrease in VOR gain.[5] Presumably, the critical stimulus for recalibration of dynamic VOR responses is not light per se but rather the presence of motion of images on the retina during head movements. A similar dependence on vision has been shown for recovery of balance in cats following vestibular neurectomy.[6]

Furthermore, the compensatory changes in the gain of the VOR that occurred after UL were lost, over the course of several weeks, following a bilateral occipital lobectomy. The occipital lobectomy itself was unlikely to have been responsible for the decrease in the gain of the VOR because there are only small alterations in the gain and in the symmetry of the VOR produced by occipital lobectomy in animals that have not undergone any prior vestibular lesions.

Taken together, these findings suggest that adaptation of VOR gain is a dynamic process, which requires visual experience for its acquisition, and depends on the posterior cerebral hemispheres for its maintenance. Presumably, the contribution of the occipital lobes is that they transmit information about image slip on the retina during head movements to the more caudal structures that, in turn, use this error information to readjust the dynamic performance of the VOR.

Recent studies have shown that recovery following unilateral labyrinthine lesions is less complete when stimuli are comprised of high accelerations or high frequencies.[7,8] Different strategies are needed, especially preprogramming of movements,[9,10] similar to those movements shown by patients who have lost labyrinthine function bilaterally.[11]

RESTORATION OF SPONTANEOUS ACTIVITY IN THE DEAFFERENTED NUCLEI

One might ask why visual experience is necessary for recalibration of dynamic VOR function, but not for restoration of static balance. Without motion of images on the retina during head movements, adaptive mechanisms do not have a reliable error signal that they can use to recalibrate the dynamic VOR. With respect to static imbalance, however, deafferentation of the vestibular nucleus might initiate alterations in the intrinsic properties of the vestibular neurons themselves, or lead to denervation hypersensitivity to remaining sensory inputs, or stimulate sprouting of extra-labyrinthine afferents.[12–14] Each process might lead to an increase in the level of the spontaneous activity of neurons on the lesioned side. Recall that restoring vestibulospinal balance also depends on rebalancing of the vestibular nuclei, and that many neurons within the vestibular nuclei have axons that bifurcate and project both rostrally, to the ocular motor nuclei, and caudally, to the spinal cord.[15] Vestibulospinal compensation would not be expected to rely solely on visual inputs for providing the necessary error signals for central readjustment of balance. Proprioceptive and somatosensory cues are probably more important, and could provide the requisite error signals leading to the static rebalancing of the vestibular nuclei that would affect both vestibulo-ocular and vestibulospinal responses.

A "CRITICAL" PERIOD FOR VESTIBULO-OCULAR REFLEX ADAPTATION?

Another finding, potentially of important clinical relevance, emerged from our study. Monkeys that had been kept in the dark for 4 days after UL, and then allowed normal visual experience, generally showed a recovery of dynamic VOR performance at about the same rate, and to the same level, as did monkeys allowed visual experience immediately following UL. There was, however, one important exception. For high-velocity rotations directed to the lesioned side, recovery was markedly delayed in the monkeys initially deprived of vision, though the final level reached was close to that of monkeys that had not been deprived of vision immediately after UL. This finding suggests that there may be a "critical period" during which, if error signals are not provided to the adaptive mechanism, and recalibration does not get underway, the rate of recovery, and perhaps the ultimate degree, may decrease. Restoration of postural control after UL also appears to be subject to a critical period.[16] If cats are immobilized for a period of days after UL, their recovery of locomotor function, even after normal activity is reinstituted, is delayed and limited. Another example of the influence on vestibular adaptation of a restriction of sensory inputs has been demonstrated in guinea pigs.[17] If their head is restrained after UL, the rate of compensation of lateral head deviation (the static VCR) is altered.

The obvious implication of these findings is that when patients incur enduring vestibular damage they should be encouraged to move about, in the light, and to try and engage their VORs and VSRs as much as possible. In this way, they will generate and experience the sensorimotor mismatches that make the central nervous system aware of a need for adaptive readjustment of its motor reflexes. As a further caveat, heavy sedation, immobilization, and restriction of activity of patients with a recent loss of vestibular function should be discouraged. Such practices may potentially retard or even limit the ultimate degree of compensation after a vestibular lesion.

In the same vein, physical exercise promotes recovery of balance function in monkeys that have undergone either unilateral or bilateral experimental vestibular ablations.[18] Although carefully controlled studies of the effects of different types of activity on vestibular compensation are sparse in human beings, physical therapy will most likely also promote recovery in patients.[19,20]

SUBSTITUTION OF SACCADES FOR INADEQUATE COMPENSATORY SLOW PHASES

Apart from readjustment of VOR gain, other mechanisms may also be invoked to help stabilize the position of the eyes during head motion after UL. Patients may learn to generate catch-up saccades (elicited, automatically, even in complete darkness) in the same direction as their inadequate compensatory slow phases.[9,10] This substitution strategy may be necessary because there appear to be inherent limitations, with respect to maximum frequency, velocity, and acceleration, in the ability of subjects with just one labyrinth to generate slow phases of the correct magnitude when the head is rotated toward the side of the lesion (Ewald's second law).[21]

RECOVERY NYSTAGMUS AND RELATED PHENOMENA

A practical clinical implication of these ideas about recovery from unilateral labyrinthine lesions relates to the phenomenon of "recovery nystagmus."[22] As indicated above, the static imbalance created by a unilateral peripheral lesions leads to a spontaneous nystagmus that is compensated by rebalancing the level of activity between the vestibular nuclei. If peripheral function should suddenly recover, central adaptation would become inappropriate, and a nystagmus would appear with slow phases directed away from the paretic side. Recovery nystagmus may confuse the clinician or therapist, who may think that the reappearance of symptoms and of a spontaneous nystagmus are due to a loss of function on the previously healthy side, rather than to a recovery of function on the previously diseased side. In either case, a spontaneous nystagmus ensues that must be eliminated, adaptively, by a further readjustment of levels of activity within the vestibular nuclei. Such a sequence of events may be a relatively common occurrence after vestibular lesions.[23]

A similar mechanism may account for some instances in which nystagmus is provoked by hyperventilation.[22] In these cases, the induced alkalosis alters the amount of calcium available for generating action potentials along the vestibular nerve, and so may lead to a restoration of function on partially demyelinated fibers (for example, due to multiple sclerosis, chronic microvascular compression, petrous bone tumors [e.g., cholesteatoma] or cerebellopontine angle tumors [e.g., acoustic neuroma]). Hyperventilation, however, may also produce nystagmus in patients with a perilymphatic fistula, by altering intracranial pressure that is then transmitted to the labyrinth. Other mechanisms for hyperventilation-induced nystagmus are possible, including alterations in compensatory mechanisms.[24]

There may even be a *dynamic* equivalent of recovery nystagmus. After sustained head shaking, patients who have a unilateral peripheral vestibular loss often develop a transient eye nystagmus with slow phases directed toward the impaired ear— so-called head-shaking nystagmus.[25] The initial phase of head-shaking nystagmus may be followed by a reversal phase in which nystagmus is directed oppositely to the initial phase. The primary phase of head-shaking nystagmus is related to a dynamic asymmetry in the VOR such that excitation (rotation toward the intact side) elicits a larger response than inhibition (rotation toward the impaired side). Head-shaking nystagmus is another manifestation of Ewald's second law. The secondary phase is often attributed to short-term (with a time constant of about 1 minute) vestibular adaptation, probably reflecting adaptive processes in both the peripheral nerve and in central structures.

If recovery occurs peripherally, however, any prior central VOR gain adaptation (which would increase the dynamic response during rotation toward the impaired side) could lead to a head-shaking–induced nystagmus with the slow phases of the primary phase directed *away* from the impaired ear. Thus, one can appreciate the pivotal role that adaptation plays in determining the particular pattern and direction of any spontaneous or induced nystagmus that may appear during the process of recovery.

Loss of Bilateral Labyrinthine Function

An even more challenging problem for the central nervous system is to compensate for a complete bilateral loss of labyrinthine function (BL). In the case of a truly complete loss, there is no labyrinthine-driven VOR to recalibrate so that alternative mechanisms—sensory substitution, motor substitution, predictive and anticipatory strategies—must be invoked.

COMPLETE VERSUS PARTIAL VESTIBULAR LOSS

Whether or not labyrinthine function is completely absent helps to determine what type of program of physical therapy should be prescribed. Because the response of the VOR to high frequencies of head rotation is usually spared until the labyrinthine loss is complete, caloric responses (which primarily simulate a low-frequency rotational stimulus) may be absent even when the patient has a relatively functional VOR. Recall the response to the high-frequency components of head rotation requires the fast-acting labyrinthine-driven VOR; visual stabilizing reflexes are only adequate to insure stabilization for the low-frequency components of head rotation. Accordingly, the results of a rotational test can help determine the degree of preservation of labyrinthine function.[26] Such information may help the therapist choose whether to prescribe a program of rehabilitation that stresses recalibration of a deficient but present VOR, or a program that emphasizes sensory substitution and alternative strategies.

EXPERIMENTAL RESULTS IN NONHUMAN PRIMATES

Dichgans et al.[27] first described compensatory mechanisms of eye-head coordination in monkeys that had undergone bilateral labyrinthine destruction. They identified three major adaptive strategies used to improve gaze stability during head movements: (1) potentiation of the COR (neck-eye loop), as reflected in slow-phase eye movements elicited in response to body-on-head (head stable in space) rotation; (2) preprogramming of compensatory slow phases in anticipation of intended head motion; and (3) a decrease in the saccadic amplitude-retinal error relationship, selectively during combined eye-head movements, to prevent gaze overshoot. With respect to the last phenomenon, saccades made with head movements would normally cause gaze to overshoot the target if there were no functioning VOR to compensate for the contribution of the movement of the head to the change in gaze. Dichgans et al.[27] also showed that saccades were programmed to be smaller when an accompanying head movement was also anticipated. When the head was persistently immobilized, however, saccades were programmed to be of their usual size.

ADDITIONAL STRATEGIES IN HUMAN PATIENTS WITH BILATERAL LOSS OF LABYRINTHINE DYSFUNCTION

The compensatory mechanisms described for monkeys without labyrinthine function have also been identified in human beings who have a complete BL.[28–31] The degree to which one or another mechanism is adopted, however, varies from patient to patient. In addition, several additional strategies have been identified in humans, which are also quite idiosyncratic from patient to patient (Box 4–2).[28,32–34] These strategies include:

1. *Substitution of small saccades* in the direction opposite to head rotation, in order to augment inadequate compensatory slow phases
2. *Enhanced* visual following reflexes
3. *Predictive strategies* to improve gaze stability during tracking of targets jumping periodically, or during self-paced tracking between two stationary targets
4. *Effort of spatial localization,* as judged by a much better compensatory response to head rotation when the patient imagines the location of stationary targets, as opposed to the response while performing mental arithmetic.

BOX 4–2   Compensatory Mechanisms Following Bilateral Vestibular Deficits

Potentiation of COR
Central preprogramming of slow phases or saccades
Decreased saccade amplitude
Enhanced visual following
Effort of spatial localization
Suppression of perception of oscillopsia

As a corollary to these last two mechanisms, responses during active (self-generated) head rotations occur at a shorter latency, and usually with a larger gain, than those during passive head rotations. Even somatosensory cues from the feet can be used to augment inadequate compensatory slow phases of the eyes—producing so-called stepping-around nystagmus.[35] Finally, perceptual mechanisms—suppression of oscillopsia (illusory movement of the environment) in spite of persistent retinal image motion—may also be part of the "compensatory" response to vestibular loss.[36]

Another example of potentiation of a reflex that is normally vestigial in human beings can be shown in the ocular motor response to static lateral tilt of the head. This presumably otolith-mediated reflex is comprised of a static torsion of the eyes, opposite to the direction of lateral head tilt—so-called ocular counter-rolling. In labyrinthine defective human beings, but not in normal subjects, ocular counter-rolling can be produced by lateral tilt of the trunk with respect to the (stationary, upright) head.[37] This response probably reflects a potentiation of a static COR in lieu of the missing otolith signals. BL patients also show an increased sensitivity to visually induced tilt. With the loss of the inertial frame of reference, normally provided by the dominating labyrinthine inputs, visual inputs become more potent stimuli to vestibular reflexes.

A new reliance on visual inputs is a necessary and useful adaptation to labyrinthine loss, although it may become a liability if visual inputs should become incongruent with the actual motion or position of the head. For example, when one is reading a newspaper in a moving elevator or escalator, visual inputs (from the motion of the image of the newspaper on the retina) provide misleading information about the position or the movement of the head, and if relied upon (as BL patients may), would lead to an inappropriate (or lack of) compensatory response, and possibly a fall.

STUDIES OF VESTIBULO-OCULAR REFLEX ADAPTATION IN NORMAL SUBJECTS

Adaptive control of the VOR has been investigated in normal subjects by artificially creating motion of images on the retina, using optical or other means, during head rotation. For example, in the pioneering experiments of Melvill Jones et al.[38] subjects wore right-left reversing prisms, which required, and led to, a reversal in the direction of the slow phase of nystagmus with respect to the direction of head motion. Likewise, magnifying and minifying spectacle lenses (used to correct for far- and near-sightedness, respectively) require and produce an adaptive increase and decrease, respectively, in VOR gain. A practical consequence of this phenomenon is that normal subjects wearing a spectacle correction undergo an adaptive change in VOR gain to meet the needs of the new visual circumstances created by their optical correction.* Such gain changes must be considered in evaluating the results of vestibular function tests in individuals who habitually wear spectacles.[39] Furthermore, if a patient does show a change in VOR gain in response to wearing spectacles, one can infer that the patient has at least some capability to undergo adaptive VOR recalibration.

---

*Note that wearing contact lenses does not require a need for an adaptive change in VOR gain because contacts rotate with the eye, and hence are unassociated with a rotational magnification effect.

VOR adaptation can also be studied by prolonged rotation of subjects while artificially manipulating the visual surround. One can use an optokinetic drum that surrounds the subject, and rotate it in phase—in the same direction as chair rotation—to produce a decrease in VOR gain, or out of phase—opposite the direction of chair rotation—to produce an increase in VOR gain. If the amplitude of drum rotation is exactly equal to that of the chair, then the required VOR gain would be 0.0 for in-phase viewing (so-called x0 viewing) and 2.0 for out-of-phase viewing (so-called x2 viewing). The usual duration for VOR training in these types of paradigms is an hour or two, although VOR adaptation can probably be detected within minutes of the onset of the change in the relationship between the visual and vestibular stimuli.[40,41]

Imagination and Effort of Spatial Localization in Vestibular Adaptation

Finally, we note that one's imagination can be a potent substitute for the real stimulus to VOR adaptation—motion of images on the retina during head rotation. Melvill Jones et al.[42] have shown that the VOR of normal subjects can be adaptively modified (as measured in darkness and tested under the same mental set) with just a few hours of imagining a visual stimulus moving in such a way that it would normally create slip of images on the retina if it were actually visible. Thus, what are usually called psychological factors—motivation, attention, effort, and interest—may actually play a more specific role in promoting adaptive recovery. The habit of professional athletes—downhill skiers or ice skaters, for example—of going through their routines in their minds as they prepare for the actual event, is probably an example of using this "cognitive" capability to create an internal model of the external environment (and the sensory consequences of moving within it) in which to rehearse their motor performance.

Similar types of paradigms, in which the motion of the visual surround is artificially manipulated with respect to the motion of the head, have been used to induce an alteration in the phase (timing) but without a change in the amplitude of the VOR,[43] and a change in the direction of the VOR, so-called cross-axis plasticity.[44–46] In the latter paradigm, the visual surround is rotated in a direction orthogonal to the direction of rotation of the head. This cross-axis plasticity accords with electrophysiological evidence that secondary neurons in the vestibular nucleus receive inputs from one, two, or all three pairs of semicircular canals.[47] Similar considerations account for the recovery in VOR function when just one single semicircular canal is plugged. The spatial tuning of information from an intact canal (as a function of the plane of rotation) is readjusted centrally so that it can provide a better signal of rotation in a plane close to that of the plugged canal.[48–52]

Furthermore, during cross-axis training, neurons in the vestibular nuclei that are normally maximally sensitive to pitch axis (vertical) stimulation increase their sensitivity to yaw axis (horizontal) rotation,[53] providing a neurophysiologic substrate for the change in direction of the VOR. A clinical consequence of a disturbance of cross-axis VOR plasticity is the occurrence of "perverted" nystagmus; nystagmus in which the slow phases are in the wrong direction relative to that of the stimulus. A strong vertical nystagmus induced during caloric stimulation is such an example, and usually occurs with central vestibular lesions.

The linear (translational) VOR, and other otolith-ocular reflexes, also appear to be under adaptive control.[54-56] The vestibular responses to translation, and their potential for rehabilitation in vestibular patients, have been largely neglected in clinical practice.

These short-term adaptation experiments probably test only one particular type of vestibular adaptation, because the learned response is not sustained in the absence of continued stimulation. There is also a long-term adaptive process, taking days to weeks, rather than just minutes to hours, which gradually supervenes and leads to a more enduring, resilient adaptive change. Thus, one must be cautious when extrapolating the results from these short-term experiments to the long-term problems of patients adapting to chronic vestibular deficits.

Adaptive capabilities have been investigated in elderly subjects,[57] by measuring changes in VOR gain after wearing of x2 (magnifying) lenses for 8 hours. At higher frequencies (above about 0.75 Hz) the ability to increase VOR gain adaptively is significantly diminished in older individuals. Because the labyrinthine-induced VOR is most needed to compensate for the high-frequency components of head rotation, a loss of adaptive capability in elderly patients could account for the more devastating and persistent symptoms after a vestibular loss.

Context Specificity

One recent finding, which may have important clinical implications, is the demonstration that VOR gain adaptation is context specific. Baker et al.[58] showed that cats can be trained to adaptively change the gain of their canal-induced (rotational) VOR in one way, when the head is oriented with respect to gravity in one particular position (e.g., right ear down), and in another way, when the head is oriented in the opposite position with respect to gravity (e.g., left ear down). Thus, even though the pattern of canal activation is the same, the pattern of static otolith inputs determines or gates different central responses to an identical input from the semicircular canals.

We have recently shown that VOR adaptation in humans also depends on the static orientation of the head in which the training of the canal-induced VOR took place.[59] Shelhamer et al.[60] have also shown that adaptation of the gain of the VOR can be made to depend on the position of the eye in the orbit in which the training took place. In their paradigm, the *horizontal* VOR gain was trained to depend on the *vertical* position of the eye in the orbit. Such a capability would be particularly useful for individuals who wear a bifocal spectacle correction. When viewing through the lower part of the lenses, which have the stronger prescription needed to overcome the effects of presbyopia, subjects require a higher VOR gain during head rotation than when viewing through the top part of the spectacles.

Potentially, then, simply putting one's glasses on (or perhaps just the frames, or putting on the glasses in complete darkness) might be enough of a cue to generate a different vestibular response. Just such an effect of spectacles has been shown for another type of ocular motor adaptation in which the eyes are required to rotate by different amounts when the two eyes have different spectacle corrections.[61]

Thus, context specificity of vestibular learning, which potentially can be derived from a variety of cues—both vestibular and nonvestibular—must be considered in the design of programs of physical therapy. Will the particular training paradigm that is being used to promote vestibular compensation "transfer" to the more natural circumstances in which the patient usually becomes symptomatic?

NEUROPHYSIOLOGIC SUBSTRATE OF VESTIBULO-OCULAR REFLEX ADAPTATION

Where might be the structures within the central nervous system that elaborate the various types of vestibular plasticity that we have discussed? First, we should remember that one must distinguish between static and dynamic VOR adaptation. The cerebellum, and especially the flocculus, seems to play an important role in the acquisition of adaptive changes in VOR gain.[62,63] The flocculus also plays a role in recovery of function after unilateral labyrinthine loss. Although restoration of relatively small degrees of imbalance between the vestibular nuclei can probably take place independently of the flocculus,[64] large amounts of spontaneous nystagmus and the recovery of amplitude and symmetry of gain during head movement probably require the flocculus.[65]

Furthermore, potentiation of the COR as an adaptive strategy during head rotation is lost in patients with bilateral vestibular loss who also have cerebellar atrophy, implying a role for the cerebellum in this aspect of vestibular adaptation.[66] The exact sites of these types of vestibular learning are still unsettled; evidence for both a cerebellar cortex and a brainstem (vestibular nuclei) locus exists.[62] Long-term, more hardwired, changes in the VOR may take place in the vestibular nuclei themselves.

Many neurotransmitters and neuropeptides have been implicated in the process of vestibular adaptation.[67–70] In the vestibulocerebellum, nitric oxide, NMDA receptors, acetylcholine and catecholamines appear to be important.[71–75] How this information can be translated into treatment should be an important focus of current research.[76]

Still unclear are the substrates for the variety of strategies and cognitive influences (e.g., context and imagination, and effort of spatial localization) that are incorporated as part of the compensatory response to vestibular damage. A possible anatomical substrate for such higher-level influences may reside in the reciprocal connections between the vestibular nuclei and the cerebral cortex.[77,78] On the other hand, it has been shown that when a rabbit is exposed to sustained sinusoidal oscillation of the head, some climbing fibers in the nodulus of the rabbit discharge in a sinusoidal fashion *after* the animal stops rotating.[79] This finding is compatible with the idea that the cerebellum can learn patterns of vestibular stimulation and generate them even after the actual stimulus has ceased.

SUMMARY

We have emphasized here that a consideration and a knowledge of the adaptive capabilities of the brain are essential to the diagnosis and management of patients with vestibular disorders. The proper interpretation of the symptoms and signs shown by patients with vestibular dysfunction, the design of an optimal plan of physical therapy to promote recovery from vestibular dysfunction, and an objective analysis of any salutary effects of physical therapy, cannot be accomplished without paying constant attention to the actions of the variety of compensatory mechanisms that are used to cope with abnormal vestibular function. Furthermore, we have reemphasized that compensation is far more than a simple readjustment of low-level, largely subconscious reflexes. The role of anticipation and prediction, altered motor strategies, sensory substitution, and cognitive factors related to mental set, psychologic effort, imagination and context, are all important in the adaptive process. We are only now beginning to identify the wide repertoire of compensatory mechanisms available to us. The challenge now is for us to learn to marshal these adaptive mechanisms to best promote recovery in our patients.

ACKNOWLEDGMENT

This research was supported by NIH Grant DC00979.

REFERENCES

1. Zee, DS, in Barber, HO, Sharpe, JA (eds): The management of patients with vestibular disorders. Vestibular Disorders. Year Book, Chicago, 1988, pp 254–274.
2. Lacour, M, et al: Sensory strategies in human postural control before and after unilateral vestibular neurotomy. Exp Brain Res 115:300–10, 1997.
3. Fetter, M, et al: Effects of lack of vision and of occipital lobectomy upon recovery from unilateral labyrinthectomy in the Rhesus monkey. J Neurophysiol 59:394–407, 1988.
4. Curthoys, IS, et al: Human ocular torsional position before and after unilateral vestibular neurectomy. Exp Brain Res 85:218–25, 1991.
5. Paige, GD: Vestibuloocular reflex and its interactions with visual following mechanisms in the squirrel monkey: II. Response characteristics and plasticity following unilateral inactivation of horizontal canal. J Neurophysiol 49:52, 1983.
6. Zennou-Azogui, Y, et al: Visual sensory substitution in vestibular compensation: neuronal substrates in the alert cat. Exp Brain Res 98:457–73, 1994.
7. Curthoys, IS, and Halmagyi, GM: Vestibular compensation: A review of the oculomotor, neural, and clinical consequences of unilateral vestibular loss. J Vestib Res 5:67–107, 1995.
8. Curthoys, IS, et al (eds): Disorders of the Vestibular System. Oxford Univ. Pr., Oxford, 1996, pp 145–54.
9. Peng, GCY, et al: Coupled asymmetries of the vestibulo-ocular (VOR) and vestibulo-collic (VCR) reflexes in patients with unilateral vestibular loss. [Abstract] Soc Neurosci Abstr 27:1294, 1997.
10. Segal, BN, and Katsarkas, A: Long-term deficits of goal-directed vestibulo-ocular function following total unilateral loss of peripheral vestibular function. Acta Otolaryngol (Stockh) 106:102–10, 1988.
11. Kasai, T, and Zee, DS: Eye-head coordination in labyrinthine-defective human beings. Brain Res 144:123–41, 1978.
12. Smith, PF, and Curthoys, IS: Mechanisms of recovery following unilateral labyrinthectomy: a review. Brain Res Rev 14:155–80, 1989.
13. Smith, PF, and Darlington, CL: Neurochemical mechanisms of recovery from peripheral vestibular lesions (vestibular compensation). Brain Res Rev 16:117–33, 1991.
14. Dieringer, N. 'Vestibular compensation': Neural plasticity and its relations to functional recovery after labyrinthine lesions in frogs and other vertebrates. Prog Neurobiol 46:97–129, 1995.
15. Minor, LB, et al: Dual projections of secondary vestibular axons in the medial longitudinal fasciculus to extraocular motor nuclei and the spinal cord of the squirrel monkey. Exp Brain Res 83:9–21, 1990.
16. Lacour, M, et al: Vestibular Compensation: Facts, Theories, and Clinical Perspectives. Elsevier, Paris, 1989.
17. Jensen, DW: Reflex control of acute postural asymmetry and compensatory symmetry after a unilateral vestibular lesion. Neuroscience 4:1059, 1979.
18. Igarashi, M, et al: Physical exercise and balance compensation after total ablation of vestibular organs. Effect of physical exercise prelabyrinthectomy on locomotor balance compensation in the squirrel monkey. Prog Brain Res 68:407–14, 1989.
19. Herdman, SJ, et al: Vestibular adaptation exercises and recovery: acute stage after acoustic neuroma resection. Otolaryngol Head Neck Surg 113:77–87, 1995.
20. Krebs, DE, et al: Double-blind, placebo-controlled trial of rehabilitation for bilateral vestibular hypofunction: Preliminary report. Otolaryngol Head Neck Surg 109:735–41, 1993.
21. Curthoys, IS, et al (eds): Disorders of the Vestibular System. Oxford Univ. Pr., Oxford, 1996, pp 145–54.
22. Leigh, RJ, and Zee, DS: The Neurology of Eye Movements. F. A. Davis, Philadelphia, 1999.
23. Lockemann, U, and Westhofen, M: On the course of early vestibular compensation after acute labyrinthine lesions. Laryngol Rhinol Otol (Stuttg) 70:326, 1991.

24. Sakellari, V, et al: The effects of hyperventilation on postural control mechanisms. Brain 120:1659–73, 1997.
25. Hain, TC, et al (eds): The Vestibulo-Ocular Reflex and Vertigo. Raven, New York, 1993, pp 217–28.
26. Tusa, RJ, et al: The contribution of the vertical semicircular canals to high-velocity horizontal vestibulo-ocular reflex (VOR) in normal subjects and patients with unilateral vestibular nerve section. Acta Otolaryngol 116:507–12, 1996.
27. Dichgans, J, et al: Mechanisms underlying recovery of eye-head coordination following bilateral labyrinthectomy in monkeys. Exp Brain Res 18:548–62, 1973.
28. Kasai, T, and Zee, DS: Eye-head coordination in labyrinthine-defective human beings. Brain Res 144:123–41, 1978.
29. Bronstein, AM, et al: The neck-eye reflex in patients with reduced vestibular and optokinetic function. Brain 114:1–11, 1991.
30. Heimbrand, S, et al: Optically induced plasticity of the cervico-ocular reflex in patients with bilateral absence of vestibular function. Exp Brain Res 112:372–80, 1996.
31. Gresty, MA, et al: Disorders of the vestibuloocular reflex producing oscillopsia and mechanisms compensating for loss of labyrinthine function. Brain 100:693–716, 1977.
32. Takahashi, M, et al: Recovery of gaze disturbance in bilateral labyrinthine loss. ORL 51:305, 1989.
33. Gresty, MA, et al: Disorders of the vestibuloocular reflex producing oscillopsia and mechanisms compensating for loss of labyrinthine function. Brain 100:693–716, 1977.
34. Huygen, PLM, et al: Compensation of total loss of vestibulo-ocular reflex by enhanced optokinetic response. Acta Otolaryngol (Stockh) 468:359–364, 1989.
35. Bles, W, et al: Somatosensory compensation for loss of labyrinthine function. Acta Otolaryngol (Stockh) 97:213, 1984.
36. Morland, AB, et al: Vision during motion in patients with absent vestibular function. Acta Otolaryngol (Stockh) 520(suppl):338–42, 1995.
37. Bles, W, and de Graaf, B: Ocular rotation and perception of the horizontal under static tilt conditions in patients without labyrinthine function. Acta Otolaryngol (Stockh) 111:456–62, 1991.
38. Gonshor, A, and Melvill Jones, G: Extreme vestibuloocular adaptation induced by prolonged optical reversal of vision. J Physiol (Lond) 256:381–414, 1976.
39. Cannon, SC, et al: The effect of the rotational magnification of corrective spectacles on the quantitative evaluation of the VOR. Acta Otolaryngol (Stockh) 100:81–8, 1985.
40. Melvill Jones, G, et al: Changing patterns of eye-head coordination during 6 h of optically reversed vision. Exp Brain Res 69:531–44, 1988.
41. Collewijn, H, et al: Compensatory eye movements during active and passive head movements: fast adaptation to changes in visual magnification. J Physiol (Lond) 340:359, 1983.
42. Melvill Jones, G, et al: Adaptive modification of the vestibulo-ocular reflex by mental effort in darkness. Exp Brain Res 56:149–53, 1984.
43. Kramer, PD, et al: Short-term adaptation of the phase of the vestibulo-ocular reflex (VOR) in normal human subjects. Exp Brain Res 106:318–26, 1995.
44. Khater, TT, et al: Dynamics of adaptive change in human vestibulo-ocular reflex direction. J Vestib Res 1:23–9, 1990.
45. Peng, GC, et al: Dynamics of directional plasticity in the human vertical vestibulo-ocular reflex. J Vestib Res 4:453–60, 1994.
46. Schultheis, LW, and Robinson, DA: Directional plasticity of the vestibulo-ocular reflex in the cat. Ann NY Acad Sci 374:504–12, 1981.
47. Baker, J, et al: Optimal response planes and canal convergence in secondary neurons in vestibular nuclei of alert cats. Brain Res 294:133–7, 1984.
48. Angelaki, DE, and Hess, BJM: Adaptation of primate vestibuloocular reflex to altered peripheral vestibular inputs. II. Spatiotemporal properties of the adapted slow-phase eye velocity. J Neurophysiol 76:2954–71, 1996.
49. Yakushin, S, et al: Semicircular canal contributions to the three-dimensional vestibuloocular reflex: A model-based approach. J Neurophysiol 74:2722–38, 1995.
50. Böhmer, A, et al: Vestibulo-ocular reflexes after selective plugging of the semicircular canals in the monkey—Response plane determination. Brain Res 326:291–8, 1985.
51. Böhmer, A, et al: Contributions of single semicircular canals to caloric nystagmus as revealed by canal plugging in rhesus monkeys. Acta Otolaryngol (Stockh) 116:513–20, 1996.
52. Angelaki, DE: Differential processing of semicircular canal signals in the vestibulo-ocular reflex. J Neurosci 15:7201–16, 1995.
53. Quinn, KJ, et al: Changes in sensitivity of vestibular nucleus neurons induced by cross-axis adaptation of the vestibulo-ocular reflex in the cat. Brain Res 718:176–80, 1996.
54. Zee, DS, et al: Adaptation of the phase of the linear VOR at low frequency. [Abstract] Soc Neurosci Abstr 25:518, 1995.
55. Wall, C III, et al: Plasticity of the human otolith-ocular reflex. Acta Otolaryngol (Stockh) 112:413–20, 1992.
56. Koizuka, I, et al: Plasticity of responses to off-vertical axis rotation. Acta Otolaryngol (Stockh) 117:321–4, 1997.

57. Paige, GD: Senescence of human visual-vestibular interactions. 1. Vestibulo-ocular reflex and adaptive plasticity with aging. J Vestib Res 2:133–51, 1992.
58. Baker, J, et al: Simultaneous opposing adaptive changes in cat vestibulo-ocular reflex direction for two body orientations. Exp Brain Res 69:220–4, 1987.
59. Tiliket, C, et al: Adaptation of the vestibulo-ocular reflex with the head in different orientations and positions relative to the axis of body rotation. J Vestib Res 3:181–96, 1993.
60. Shelhamer, M, et al: Context-specific adaptation of the gain of the vestibulo-ocular reflex in humans. J Vestib Res 2:89–96, 1992.
61. Oohira, A, et al: Disconjugate adaptation to long-standing, large-amplitude, spectacle-corrected anisometropia. Invest Ophthalmol Vis Sci 32:1693–703, 1991.
62. du Lac, S, et al: Learning and memory in the vestibulo-ocular reflex. Annu Rev Neurosci 18:409–41, 1995.
63. Cohen, H, et al: Habituation and adaptation of the vestibulo-ocular reflex; a model of differential control by the vestibulo-cerebellum. Exp Brain Res 110:110–20, 1993.
64. Haddad, GM, et al: Compensation of nystagmus after VIIIth nerve lesions in vestibulo-cerebellectomized cats. Brain Res 135:192–6, 1977.
65. Kitahara, T, et al: Role of the flocculus in the development of vestibular compensation: immunohistochemical studies with retrograde tracing and flocculectomy using fos expression as a marker in the rat brainstem. Neuroscience 76:571–80, 1997.
66. Bronstein, AM, et al: The neck-eye reflex in patients with reduced vestibular and optokinetic function. Brain 114:1–11, 1991.
67. Darlington, CL, et al: Molecular mechanisms of brainstem plasticity: the vestibular compensation model. Molec Neurobiol 5:355–68, 1991.
68. Smith, PF, and Darlington, CL: Neurochemical mechanisms of recovery from peripheral vestibular lesions (vestibular compensation). Brain Res Rev 16:117–33, 1991.
69. du Lac, S: Candidate cellular mechanisms of vestibulo-ocular reflex plasticity. Ann NY Acad Sci 781:489–98, 1996.
70. Peterson, BW, et al: Potential mechanisms of plastic adaptive changes in the vestibulo-ocular reflex. Ann NY Acad Sci 781:499–512, 1996.
71. McElligott, JG, and Freedman, W: Vestibuloocular reflex adaptation in cats before and after depletion of norepinephrine. Exp Brain Res 69:509–21, 1988.
72. Van Neerven, J, et al: Injections of noradrenergic substances in the flocculus of rabbits affect adaptation of the VOR gain. Exp Brain Res 79:249–60, 1990.
73. Li, J, et al: Cerebellar nitric oxide is necessary for vestibulo-ocular reflex adaptation, a sensorimotor model of learning. J Neurophysiol 74:489–94, 1995.
74. Kim, MS, et al: Role of vestibulocerebellar N-methyl-D-aspartate receptors for behavioral recovery following unilateral labyrinthectomy in rats. Neurosci Lett 222:171–4, 1997.
75. McElligott, JG, et al (eds): Neurochemistry of the Vestibular System. Pergamon, London, 1997.
76. Smith, PF, and Darlington, CL: Can vestibular compensation be enhanced by drug treatment? A review of recent evidence. J Vestib Res 4:169–80, 1994.
77. Fukushima, K: Corticovestibular interactions: Anatomy, electrophysiology, and functional considerations. Exp Brain Res 117:1–16, 1997.
78. Guldin, W, et al (eds): Le Cortex Vestibulaire. Editions IRVINN, Paris, 1996, pp 17–26.
79. Barmack, NH, and Shojaku, H: Vestibularly-induced slow phase oscillations in climbing fiber responses of Purkinje cells in the cerebellar nodulus. Neuroscience 50:1–5, 1992.

CHAPTER 5

Vestibular System Disorders

Michael Fetter, M.D.

Peripheral vestibular dysfunction, which involves the vestibular end organs and/or the vestibular nerve, can produce a variety of signs and symptoms. A thorough evaluation by a physician is needed to identify the specific pathology behind the patient's complaints of vertigo or disequilibrium. Patient history is the main key for diagnosis, supported by a careful otoneurologic examination. Determining whether vestibular rehabilitation is appropriate and, if it is, which approach should be used is based in part on the patient's diagnosis. This chapter describes the clinical presentation of the more common peripheral vestibular disorders. The results of diagnostic tests, and the medical, surgical, and rehabilitative management of each of these disorders is presented as an overview only, because this material is covered in detail in other chapters.

BENIGN PAROXYSMAL POSITIONAL VERTIGO

Benign paroxysmal positional vertigo (BPPV) is the most common cause of vertigo. Typically, a patient with BPPV will complain of brief episodes of vertigo precipitated by rapid change of head posture. Sometimes symptoms are brought about by assuming very specific head positions. Most commonly these head positions involve rapid extension of the neck, often with the head turned to one side (as when looking up to a high shelf or backing a car out of a garage) or lateral head tilts toward the affected ear. The symptoms are often encountered while rolling from side to side in bed. Patients can usually identify the offending head position, which they often studiously avoid. Many patients also complain of mild postural instability between attacks. The vertigo will last only 30 seconds to 2 minutes (usually less than 1 minute), and will go away even if the precipitating position is maintained. Hearing loss, aural fullness, and tinnitus are not seen in this condition, which most commonly occurs spontaneously in the elderly population but can be seen in any age group after even mild head trauma. Women are more commonly affected than men. Bilateral involvement can be found in 10 percent of the spontaneous cases and 20 percent of the traumatic cases. Spontaneous remissions are common, but recurrences can occur, and the condition may trouble the patient intermittently for years.

Evaluation should include a careful otoneurologic examination, the most important part being the history. A key diagnostic maneuver is the Dix-Hallpike positioning test[1] while observing the eyes with a pair of Frenzel lenses or in combination with electronystagmography (ENG) monitoring. A typical response is induced by rapid position changes from the sitting to the head-hanging right or left position. Vertigo and nystagmus begin with a latency of 1 or more seconds after the head is tilted toward the affected ear and increase in severity within about 10 seconds to a maximum accompanied by a sensation of discomfort and apprehension that will sometimes cause the patient to cry out and attempt to sit up. The symptoms reduce gradually after 10 to 40 seconds and ultimately abate, even if the precipitating head position is maintained. The nystagmus is mixed upbeat and torsional with a slight horizontal component: the direction corresponds very closely with the plane of the offending semicircular canal, very similar to experimental stimulation of the afferents of the posterior semicircular canal of the dependent ear.[2] The nystagmus changes with the direction of gaze, becoming more torsional on looking toward the dependent ear and becoming more vertical on looking toward the higher ear.

Sometimes, a low-amplitude, secondary nystagmus, directed in the opposite direction, may occur. If the patient then quickly sits up, a similar but usually milder recurrence of these symptoms occurs, the nystagmus being directed opposite to the initial nystagmus. Repeating this procedure several times will decrease the symptoms. This adaptation of the response is of diagnostic value because a clinical picture similar to that of BPPV can be created by cerebellar tumors. In the latter, though, there is no habituation of the response with repetitive testing. Further diagnostic criteria indicating a central positional nystagmus is that the condition does not subside with maintenance of the head in the precipitating position; the nystagmus may change direction when different head positions are assumed; or it may occur as downbeat nystagmus only in the head-hanging position. BPPV must be differentiated from positional nystagmus in Ménière's disease, perilymph fistulas, and alcohol intoxication.

A few patients do not display the typical torsional upbeat nystagmus but, for example, show a strong horizontal nystagmus, which, nevertheless, follows a similar pattern of buildup and decline but often over a longer period. This horizontal nystagmus may indicate a lateral canal variant of BPPV.

The classic explanation of the underlying pathophysiology (cupulolithiasis) was first described by Schuknecht[3] in 1969. His study of the temporal bones of two patients afflicted with this disorder showed deposition of otoconial material in the cupula of the posterior semicircular canal. The cupulolithiasis theory suggests that the debris adheres to the cupula, making it denser than the surrounding endolymph and thereby susceptible to the pull of gravity. This theory, however, implies that a positioning maneuver should result in an enhanced positioning response with a nystagmus initially beating in the direction of an ampullopetal stimulation. This nystagmus should occur immediately after the positioning maneuver, and should change direction as gravity drags the cupula down. The nystagmus, however, should not subside as long as the head down position is maintained. That is, one would expect positional instead of positioning nystagmus. None of these features is typically seen.

Brandt and Steddin[4] recently emphasized a second theory, canalithiasis, which better explains the typical features of BPPV. It suggests that the debris of a higher density than the endolymph is free-floating in the long arm of the canal. When the head is moved in the plane of that canal, the debris sinks to the lowest point in the canal, causing the endolymph to move and deflecting the cupula by suction or pressure (like a plunger), depending on the direction it moves. This theory is in accordance with the direction of the nystagmus and also allows for a latency.

If symptoms persist longer than expected, then further investigation such as a magnetic resonance imaging (MRI) scan should be done to assess for unusual causes of positional vertigo such as acoustic neuroma or tumors of the fourth ventricle.

BPPV is usually a self-limiting disorder and will commonly resolve spontaneously within 6 to 12 months. Simple vestibular exercises or maneuvers aimed at dispersing the otolithic debris from the cupula can speed recovery; antivertiginous drugs are not helpful. One approach is to instruct the patient to assume repeatedly the positions that bring on the symptoms.[5] In 1988, Semont et al.[6] introduced a single liberatory maneuver, and Epley,[7] in 1992, proposed a variation, later modified by Herdman et al.[8] (see also Chapter 16). The period of recovery varies from immediate recovery after one positioning maneuver (physical displacement) to usually 6 weeks to 6 months. Only in a few patients, usually the more elderly, will the symptoms persist in spite of compliance with vestibular exercises. For more severe symptoms unresponsive to exercises, three surgical options are available for relief. The first is transmeatal posterior ampullary nerve section (also known as singular neurectomy). The other two options are partitioning of the labyrinth using a laser technique and nonampullary plugging of the posterior semicircular canal. Nonampullary plugging seems to be a safe and effective alternative to singular neurectomy for the small group of patients with physically intractable BPPV.

VESTIBULAR NEURITIS

Acute unilateral (idiopathic) vestibulopathy, also known as vestibular neuritis, is the second most common cause of vertigo. Although in most cases a definitive etiology is never proved, evidence to support a viral etiology (similar to Bell's palsy or sudden hearing loss) comes from histopathologic changes of branches of the vestibular nerve in patients who have suffered such an illness[9] and the sometimes epidemic occurrence of the condition. Onset is often preceded by the presence of a viral infection of the upper respiratory or gastrointestinal tracts. The associated viral infection may be coincident with the vestibular neuritis or may have preceded it by as long as 2 weeks. The chief symptom is the acute onset of prolonged severe rotational vertigo that is exacerbated by movement of the head, associated with spontaneous horizontal-rotatory nystagmus beating toward the good ear, postural imbalance, and nausea. Hearing loss is not usually present, but when it is then mumps, measles, and infectious mononucleosis, among other infections, have been implicated. The latter condition should also alert the physician to consider other diagnoses (i.e., ischemia of labyrinth artery, Ménière's disease, acoustic neuroma, herpes zoster, Lyme disease, or neurosyphilis). The condition mainly affects those aged between 30 and 60 years, with a peak for women in the fourth decade and men in the sixth decade.

If examined early, the patient may manifest an irritative nystagmus from the acute phases of the inflammation. Usually the patient is examined after these initial findings have given way to a more paralytic, or hypofunctional, pattern. Caloric testing invariably shows ipsilateral hyporesponsiveness or nonresponsiveness (horizontal canal paresis). The possibility that the three semicircular canals and the otoliths (utricle and saccule) may be separately involved in partial labyrinthine lesions is suggested by the occasional observation of an acute unilateral vestibulopathy and a benign paroxysmal positioning vertigo simultaneously in the same ear of a patient.[10] With three-dimensional measurements of the vestibulo-ocular reflex in patients with vestibular neuritis this notion could be confirmed. Patients with this condition most often showed a partial involvement of only the superior vestibular nerve portion (subserving the anterior and lateral semicircular canals, the utricle, and a small part of the saccule) leaving part of the saccule and the posterior semicircular canal afferents intact.[11] The symptoms usually abate after a period of 48 to 72 hours, and gradual return to normal balance occurs over approximately 6 weeks. Rapid head movements toward the lesioned side, however, can still cause slight oscillopsia of the visual scene and impaired balance for a short moment. Recovery is produced by the combination of central compensation of the vestibular tone imbalance, aided by physical exercise, and peripheral restoration of labyrinthine function. The latter is found in about two-thirds of the patients.

The differential diagnosis should initially include other causes of vertigo, and careful history taking, physical examination, and an audiogram are required. Physical examination should include a neurological examination with attention to cranial nerve findings and cerebellar testing. Careful otoscopy is performed to rule out the presence of a potential otologic infectious process as the source of a toxic serous labyrinthitis. Fever in the presence of chronic ear disease and labyrinthitis suggests suppuration and meningitis. Commonly, a toxic labyrinthitis is the result of a well-defined event such as surgery or trauma.

Initial treatment is accomplished with the use of vestibular suppressants such as the antihistamine dimenhydrinate or the anticholinergic scopolamine. In addition, bed rest is very helpful early on in the course of the disease. After the most severe vertigo and nausea have passed (after 24 to 72 hours), then ambulation may resume with assistance; independent ambulation may be achieved over the next few days. At the same time, the administration of vestibular suppressants should be greatly diminished or, even better, stopped completely because they prolong the time required to achieve central compensation. To further speed up the process of recuperation, vestibular exercises challenge the compensatory mechanisms of the central nervous system (CNS), stimulating adaptation. These exercises are designed to improve both gaze stability and postural stability (see Chapter 14). The symptomatology is usually self-limited to a course of approximately 6 weeks.

Animal experiments have shown that alcohol, phenobarbital, chlorpromazine, diazepam, and ACTH antagonists retard compensation; caffeine, amphetamines, and ACTH accelerate compensation. The use of drugs for acceleration of compensation in patients has still to be proven.[12]

MÉNIÈRE'S DISEASE AND ENDOLYMPHATIC HYDROPS

Ménière's disease is a disorder of inner ear function that can cause devastating hearing and vestibular symptoms. The typical attack is experienced as an initial sensation of fullness of the ear, a reduction in hearing, and tinnitus, followed by rotational vertigo, postural imbalance, nystagmus, and nausea and vomiting after a few minutes. This severe disequilibrium (vertigo) will persist anywhere from approximately 30 minutes to 24 hours. Gradually, the severe symptoms will abate, and the patient is generally ambulatory within 72 hours. Some sensation of postural unsteadiness will persist for days or weeks, and then normal balance will return. During this recuperation time, hearing gradually returns. Hearing may return to the pre-attack baseline or there may be residual permanent sensorineural hearing loss, most commonly in the lower frequencies. The rare transient improvement of hearing during the attack is known as the *Lermoyez phenomenon*. Tinnitus will also usually diminish as hearing returns. As the disease progresses, hearing fails to return after the attack, and after many years, the symptoms of vertigo may gradually diminish in frequency and severity. Some patients may suddenly fall without warning; these events, which may occur in later stages of the disease, are referred to as *Tumarkin's otolithic crisis* and should be differentiated from other forms of drop attack.

The typical form of Ménière's disease is sometimes not complete and is called vestibular Ménière's disease, if only vestibular symptoms and aural pressure are present, or cochlear Ménière's disease, if only cochlear symptoms and aural pressure are encountered.[13]

The disease is about equally distributed between the sexes and usually has its onset in the fourth to sixth decades of life. However, there are reports of children as young as 6 years of age with classical Ménière's disease.[14] About 15 percent of the patients have blood relatives with the same disease, suggesting genetic factors. The incidence of bilaterality of involvement ranges between 33 and 50 percent.[15]

A phenomenon fundamental to the development of Ménière's disease is *endolymphatic hydrops*. Whether endolymphatic hydrops itself is the cause of the symptoms characteristic of Ménière's disease or whether it is a pathologic change seen in the disease is still unclear. The development of hydrops is generally a function of malabsorption of endolymph in the endolymphatic duct and sac. Malabsorption may itself be a result of disturbed function of components comprising the endolymphatic duct and sac, mechanical obstruction of these structures, or altered anatomy in the temporal bone. Endolymph is produced primarily by the stria vascularis and flows both longitudinally (along the axis of the endolymphatic duct toward the endolymphatic sac) and radially (across the membrane of the endolymphatic space into the perilymph system). Ménière's disease is generally a consequence of altered longitudinal flow, usually evolving over a course of many years. Experimental obstruction of the endolymphatic duct will routinely result in endolymphatic hydrops in many animal models.[16] Lesions in the temporal bone that have been associated with the development of hydrops include fractures of the temporal bone, perisaccular fibrosis, atrophy of the sac, narrowing of the lumen in the endolymphatic duct, otitis media, otosclerotic foci enveloping the vestibular aqueduct, lack of vascularity surrounding the endolymphatic sac, syphilitic osteitis of the otic capsule, and leukemic infiltrations, to name just a few. Anatomically, ears affected by Ménière's disease are likely to demonstrate hypodevelopment of the endolymphatic duct and sac, periaqueductal cells, and mastoid air cells. Therefore, one can postulate a cause-and-effect relationship between constricted anatomy in the temporal bone and malabsorption of endolymph.

Any explanation of the clinical symptoms of Ménière's disease should account for all of the symptoms, including rapid or prolonged attacks of vertigo, disequilibrium, positional vertigo during and between attacks, fluctuating progressive sensorineural hearing loss, tinnitus, aural pressure, inability to tolerate loudness, and diplacusis. These symptoms probably result from both chemical and physical mechanisms. Physical factors can tamponade the cochlear duct, contributing to fluctuating progressive sensorineural hearing loss and other cochlear symptoms, whereas distension of the otolithic organs can physically affect the crista ampullaris, resulting in vestibular symptoms. The prolonged nystagmus and vertigo are commonly believed to be caused by periodic membrane ruptures with subsequent transient potassium palsy of vestibular nerve fibers.

Useful diagnostic tests include the audiogram and ENG. Typically, the audiogram displays an ipsilateral sensorineural hearing loss involving the lower frequencies. Fluctuation in discrimination scores is often seen, with a long-term trend toward poor scores. ENG may demonstrate a unilateral vestibular weakness on caloric testing, again involving the ear symptomatic for pressure, hearing loss, and tinnitus. Electrocochleography is useful in cases that are unclear. The finding of enlarged summating potentials in the suspected ear is diagnostic of endolymphatic hydrops.

A brainstem-evoked acoustic response (BEAR) must be done in those cases with findings of retrocochlear pathology on routine audiometry to screen for cochlear nerve or brainstem pathology. If the BEAR is found to be positive, then MRI scanning with the use of intravenous gadolinium should be done to assess for central nervous system pathology or eighth-nerve schwannoma.

Treatment in the remission phase aims to reduce the frequency of the attacks and preserve hearing without distressing tinnitus. Dietetic programs, including restriction of salt, water, alcohol, nicotine, and caffeine, are as valueless in treating the disease as are physical exercise or avoidance of exposure to low temperatures. Stellate ganglion blocks, diuretics, vasoactive agents, tranquilizers, neuroleptics, and lithium have been employed under the mistaken assumption that diminishing endolymphatic hydrops is possible by changing inner-ear blood flow, osmotic diuresis, or central sedation. There has never been prospective proof of the efficiency of these therapies. The histamine derivative betahistine has been advocated as the drug of first choice. Findings from a 1-year prospective double-blind study showed that this treatment is preferable to leaving the disease untreated.[17] The action is attributed to improvement of microcirculation of the stria vascularis, but betahistine also has inhibitory effects on polysynaptic vestibular neurons. Adjunct medications in the form of vestibular suppressants other than betahistine are to be used primarily during the acute episodes of vertigo and should be discouraged as a chronic daily medication.

In addition to pharmacologic therapies, many patients with Ménière's disease require psychologic support to help cope with the frustrations and changes brought about by their medical condition. Those patients in whom the vertigo becomes disabling by virtue of increased severity or frequency of attacks despite maximal medical therapy would be considered candidates for surgical intervention. Only about 1 to 3 percent of patients ultimately require surgical treatment, because the success of regular endolymphatic sac shunt operations has been shown to be a placebo effect.[18]

Sacculotomy has been proposed by a variety of authors as a method of relieving the pressure build-up in the endolymphatic chamber. Long-term success rates for this procedure are not yet available, but significant hearing loss is observed in 50 percent of patients undergoing cochleosacculotomy. Advantages are ease of performance, utility in elderly patients as a first procedure under local anesthesia, and little risk other than hearing loss.

Intratympanic treatment with ototoxic antibiotics such as gentamicin sulfate, 8 to 24 mg instilled daily via a plastic tube inserted behind the annulus via the transmeatal approach, is obviously able to damage selectively the secretory epithelium (and thereby improve endolymphatic hydrops) before significantly affecting vestibular and cochlear function.[19] Instillation (up to 10 days) should be stopped when daily audiograms or a check of spontaneous nystagmus indicate end-organ dysfunction.

The current treatment most successful is vestibular nerve section. This procedure is indicated in individuals with serviceable hearing in whom maximal medical therapy has been unsuccessful in controlling vertigo. Success rates in the range of 90 to 95 percent have been reported by numerous authors. The newer technique of focused ultrasound seems to have an advantage over open surgery in that partial ablation of vestibular function (with preservation of hearing) can be performed without invading the labyrinth.

Surgical fistulization in various parts of the membranous labyrinth has been used in patients with Ménière's disease. Cochlear endolymphatic shunt operation is the current solution, and Schuknecht and Bartley[20] report that 72 percent of cases were relieved of vertigo, but hearing was worse in 45 percent of cases.

In patients with hearing loss, destructive procedures are also possible, such as transmeatal, transmastoid, or translabyrinthine labyrinthectomy. The success rate is 95 percent. An extension of this surgery is the translabyrinthine vestibular nerve section, shown to eliminate vertigo in 98 percent of cases. However, particularly in elderly patients, ablative surgical procedures may cause long-lasting postural imbalance because of the reduced ability of central mechanisms to compensate for the postoperative vestibular tone imbalance.

Vestibular exercises are not appropriate in patients with Ménière's disease unless there is permanent loss of vestibular function. Vestibular exercises are designed to induce long-term changes in the remaining vestibular system or to foster the substitution of other strategies to compensate for the loss of vestibular function. In Ménière's disease, the vestibular dysfunction is episodic and between episodes, the system usually returns to normal function. Some patients developed a loss of vestibular function at the end stages of the disease, and for those patients, vestibular rehabilitation may be appropriate. Vestibular exercises are also beneficial in those patients who have surgical destruction of the inner ear.

PERILYMPHATIC FISTULA

Perilymphatic fistula may lead to episodic vertigo and sensorineural hearing loss owing to the pathologic elasticity of the bony labyrinth. Most commonly, these fistulas occur at the round and oval windows of the middle ear. Classically, a history of (often minor) head trauma, barotrauma, mastoid or stapes surgery, penetrating injury to the tympanic membrane, or vigorous straining precedes the onset of sudden vertigo, hearing loss, and loud tinnitus. The patients often report a "pop" in the ear during the precipitating event. Later on, patients with fistula may complain of imbalance, positional vertigo, and nystagmus as well as hearing loss. Tullio phenomenon, vestibular symptoms that include vertigo, oscillopsia, nystagmus, ocular tilt reaction, and postural imbalance induced by auditory stimuli, is usually due to perilymph fistula, but subluxation of the stapes foot plate and other ear pathology may be responsible. The symptoms will often subside while at rest only to resume with activity. Sneezing, straining, nose blowing, and other such maneuvers can elicit the symptoms after the initial event. Perilymph fistulas probably account for a considerable proportion of those patients presenting with vertigo of unknown origin. Diagnosing perilymph fistula is difficult because of the great variability of signs and symptoms and the lack of a pathognomonic test. In the acute phase, medical treatment is universally recommended because these fistulas usually heal spontaneously, and the results of surgical interventions are not encouraging.[21]

Physical examination, particularly otoscopy, is important. In the cases of head trauma and barotrauma, hemotympanum is often seen as an early finding. In cases of penetrating injury to the ear, a tympanic membrane perforation makes the likelihood of ossicular discontinuity with fistula very high. A useful clinical test consists of applying manual pressure over the tragus or applying pressure to the tympanic membrane with the pneumatic otoscope; a positive test is indicated by the evocation or exacerbation of vertigo (Hennebert's sign) or the elicitation of nystagmus. Audiometric findings usually demonstrate a mixed or sensorineural hearing loss, depending on the mechanism of injury. This loss may be quite severe and usually involves the high frequencies more than the low frequencies. ENG with caloric testing may be normal or show a unilateral weakness in the affected ear. The specificity of the clinical fistula tests can be augmented by recording eye movements or measuring body sway as pressure on the tympanic membrane is increased. Despite refinements, these tests remain unreliable in detecting all fistulas. The diagnosis remains essentially a historical one, and in those patients with a suggestive history and symptoms treatment is indicated. Often the only manner in which the diagnosis is made definitively is at the time of surgical exploration by tympanoscopy as the patient performs Valsalva maneuvers.

Medical treatment consists of absolute bed rest with the head elevated for 5 to 10 days. Mild sedation with tranquilizers; avoidance of straining, sneezing, coughing, or head-hanging positions; and the use of stool softeners is important for reduction of further explosive and implosive forces that may activate perilymph leakage.[22]

When symptoms persist for longer than 4 weeks, or if hearing loss worsens, exploratory tympanotomy is indicated. Considerable controversy persists surrounding the frequency with which perilymph fistulas are found at surgery. Surgical management consists of middle ear exploration and packing of the oval and round window areas with fat, Gelfoam, and areolar and/or fibrous tissue. These areas are packed whether or not a clear-cut fistula is demonstrated. Reported success rates for this treatment vary between 50 and 70 percent and likely reflect some element of variable patient selection.

VESTIBULAR PAROXYSMIA (DISABLING POSITIONAL VERTIGO)

Neurovascular cross-compression of the root entry zone of the vestibular nerve can elicit disabling positional vertigo.[23] The term describes a heterogeneous collection of signs and symptoms rather than a reliable diagnosable disease entity. Brandt and Dieterich[24] proposed the following criteria: (1) short and frequent attacks of rotational or to-and-fro vertigo lasting from seconds to minutes; (2) attacks frequently dependent on particular head positions and modification of the duration of the attack by changing head position; (3) hypacusis and/or tinnitus permanent or during the attack; (4) measurable auditory or vestibular deficits by neurophysiological methods; (5) positive response to antiepileptic drugs (carbamazepine).

Neurovascular cross-compression can cause local demyelinization of the root entry zone of the eighth nerve. Ephaptic transmission between bare axons or central hyperactivity initiated and maintained by the peripheral compression are the suggested mechanisms. Analogous to trigeminal neuralgia, antiepileptic drugs are the first choice of medical treatment of the condition before surgical microvascular decompression is contemplated.

BILATERAL VESTIBULAR DISORDERS

Bilateral vestibulopathy may occur secondary to meningitis, labyrinthine infection, otosclerosis, Paget's disease, polyneuropathy, bilateral tumors (acoustic neuromas in neurofibromatosis), endolymphatic hydrops, bilateral sequential vestibular neuritis, cerebral hemosiderosis, ototoxic drugs, inner-ear autoimmune disease, or congenital malformations. Autoimmune conditions affecting the inner ear are rare but distinct clinical entities,[25] characterized by a progressive, bilateral sensorineural hearing loss often accompanied by a bilateral loss of vestibular function. Other autoimmune-mediated disease is often present in the afflicted patients; examples include rheumatoid arthritis, psoriasis, ulcerative colitis, and Cogans's syndrome (iritis accompanied by vertigo and sensorineural hearing loss). The history is the most useful diagnostic tool. Support for the diagnosis can be obtained by blood testing for complete blood count, erythrocyte sedimentation rate, rheumatoid factor, and antinuclear antibodies. Western-blot precipitation studies to look for anticochlear antibodies can be done in some research centers and may be the future definitive test of choice in these cases.

Little is known about how autoimmune disorders cause otologic symptoms. As with other autoimmune conditions, the otologic symptoms may occur as a direct assault by the immune system in the form of humoral and cellular immunity directed at the inner ear. Another mechanism of injury may be related to the deposition of antibody-antigen complex in capillaries or basement membranes of inner ear structures. Further immunologic studies of temporal bones harvested from deceased patients who had clinical evidence of autoimmune inner ear involvement may shed some light on the underlying process.

Because autoimmune vestibulopathy usually affects both ears, therapy is almost exclusively medical. Vestibular suppressants are most useful in controlling the more severe exacerbations of vertigo. The use of corticosteroids and some cytotoxic agents (cytoxan, methotrexate) has been shown to provide relief in some patients. There is some newer evidence to suggest that serum plasmapheresis may play a more prominent role in controlling this disease in the future. The natural history of the disease leads to eventual bilateral vestibular ablation. This end result is almost inevitable unless the underlying process can be arrested with treatment or arrests spontaneously.

The most common toxic cause of acute vertigo is ethyl alcohol. We know that positional changes exacerbate the vertigo of a hangover. The reason may be that alcohol diffuses into the cupula and endolymph at different rates and so creates a density gradient, making the cupula sensitive to gravity.[26] Other agents that may produce vertigo include organic compounds of heavy metals and aminoglycosides. The aminoglycosides are notorious for causing irreversible failure of vestibular function without vertiginous warning or hearing loss. Thus, monitoring of vestibular function may be necessary during such therapy.

Independent of vestibulopathies produced by ototoxins, single cases of "progressive vestibular degeneration" of unknown origin have been described, with the following factors in common: repeated episodes of dizziness relatively early in life, bilat-

TABLE 5-1 Summary of Vestibular System Disorders

	BPPV	Vestibular Neuritis	Ménière's Disease	Fistula	Nerve Compression	Bilateral Vestibular Disorder
Vertigo	+	+	+	+	+	–
Type	Rotational	Rotational	Rotational	Rotational/ linear	Rotational/ linear	–
Nystagmus	+	+	+	+	+	–
Duration	30 sec–2 min	48–72 hr	30 min–24 hr	Seconds	Seconds to minutes	Permanent
Nausea	–/(+)	+	+	–	+	–
Postural Ataxia	–/(+)	+	+	+	+	++
Specific symptoms	Onset latency, adaptation	Acute onset	Fullness of ear, hearing loss, tinnitus	Loud tinnitus, Tullio sign, Hennebert sign	Frequent attacks, tinnitus, hypacusis	Gait ataxia
Precipitating action	Positioning, turning in bed	–	–	Head trauma, ear surgery, sneezing, straining, nose blowing	Changing head position	–

Key: – absent, + present, ++ very strong.

eral loss of vestibular function with retention of hearing, and freedom from other neurological disturbances.[27]

Alport's (inherited sensorineural deafness associated with interstitial nephritis), Usher's (inherited sensorineural deafness associated with retinitis pigmentosa) and Waardenburg's syndromes (inherited deafness associated with facial dysplasia) usually cause bilateral labyrinthine deficiency when they affect the vestibular system. Congenital vestibular loss is secondary to either abnormal genetic or intrauterine factors including infection (most commonly rubella and cytomegalo virus); intoxication (thalidomide); or anoxia.

Controlled physical exercises can improve the condition in patients with permanent bilateral vestibulopathy by recruiting nonvestibular sensory capacities such as the cervico-ocular reflex and proprioceptive and visual control of stance and gait (see Chapter 15).

SUMMARY

This chapter describes the clinical presentation of the more common peripheral vestibular disorders and the differential diagnosis to central origins of vertigo. Although the symptomatology of a certain peripheral vestibular disorder might be rather specific, as in acute unilateral vestibular loss, the cause can be rather different, ranging from infection to ischemia to traumatic lesions. A thorough evaluation, therefore, should, in addition to the specific otoneurological investigation, always include a detailed history and a general physical examination. For a quick review, Table 5–1 summarizes the hallmarks of the peripheral vestibular disorders treated in this chapter.

REFERENCES

1. Dix, R, and Hallpike, CS: The pathology, symptomatology and diagnosis of certain common disorders of the vestibular system. Ann Otol Rhinol Laryngol 6:987, 1952.
2. Fetter, M, and Sievering, F: Three-dimensional eye movement analysis in benign paroxysmal positioning vertigo and nystagmus. Acta Otolaryngol (Stockh) 115:353, 1995.
3. Schuknecht, HF: Cupulolithiasis. Arch Otolaryngol 90:765, 1969.
4. Brandt, T, and Steddin, S: Current view of the mechanism of benign paroxysmal positioning vertigo: Cupulolithiasis or canalolithiasis? J Vestib Res 3:373, 1993.
5. Brandt, T, and Daroff, RB: Physical therapy for benign paroxysmal positional vertigo. Arch Otolaryngol 106:484, 1980.
6. Semont, A, et al: Curing the BPPV with a liberatory maneuver. Adv Oto-Rhinol-Laryngol 42:290, 1988.
7. Epley, JM: The canalith repositioning procedure: For treatment of benign paroxysmal positional vertigo. Otolaryngol Head Neck Surg 107:399, 1992.
8. Herdman, SJ, et al: Single treatment approaches to benign paroxysmal vertigo. Arch Otolaryngol Head Neck Surg 119:450, 1993.
9. Schuknecht, HF, and Kitamura, K: Vestibular neuritis. Ann Otol Rhinol Laryngol 90(suppl 79):1, 1981.
10. Büchele, W, and Brandt, T: Vestibular neuritis—A horizontal semicircular canal paresis? Adv Oto-Rhinol-Laryngol 42:157, 1988.
11. Fetter, M, and Dichgans, J: Vestibular neuritis spares the inferior division of the vestibular nerve. Brain 119:755, 1996.
12. Zee, DS: Perspectives on the pharmacotherapy of vertigo. Arch Otolaryngol 111:609, 1985.
13. Paparella, MM, and Kimberley, BP: Pathogenesis of Ménière's disease. J Vestib Res 1:3, 1990.
14. Paparella, MM, and Meyerhoff, W: Ménière's disease in children. Laryngoscope 88:1504, 1978.
15. Balkany, T, et al: Bilateral aspects of Ménière's disease: An underestimated clinical entity. Otolaryngol Clin North Am 13:603, 1980.
16. Kimura, R: Animal models of endolymphatic hydrops. Am J Otol 3:447, 1982.

17. Meyer, ED: Treatment of Ménière's disease with betahistin-dimesilate—a double blind, placebo con-
    trolled study. Laryngol Rhinol Otol 64:269, 1985.
18. Thomson, J, et al: Placebo effect in surgery for Ménière's disease. Arch Otolaryngol 107:271, 1981.
19. Lange, G: Intratympanic treatment of Ménière's disease with ototoxic antibiotics. Laryngol Rhinol
    56:409, 1977.
20. Schuknecht, HF, and Bartley, M: Cochlear endolymphatic shunt for Ménière's disease. Ann J Otol Suppl
    20, 1985.
21. Singleton, GT, et al: Perilymph Fistulas. Diagnostic criteria and therapy. Ann Otol Rhinol Laryngol 87:1,
    1978.
22. Brandt, T: Episodic vertigo. In Rakel, RE (ed): Conn's Current Therapy. WB Saunders, Philadelphia,
    1986, p 723.
23. Jannetta, P, et al: Disabling positional vertigo. N Engl J Med 310:1700, 1984.
24. Brandt, T, and Dieterich, M: Vestibular paroxysmia: Vascular compression of the VIII nerve? Lancet i:798,
    1994.
25. Hughes, GB, et al: Clinical diagnosis of immune inner ear disease. Laryngoscope 98:251, 1988.
26. Brandt, T: Positional and positioning vertigo and nystagmus. J Neurol Sci 95:3, 1990.
27. Baloh, RW, et al: Idiopathic bilateral vestibulopathy. Neurology 39:272, 1989.

SECTION II

Medical Assessment

CHAPTER 6

Quantitative Vestibular Function Tests and the Clinical Examination

Vicente Honrubia, MD, DMSc

The maintenance of equilibrium, posture, and gaze, and the awareness of spatial orientation are complex functions depending on multiple peripheral organs and neural centers in addition to the labyrinthine end organs and nerves. Visual and proprioceptive information must be integrated with vestibular sensory inputs for gaze and body stability in the vestibular nuclei (Fig. 6–1).[1,2] Consequently, evaluation of the "vestibular system" requires the study of the function of all these systems, in addition to that of the vestibular organs. The physician must investigate, through medical history and physical evaluation, every aspect relevant to this contemporary view of vestibular function. His or her first objective is the identification of the site of lesion, and subsequently the characterization of the disease process.

Clinical evaluation of the patient remains the most important aspect of the vestibular diagnosis. The most common symptom of vestibular dysfunction is dizziness, and the most common signs are spontaneous nystagmus and abnormal voluntary eye movements. Dizziness or some form of disequilibrium or disorientation can be produced by lesions in sites other than the vestibular system. The patient's history provides many clues to the cause of symptoms, and the physical examination provides objective data about the operation of various components of the vestibular system. Careful evaluation of information obtained from the medical history and physical examination is necessary to complement the laboratory objective and quantitative data obtained from the various reflexes. The associated evidence makes it possible in many instances to determine if the site of the lesion is the inner ear, the eyes, or the vestibular and visual centers or pathways in the central nervous system (CNS).

Significant improvement in patient management has occurred during the last 10 years with the creation of technology that has led to new tests for differential diagnosis

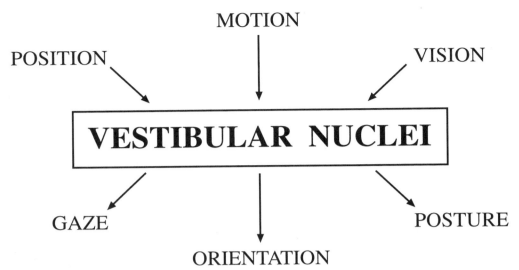

FIGURE 6–1. Euristic model of vestibular system organization. Information from head position, motion, and vision converge in the vestibular nuclei where signals are generated to facilitate vestibular function.

and evaluation of treatment of vestibular patients. The most often used vestibular tests are those evaluating maintenance of gaze, because this is one of the primary functions of the vestibular system. Eye movements produced for this purpose are the result of three basic systems with different physiological characteristics and neuroanatomic pathways: the *saccadic system*, the *smooth-pursuit and optokinetic systems*, and the *vestibulo-ocular system*. Tests for independent evaluation of eye movements associated with each system have become important parts of the modern neurotological examination. The contribution of these tests goes beyond their individual intrinsic value, because their combined information represents a powerful method for evaluating the state of large parts of the CNS and diagnosing many neurological disorders.

CLINICAL EVALUATION OF VESTIBULAR PATIENTS

The neurotological evaluation consists of a detailed history to ascertain the character of dizziness, physical examination of the ear, evaluation of the function of vestibulo-visual-ocular and equilibrium reflexes and hearing, as well as an overall neurological assessment. This section emphasizes the more "vestibular" aspects of the examination during the first interaction between patient and clinician, and describes the most important details of the history of dizziness and the clinical evaluation of vestibular- and visual-dependent eye movements.

Dizziness and Vertigo

The individual's description of the nature of dizziness can be helpful in determining which of the systems involved in orientation is responsible for the symptoms. **Vertigo** is an illusion of movement that is specific to vestibular system disease, and rotation is the most commonly described experience. The illusion of linear displacement, or rocking, is less frequently noted and suggests otolithic organ involvement. Other terms frequently used to describe dizziness are less specific and include giddiness, that "one's head is swimming," light-headedness, floating, a feeling of drunkenness, or weakness of lower extremities. These sensations can be associated with disorders of other parts of the nervous system, such as hemodynamic brain insufficiencies, including transient ischemic episodes even with loss of consciousness, which is not typical of peripheral vertigo.

Vertigo always indicates an imbalance within the vestibular system, although the symptom per se does not indicate where in the system the imbalance originates, whether in the inner ear, the deep paravertebral stretch receptors of the neck, the vestibular centers, the cerebellum, or the upper cerebral pathways and cortex. The distinction between peripheral and central causes of vertigo can be suspected on the basis of history. Vertigo of peripheral origin is often severe, rotatory, and associated with other physiological changes, such as hearing loss, ear pathology, and with autonomic symptoms, such as nausea. Vertigo of central origin is more moderate and more persistent. It is often referred to as disequilibrium, a tendency to fall, and is associated with generalized weakness of the extremities.

THE CHARACTERISTICS OF VERTIGO

Intensity, duration, and frequency of vertigo attacks, precipitating or relieving factors, and characteristics of associated symptoms (tinnitus, hearing loss, ear pain, and infections) are all important elements in elucidating the underlying cause of dizziness. The *intensity* of peripheral vestibular vertigo is usually abrupt in onset and of a variable degree. It can be completely disabling (Ménière's attack) or very mild, as a slight disequilibrium associated with quick head movements in normal elderly subjects. The *duration* of vertigo with peripheral disorders varies from seconds, as in benign paroxysmal postural vertigo, to minutes and hours as in Ménière's disease, or even days following a vascular compromise or inflammation of the inner ear. In the latter case, the intensity decreases as the precipitating factor disappears. In severe cases, the episode is followed by lightheadedness, fatigue, and generalized weakness that subside with time. Recovery may take several days to a week if peripheral vestibular damage is severe. Even at such times it is important to differentiate spontaneous episodes of vertigo, as may occur in Ménière's disease, from the rather brief episodes or disorientation provoked by quick head movements due to deficient function of a damaged vestibular receptor. Peripherally induced vertigo, even in the case of severe damage, invariably resolves gradually as central compensation occurs, although the duration of symptoms depends on the extent of damage. Vertigo without fluctuation for long periods of time is not typical of vestibular disorders of peripheral origin.

The *frequency* of vertigo provides information about its cause. Repeated episodes associated with specific head movements or positions suggest benign paroxysmal or positional vertigo. An episode with several days of severe associated symptoms indicates some permanent and repeated damage to the inner ear. Isolated episodes lasting several minutes or hours are most likely due to Ménière's disease.

The *precipitating* or *associated factors* of vertigo help to diagnose the specific disease process. Fluctuating hearing loss, earache, and appearance of or increase in tinnitus are typical of Ménière's disease. Positional vertigo may be precipitated by turning over in bed, sitting up from a prone position, extending the neck to look upwards, or bending over and straightening up. Patients with Ménière's disease find relief by lying motionless in bed. Patients with perilymph fistulae develop brief episodes of vertigo precipitated by changes in middle ear pressure, such as when coughing, sneezing, quickly changing altitude, or engaging in vigorous physical activities. Occasionally, loud noises can produce vertigo when a fistula is present or when there is inner ear pathology (syphilis, advanced Ménière's disease). Ear discharge and upper respiratory symptoms may be significant in the diagnosis of labyrinthitis.

The medical history may also point out a *contributing factor* in the use of drugs such as alcohol, tranquilizers, anticonvulsants, or barbiturates. A compromised cardiovascular, metabolic, or immunological condition, impaired vision, or generalized neuropathies may be associated with dizziness. Severe headaches associated with vertigo may suggest it is a complication of migraines; there is often a similar history in other members of the family. If headaches are associated with ataxia, one should inquire whether other family members experience the same symptoms. Episodes of vertigo can occur from decreased cerebral blood flow, as occurs during changes in position of the body and head in hypotensive conditions and cardiac insufficiency, or spontaneously during transient ischemic episodes in basilar vertebral insufficiency. The latter should be differentiated from Tumarkin episodes occurring in patients with Ménière's disease. Patients with handicapped brain blood flow experience generalized weakness, particularly of the lower extremities, transient neural symptoms, diplopia, amaurosis fugax, desartria, brief disorientation, and finally near or complete loss of consciousness. Patients undergoing Tumarkin crises feel irresistibly catapulted to the ground without loss of consciousness. Both conditions can occur in elderly patients with Ménière's disease. Dizziness in a continuous static fashion without episodic vertigo has a central origin and should lead to inquiry about other CNS symptoms or signs (e.g., cranial nerve function evaluation and possibly imaging studies of the brain).

Finally, the *association* of dizziness or vertigo with psychological conditions such as panic attacks, agoraphobia, anxiety, or hyperventilation should be considered. Anxiety is also an important component of the status of the patient at the time of clinical examination, and should be differentiated from other conditions in which it is the primary cause of dizziness. A proportion of vestibular patients express fear and/or clinical psychological distress that are different than those of patients with psychological dizziness.[3] A brief hyperventilation test may be most helpful to direct the history to the cause of psychological stress (Box 6–1).

Nystagmus

Nystagmus can be defined as nonvoluntary rhythmic oscillation of the eyes. It usually has clearly defined fast and slow components beating in opposite directions. Figure 6–2 shows diagrammatically the various components of typical horizontal nystagmus. By convention, the direction of the fast component defines the direction of nystagmus.

CLASSIFICATION OF NYSTAGMUS

Physiological nystagmus can be induced with natural or experimental stimuli in normal subjects; pathological nystagmus can appear with or without external stimulation in patients with vestibular disorders. Physiological nystagmus is produced by vestibular (caloric, rotatory or linear acceleration) or visual (optokinetic) stimulation,

---

BOX 6–1 **Differential Characteristics of Dizziness in Peripheral Vestibular Disorders**

Sensation

Illusion of translational or rotatory motion

Intensity

Disabling; minutes, hours

Duration

Seconds or days, but in declining intensity

Frequency

Episodic

Precipitating Factors

Head movements with angular accelerations, loud sounds, changes in middle ear pressure

Associated Symptoms

Hearing loss, tinnitus, earaches, fear

---

or it can occur on extreme lateral gaze (end-point nystagmus). The characteristics (direction, intensity, shape) of pathological nystagmus and the method used to induce it often offer clues to the underlying pathology. Pathological nystagmus can be spontaneous (present with head erect and gaze centered), positional (induced by change in head position), or gaze-evoked (induced by change in eye position or congenital).

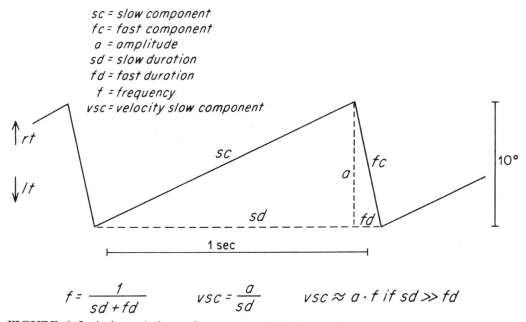

$$f = \frac{1}{sd + fd} \qquad vsc = \frac{a}{sd} \qquad vsc \approx a \cdot f \text{ if } sd \gg fd$$

FIGURE 6–2. A theoretic beat of nystagmus, indicating major components and their approximated values. (From Baloh, RW, and Honrubia, V: Clinical Neurophysiology of the Vestibular System, ed. 2. FA Davis, Philadelphia, 1990, p 132, with permission.)

BOX 6–2   Types of Nystagmus

Physiologic
- Rotational-induced
- Caloric-induced
- Optokinetic
- End-point

Pathologic
- Spontaneous
- Gaze-evoked
- Positional
- Congenital

It can be affected by interference with fixation (darkness, use of special lenses) and gaze position (e.g., congenital) (Box 6–2; Fig. 6–3). The causes of pathological nystagmus can be lesions of the peripheral or central vestibular system as well as lesions of other CNS pathways (e.g., medial longitudinal fascicles) involved in the control of eye movements, or it can be visual-ocular in origin (congenital). The nystagmus characteristics (amplitude, frequency, shape) and the combined effects on nystagmus of vision (or its absence), position of the head, and direction of gaze are helpful in elucidating its origin.[1]

METHODS OF CLINICAL EXAMINATION OF PATHOLOGICAL NYSTAGMUS

The search for pathological nystagmus can be accomplished during clinical examination of the patient, and should always be part of the laboratory evaluation of vestibular function. The clinical examination search for pathological nystagmus should include a systematic study of the eye during changes in (1) fixation, (2) eye position, and (3) head position. In addition, a "fistula" test should be conducted to determine the possibility of inducing nystagmus associated with slow pressure variation in the external ear canal.

The control of *fixation* during physical examination is accomplished with Frenzel glasses, which consist of +30 lenses mounted in a frame. A battery-powered internal light or an external flashlight held by the examiner enables observation of the patient's eyes. Examination with Frenzel glasses in a darkened room is easier to accomplish and prevents the patient from fixating (at least partially) through the lenses on lighted objects. Clinical examination without the ability to control fixation is of very little help in determining differential diagnosis. Recently, the availability of small infrared cameras has been making it possible to obtain video images of the eye for a clinical examination of nystagmus, which is most helpful.

The effect of changes in *eye position* is evaluated by having the patient fixate on a target 30° to the right, left, up, and down from center. Because horizontal eye deviation beyond 40° may result in low-amplitude, high-frequency torsional nystagmus in normal subjects (end-point nystagmus), extreme eye positions should be avoided. Each eye position is held for at least 20 seconds and should be repeated at least once. First-degree nystagmus refers to nystagmus present only on gaze in the direction of the fast

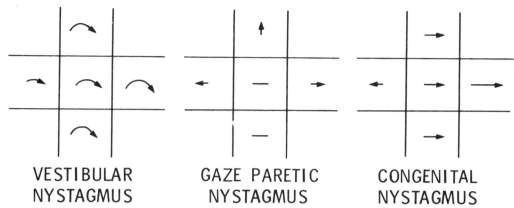

FIGURE 6–3. Method for describing the effect of eye position on nystagmus amplitude and direction. Arrows indicate direction of nystagmus (direction of fast eye component) and its relative magnitude in each of five primary eye positions. (From Baloh, RW, and Honrubia, V: Clinical Neurophysiology of the Vestibular System. FA Davis, Philadelphia, 1979, p 109, with permission.)

component. Second-degree nystagmus is present in the midposition, and third-degree nystagmus is present even on gaze in the direction opposite to the fast component. These terms, however, are not applicable to all varieties of nystagmus and, therefore, can lead to confusion. A simple description can be summarized with a box diagram as illustrated in Figure 6–3. The size, shape, and direction of the arrow provide information about the amplitude and direction of the fast component of nystagmus in the five primary eye positions.

The effect of *head position* is evaluated with two types of positional testing—slow and rapid. First, the patient is slowly placed into supine, right lateral, and left lateral positions. The nystagmus is observed for 20 to 60 seconds as the patient looks straight ahead. Rapid positional changes are used to induce paroxysmal positional nystagmus, which, owing to the moving maneuver, should not be confused with the physiological nystagmus. Both tests can be conducted with fixation and, using Frenzel glasses or infrared video cameras, without fixation. The ability to inhibit nystagmus with fixation on center or lateral gaze is essential information during the search for nystagmus.

The *fistula test* is easily performed during otoscopic examination with the aid of a pneumatic otoscope. After a speculum that tightly fits the canal is selected, pressure is applied (approximately 200 to 300 cc H_2O) while the tympanic membrane and the skin of the auditory meatus are observed to verify the effect of successive periodic pressure variations of about 2- to 3-second cycles. In our clinic, a Siegle speculum is mounted on the regular otoscope by means of an adapter. Tympanic membrane motion and changes in the external canal skin color owing to interference with blood flow are good indications of the use of adequate pressure. Corroboration of tympanic membrane motion with an otological microscope is preferred. It is helpful to have an assistant observe the eyes, which are behind Frenzel glasses, to prevent fixation while the physician executes the test; the patient should be asked to describe any unusual sensations, mainly the illusion of motion, during the test. The resulting eye movement is not necessarily a burst of nystagmus; it can be a back-and-forth motion related to the pressure variation, and it can be in either the horizontal or vertical plane. If the test is positive, the nystagmus should be documented with electronystagmographic recordings at a later time.

CLINICAL EXAMINATION OF VISUAL-OCULAR MOTOR FUNCTION

Together with the vestibular system, the visual system provides information about the perception of object motion in relation to self as well as the relative motion between objects and subjects. The visual system's contribution to gaze maintenance depends on two ocular stabilizing systems, the saccadic and the smooth-pursuit systems. The *saccadic system* produces ballistic movement of the eye to bring a peripheral visual object to the fovea in the shortest possible time. The intrinsic stimulus is a position error. The *smooth-pursuit system* maintains gaze on a moving target by generating a continuous tracking motion. The intrinsic stimulus is the object velocity. The smooth-pursuit system has two subsystems: the cortical smooth-pursuit system, which depends on foveal function, and the optokinetic system, which depends on the retinal periphery. Objective and quantitative evaluation of these systems can be easily obtained as part of the vestibular laboratory evaluation. However, gross evaluation can be made in the clinic or at the bedside by asking the subject to execute eye movements that are appropriate for testing either the saccade or tracking systems, or, with the aid of a patterned cloth, the optokinetic system. For saccades the examiner places the index finger of each hand about 40° from center and asks the subject with head at rest to fixate on command on either the left or the right index and wait for several (3 to 10) seconds before repeating the test. For smooth pursuit testing the subject is asked to follow the index finger of one hand in a 30° to 40° arc for 2 to 3 seconds in each direction—left, right, up, and down. Because of the similarities between smooth-pursuit and optokinetic system findings in patients, the latter may be postponed for the laboratory's vestibular evaluation tests. These visual oculomotor tests are normal for patients with peripheral lesions, except for the influence of spontaneous nystagmus, if present. Tests can be undirectionally or bidirectionally abnormal on CNS lesions involving a variety of locations, as will be shown later.[1]

Recording Pathological Nystagmus

In addition to clinical observations, the recording and quantitative measurements of nystagmus form the ideal basis of many vestibular tests and provide objective documentation of vestibular function. The search for nystagmus in the laboratory is made with the aid of electro-oculography, which is the simplest and most readily available method for recording many eye movements.[4,5] With this technique, a voltage surrounding the orbit, whose magnitude is proportional to the amplitude of eye movement, is measured. When used for evaluating vestibular function, the technique has also been termed electronystagmography (ENG).[6,7] ENG provides a permanent record for comparison with eye movement and nystagmus findings from other patients. Because of the transient nature of many types of nystagmus, a permanent record is invaluable.

A systematic search for pathological nystagmus should be conducted during ENG examination. Recording with eyes closed or open in darkness is more effective than the use of Frenzel glasses for identifying spontaneous and positional nystagmus of peripheral origin. Even with the use of Frenzel glasses to prevent fixation, patients can inhibit spontaneous nystagmus by converging on the light inside the lenses or on other unexpected references. Approximately 20 percent of normal subjects have spontaneous nystagmus and as many as 75 percent have positional nystagmus when tested with eyes closed or with eyes open in darkness.[8,9] Apparently, in many otherwise normal individuals, the vestibular system alone is unable to stabilize the position of the eyes when visual signals are removed. In our clinic, if the average slow component velocity of spontaneous or positional nystagmus exceeds 4° per second, it is considered a sign of vestibular impairment.[9,10]

THE PRINCIPLE OF ELECTRONYSTAGMOGRAPHY

The principle of ENG is illustrated in Figure 6–4. A potential difference exists between the cornea and the retina, oriented in the direction of the long axis of the eye. In relation to an indifferent remotely located electrode, an electrode placed in the vicinity of the eye becomes more positive when the eye rotates toward it and less positive when the eye rotates in the opposite direction. Recordings are usually made with a three-electrode system, using differential amplifiers. Two of the electrodes (active) are placed on each side of the eye and the reference electrode (ground) in a remote location (e.g., on the forehead). The difference in potential between the active electrodes is am-

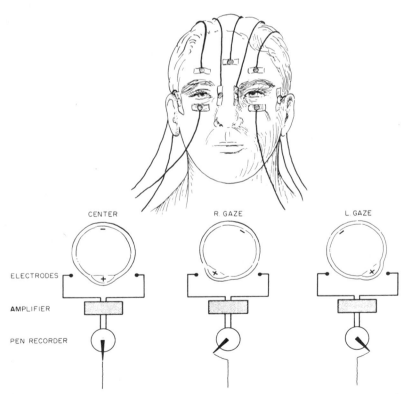

FIGURE 6–4. Recording of eye movements with ENG. See text for details. (From Baloh, RW, and Honrubia, V: Clinical Neurophysiology of the Vestibular System, ed 2. FA Davis, Philadelphia, 1990, p 131, with permission.)

plified and used to produce a permanent record with the aid of a polygraph or similar device.

With properly designed amplification, ENG can consistently record eye rotation of 0.5°, although one occasionally encounters patients (particularly elderly patients) with a high noise-to-signal ratio, limiting the sensitivity from 1° to 2°. Even at its best, the sensitivity of ENG is less than that of direct visual inspection (approximately 0.1°) and therefore visual search for small amplitude eye movements (i.e., gaze-evoked vertical nystagmus) remains an important part of the examination.

ELECTRODE PLACEMENT

Because of the genesis of the corneoretinal potential, ENG can monitor horizontal and/or vertical eye movements. Unfortunately, vertically aligned electrodes sense the voltage changes associated with both the lid movement, as well as the modification of the vertical corneoretinal potential produced by the closure of the eye during blinking or changes in lid position.[11] Thus, ENG is not suitable for quantitative analysis of vertical eye movements, for which purpose other methods must be used. Alternatively, vertical ENG recordings are useful in recognizing the existence of eye blinks, which can affect the characteristics of horizontally recorded eye movements.

INTERPRETING THE RECORDING

By convention, for horizontal recordings, the voltage changes produced by eye movements to the right are displayed in a moving chart recorder (e.g., 1 mm per second) so that they produce upward pen deflections and those to the left produce downward pen deflections. For vertical recordings, upward and downward eye movements are made to produce upward and downward deflections, respectively. To interpret ENG recordings, a standard angle of eye deviation is represented by a known amplitude of pen deflection associated with the recorded change in ENG voltage. To calibrate ENG, the patient is asked to look at a series of dots or lights 10° to 15° on each side of, and above and below, a reference central fixation point. The calibration should be performed frequently because the magnitude of the corneoretinal potential is affected by ambient light and changes in skin resistance. Once calibration is established, the precise value of various nystagmus parameters, such as amplitude, duration, and velocity of recorded eye movements, can be easily calculated. The relationship between components of a typical beat of nystagmus is illustrated in Figure 6–2. Scale values chosen for duration and amplitude are those commonly seen with vestibular nystagmus recorded in the dark. The fast component of the illustrated nystagmus moves to the left, so by convention the direction assigned to this nystagmus is the left. A 10° fast component would have an average velocity of approximately 100° per second. The slow component velocity is usually much slower, in this case, 10° per second. It is approximately the product of amplitude and frequency, as long as the fast duration is small compared to the slow duration. Although the magnitude of each nystagmus measurement, as shown in Figure 6–2, can be calculated directly from the polygraph recording, such a procedure is very tedious and time consuming, and therefore subject to error. Computers are ideally suited for making such measurements. After analog-to-digital conversion of the data, a computer, using a programmed algorithm, can measure the point-by-point position and velocity of the eye, or can calculate the amplitude, duration and velocity of each of the slow and fast components.[2,12,13] Plots of the nystagmus slow component velocity versus time are particularly useful for quantifying the magnitude of induced nystagmus (as will be shown later).

Characteristics of Different Types of Pathological Nystagmus

SPONTANEOUS NYSTAGMUS

Spontaneous nystagmus results from an imbalance of neural signals arriving at the oculomotor neurons. Because the vestibular system is a main source of tonic and phasic neural inputs to the oculomotor neurons, it is the driving force of most types of spontaneous nystagmus (tonic signals arising in the smooth-pursuit and optokinetic systems may also play a role, particularly with congenital nystagmus).[14,15] Vestibular imbalance produces a constant drift of the eyes in one direction interrupted by fast components in the opposite direction. If the imbalance results from a peripheral vestibular lesion, the pursuit system can be used to cancel it. In the light the spontaneous nystagmus activates the smooth-pursuit system owing to the slip of images in the retina. If it results from a central vestibular lesion, the pursuit system cannot suppress it because visual signals share some of the pathways of the vestibular signals in the vestibular nuclei.

PERIPHERAL SPONTANEOUS NYSTAGMUS

Lesions of the peripheral vestibular system (labyrinth or eighth nerve) typically interrupt or diminish tonic afferent signals originating from all of the receptors of one labyrinth, so that the resulting peripheral vestibular spontaneous nystagmus has combined horizontal and minor vertical or torsional components. The horizontal component dominates, suggesting that the tonic activities from the intact vertical canals and otolith partially cancel one another. The fast component is directed to the healthy ear, and gaze deviation in the direction of the fast component increases frequency and velocity, whereas gaze in the opposite direction has the reverse effect (Alexander's law). As noted above, peripheral spontaneous nystagmus is strongly inhibited by fixation. Unless the patient is seen within a few days of the acute episode, spontaneous nystagmus will not be present when fixation is permitted (Fig. 6–5), even when gaze is deviated in the direction of the fast component. On the other hand, when the slow component of spontaneous nystagmus is greater than 20° to 40° per second, it is difficult to demonstrate any effect on the peripheral spontaneous nystagmus with any of the maneuvers. In addition, patient cooperation may be lacking because of the severity of symptoms.

CONGENITAL NYSTAGMUS

One type of spontaneous nystagmus is congenital nystagmus, which is almost always highly dependent on fixation, disappearing or decreasing with loss of fixation.[16] The nystagmus waveform is variably triangular, or with small humps. In some instances, a slow nystagmus in the reverse direction is recorded with eyes closed. One common variety, so-called latent congenital nystagmus, occurs only when either eye is

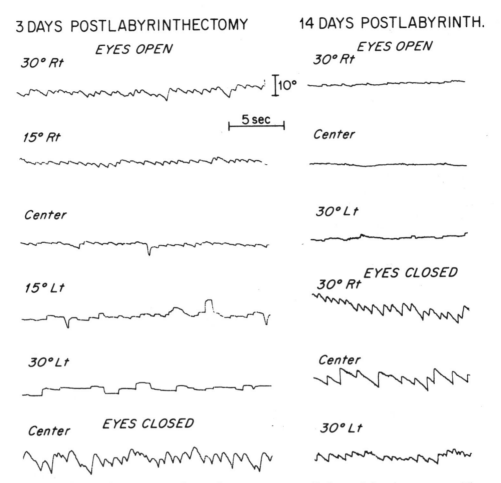

FIGURE 6–5. Sample ENG recordings of spontaneous vestibular peripheral nystagmus. The various record sequences illustrate the effect of gaze, vision, and compensation.

covered, permitting monocular fixation. The resulting nystagmus beats toward the fixating eye. The frequency of congenital nystagmus is usually greater than 2 beats per second and at times reaches 5 to 6 beats per second. Such a high frequency is unusual in other types of nystagmus. Of course, most patients are aware that the nystagmus has been present since infancy. There is a position of gaze where the nystagmus is minimal and patients tend to turn the head to look in front with the eyes deviated at the most neutral orbital position.

Another form of spontaneous nystagmus is periodic alternating nystagmus (PAN), which changes direction periodically without a change in eye or head position.[17] Cycle length varies between 1 and 6 minutes, with null periods between each half-cycle varying from 2 to 20 seconds. The nystagmus slowly builds in intensity, reaching a peak slow component velocity near the center of each half-cycle before slowly decreasing. PAN has been reported to be a congenital disorder, but has also been found in association with such varied conditions as encephalitis, brainstem ischemia, demyelinating disease, syringobulbia, syphilis, and trauma.[17,18]

CENTRAL SPONTANEOUS NYSTAGMUS

Central spontaneous nystagmus is as prominent with as without fixation, as opposed to peripheral spontaneous nystagmus. It may be purely vertical, horizontal, or torsional, or have some combination of torsional and linear components. As with peripheral spontaneous nystagmus, gaze in the direction of the fast component usually increases nystagmus frequency, but, unlike peripheral spontaneous nystagmus, gaze away from the direction of the fast component often changes the direction of nystagmus. In this case, there is a null region several degrees off center in the direction opposite to that of the fast component where nystagmus is minimal or absent. Gaze beyond this null region results in reversal of nystagmus direction.

Lesions involving the vestibular nuclear region can produce horizontal torsional nystagmus similar to that seen with peripheral lesions, but unlike the latter, the direction of nystagmus does not reliably indicate the side where the lesion is located, and the nystagmus persists with fixation owing to damage of visual vestibular interaction pathways.[19] Vertical nystagmus is of central origin and can have different presentations. Spontaneous vertical downbeat nystagmus may result from cerebellar atrophy, vertebrobasilar ischemia, multiple sclerosis, or Arnold-Chiari malformation.[20,21] Spontaneous upbeat nystagmus usually results from lesions of the dorsal central medulla in the region of the medial vestibular and propositus hypoglossi nuclei.[20,22] Common causes include infarction, infiltrating tumors, and multiple sclerosis. Pure torsional spontaneous nystagmus is frequently associated with syringomyelia and syringobulbia. High-frequency, small-amplitude pendular spontaneous nystagmus commonly occurs in the late stages of multiple sclerosis.[23] This pendular nystagmus converts to a sawtooth pattern on lateral gaze to either side.

GAZE-EVOKED NYSTAGMUS

Patients with gaze-evoked nystagmus are unable to maintain stable, conjugated eye deviation away from the primary position. The eyes drift back toward the center with an exponentially decreasing waveform; corrective saccades (fast components) constantly reset the desire gaze position. Gaze-evoked nystagmus is therefore always in the direction of gaze. The site of abnormality can be anywhere from the neuromuscular junction to the multiple brain centers controlling conjugated gaze. Dysfunction of the so-called oculomotor integrator may be a common mechanism causing several types of gaze-evoked nystagmus.[14]

Symmetric gaze-evoked nystagmus (equal amplitude to the left and right) is most commonly produced by ingestion of drugs such as phenobarbital, phenytoin, diazepam, and alcohol. Symmetric gaze-evoked nystagmus can occur in patients with myasthenia gravis, advanced multiple sclerosis, and cerebellar atrophy.

Asymmetric horizontal gaze-evoked nystagmus always indicates a structural brain lesion. When it is caused by a focal lesion of the brainstem or cerebellum, the larger-amplitude nystagmus is usually directed toward the side of the lesion.[24] Large cerebellopontine angle tumors commonly produce asymmetric gaze-evoked nystagmus from compression of the brain stem and cerebellum (Bruns' nystagmus). Some patients with large acoustic neuromas develop a combination of symmetric gaze-evoked nystagmus from brainstem compression, and peripheral spontaneous nystagmus from eighth nerve damage. Asymmetric gaze-evoked nystagmus may be present during the recovery from gaze paralysis (either cortical or subcortical in origin), in which case it is large in amplitude, low in frequency, present in only one direction of gaze (the direction of the previous gaze paralysis).[24]

A special type of gaze nystagmus is rebound nystagmus. When the eyes return to the primary position, a burst of nystagmus occurs in the direction of the return saccade. Rebound nystagmus occurs in patients with cerebellar atrophy and focal structural lesions of the cerebellum; it is the only variety of nystagmus thought to be specific for cerebellar involvement.[25]

Lesions of the medial longitudinal fasciculus (MLF), so-called internuclear ophthalmoplegia, produces dissociated or disconjugated gaze-evoked nystagmus. With early MLF lesions the eyes appear to move conjugatedly, but the abducting eye on the side opposite the MLF lesion develops regular, small-amplitude, high-frequency nystagmus in the direction of gaze. With more extensive MLF lesions, the abducting eye fast component develops large-amplitude nystagmus that has a characteristic "peaked waveform."[26] MLF nystagmus can be bilateral or unilateral, depending on the extent of MLF involvement. Bilateral MLF nystagmus is most commonly seen with demyelinating disease, whereas unilateral MLF nystagmus most often accompanies vascular disease of the brainstem.[27] Patients with myasthenia gravis develop dissociated gaze-evoked nystagmus, similar to MLF nystagmus (pseudo-MLF nystagmus), because of unequal impairment of neuromuscular transmission in adducting and abducting muscles. Unlike MLF nystagmus, the dissociated nystagmus with myasthenia gravis progressively increases in amplitude as gaze position is maintained.[28]

POSITIONAL NYSTAGMUS

Position-induced static nystagmus has been attributed to lesions of the otoliths and their connections in the vestibular nuclei and cerebellum, because these are the receptors that are sensitive to change in the direction of gravity.[29-31] Recently, other mechanisms for the production of positional nystagmus have been proposed, forcing reexamination of traditional concepts. If the semicircular canal endolymph or cupula were altered so that their specific gravity no longer equaled that of the surrounding endolymph, the organ would become sensitive to changes in the direction of gravity and would produce positional nystagmus.

Traditional classifications of positional nystagmus are often confusing and can be difficult to apply in clinical practice. Some classifications have been based on clinical observations obtained while the patient is fixating, whereas others have been based on ENG recordings with eyes closed or with eyes open in darkness. Some investigators use slow positioning maneuvers; others employ only rapid positioning. These different methods make it difficult to compare classifications. Nylen[31] initially described three types of positional nystagmus based on visual inspection of nystagmus direction and regularity. Type I, direction-changing, and type II, direction-fixed, remained constant as long as the position was maintained. Type III was less clearly defined, comprising all paroxysmal varieties of positional nystagmus and some persistent varieties that did not fit into types I and II. Numerous modifications of Nylen's original classifications have subsequently been proposed, and the definition of each type has changed.

Most investigators do agree that two general categories of positional nystagmus can be identified: paroxysmal and static.

PAROXYSMAL POSITIONAL NYSTAGMUS

Paroxysmal positional nystagmus is induced by a rapid change from erect torso and head while sitting, to a supine head-hanging-left, -center, or -right position, the so called Dix-Hallpike maneuver (Fig. 6–6).[32] The provocative movement is in the plane of the posterior semicircular canal of the ear on the lower side of the head. Schuknecht[33] proposed that benign paroxysmal positional nystagmus is caused by a lesion in the posterior semicircular canal resulting in the formation of a precipitate in the cupula of density greater than that of the surrounding fluid. It is a common sequela of head concussion, viral labyrinthitis, and occlusion of the vasculature of the inner ear.

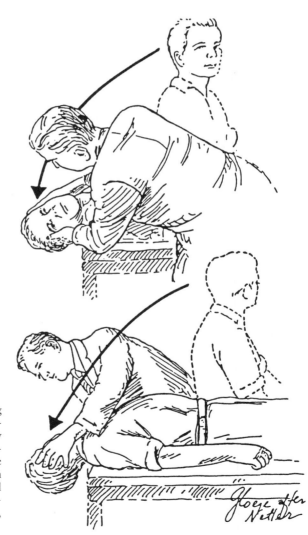

FIGURE 6–6. Technique for inducing paroxysmal positional nystagmus (Hall-pike maneuver). Patient is taken rapidly from the sitting to head-hanging position. Note that head is turned 45° to the side of the examiner for each test. (From Baloh, RW, and Honrubia, V: Clinical Neurophysiology of the Vestibular System, ed 2. FA Davis, Philadelphia, 1990, p 124, with permission.)

In the majority of cases, however, it occurs as an isolated sign. The nystagmus response is consistent with the contraction of the primary muscles innervated by the posterior semicircular canal (PSC), the ipsilateral superior oblique, and the contralateral inferior rectus (Fig. 6–7).

A significant observation was made by Parnes that impacted the understanding of the pathophysiology of the disease. At the time of fenestration surgery of the PSC for the purpose of occluding the membranous endolymphatic canal to prevent stimulation of its cristae by endolymph motion, free-moving particles were seen inside the endolymphatic space resting on the lower arch of the canal. The condition is now believed to represent a PSC organ fluid disorder owing to the presence of otoliths detached from the maculae that enter the ductus reuniens, driven by gravity toward the ampulla where they become trapped by the cupula shielding the ampulla.[34-36] Once the otoliths reach a critical mass, they affect the physiological fluid motion and create intense abnormal stimulation during the Dix-Hallpike tests. Parnes' "live" observation led to the design of a new treatment modality, namely, the canal repositioning procedure (CRP), also known as the Epley Maneuver, designed to remove the loose calcium carbonate particles from their location in the canal toward the vestibule.[37] The affected

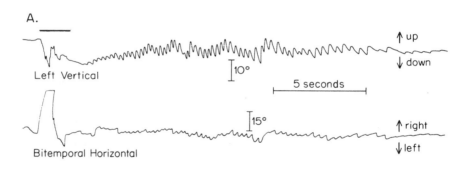

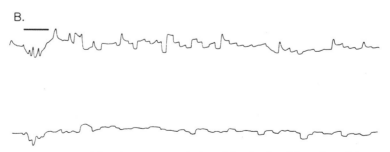

FIGURE 6–7. Benign positional nystagmus induced in the head-hanging-right position (vertical monocular and horizontal temporal recording). (*A*) Sitting to head-hanging. (*B*) Head-hanging to sitting. Solid bar indicates duration of rapid positioning maneuver. (From Baloh, RW, Honrubia, V, and Jacobson, K: Benign positional vertigo: Clinical and oculographic features in 240 cases. Neurology 37:137, 1987, with permission.)

TABLE 6–1 Characteristics of Nystagmus

Organ	PSC-Can	ASC-Can	HSC-Can	HSC-Cup
Stimulus: angular acceleration and gravity	Synergistic	Antagonistic	Synergistic	Antagonistic
Duration	Paroxysmal	Paroxysmal	Paroxysmal	Continuous
Stimulated muscles	SO ipsilateral IR contralateral	IO ipsilateral SR contralateral	MR ipsilateral LR contralateral	MR ipsilateral LR contralateral
Eye movement	Dissociated	Dissociated	Conjugated	Conjugated
Direction of fast-component ipsilateral eye	Outtorsional Up/adduction	Intorsional Down/adduction	Horizontal Geotropic	Antigeotropic
contralateral eye	Up/adduction	Outtorsional Down	Horizontal Geotropic	Horizontal Antigeotropic
Delayed	Yes	Yes	Yes	No
Treatment	Epley	Reverse Epley	Rotation to healthy ear	Rotation to healthy ear

Abbreviations: PSC-Can, posterior semicircular canal-canalithiasis; ASC-Can, anterior semicircular canal-canalithiasis; HSC-Can, horizontal semicircular canal-canalithiasis; HSC-Cup, horizontal semicircular canal-cupulolithiasis; SO, superior oblique; IO, inferior oblique; MR, medial rectus; IR, inferior rectus; SR, superior rectus; LR, lateral rectus.

canals are slowly rotated, changing the direction of the gravitational vector inside the endolymphatic canal to inertially draw the otoliths in an ampullofugal direction toward the utricle and away from the cupula itself.

More recently it has been proposed that other semicircular canals can be affected, not only the PSC. The unique situation created by the presence of otoliths inside the canals leads to the production of vertigo with distinctive characteristics, depending on the organ affected. Because the primary neural excitatory connectivity of each canal with two extraocular muscles is well known, it is possible to identify the site of pathology from the analysis of the induced eye movements.[38–40]

Furthermore, two different pathophysiological mechanisms have been proposed to account for diverse clinical presentations. For example, following the Dix-Hallpike type stimulation of the horizontal semicircular canal (HSC), two varieties of abnormal eye movements have been demonstrated that are consistent with the presence of otoliths in the endolymphatic lumen of the canal (HSC-canalithiasis; HSC-Can), or with deposits of particles in the cupula itself (HSC-cupulothiasis; HSC-Cup).[41] Also, following the Dix-Hallpike maneuver for the ipsilateral PSC, in a smaller percentage of patients the eye movements were consistent with activation of the contralateral anterior semicircular canal (ASC). Furthermore, occasionally more than one organ might be involved.[37,41–46]

The pertinent epidemiologic characteristics of the 290 patients recently studied by Honrubia et al[47,48] are summarized in Tables 6–1 and 6–2. The majority of patients (93 percent) presented with eye movement responses corresponding to canalithiasis of the PSC (PSC-Can). Movement of the head during the downward Dix-Hallpike test produced immediate ampullofugal motion of the fluid of the PSC, as well as a delayed synergistic mobilization of the particles due to the effect of changes of the gravity vector in the canal (Fig. 6–8, top left). Of these, 85 percent were unilateral and 8 percent bilateral. The characteristics of the eye movements of these patients suggest that the condition is consistent with excitatory stimulation of the PSC resulting in contraction of the ipsilateral superior oblique and the contralateral inferior rectus muscles. The action of these muscles cause the ipsilateral eye to move with large inward torsional (eye upper pole motion toward the nose) and smaller downward and abduction trajectories.[47–49] The contralateral eye trajectory is clearly downward, and has a minor outtorsional adduction motion (see Fig. 6–7, bottom). The resulting nystagmus fast component in the ipsilateral eye has an outtorsional and small upward direction, and a

TABLE 6–2 CRP Treatment Results

Diagnosis	Patients (*n*)	Positive Canal Repositioning Procedure	Percentage
Posterior semicircular canal-canalithiasis unilateral	250	221	88
Posterior semicircular canal-canalithiasis bilateral	23	16	69
Horizontal semicircular canal-canalithiasis	9	3	33
Horizontal semicircular canal-cupulolithiasis	6	3	50
Anterior semicircular canal-canalithiasis	4	2	50
Totals	292	245	84

PSC-Can

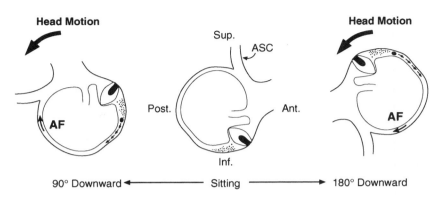

PSC-Can (Rt)

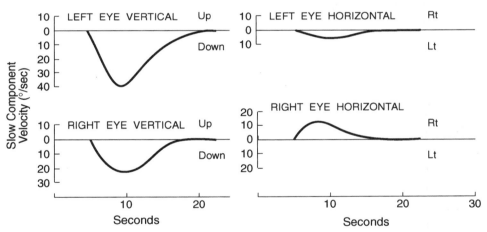

FIGURE 6–8. *Top:* Theoretical mechanisms of abnormal crista stimulation of the posterior semicircular canal. Canalith particles are driven by both angular acceleration and gravity in the ampullofugal direction during backward head rotation, as in the Fitzgerald-Hallpike right-side-down test. *Bottom:* Traces of typical eye velocity of the nystagmus slow component resulting from the excitatory (ampullofugal) stimulation of the right posterior semicircular canal. Note the significant delay of the response to the physical stimulation and the dissociated eye movements.

horizontal (toward the nose) component. The fast component of the contralateral eye has a predominant upward motion (see Table 6–1).

Other canal presentations found in this study include four patients with ASC of the canalithiasis variety (ASC-Can), not described earlier. This canal's cupula is physiologically inhibited; that is, ampullopetally deviated during the downward Dix-Hallpike test for excitatory stimulation of the contralateral PSC. As the head continues to be rotated backward by more than 90°, the particles are displaced by gravity in a direction opposite to the force associated with the head angular acceleration, producing

ASC-Can

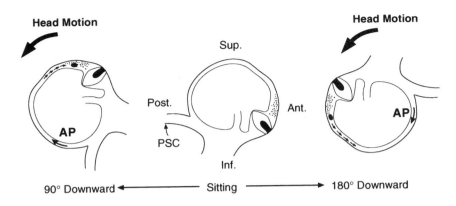

ASC-Can (Lt)

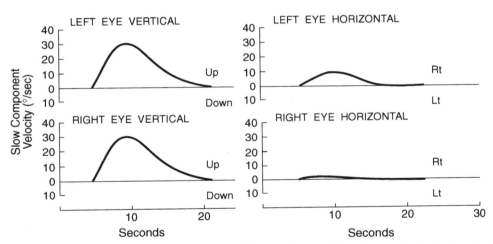

FIGURE 6–9. *Top:* Theoretical mechanisms of the anterior semicircular canal stimulation during the same head rotation as Figure 6–8. *Bottom:* Traces of typical eye velocity of the nystagmus slow component resulting from "excitatory" ampullofugal canal stimulation of the left anterior semicircular canal. Note that gravity is the force that drives the displacement of the canalith particles.

excitatory ampullofugal stimulation of the crista as shown in Figure 6–9 (top left). The reflex response produces a compensatory contraction of the ipsilateral inferior oblique and the contralateral superior rectus muscles resulting in eye movements opposite to the ones induced by stimulation of the PSC-Can in the ear downside condition. The fast component nystagmus in the ipsilateral eye is intorsional, down, and has a smaller inward component, whereas the contralateral eye is outtorsional and mainly down (see Table 6–1). The nystagmus usually has a 3 to 10 second latency and rarely lasts more than 30 seconds. The direction of the nystagmus reverses when the patient moves back to the sitting position (see Fig. 6–11).

HSC-Can

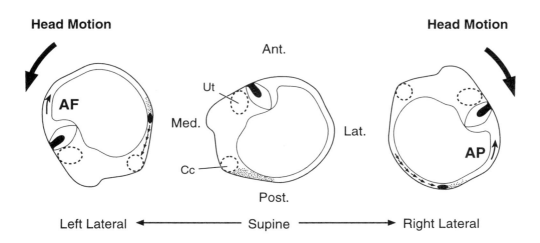

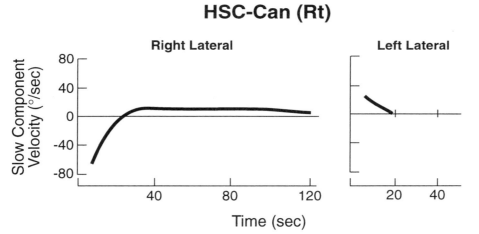

FIGURE 6–10. *Top:* Theoretical mechanism of abnormal crista stimulation of the right horizontal semicircular canal crista during head rotation in the plane of the canal toward the right and left as indicated below, on the left and right sides, respectively. *Bottom:* Traces of typical eye velocity of the nystagmus slow component resulting from right crista excitatory ampullopetal stimulation (*right*) and of inhibitory ampullofugal stimulation (*left*). Note that angular acceleration and gravity forces act synergistically to drive the canalith particles.

A group of patients (*n* = 15 or 5 percent) presented with HSC dysfunction, all unilateral. The provoking maneuver consisted of rotating the head around the cephaloacaudal axis while the patient was in a supine position. Nine patients corresponded to the HSC-Can and six to the HSC-Cup varieties. The induced eye movements in these patients, under visual inspection or when recorded with ENG, were conjugated and pure horizontal. These findings are consistent with the vector of force produced by the synergistic contractions of the lateral rectii muscles on the contralateral eye and medial

HSC-Cup

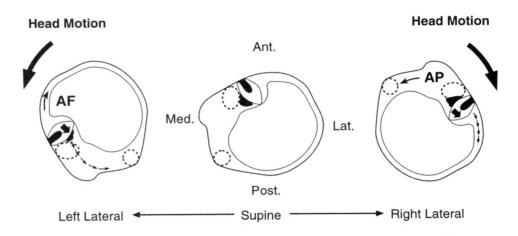

HSC-Cup (Rt)

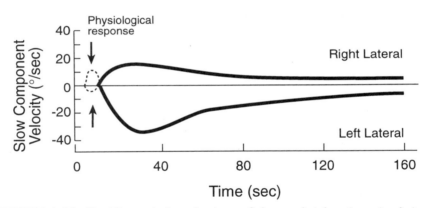

FIGURE 6–11. *Top:* Theoretical mechanisms of abnormal right crista stimulation in the case of true cupulolithiasis condition. During rotation to the right, particles loaded in the crista produce a deflection of the cupula in the direction opposite to that expected from the angular acceleration of the canal. *Bottom:* Traces of typical eye velocity of the nystagmus slow component resulting from motion to the right (ampullofugal stimulation, *top*) and to the left (ampullopetal stimulation, *bottom*). Note that the physiologic stimuli produces a physiologic brief instantaneous response in the direction opposite to the pathological response. The time course of the eye velocity suggests that the cupula deflection takes place with a rather long time constant, as during constant angular accelerations, and remains deflected, suggesting that the "load" must remain attached to the cupula.

rectii muscles in the ipsilateral eye. Of note is the opposite direction of the eye movement in the HSC-Can to that of the HSC-Cup group (Fig. 6–10 and Fig. 6–11). In patients with HSC-Can, the eye movements were qualitatively the same as during physiological stimulation of the end organ. When the affected canal was activated by the ampullopetal endolymph motion, induced by a sudden rotation to the side of lesion, the slow eye movements were compensatory toward the contralateral side and transient with the nystagmus fast component beating toward the ground (geotropic). Rotation to the opposite direction produced ampullofugal stimulation of the cupula slow component to the healthy side and therefore antigeotropic nystagmus. As expected from Ewald's law of vestibular function,[1] the magnitude of the ampullopetal reaction was greater than the ampullofugal. In these tests the angular acceleration force and gravity acted synergistically.

In HSC-Cup patients, the eye movements were consistent with the notion that they are due mainly to the effect of gravity on the cupula because they are in the direction opposite to that expected by the force associated with angular acceleration. Head rotation to the affected side produced ampullofugal inhibition, not excitation, of the crista, because of the weight of the otoliths resting over the cupula. In fact, the nystagmus can be produced without angular acceleration by slowly placing the head toward the affected side while the patient is in supine position. The postulated location of the otoliths is depicted in Figure 6–11 on the utricular side of the cupula, although the stimulatory effect will be similar whether the particles are attached to the cupula or resting in the utricular entrance of the canal. The resulting compensatory eye movements, consequently, are greater when the head is rotated toward the contralateral side. The fast component of the nystagmus is antigeotropic in the HSC-Cup group (see Table 6–2).

The results of the CRP treatments are summarized in Table 6–2. The great majority (88 percent) of PSC unilateral patients were relieved of their symptoms. The ASC-Can group experienced about 50 percent success. The HSC variety was less successfully treated: 33 percent of the HSC-Can and 50 percent of the HSC-Cup. The overall success rate for the 292 patients was 84 percent, but clearly more experience is necessary in the HSC and ASC varieties. The initial presentation of these patients was clear indication of the pandemic involvement of all the semicircular canal organs.

Benign paroxysmal positional nystagmus of different modalities is a reliable sign of vestibular end-organ disease. It can be the only finding in an otherwise healthy individual or it may be associated with other signs of peripheral vestibular damage, such as peripheral spontaneous nystagmus and unilateral caloric hypoexcitability.[50] In those instances of PSC-Can where abnormality is identified on caloric testing, nystagmus usually occurs when the patient is positioned with the damaged ear down.

Another type of paroxysmal positional nystagmus can also result from brainstem and cerebellar lesions.[51,52] Central paroxysmal positional nystagmus does not decrease in amplitude or duration with repeated positioning, does not have a clear latency, and usually lasts longer than 30 seconds.[53] The direction is unpredictable and may be different in each position. It is often purely vertical, with the fast components directed downward (i.e., toward the cheeks). The presence or absence of associated vertigo is not a reliable differential feature.

STATIC POSITIONAL NYSTAGMUS

When the position of the head in relationship to gravity is changed, nystagmus may be produced that remains as long as the position is held, although it may fluctuate in frequency and amplitude. It may be in the same direction in all positions or change directions in different positions. Not infrequently, patients with paroxysmal positional nystagmus will have static positional nystagmus after the paroxysmal positional nystagmus has disappeared. In the past, this category may have included patients with paroxysmal vertigo of the cupulolithiasis variety that was not recognized until recently. It is nevertheless accepted that the two types, direction changing and direction fixed static positional nystagmus, are most commonly associated with peripheral vestibular disorders, although both occur with central lesions.[10,54] Their presence indicates only a dysfunction in the vestibular system without localizing value. As with spontaneous nystagmus, however, lack of suppression with fixation and signs of associated brain stem dysfunction suggest a central lesion.

QUANTITATIVE VESTIBULAR OCULAR TESTS

Vestibular function, as indicated earlier, is a complex sensorimotor integration process that makes possible the perception of motion of objects relative to subjects (orientation) and the maintenance of balance. The vestibular evaluation includes both methods to obtain psychophysical information about the perception of motion and tests for evaluating motor function of the various vestibular dependent reflexes. Of these reflexes, the two that have received the most attention and are best understood are those involved in the maintenance of gaze and balance.

The maintenance of gaze is one of the most important functions of human orientation and a relatively simple one to measure. Vestibular and visual-dependent reflexes contribute to preserve gaze; those stemming from the inner ear, with its receptors for the perception of linear and angular acceleration constitute the vestibulo-ocular reflex (VOR) arc, and those from the visual system, with the three visual oculomotor systems—saccadic, smooth-pursuit, and optokinetic—comprise the visual ocular reflex. Hence, measurement of gaze following reflex stimulation is the ideal method to evaluate the function of these reflexes, and the study of vestibular disorders includes tests for their evaluation independently and during their interaction. For this purpose, a standardized "vestibular test battery" has been developed in the laboratories at the University of California, Los Angeles, to quantify functions of the various oculomotor systems in patients (Box 6–3).[1] It is also generally accepted for evaluation of normal function. The vestibular test battery takes advantage of the computerized ENG capability of quantifying the characteristics of the reflexes. It allows the differentiation of

---

BOX 6–3   UCLA ENG Test Battery

Recording for pathologic nystagmus
  Fixation at midposition
  Fixation inhibited with eyes open in darkness (constant mental alerting)
  Gaze held 30° right, left, up, and down
  Rapid and slow positional changes
Visual tracking tests
  Saccades: 5° to 40°; target can be a series of dots or lights
  Smooth pursuit: target velocity 20° to 40° per second
  Optokinetic nystagmus: stripe velocity 20° to 40° per second
  Optokinetic after nystagmus: lights turned off after 1 min, constant velocity
    optokinetic nystagmus in each direction
Bithermal caloric test
  30° C and 44° C water infused into each ear, eyes open in darkness, continuous mental
    alerting; allow at least 5 min between each
Physiological vestibular test
Vestibular-visual interaction test

pathology affecting peripheral vestibular end organs from that affecting vestibular pathways in the CNS, and that of patients with a wide range of disease processes at different locations in the visual oculomotor system. In many cases, the tests make it possible to identify the precise location of the lesion.

One benefit derived from the distributed nature of the reflexes is the opportunity to obtain information about pathological changes in a large extent of the brain that includes the eye, visual sensory pathways, efferent visual motor pathways in the parietal and frontal cortex, the midbrain, and cerebellum, as well as the operation of neurons in the inner ear, brainstem, and oculomotor nuclei and nerves (Fig. 6–12). The clinical

ANATOMICAL BASES OF FUNCTION AND LOCATION OF LESIONS

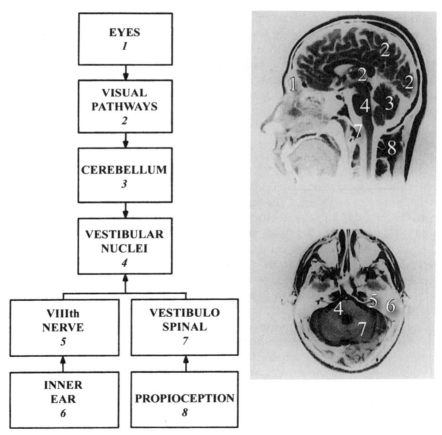

FIGURE 6–12. Reproduction of a human brain MRI to indicate the most frequent locations of lesions that affect vestibular patients (e.g., #1-8). Given the wide distribution of nerve pathways, vestibular tests allow the evaluation of the functional integrity of large segments of the central nervous system.

evaluation of these reflexes is accomplished using principles of physiology whereby the results of the reflex output are compared with normative values from the use of standard controlled stimuli. The selection of these stimuli is likewise based on physiological principles. Reports of measurement results are interpreted in the context of parametric information using concepts borrowed from the field of control theory and the implications of heuristic physiological models for description of various system reflex functions.[55,56]

Even the caloric tests, based on the use of an unnatural stimulus whose design and interpretation were of empirical nature, can now be interpreted in the context of physiological principles. For example, contemporary understanding of VOR function substantiates the hypothesis initially advanced by Henriksson[57] that the velocity of the slow component is the relevant vestibular parameter to evaluate the caloric test. The caloric test stimulates mainly the horizontal semicircular canals, and because the function of the horizontal canal ocular reflex is the production of eye movements to compensate for the horizontal angular rotation of the head, theoretically the caloric test results should be interpreted in physiological terms. Indeed, it has been shown that the magnitude of the reaction reflects sensitivity of the semicircular canals to a low-frequency physiological stimulus of a period twice the duration of the irrigation.[58] Thus it is possible to interpret the caloric responses in terms of physiological mechanisms when using the velocity of the slow component of the nystagmus. Measurements of the duration of the response or frequency of nystagmus have no direct physiological correspondence and are only of empirical value. Measurements of the cumulative amplitude of the nystagmus are equivalent to velocity measurements.[59] They have been relegated because computation of the eye velocity was easiest with the oldest electronic analysis of the ENG.

Tests of Visual-Ocular Control

Each of three major visual oculomotor systems contribute to the production of different types of eye movements. The saccadic system responds to an error in the direction of gaze with respect to the position of an object of interest in initiating a rapid eye movement—a saccade—to bring objects into the fovea in the shortest possible time. The reflex arc involves cortical centers as well as centers in the midbrain and brainstem. Saccades are stereotyped in that their trajectory and velocity cannot be voluntarily altered.[1,14,60]

The two other systems allow the eye to maintain gaze on moving objects. The smooth-pursuit system has rapid dynamics, depends primarily on foveal activation, and requires voluntary participation involving the cerebral cortex.[61] It is a negative feedback system that minimizes velocity difference between the eye and the object selected for fixation. It operates quite effectively to maintain objects within a visual angle even smaller than that of the fovea for object velocities below 90° per second. The optokinetic system has rather sluggish dynamics, depending mainly on activation of direction-sensitive neurons scattered through the retina. It produces involuntary, reflexive fixation eye movements—more effective with objects that cover large portions of the visual field and that move with velocities of less than 20° to 30° per second. Visually generated signals of the optokinetic system travel through short subcortical neural pathways—the accessory optic system—to reach the vestibular nuclei. Here they are integrated with afferent vestibular signals[2,61] to participate in the maintenance of gaze and equilibrium.

Central vestibulo-ocular connections are highly integrated with visual-ocular stabilizing pathways, and both systems share the final common pathway of oculomotor neurons. If the efferent limb of the VOR arc is damaged, visually and vestibularly controlled eye movements are abnormal, whereas if the vestibular afferent limb of the reflex is damaged, visually controlled eye movements are usually normal, but vestibular-dependent eye movements are abnormal.

Saccadic Eye Movements

METHODS OF TESTING AND RESULTS IN NORMAL SUBJECTS

Saccadic eye movements can be induced by asking the subject to fixate gaze on a series of dots or lights separated by specific angular distances, or on a dot or light moving on a neutral screen through a series of jumps of different amplitudes. Tests in our laboratory are conducted, on this part of the battery, with monocular recordings to independently document the ability of each eye to maintain gaze and produce conjugated eye movements. Recordings are made with DC preamplifiers, which have a sensitivity that makes possible the recognition of eye movements of less than 1° and do not require adjustments on the chart recorder trace for several minutes, thus allowing proper documentation of the ability of the eyes to maintain a steady position. Once the recording system proves to be operational and calibrated, the saccadic eye movement test is initiated.

The ENG recording in Figure 6–13A illustrates the high speed and accuracy of saccadic eye movements induced in a normal subject by a target moving in steps of random amplitude. Normal subjects consistently undershoot the target for jumps larger than 20°, requiring a small corrective saccade to achieve the final position.

Computer algorithms have been developed to rapidly quantify these saccade parameters.[13,62] Saccades are easily evaluated based on the characteristics relationship between peak velocity and amplitude (the so-called main sequence). This relationship is nonlinear, with larger but relatively decreasing peak velocities for higher amplitude saccades (Fig. 6–13B).[62] For example, the average peak velocity for a 15° saccade is 400° per second whereas that for a 30° saccade is only 550° per second. Saccade accuracy is defined as the ratio of the initial saccade amplitude to target displacement amplitude times 100. Mean saccade accuracy for normal subjects on the random saccade test is 88 percent. Overshooting of the target rarely occurs in normal subjects. The mean delay time on the same test is 0.180 of a second.

RESULTS IN PATIENTS

Slowing of saccadic eye movements can be caused by lesions anywhere in the widely scattered central pathways involved in their generation. The most pronounced slowing occurs with lesions of pretectal and paramedian pontine gaze centers, oculomotor neurons, and extraocular muscles. Lesions involving these pathways impair both voluntary and involuntary saccades. Damage to oculomotor neurons, oculomotor

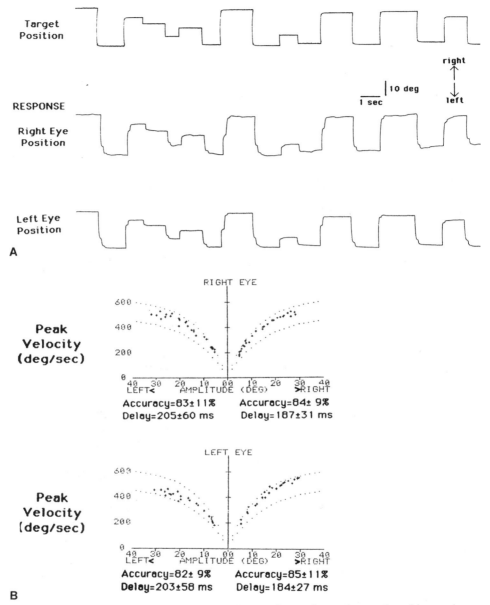

FIGURE 6–13. (*A*) Sample of monocular ENG recordings of saccades produced by random steps of target position in a normal subject. (*B*) Graphs showing the relationship between the saccade maximum velocity and its amplitude from the same subject.

nerves, and extraocular muscles causes slowing of saccades when the paretic muscle is the agonist required to generate the sudden force necessary to move the globe rapidly. In early lesions of the MLF, saccade slowing is identified on ENG testing,[63,64] before clinical examination reveals any abnormality in gaze (Fig. 6–14).[65,66] In myasthenia gravis, saccades begin with normal velocity, but within a short time the neurotransmit-

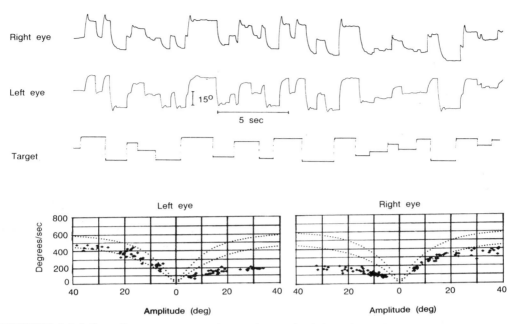

FIGURE 6–14. Saccadic eye movements in a patient with a bilateral MLF lesion caused by multiple sclerosis. Recordings as in Figure 6–13. Adducting saccades are markedly slow; abducting saccades have normal velocity but overshoot the target. (From Baloh, RW, and Honrubia, V: Clinical Neurophysiology of the Vestibular System, ed 2. FA Davis, Philadelphia, 1990, p 145, with permission.)

ters at the myoneural junction are depleted, and the remainder of the saccade is markedly slow.[67] Patients with Huntington's disease and progressive supranuclear palsy develop slowing saccades, apparently owing to diffuse degeneration of supranuclear pathways.[68,69] Lesions of one paramedian pontine center produce ipsilateral saccade slowing. Reversible saccade slowing is produced by fatigue or by ingestion of alcohol or tranquilizers.[70–72]

The accuracy of saccades is commonly impaired with cerebellar disorders.[72,73] Overshooting of the target (saccade overshoot dysmetria) is apparent; overshoots rarely occur in normal subjects. Saccade dysmetria is most prominent with Friedreich's ataxia.[74] Monocular overshoots in the abducting eye are characteristic of MLF lesions. Disorders of cortical and subcortical supranuclear centers also affect accuracy of saccades.[75,76] Patients with Parkinson's disease exhibit delayed saccade reaction time and hypometria of voluntary saccades.

Complete removal of one hemisphere or the presence of a large frontal parietal lesion results in hypometria of horizontal saccades in the contralateral direction.[77] Vertical saccades are unaffected. Impaired reaction time for initiation of voluntary saccades occurs in patients with acquired and congenital oculomotor apraxia[78] and ataxia telangiectasia.[79] Nystagmus fast components (involuntary saccades) are also abnormal, so that the eyes deviate in the direction of the slow component rather than in the direction of the fast component.

Smooth Pursuit

METHODS OF TESTING AND RESULTS IN NORMAL SUBJECT

Precise control of a visual target can be achieved over a series of velocities by projecting a dot on a screen with a motor-controlled device. Figure 6–15A is a reproduction of a polygraph recording of smooth pursuit in a normal subject who follows a sinusoidally moving dot on a white screen (0.2 Hz, maximum amplitude 18°). Accuracy of smooth pursuit is quantified by repeatedly sampling eye and target velocity and plotting the two values against each other (Fig. 6–15B) after saccade waveforms have been removed, if necessary by a computer algorithm.[12,13] The slope of this eye-target velocity relationship represents the gain of the smooth pursuit system. The mean gain determined from similar plots in 25 young normal subjects was 0.95 ± 0.7. Elderly normal subjects (more than 70 years of age) show marked variability in pursuit ability, and therefore pursuit testing must be interpreted with caution in elderly patients.[80,81] Also, smooth-pursuit

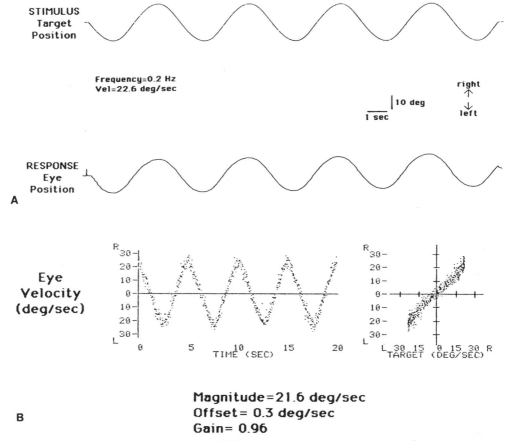

FIGURE 6–15. (*A*) Sample of binocular ENG recordings of smooth pursuit reflex response to a sinusoidally moving light at 0.2 Hz and ±18° amplitude. (*B*) Graphs illustrating eye velocity during four consecutive cycles of target trajectory, as in Figure 6–15A (*left*), and of the relationship between eye and target velocity (*right*).

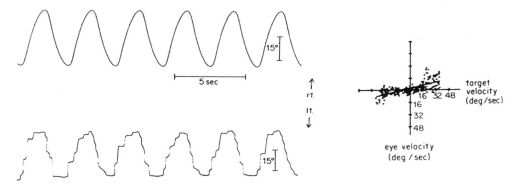

FIGURE 6–16. Smooth pursuit of a target moving with a sinusoidal waveform in a normal subject and in a patient with cerebellar atrophy. Eye velocity is plotted against target velocity (both samples 10 times per second) after saccades have been removed for the normal subject and the patient, respectively. (From Honrubia, V, and Luxon, L: Optokinetic nystagmus with reference to the smooth-pursuit system. In Oosterveld, WJ (ed): Otoneurology. Wiley, Chichester, 1984, p 195. ©1984 John Wiley & Sons. Reprinted by permission of John Wiley & Sons, Ltd.)

gain decreases with both increasing frequency and increasing velocity of the target. Each laboratory must establish normative data for their standard test protocol.

RESULTS IN PATIENTS

Patients with impaired smooth pursuit require frequent corrective saccades to keep up with the target, producing so-called cogwheel or saccadic pursuit (Fig. 6–16). As expected, gain (given by the slope of the plot of eye velocity versus target velocity) of the smooth-pursuit system is markedly decreased in such patients.

Abnormalities of smooth pursuit occur with disorders throughout the CNS. Acute lesions of the peripheral labyrinth or vestibular nerve transiently impair smooth pursuit contralateral to the lesion when the eyes are moving against the slow component of spontaneous nystagmus. This asymmetry in smooth pursuit disappears within a few weeks despite the continued presence of spontaneous nystagmus in darkness. Just as they affect saccadic eye movements, tranquilizing drugs, alcohol, and fatigue impair smooth pursuit eye movements.[82,83] Smooth pursuit is also affected by retinal lesions.[84] Patients with diffused cortical disease (degenerative or vascular), basal ganglia disease[68,75] (Parkinson's and Huntington's disease), and diffuse cerebella disease,[73,85] consistently have bilaterally impaired smooth-pursuit eye movements. Focal disease of one cerebellar hemisphere or one side of the brainstem usually produces ipsilateral impairment of smooth pursuit, although large cerebellopontine angle tumors are frequently associated with bilaterally impaired smooth pursuit. Focal cortical lesions in the parieto-occipital region impair ipsilateral smooth pursuit (Fig. 6–17).[86,87]

Optokinetic Nystagmus

METHODS OF TESTING AND RESULTS IN NORMAL SUBJECTS

Optokinetic testing should be conducted by using a full visual field optokinetic drum moving at constant or sinusoidal velocities. Figure 6–18A shows such a record-

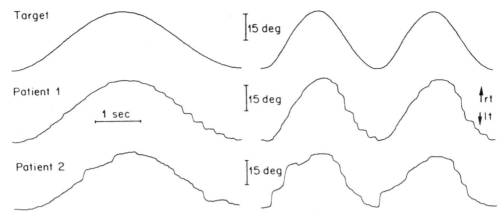

FIGURE 6–17. Smooth pursuit records of patients with left temporal lesions. Tests were conducted at two frequencies: 0.4 and 0.2 Hz. Stimulus excursions are of equal amplitude (±18°) (*upper trace*) and hence the stimuli have different peak velocities: 45 and 22.5° per second nystagmus with reference to the smooth-pursuit system. (From Honrubia, V, and Luxon, L: Optokinetic nystagmus with reference to the smooth-pursuit system. In Oosterveld, WJ (ed): Otoneurology. Wiley, Chichester, 1984, p 195. ©1984 John Wiley & Sons. Reprinted by permission of John Wiley & Sons, Ltd.)

ing of optokinetic nystagmus (OKN) induced by a striped drum, completely surrounding a subject and moving at a constant velocity of 30° per second (*top*) and with a sinusoidal trajectory of 60° per second peak velocity (*bottom*). A plot of nystagmus slow component velocity is provided in Figure 6–18B. Typically, OKN slow component velocity approaches that of drum velocity as long as the latter does not exceed 30° to 40° per second. Following constant velocity stimulation, if the lights are extinguished and optokinetic after nystagmus (OKAN) is recorded after an initial rapid drop-off followed by an exponential decay, the velocity of the OKAN is more variable than that of the OKN, even in young normal subjects. After 1 minute of 30° per second optokinetic stimulation, the mean maximum OKAN slow component velocity was 6.3° ± 4.5° per second and the mean total duration 23.75 ± 23.1 seconds (*n* = 20).[88]

RESULTS IN PATIENTS

As a general rule, abnormalities of optokinetic slow components parallel abnormalities of smooth pursuit, whereas abnormalities of fast components parallel abnormalities of voluntary saccades. Symmetrically decreased slow component velocity is produced by diffused lesions of the cortex, diencephalon, brainstem, or cerebellum (Fig. 6–19).[75,78,84–86,89] As with smooth pursuit, focal lateralized disease of the parietal region, brainstem, and cerebellum, results in impaired OKN when the stimulus moves toward the damaged side.[1,14] Lesions of the occipital lobe, even though they may produce hemianoptic visual field defects, are not associated with impaired smooth pursuit or OKN, presumably because each parietal lobe receives oculomotor signals from the two occipital lobes. Some patients with severely impaired smooth pursuit exhibit gradual build-up in OKN slow component velocity (Fig. 6–20).[90] This feature of OKN normally occurs in afoveate animals, which have only a subcortical OKN system. Presumably, in normal humans, the cortical pursuit system dominates the subcortical OKN system so that normal OKN exhibits features of normal pursuit. When the corti-

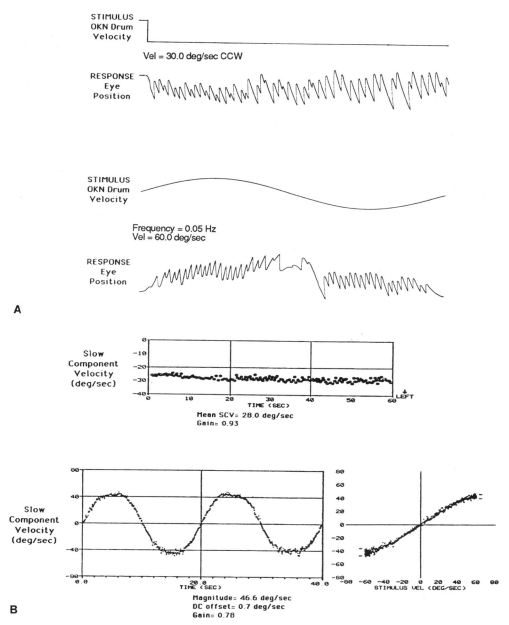

FIGURE 6–18. (A) Sample of binocular ENG recordings of optokinetic reflex responses to constant (*top*) and sinusoidal (*bottom*) stimuli of the specified characteristics as indicated. (B) Graphs showing the results of analysis of the data shown in (A). Top plot shows slow component eye velocity in response to the constant OK stimulus. Bottom plots show the eye velocity during two cycles of stimulus (*left*) and the relationship between eye and stimulus velocity (*right*). Note the amplitude saturation of the response to the large stimulus (60° per second).

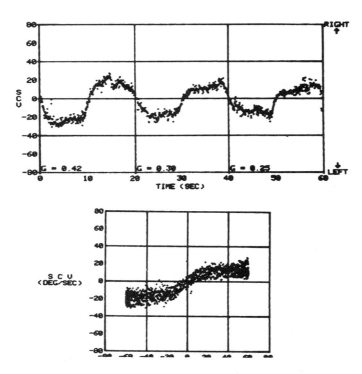

FIGURE 6–19. (*A*) Sinusoidal OKN in patient with cerebellar degeneration, slow component velocity (SCV) versus time. Drum is rotating at 0.05 Hz and 60° per second peak velocity. Note that peak SCV is low compared with peak drum velocity. G is peak SCV gain. (*B*) Sinusoidal OKN in patient with cerebellar degeneration, SCV versus drum velocity. Drum is rotating at 0.05 Hz and 60° per second peak velocity. Three cycles are overlaid. Velocity + (*right*); − (*left*). Note that SCV increases to a peak of only 20° per second. (From Yee, RD, et al: Pathophysiology of optokinetic nystagmus. In Honrubia, V, and Brazier, MAB (eds): Nystagmus and Vertigo: Clinical Approaches to the Patient With Dizziness. UCLA Forum in Medical Sciences, No. 24. Academic Press, New York, 1982, pp 256–257, with permission.)

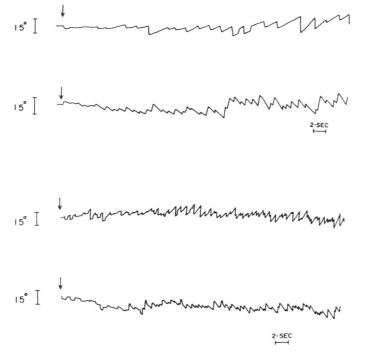

FIGURE 6–20. Slow build-up of OKN in two patients with down-beat vertical nystagmus. Deflection upward are to the right, downward to the left. Lights were turned on at arrows. Drum velocity was always 30° per second whether in the clockwise or counterclockwise direction. (From Honrubia, V, and Luxon, L: Optokinetic nystagmus with reference to the smooth-pursuit system. In Oosterveld, WJ (ed): Otoneurology. Wiley, Chichester, 1984, p 195. © 1984 John Wiley & Sons. Reprinted by permission of John Wiley & Sons, Ltd.)

cal pursuit system is lesioned, however, the remaining OKN may exhibit features of the subcortical system. In humans, the precise anatomic and physiological mechanisms of such distinct behavior in the reflexes are yet to be elucidated.

Patients who are unable to produce saccadic eye movements can produce slow tonic deviation of the eyes. Thus, when patients with slow saccades are stimulated with optokinetic stimuli, their nystagmus has a rounded waveform, and its amplitude and slow component velocity are also affected. The delayed ending of the impaired fast component subtracts from the initial part of the slow component in the opposite direction.

Abnormalities of OKAN typically occur with acute peripheral vestibular lesions, especially if the spontaneous nystagmus is strong (at least 10° per second).[91] The OKAN might be present only in the direction of spontaneous nystagmus while bilateral lesions (e.g., owing to ototoxic drugs) result in normal OKN but diminished or absent OKAN.[92]

Test of Vestibulo-Ocular Reflex Function

THE BITHERMAL CALORIC TEST

The caloric test, introduced by Robert Barany, uses a nonphysiological stimulus (water or air) to induce endolymphatic flow in the semicircular canals by creating a temperature gradient from one side of the semicircular canal, the closest to the temperature source, to the other side (Fig. 6–21).[93] For this purpose the external auditory canal is irrigated with water or filled with air that is below or above ear canal temperature. Of the three semicircular canals, the largest temperature gradient develops in the HSC. Following temperature changes in the external ear canal, when the HSC is placed in the vertical plane, the endolymphatic fluid circulates, because of the difference in its specific gravity, between the two-sided arms of the HSC system—the space of the long arc versus the utricular-cupular cavity—owing to heat expansion. Because the vertical canals are relatively remote from the external ear, the intensity of the heat is lower. Furthermore, they are oriented with the two arms of the canal about the same distance from the heat front, whereby no temperature gradient is created across the cupula. The caloric stimulation of the vertical canals has proved to be unreliable.

Mechanism of Stimulation

Caloric testing of HSC function is usually performed with the patient in the supine position, head tilted 30° up, so that the HSCs are in the vertical plane. With warm caloric stimulation, the column of endolymph in the canal nearest the middle ear rises because of its decreased density. This movement causes the cupula to deviate towards the utricle, with an ampullopetal flow (excitatory), and produces horizontal nystagmus, with the fast component directed toward the stimulated ear. A cold stimulus produces the opposite effect on the endolymph column, causing ampullofugal endolymph flow with nystagmus directed away from the stimulated ear (cold opposite, warm same; COWS). If the same test is repeated with the patient lying on his or her abdomen, so that the HSC is reversed in the vertical plane (the direction of the gravity vector with relation to the head is reversed), the direction of nystagmus induced by warm and cold stimulation is reversed.[93]

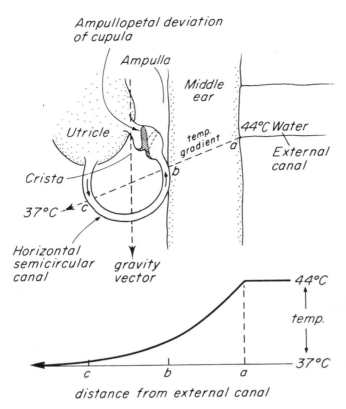

FIGURE 6–21. Mechanism of caloric stimulation of the horizontal semicircular canal. (From Baloh, RW, and Honrubia, V: Clinical Neurophysiology of the Vestibular System, ed 2. FA Davis, Philadelphia, 1990, p 138, with permission.)

Other mechanisms, including differential pressure, electrokinetic effects from the temperature gradient, direct thermal effect on the nerve, and central otolith-canal interactions, have also been proposed as influencing caloric responses in abnormal situations.[94,95] From a clinical point of view, however, gravity is the main driving force behind the caloric response. The response can be effectively shut off (in instances when the patient becomes extremely uncomfortable) simply by positioning the head so that the HSCs are horizontal, that is, tilted approximately 30° downward while the patient sits on the examination table.[96]

The caloric test is the most widely used clinical test of the VOR for two major reasons: (1) each labyrinth can be stimulated individually, and (2) the stimulus is easy to apply without requiring complex equipment. Several limitations of the test must be appreciated, however, if one is to assess the results properly. Slow component velocity and duration of caloric-induced nystagmus are dependent not only on the relationship between the temperature gradient vector and the gravity vector but also on blood flow to the skin, length of transmission pathway from the tympanic membrane to the HSC, and heat conductivity of the temporal bone.[95–97] If local blood flow in the skin is decreased (from vasoconstriction owing to pain or anxiety), the velocity of the maximum slow component of the response decreases (from decreased heat conductivity through skin), but the duration is prolonged (from delayed heat dissipation). Patients with infection or fluid in the middle ear and mastoid air cells may have increased caloric response (increased maximum slow component velocity) because of increased heat conductivity from the external to the inner ear. Similarly, patients who have undergone mastoid surgery and reconstruction of the middle ear may have increased responses owing to shortening of the conduction pathway. A thickened temporal bone, on the other hand, would produce the opposite effect because of decreased bone heat conductivity. Some of these factors no doubt play a role in the large variability of caloric responses in normal subjects, and may explain the occasional unexpected increase or decrease in caloric responses from patients with temporal bone disease.

Test Methodology

With the bithermal caloric test introduced by Fitzgerald and Hallpike, each ear is irrigated with about 250 cc of water for a fixed duration (30 to 40 seconds) with constant flow-rate of water that is 7° below body temperature (30°C) and 7°C above body temperature (44°C).[98] A minimum of 5 minutes must elapse from the end of one response to the beginning of the next stimulus to avoid additive effects. The major advantages of this test methodology are that: (1) both the ampullopetal and ampullofugal endolymph flow are serially induced in each horizontal semicircular canal, (2) the caloric stimulus is highly reproducible from patient to patient, and (3) the test is tolerated by most patients. The major limitation is the need for constant temperature baths and plumbing to maintain continuous circulation of water through the infusion hose.

The maximum magnitude of the caloric-induced nystagmus slow component velocity is highly dependent on the degree of fixation permitted during the test procedure. Four different fixation conditions have been used for caloric testing: (1) eyes open, fixating; (2) eyes open, Frenzel glasses; (3) eyes open, total darkness; and (4) eyes closed. Without eye movement recording devices, obviously only the first two conditions can be used. Comparison of these four conditions in normal subjects reveals a consistently lower coefficient of variation (expressed as 100 × standard deviation of the mean value) for response measurements when the test is performed with eyes open, either behind Frenzel glasses or in total darkness.[98]

When caloric testing is performed with fixation (as initially described by Fitzgerald and Hallpike), two separate systems are being evaluated—the VOR and smooth-pursuit system. Some normal subjects are very efficient in suppressing caloric-induced nystagmus with fixation; others are not. Patients with impaired smooth pursuit (such as those with cerebellar atrophy) may show no difference in caloric-induced nystagmus with or without fixation.[99] When measured with fixation, responses in these patients will appear hyperactive compared with those of subjects having a normal smooth-pursuit system. Eye closure and the associated upward deviation of the eyes can lead to suppression of both spontaneous and induced nystagmus,[98] or can alter the nystagmus waveform, which then becomes more difficult to quantify with ENG. Patients with CNS lesions often have horizontal deviation of the eyes on closure, which can also change the waveform of induced nystagmus.[100] To avoid these uncontrollable variables, we recommend that in such patients caloric testing be performed with eyes open, preferably in total darkness. For a brief period during the test, fixation can be permitted so that the functional status of the smooth pursuit system can be evaluated.

Normative Data

With the application of computerized technology, it is possible to accurately record multiple response measurements. The most useful information, however, is derived from measurements of the velocity of the slow component of nystagmus.[57,59] An ENG recording of a normal caloric response is illustrated in Figure 6–22. The subject was supine, with head elevated 30° and eyes open behind Frenzel glasses in a dark-

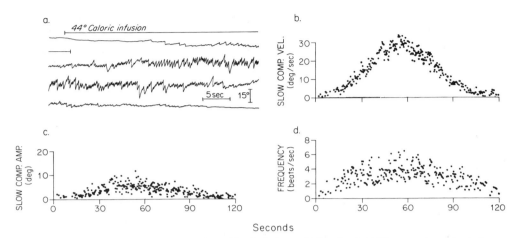

FIGURE 6–22. Caloric response produced by infusion of 20 mL of 44°C water into the left ear of a normal subject. (*A*) Bitemporal ENG recording. Horizontal bar indicates duration of infusion. Plots of slow component velocity (b), slow component amplitude (c), and frequency (d) versus time generated by a digital computer. (From Baloh, RW, and Honrubia, V: Clinical Neurophysiology of the Vestibular System, ed 2. FA Davis, Philadelphia, 1990, p 140, with permission.)

ened room. Water (250 cc at 44°C) was infused into the left ear during 40 seconds at the time indicated in the figure, resulting in ampullopetal endolymph flow in the left horizontal semicircular canal, and producing left-beating horizontal nystagmus. The nystagmus began just before the end of stimulation, reached a peak approximately 60 seconds poststimulus and then slowly decayed over the next minute (Fig. 6–22*A*). Shown next to the ENG tracing is a record of the velocity of the nystagmus slow component, and below, its amplitude and frequency (Fig. 6–22–*B,C,D*, respectively) all plotted versus time. Each measurement demonstrates beat-to-beat variability, but the velocity of the slow components shows the least amount of irregularity between successive nystagmus beats.

As suggested earlier, the absolute magnitude of caloric response depends on several physical factors unique to each subject that are unrelated to actual semicircular canal function. Maximum slow component velocity (MxSCV) after caloric stimulation can be as low as 5° per second and as high as 75° per second and still be within the 95 percent confidence interval for normal subjects.[1] Mean values in our laboratory are 21° ± and 19° ± per second[59] for warm and cold irrigation, respectively. Because of the large intrasubject variability, intrasubject measurements have been found to be more useful clinically, as shown in Figure 6–23.

To quantify caloric tests, two formulas are used. One is the *vestibular paresis formula:*

$$\frac{(R\,30° + R\,44°) - (L\,30° + L\,44°)}{R\,30° + R\,44° + L\,30° + L\,44°} \times 100,$$

which compares MxSCV of right-sided responses with that of left-sided responses. The second is the *directional preponderance formula:*

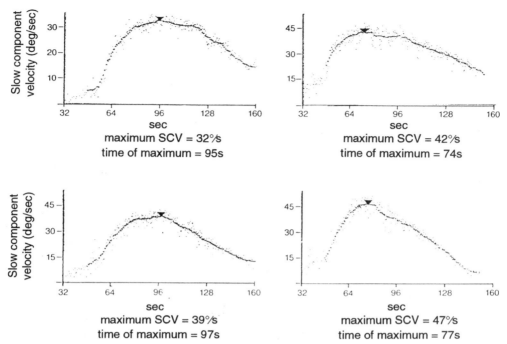

FIGURE 6–23. Plots of eye velocity during the slow component of the nystagmus reaction to caloric irrigation in a normal subject. The four traces correspond to irrigation of the left (*L*) and right (*R*) ears, each at water temperatures of 30°C and 40°C (86°F and 104°F). Arrows point to maximum intensity of each response. (From Honrubia, V: Auditory disorders, evaluation and diagnosis of: Vestibular examination. In Gaullaudet Encyclopedia of Deaf People and Deafness, vol 1. McGraw-Hill, New York, 1986, p 83, with permission.)

$$\frac{(R\,30° + L\,44°) - (R\,44° + L\,30°)}{R\,30° + L\,44° + R\,44° + L\,30°} \times 100,$$

which compares MxSCV of nystagmus beating to the right with that of nystagmus to the left in the same subject.

A *caloric fixation-suppression index* is obtained by having the patient fixate on a target during the middle of the response. Because the slow component velocity of caloric-induced nystagmus is constantly changing, it is important that the fixation period occurs near the time of maximum response to obtain the best estimate of fixation suppression. The fixation-suppression index is defined as (MxSCV with fixation directed by MxSCV without fixation) times 100. With each of these formulas, the result is reported as a percentage of the total response. Dividing by the total response normalizes measurements to remove the large variability in absolute magnitude of normal caloric responses.

In our laboratory, vestibular paresis is defined as a difference between each ear's response of at least 25 percent and directional preponderance as a difference between left- and right-beating nystagmus of at least 30 percent; a fixation suppression index of at least 70 percent is abnormal, but we favor the evaluation of this index with rotational testing when it is suspected to be abnormal (i.e., when visual ocular reflexes are suspected or found to be abnormal during clinical evaluation). These values are comparable to those reported by other investigators, but it must be emphasized that each laboratory should establish its own normal range because of the many methodologic variables discussed earlier.[101]

Results in Patients

The abnormalities found in caloric testing, their meaning in terms of location of lesion, and the mechanism by which each abnormality is produced are summarized in Table 6–3.

Peripheral Lesions. The findings of significant vestibular paresis with bithermal caloric stimulation suggests damage to the peripheral vestibular system that can be located anywhere from the end-organ to the vestibular nerve root entry zone in the brainstem. It is almost certainly a sign of unilateral peripheral vestibular disease if there are no associated brainstem signs. Directional preponderance on caloric testing can occur with peripheral end-organ and eighth nerve lesions as well as with CNS lesions (from brainstem to cortex). It indicates an imbalance in the vestibular system and is usually associated with spontaneous nystagmus; often, the velocity of slow components of spontaneous nystagmus adds to that of caloric-induced nystagmus in the same direction and subtracts from that of caloric-induced nystagmus in the opposite direction.[102] These interactions are nonlinear and unpredictable. Occasionally, directional preponderance will occur in patients without spontaneous nystagmus; in this case a central lesion is more likely.

The vestibular paresis and directional preponderance formulas are of little use in evaluating patients with bilateral peripheral vestibular lesions, because caloric responses can be symmetrically highly depressed. Because of the wide range of normal values for MxSCV, the patient's value may decrease severalfold before falling below the normal range. Serial measurements in the same patient are needed if one hopes to identify bilateral vestibular impairment, such as that produced by ototoxic drugs.

Central Lesions. As suggested earlier, patients with CNS lesions may exhibit vestibular paresis on caloric testing if the lesion involves the root entry zone of the vestibular nerve. The most common neurological disorders associated with this finding are multiple sclerosis, lateral brainstem infarction, and infiltration gliomas. Each disease produces other brainstem signs so that the finding of vestibular paresis is not likely to be misinterpreted as a sign of peripheral vestibular disorder. In rare cases, massive

TABLE 6–3 Interpreting the Results of Bithermal Caloric Testing

	Location of Lesion	Mechanism
Vestibular paresis	Labyrinth, eighth nerve	Decreased peripheral sensitivity
Directional preponderance	Not localizing	Tonic bias in vestibular system
Hyperactive responses	Cerebellum	Loss of inhibitory influence on vestibular nuclei
Dysrhythmia	Cerebellum	Loss of inhibitory influence on pontine nuclei
Impaired fixation suppression	CNS pursuit pathways	Interruption of visual signals on way to oculomotor neurons
Perverted nystagmus	Fourth ventricular region	Disruption of vestibular commissural fibers

brainstem infarction or diffusely infiltrating glioma leads to bilaterally decreased caloric responses.

Lesions of the cerebellum can lead to heightened caloric responses. Because of the wide range of normal caloric responses, however, it is unusual for any of the responses to statistically exceed the upper normal range. Patients with cerebellar atrophy syndromes demonstrate a wide range of caloric responses.[85] Those with Friedreich's ataxia often have bilaterally decreased responses because of associated atrophy of the vestibular nerve and ganglia, whereas those with olivopontocerebellar atrophy have decreased, normal, or even increased responses, depending on which areas of the medulla and pons are involved. Increased caloric responses, when they do occur, are usually found in patients with clinically pure cerebellar atrophy.

An abnormal fixation-suppression index on caloric testing typically occurs with lesions involving the smooth pursuit system (from the parietal-occipital cortex to the pons and cerebellum).[99] Lesions of the midline cerebellum produce the most profound impairment of fixation suppression. When they are asymmetric, pursuit deficits in one direction correlate with suppression deficits in the opposite direction.

Dysrhythmia refers to a marked beat-to-beat variability in caloric-induced nystagmus amplitude without any change in slow component velocity profile. This phenomenon has often been attributed to CNS lesions, mainly in the cerebellum. Unfortunately, from a diagnostic point of view, caloric dysrhythmia also occurs in normal subjects when they are tired and inattentive. As will be shown, rotatory stimuli are better suited than caloric stimuli for examining the pattern of induced nystagmus.

Vertical or oblique nystagmus produced by caloric stimulation of the horizontal semicircular canals is called perverted nystagmus. Normal subjects commonly exhibit a small vertical component on ENG recordings of caloric-induced nystagmus, but vertical components larger than horizontal components are clearly abnormal.[103] Perverted nystagmus with caloric stimulation has been reported with both peripheral and central lesions, the latter usually in the region of the floor of the fourth ventricle (near the vestibular nuclei).[104] Uemura and Cohen[105] found perverted caloric nystagmus in rhesus monkeys after producing unilateral focal lesions in the rostromedial vestibular nucleus. Warm caloric stimulation on the intact side produced downward nystagmus and cold stimulation produced upward diagonal nystagmus. The investigators attributed their findings to disturbance of commissural fibers between vestibular nuclei.

ROTATIONAL TESTING OF THE HORIZONTAL SEMICIRCULAR CANAL

The most often used quantitative tests of vestibular function concentrate on the HSC ocular reflex because it is the easiest reflex to induce and record. Tests of other VORs (from vertical semicircular canals and otolith organs) have yet to be shown useful and practical in the clinical setting.[106] Tests of several vestibulospinal reflexes are described in other chapters.

Rotational testing of the horizontal semicircular canal offers several advantages over caloric testing. Multiple graded stimuli can be applied in a relatively short period of time and the testing is usually well tolerated by patients. Unlike caloric testing, rotatory stimulation of the semicircular canals is unrelated to physical features of the external ear or temporal bone, so that a more exact relationship between stimulus and response can be established. On the other hand, rotatory stimuli affect both labyrinths simultaneously, compared with the selective stimulation of one labyrinth with caloric testing.

Mechanisms of Stimulation

According to the pendulum model of vestibular function, slow component velocity of rotational-induced nystagmus should be proportional to deviation of the cupula, which, in turn, is proportional to magnitude of the angular velocity of the head movement. As will be demonstrated in the following sections, this model's applicability to different forms of stimulation is remarkably consistent and provides a rational approach to the evaluation of clinical rotational testing.

Three types of angular accelerations have been used to clinically evaluate the HSC ocular reflex: (1) impulsive, (2) constant, and (3) sinusoidal. Historically, each type of stimulation has been popular at different times for different reasons. Barany,[107] in 1907, introduced an impulsive rotational test in which the chair in which the patient was seated was manually rotated 10 turns in 20 seconds and then suddenly brought to a standstill with the patient facing the observer. The function of the HSCs was assessed by measuring the duration of visually monitored nystagmus after clockwise and counterclockwise rotations. Montandon[108] introduced a constant-acceleration test to investigate nystagmus threshold as the smallest stimulus at which nystagmus was first observed, a measure of the fast component generating system rather than that of the end organs.

A simple, reproducible method of generating sinusoidal angular acceleration in a clinical setting, the torsion swing test, was popularized in France as another method of rotatory stimulation. With this test, the patient was seated in a chair, the rotation of which was mechanically controlled by the action of a calibrated spring. Because of technical limitations and limited understanding of the relevant physiology at the time, the most effective parameter for evaluation of vestibular reflex function (eye velocity) was not used. Instead, frequency of nystagmus or threshold of fast component production were the parameters measured. These test results, as could be anticipated by presently known mechanisms of vestibular function, were rather empirical and of limited quantitative physiological value, but are still being used in some clinics.

Contemporarily, among the various modalities of rotatory stimulation, impulsive and sinusoidal angular acceleration stimuli are preferred over constant accelerations because of the long duration of the test. Sinusoidal stimulation is the most widely used because it is reproducible and easy to generate, and can be defined by the period and the maximum amplitude of oscillation. The first parameter defines the frequency and the second can be selected within a wide range of velocity magnitudes. The characteristics of the responses produced by different directions and magnitudes of rotation for each stimulus allow for additional comparison, not only with normal subjects, but within response directions in the same subject.

Test Methodology

For rotational testing of the horizontal canal-ocular reflex, the patient is seated in a chair mounted on a motorized rotating platform, which is under computer control, inside a dark, acoustically and electrically shielded room.[109,110] An array of three lights (light-emitting diodes) spaced 10° or 15° apart is attached to the chair directly in front of the subject. Frequent electro-oculographic (EOG) calibrations are conducted throughout the testing procedure to correct for any fluctuations in corneoretinal potential. The EOG signals can be displayed on a polygraph recorder or the equivalent and digitized by a small laboratory computer for analysis. The patient is constantly questioned to maintain alertness. For sinusoidal testing, we use stimulus signals at frequencies ranging from 0.0125 Hz to 1.6 Hz and several peak velocities with a maximum of

120° per second. Impulse changes in velocity of 256° per second can be produced with an acceleration of 140° per second. This wide range of stimuli provides comprehensive information, but the procedure is time consuming and tiring for most patients. Therefore, for screening purposes and before exploring responses to other stimuli, we routinely use sinusoidal frequencies of 0.0125, 0.05, and 0.2 Hz, peak velocity of 60° per second, and step change in velocity of 100° per second. An example of pairs of responses obtained in a patient before and 1 month after left vestibular nerve section is shown in Figure 6–24 (*top trace*, before; *bottom trace*, after).

Two types of measurements are typically used to quantify the response to rotational stimulation: *delays* (phase) and *magnitude* (gain) measurements. The phase measurement corresponds to evaluation of timing relationships between the response and the stimuli. This information reflects two major factors, the times of the mechanical bilogical transduction in the inner ear and the so-called storage capabilities of the central vestibular system reflex. In terms of the pendulum model, the phase measurement allows evaluation of the long time constant of the VOR reflex (T_{vor}). The phase angle (ϕ) at low frequencies of sinusoidal rotation, and the T_{vor} are related by the following equation:

$$T_{vor} = \frac{1}{\omega \tan \phi},$$

where $\omega = 2\pi f$ is the angular frequency of rotation.

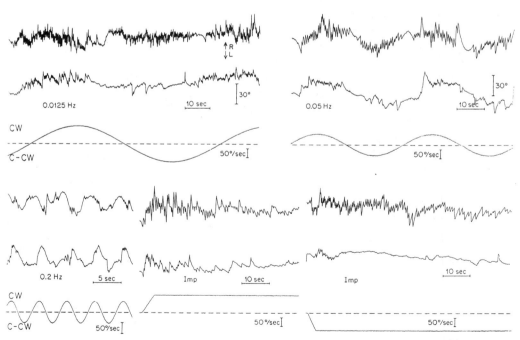

FIGURE 6–24. Records of various sinusoidal rotatory and impulse tests. Nystagmus traces were obtained before (*top*) and 1 month after (*bottom*) surgery for removal of a left acoustic neuroma. Stimulus velocity is indicated by the sinusoidal or step trajectory of the rotating platform. (From Honrubia, V, et al: Vestibulo-ocular reflexes in peripheral labyrinthine lesions: I. Unilateral dysfunction. Am J Otolaryngol 5:16, 1984, with permission.)

For a sinusoidal stimulus, the phase measurement is obtained by comparing the time of maximum head velocity (stimulus) with the time of maximum slow component eye velocity (response). The same results will be obtained by comparing responses at equivalent moments of the sinusoidal stimulus and response (e.g., zero crossings). Responses from normal subjects show that maximum slow component eye velocity leads to maximum head velocity at low frequencies of sinusoidal rotation. This is an awkward notion for health professionals to accept, a response that precedes the stimulus. To be more precise, the response lags the natural physiological stimulus, head angular acceleration, which is the first derivative of velocity, hence leading by 90° or a quarter cycle the head velocity. Thus, the low-frequency VOR response in reality lags head acceleration stimulus by less than 90° (e.g., 30° at 0.0125 Hz) or would appear to lead head velocity (e.g., 60° at 0.0125 Hz). For higher frequencies (over 0.2 Hz), which correspond to the natural head movements, the response delay increases to the point that the stimulus and response are of approximately opposite phases. This cumulative delay has the effect of making the VOR response eye velocity compensate for the head velocity to maintain gaze. Such arbitrary practices are most confusing to the initiate, but, unfortunately, are common practice and require some small effort to be understood.

Another measure of the long time constant T_{vor} can be obtained from the response to impulse rotatory stimuli in the dark which is the time required for the response to decay to $1/e$ or to 37 percent of the maximum value. These values of T_{vor} are smaller than those obtained with sinusoidal data.[111]

Magnitude is traditionally defined as gain, which is obtained by dividing maximum slow component eye velocity by maximum stimulus magnitude. The coefficient of variation for gain values after sinusoidal and impulsive rotatory stimulation is about one-half the coefficient of variation after caloric stimulation.[89,112] Even with this increased precision, however, there is still a large coefficient variation (approximately 30 percent) in rotational responses of normal subjects. Factors such as stress, fatigue, level of mental alertness, and habituation contribute to variability.

Sinusoidal Rotational Tests. With sinusoidal rotational testing, gain of the canalocular reflex can be measured at multiple cycles after the subject has attained a "steady-state" response (i.e., after a half-cycle of low frequency rotation). Because of the several values obtained for each cycle, sinusoidal rotational testing usually provides a more accurate assessment of gain than does impulsive testing. Its main disadvantage is the lengthy procedure required to test a broad frequency range to precisely determine the complete frequency response of the system.

Two standard computer plots generated during sinusoidal rotational testing in a normal subject are shown in Figure 6–25. The subjects were rotated at 0.05 Hz (peak velocity 60° per second) with eyes open in the dark while performing continuous mentally-alert tasks. Each dot represents the average slow component velocity sample at 25-ms intervals. The plot on the left shows slow component velocity versus time for two complete cycles of response. The magnitude of the response in each direction can be read directly from these plots. A more precise estimate can be obtained by performing a curve-fitting using discrete Fourier analysis with computer assistance, which allows the alignment of the response and stimulus. From this analysis, one obtains information about timing, the phase relationship between the fundamental of slow component velocity and chair velocity, gain, the ratio of the magnitude of the stimulus to that of the response, and symmetry between response to opposite directions, and a dc bias if any exists.[109,111,113,114] If slow component velocity data are symmetrical (as in

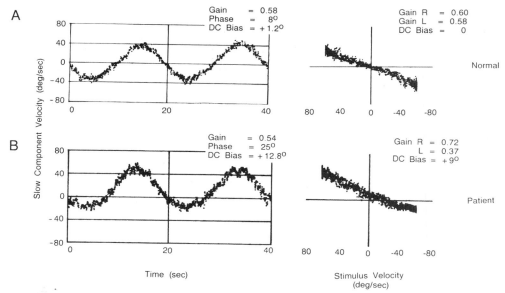

FIGURE 6–25. Plots of nystagmus slow component velocity versus time (*left*) and versus chair velocity (*right*) during sinusoidal angular rotation (0.05 Hz, 60° per second peak velocity). The horizontal axis on the left indicates the time after the beginning of the cycle of stimulus velocity (period, 20 seconds), and on the right, the magnitude of the stimulus. The data in (*A*) are from a normal subject and in (*B*) from a patient with an acute right peripheral vestibular lesion. Gain, phase (lead), and dc bias (+rightward bias) were determined from frequency analysis (Fourier analysis) of the data. (From Baloh, RW, and Honrubia, V: Clinical Neurophysiology of the Vestibular System, ed 2. FA Davis, Philadelphia, 1990, p 158, with permission.)

normal subjects), phase can be read directly from these plots by comparing the time of zero eye velocity with that of zero chair velocity. The time difference (t), multiplied by 360° and by the frequency (fr) of the stimulus, gives the phase

$$\phi(\phi = t \cdot 360° \cdot fr).$$

If, however, responses are asymmetric (as in Fig. 6–25B), the computations should be cautiously examined because often cycles also have asymmetrical durations.[115]

Gain and phase of the canal-ocular reflex vary with frequency in normal subjects,[56,113] consistent with the pendulum model. Normal subjects exhibit approximately a 40° phase lead of eye velocity relative to chair velocity at 0.0125 Hz, but this phase lead is near zero by 0.2 Hz. Likewise, response gain is frequency dependent (Table 6–4).

Variance associated with measurements comparing clockwise and counterclockwise responses in the same subject is less than variance between subjects which makes useful the computation of a normalized difference formula:

(clockwise − counterclockwise) ÷ (clockwise + counterclockwise) × 100.

Impulse Rotational Tests. The main advantage of the impulse stimulus is that it provides rapid assessment of gain and time constant of the canal-ocular reflex inde-

TABLE 6-4 Gain, Phase, and Time-Constant Measurements for Sinusoidal (0.0125 to 2.0 Hz) and Impulse Rotation in Normal Subjects

Measurement	Frequency (HZ)*							Impulse[a]
	0.0125[a]	0.05[b]	0.2[b]	0.4[c]	1.0[d]	1.5[d]	2.0[d]	
Gain	0.40 ± 0.07	0.50 ± 0.15	0.59 ± 0.19	0.59 ± 0.18	0.94 ± 0.16	1.01 ± 0.12	1.14 ± 0.11	0.63 ± 0.18
Phase (degrees)	−39 ± 7	−10 ± 4	−1 ± 4	0 ± 3				12.2 ± 3.6

Values are mean ± standard deviation.

*Stimulus magnitude in degrees per second: [a]100, [b]60, [c]30, [d]20.

Impulse time constant, equivalent to the time needed for the response to decline $1/e$ (i.e., as in a first-order system).

pendently in each direction. Sinusoidal testing, on the other hand, provides a measure of only a single time constant, which represents the average value for responses in both directions of rotation. The impulse stimulus is so brief that if the subject is not maximally alert or attempts to suppress the response, the initial peak will be blunted and the estimate of gain inaccurate. The results of typical impulse responses in a normal subject are shown in Figure 6–26. Slow component velocity is plotted versus time for four different stimuli of the indicated magnitudes; each dot in this illustration represents average slow component velocity of one nystagmus beat. From these plots peak slow component velocity to compute gain can be read directly, as well as the time required for slow component velocity to fall to 37 percent of its initial value, and gain and time constant can be computed. In our laboratory, these parameters are obtained by plotting the logarithm of the slow component velocity versus time after start of the stimulus, and curve-fitting the data to a straight line with a least-squares method. An example is shown in Figure 6–27B. Normal mean gain and T_{vor} values calculated from similar plots in 20 normal subjects using step of velocity of 100° per second were gain,

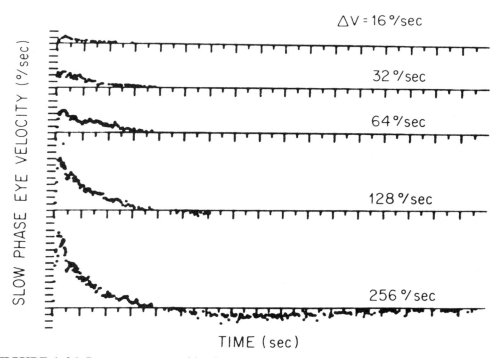

FIGURE 6–26. Responses measured by slow component eye velocity of nystagmus shown for progressively greater impulse stimuli (ΔV). Horizontal axis is marked every 5 seconds, and vertical axis is marked every 10° per second. Axes are the same for all responses. Up to impulses of 64° per second, responses behave as predicted by the dampled pendulum model; above this, after nystagmus disappears, beating in the direction opposite to that of the postrotatory response, as noted by change in signs of the last part of the eye velocity records. (From Sill, AW, and Honrubia, V: A new method for determining impulsive time constraints and their application to clinical data. Otolaryngology 86:81, 1978, with permission.)

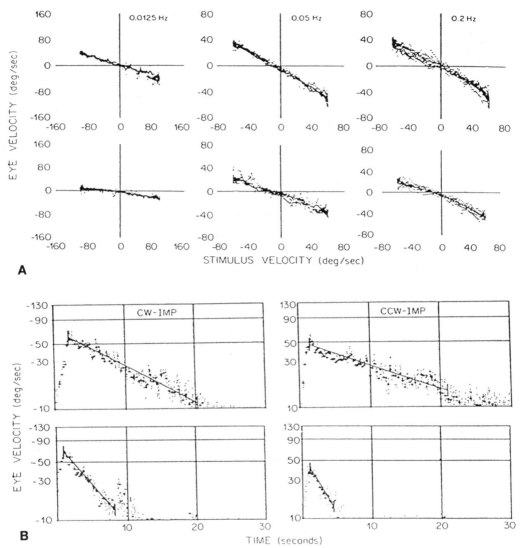

FIGURE 6–27. Computer outputs used to quantify results of sinusoidal and impulse tests. (*A*) Scatter plots of the relationship between slow component eye velocity and table velocity for three frequencies after the phases of the two signals were aligned. The set of records shown in the top row was obtained before surgery; that shown in the bottom row, after surgery. (*B*) Scatter plots, using semilog coordinates, of the magnitude of slow component eye velocity during the postrotatory nystagmus response following an impulse of acceleration. (From Honrubia, V, et al: Vestibulo-ocular reflexes in peripheral labyrinthine lesions: I. Unilateral dysfunction. Am J Otolaryngol 5:17, 1984, with permission.)

0.63 + 0.18 and T$_{vor}$, 12.2 + 3.6 seconds, respectively. Asymmetry of more than 20 percent on the standard directional preponderance formula is considered abnormal for all frequencies and amplitudes of stimulation.

Results in Patients

Unilateral Peripheral Lesions. Patients who suddenly lose vestibular function on one side have asymmetric responses to rotational stimuli because of (1) the dc bias resulting from spontaneous nystagmus, and (2) the difference in response to ampullopetal and ampullofugal stimulation of the remaining intact labyrinth as predicted by Ewald's second law of labyrinthine function.[111,113,114,116,117] These features are readily seen in impulsive and sinusoidal data in the records of eye movements and in the reproduction of computerized data analysis from the same patient whose data is shown in Figure 6–24. The data were obtained shortly before and after surgery for removal of a left acoustic nerve tumor. At the time of postoperative testing the patient exhibited spontaneous nystagmus (with eyes open in the dark), with average slow component velocity of 7° per second. This spontaneous nystagmus was added to rotational-induced nystagmus in the same direction and subtracted from that in the opposite direction, contributing to asymmetry in the response, or the dc bias. That is, peak values are different, and the data do not cross the cartesian coordinates of the plot at the intersection. Another effect, however, is shown in the difference in gain of the responses obtained from ampullopetal and ampullofugal stimulation. This gain asymmetry is particularly obvious in differences in the slopes of the lines describing the relationship between eye velocity and stimulus velocity (Fig. 6–27A). Following rotations at 0.0125 Hz and 0.2 Hz, counterclockwise-induced rotations produced smaller responses than those of clockwise-induced rotations. On impulse stimulation, changes in gain and time constant of responses resulting from unilateral lesions are evident in this patient (Fig. 6–27B).

After compensation by the CNS for vestibular loss, clinically important changes take place in VOR responses, even in patients with complete unilateral paralysis. An example is illustrated in Figure 6–28. These responses were obtained 1 year after surgical resection of the vestibular nerve. With compensation, spontaneous nystagmus diminishes, dc bias gradually disappears, gain asymmetry between ampullopetal and ampullofugal stimulation decreases, and responses to low frequencies of rotation become symmetrical.[56,114] Of note is that differences in impulse stimuli responses are more resistant to change than are differences in sinusoidal stimuli responses.

Theoretical computations based on the pendulum model of vestibular function postulate four conditions following unilateral labyrinthectomy that contribute to asymmetrical responses.[111,114,116,118–120] First, a decrease of pain of approximately 50 percent should occur owing to removal of input from one ear. Second, asymmetry should occur in responses to each of the half-cycles of stimuli with magnitude much less than 100° per second owing to the difference in sensitivity of primary neurons to excitatory and inhibitory stimulation. The vestibular fibers have a spontaneous activity of 100 spikes per second and theoretically, during stimulation the ratio of ampullopetal increase to ampullofugal decrease responses should be 1.3 at low frequencies but less at higher frequencies. Thus there will be asymmetry due to differences in sensitivity. Third, for higher stimulus magnitudes, there should be differences among ampullofugal and ampullopetal responses of another nature. With ampullofugal inhibitory stim-

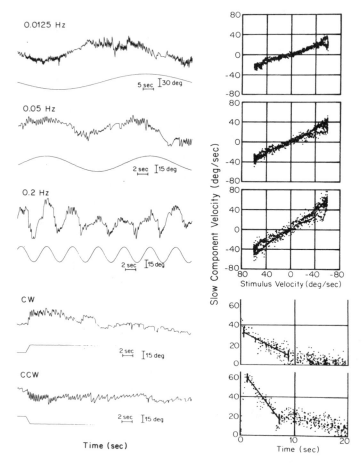

FIGURE 6–28. Responses of a patient (history of Ménière's disease, 1 year postoperative, right vestibular nerve section) to different vestibular rotatory stimulations. (From Honrubia, V, et al: Evaluation of rotatory vestibular tests in peripheral labyrinthine lesions. In Honrubia, V: UCLA Forum in Medical Sciences, No 24. Academic Press, New York, 1982, p 66, with permission.)

uli of large magnitude, the response can reach only a limit value of zero when the spontaneous activity is eliminated. On the other hand, the ampullopetal response will increase with increased stimulus until reaching the maximum capability of the organ (up to 500 spikes per second). Because the canal's transduction process for high frequencies is more than twice as sensitive (relative to velocity) than to low frequencies of rotation,[121] it takes smaller stimulus amplitudes to completely inhibit the vestibular nerve's spontaneous activity and to create the asymmetrical response. This amplitude dependent asymmetry will be more noticeable for high frequencies of stimulation at stimulus velocities of at least approximately 50° per second; at frequencies equal to or lower than 0.05 Hz, it will require velocities twice or three times bigger to produce asymmetrical responses (see Fig. 6–29). Instead, with the use of a brief impulse representative of a high frequency signal, the asymmetry is clearly evident (see Fig. 6–27 and Fig. 6–28) with the smaller stimulation. These three theoretical predictions have been demonstrated experimentally also.[118,119]

Although time constants and phase relationships should be expected to remain approximately constant, reflecting the normal ear function, the data show instead changes that continue for years, namely a shortening of the time constants (see Fig. 6–27). The reason for the above findings is unclear. First, the process of symmetry re-

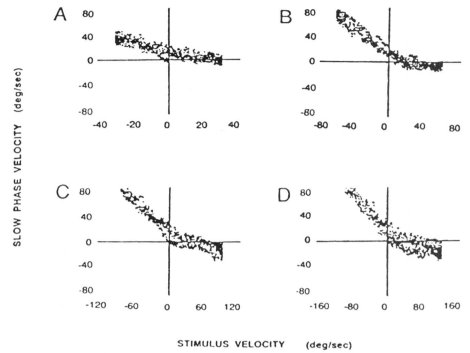

FIGURE 6–29. Plots of slow component eye velocity versus stimulus velocity from one patient (right-sided lesion) at four peak stimulus velocities (30°, 60°, 90°, and 120° per second, 0.05 Hz). (From Baloh, RW, et al: Horizontal vestibulo-ocular reflex after acute peripheral lesions. Acta Otolaryngol (Stockh) 468(suppl):323, 1989, with permission.)

covery is known to be highly dependent on visual-vestibular interactions. The gain of the VOR is modifiable by vision as with the use of magnifying or reducing lenses.[60] It involves visual feedback action between the vestibular-induced eye movements and the head movements to minimize the difference. It represents an adaptive change in the CNS associated even with complete unilateral disappearance of inputs to the second order neurons in the vestibular nuclei, referred to as vestibular compensation.[56,118,119] The end-organ conditions mentioned above continue to operate in the normal ear because there is no evidence that compensation affects vestibular nerve and hair cell function in the intact organ; thus, compensation is a central process.

In a study of rotatory responses from two groups of patients, one with total unilateral labyrinthine paralysis, as judged by caloric testing, and another with partial but statistically significant (greater than 20 percent) paralysis, it was found that only in the first group were there some patients with differences in gain and phase from those of normal subjects significant.[112] In patients with a partial unilateral lesion, as would be expected, the changes depend on the degree of inner ear pathology and the time since the inception of the lesion when vestibular plasticity becomes operative and the group differences were not statistically significant.[56] The vestibular compensation process remains the least understood vestibular phenomenon in spite of its clinical relevance.

Bilateral Peripheral Lesions. Rotational stimuli are ideally suited for testing patients with bilateral peripheral vestibular lesions; because both labyrinths are stimu-

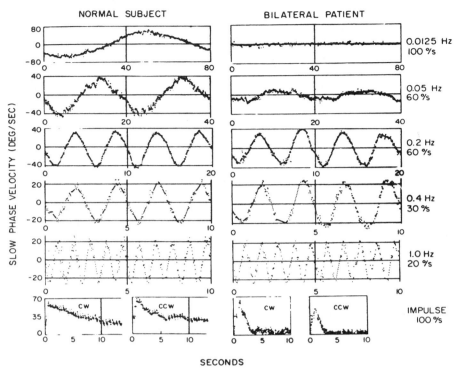

FIGURE 6–30. Plots of slow component eye velocity versus time for sinusoidal (0.125 to 1.0 Hz) and impulse stimulation in a normal subject and a patient with bilateral peripheral vestibular lesion. (From Baloh, RW, et al: Changes in the human vestibulo-ocular reflex after loss of peripheral sensitivity. Ann Neurol 16:222–228, 1984. Reprinted with permission from the Annals of Neurology.)

lated simultaneously, the degree of remaining physiological function can be accurately quantified (Fig. 6–30).[110,111] Several other observations support the value of rotational tests in these patients. Frequently, patients with absent response to bithermal caloric stimulation have decreased but recordable rotational-induced nystagmus, particularly at higher frequencies of sinusoidal rotation. Diminished bilateral function is identified earlier because variance associated with normal rotational responses is less than that associated with caloric responses. Changes in gain are also associated with changes in phase, an important parameter which has the smallest variance among normal subjects and contributes to identification of abnormality. Furthermore, artifactually decreased caloric responses occasionally occur in patients with angular, narrow external canals or with thickened temporal bones, whereas the intensity of rotational stimuli is unaffected by these physical features. Results of rotatory responses in two groups of patients with bilateral labyrinthine disorders are shown in Figure 6–31. Patients in the first group (•) had received ototoxic drugs for the treatment of bacterial infections. The second group (o) consisted of patients with various inner ear pathologies. *All* patients had either complete absence of caloric response to ice water or responses to the four caloric irrigations that averaged less than 20 percent of normal, below the 95 percent confidence limits from our laboratory. None had spontaneous nystagmus with eyes open in the dark.

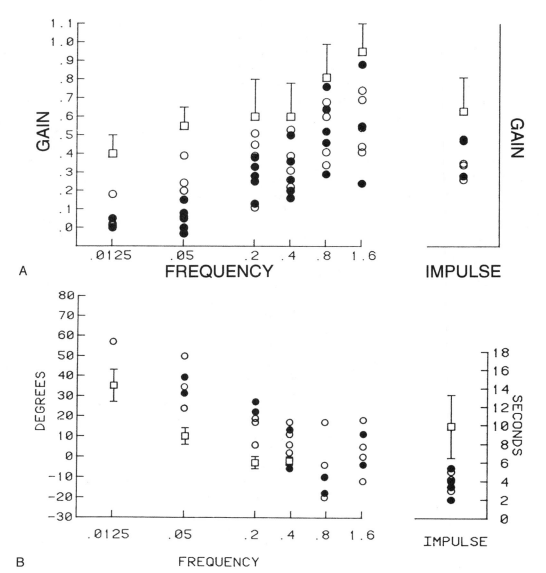

FIGURE 6–31. (*A*) Scatter plot showing normal subjects' mean and standard deviation values (*squares*) and data from individual patients (*circles*). In the plot on the left, the ordinate indicates the gain of the VOR. In the plot on the right, the ordinate indicates the gain for the single impulse of 100° per second. Gain is defined as the ratio of the response amplitude to the stimulus amplitude. Filled circles represent data from ototoxic patients. Frequency is in Hz. (*B*) Scatter plot displaying the results of phase angle measurements (*left*) and the time constant following impulse testing (*right*). Phase was measured in relation to the velocity of the rotation of the table. For convenience, 180° have been subtracted from the data. Frequency is in Hz. (From Honrubia, V, et al: Vestibuloocular reflexes in peripheral labyrinthine lesions: III. Bilateral dysfunction. Am J Otolaryngol 6:345, 1985, with permission.)

The ability to identify remaining vestibular function, even if minimal, is an important advantage of rotational testing, particularly when the physician is contemplating ablative surgery or monitoring the effects of ototoxic drugs. Ototoxic effects are recognized earlier and better by using precisely graded rotational stimuli on a serial basis, than by using the quantitatively less precise caloric stimulus.

The patients whose VOR responses are shown in Figure 6–24, had normal OKN and smooth-pursuit responses; consequently, when they were rotated in the light, their vestibulo-visual ocular responses were perfectly normal—a finding of significant behavior difference. Because of the normal visual oculomotor responses, most of these patients were able to maintain fixation during head rotations and were unaware of their VOR pathology.

Central Vestibular Lesions. As with lesions of peripheral vestibular structures, lesions of central VOR pathways can lead to a variety of abnormalities, including asymmetries in gain of rotational-induced nystagmus. Lesions involving the nerve root entry zone and vestibular nuclei may produce responses indistinguishable from those produced by peripheral vestibular lesions. The spectrum of abnormalities associated with central lesions, however, is much more diverse than a simple decrease in slow component velocity. On the contrary, gain may be increased in some patients with cerebellar lesions.[122] The highly organized pattern of the nystagmus seen in normal subjects may be disorganized, resulting in so-called dysrhythmic nystagmus.[123] If the production of fast components is impaired, the nystagmus waveform is distorted or there may be only a slow tonic deviation of eyes from side to side. Finally, central lesions often interfere with the integration of visual and vestibular signals, producing abnormalities on tests of visual-vestibular interaction.

Sinusoidal rotational tests are ideally suited for studying the specific pattern of induced nystagmus because they produce nystagmus beating in opposite directions during each half cycle, enabling immediate comparison. Figure 6–32 illustrates responses to sinusoidal rotation (eyes open in darkness) in a normal subject (*A*), a patient with cerebellar atrophy (*B*), left pontine lesion (astrocytoma) (*C*), and bilateral lesion of the MLF (*D*). In the normal subject the eyes alternately deviate in the direction of the slow component for each half cycle of induced nystagmus. In humans, the average eye position in the orbit for initiation of fast components is near the midline, from which the eyes take a countercompensatory direction (see Fig. 6–32*A*), contrary to what happens in afoveate animals (e.g., rabbits).[124] Fast components (saccades) are generated in the paramedian pontine reticular formation, and the cerebellum controls (finetunes) the amplitude of both voluntary and involuntary saccades. In the patient with cerebellar atrophy (Fig. 6–32*B*) the nystagmus pattern is disorganized, with fast component occurring in random fashion, causing marked beat-to-beat variability in amplitude. This type of abnormality has been termed dysrhythmia and commonly occurs in patients with varieties of cerebellar lesions. Patients with dysrhythmic vestibular nystagmus also demonstrate dysmetria of voluntary saccades.

The patient with a left pontine lesion (Fig. 6–32*C*) could not produce voluntary or involuntary saccades (fast components) to the left, so that during the half-cycle that normally produces left-beating nystagmus the eyes tonically deviated to the right. In patients with bilateral pontine lesions, the eyes tonically deviate to the right and left with each half-cycle of rotation because of the complete absence of fast components.[125] One might mistakenly interpret this abnormality as an absent vestibular response.

The patient with a bilateral MLF lesion (Fig. 6–32*D*) demonstrates dissociation in fast components between the two eyes. When either "paretic" abducting eye is re-

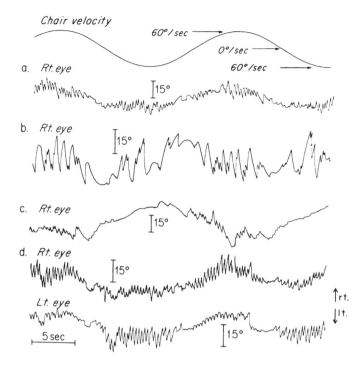

FIGURE 6–32. ENG recordings of nystagmus response to sinusoidal rotation at 0.05 Hz, peak velocity 60° per second in normal subject (*A*) and in patients with cerebellar atrophy (*B*), left pontine glioma (*C*), and bilateral MLF lesions caused by multiple sclerosis (*D*). (From Baloh, RW, and Honrubia, V: Clinical Neurophysiology of the Vestibular System, ed 2. FA Davis, Philadelphia, 1990, p 162, with permission).

quired to produce a fast component, nystagmus beats are rounded because of decrease in frequency of action potentials arriving at the medial rectus motor neurons via the damaged MLF. Abducting fast components, however, are normal, because the abducting muscles (abducens nuclei) receive their innervation for fast components directly from the paramedian pontine reticular formation, with no involvement of the MLF. Frequently, the abducting fast components are actually too large, and the oculomotor control centers attempt to overcome the block at the MLF by increasing the innervation transmitted from the paramedian pontine region to the paretic oculomotor neurons.[26,126] Because, according to Herring's law, this increased innervation is transmitted equally to the two synergistic muscles—the medial and lateral rectus—the difference in amplitude between adducting and abducting fast components is further magnified.

Tests of Visual Vestibular Interaction

The maintenance of gaze and posture is accomplished by interaction of inputs from the vestibular, visual, and proprioceptive systems. Daily activity requires normal functioning of the three reflexes. The vestibular nucleus is the crucial center where interaction takes place among these multiple sensory inputs. The same vestibular neurons that respond to vestibular stimulation also respond to smooth-pursuit and optokinetic stimuli.[127] The interaction of the reflexes is the result of complex mechanisms that can be explained on the basis of elementary control-theory principles. The VOR is an open-loop reflex; that is, it does not have the capacity to monitor and appropriately adjust its own performance when a subject is rotated in the dark. The smooth pursuit and optokinetic systems function as closed-loop reflexes. An example of the interaction occurs during low-frequency head movements. Below about 0.5 Hz, visual reflexes are dominant; at higher frequencies input from the vestibular system alone is sufficient to maintain retinal stability.

There is clear experimental evidence of how these interactions take place. The optokinetic and smooth pursuit signals reach vestibular nuclei converging with peripheral vestibular inputs in second-order neurons. Visual inputs arrive by different pathways that involve several brain centers from the cerebral cortex to the medulla. Among these, the cerebellar flocculus is known to relay smooth-pursuit signals to vestibular nucleus cells. For a recent review of this problem see related publications from the University of California, Los Angeles, Vestibular Adaptation Symposium.[128] Tests of visual vestibular interaction take advantage of these different anatomic connections in acquiring data for the purpose of topological diagnosis. Diagnostic interpretation of the results should be based on and is strengthened by using predictions of heuristic models of visual vestibular interactions, as described.[1,55]

METHODS OF TESTING AND RESULTS IN NORMAL SUBJECTS

In spite of some theoretical limitations, clinical experience since the 1980s has demonstrated important applications of tests of visual vestibular interaction. Of the many possible combinations of stimuli, the one most commonly used in our laboratory is the following. The patient is first tested independently for smooth-pursuit, optokinetic, and VOR functions, as described earlier in this chapter, and then with synergistic and antagonistic vestibular and visual stimuli. For these the subject is rotated either sinusoidally or with a step change in velocity while (1) the surrounding optokinetic drum is stationary (to induce the visual VOR [VVOR], a synergistic interaction of visual and vestibular systems) or (2) drum and chair are coupled so that they move together to accomplish fixation suppression (VOR-FIX) that is, creating an antagonistic interaction between visual and vestibular systems. Fixation suppression can also be tested by rotating the subject in the dark with a single fixation light attached to the chair.

Typical responses of a normal subject to low-frequency sinusoidal (0.05 Hz) VOR, VVOR and VOR-FIX stimulation are shown in Figure 6–33. In each case, peak stimulus velocity is 60° per second. At this low frequency and peak velocity the normal subject has a VVOR gain of one (i.e., slow component eye velocity is equal and opposite to head velocity) and a VOR-FIX gain of zero (i.e., the subject is able to suppress completely the VOR with fixation). Gain (mean ± standard deviation) for the complete test battery in 20 normal subjects was: smooth pursuit, 0.96 ± 0.06 (0.2 Hz ± 18°); OKN, 0.83 ± 0.13; VOR, 0.50 ± 0.15; VVOR, 0.99 ± 0.05; VOR-FIX, 0.03 ± 0.02.

RESULTS IN PATIENTS

Examples of responses from tests of visual-vestibular interaction reflexes in patients with different inner ear pathologies are shown in Figure 6–34. Patients with peripheral vestibular lesions have decreased and/or asymmetric VOR gain, but visual vestibular responses are usually normal at low stimulus frequencies and velocities (see Fig. 6–34, center and right). Even with complete bilateral loss of vestibular function, the visual motor system can provide good ocular stability. At high frequencies and velocities, however, VVOR gain decreases if VOR gain decreases.[129]

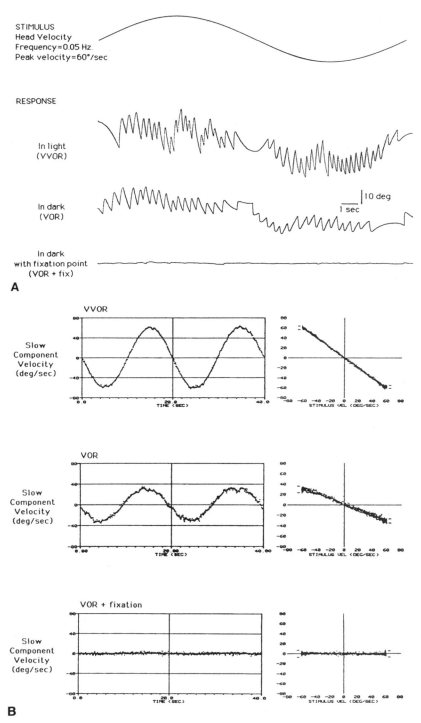

FIGURE 6–33. (*A*) Three typical eye movement responses to a sinusoidal rotatory stimulus as indicated in the frequency under three test conditions: in the light (VVOR), in the dark (VOR), and in the dark with a fixation point that moves with the subject (VOR+FIX). (*B*) Computer analysis of the slow component velocity for the three responses during the rotatory test illustrated in *A*.

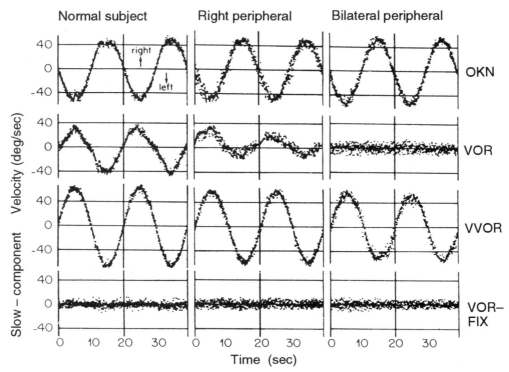

FIGURE 6–34. Plots of slow component velocity versus time from the first four standard sinusoidal rotatory tests (0.05 Hz, peak velocity 60° per second) in a normal subject and patients with peripheral vestibular lesions. (From Baloh, RW, et al: Quantitative assessment of visual-vestibular interaction using sinusoidal rotatory stimuli. In Honrubia, V, and Brazier, MAB (eds): Nystagmus and Vertigo: Clinical Approaches to the Patient with Dizziness. UCLA Forum in Medical Sciences, No 24. Academic Press, New York, 1982, p 233, with permission.)

In patients with central lesions, three abnormal patterns of visual vestibular interaction seen on low frequency sinusoidal testing are shown in Figure 6–35.[110] Patients with lesions involving the vestibular nucleus region (e.g., with Wallenberg's syndrome) exhibit prominent oculomotor abnormalities. OKN and VOR responses are asymmetric but in opposite directions. Despite decreased OKN gain, VVOR gain is normal in both directions. Fixation suppression of VOR slow components toward the side of the lesion is impaired. A similar pattern of abnormalities was found in six other patients with infarction in the lateral medulla.[126]

Patients with lesions involving the vestibulocerebellum are unable to modify vestibular responses with vision. This inability is illustrated by the patient data shown in Figure 6–35 (*center*), in which VOR, VVOR, and VOR-FIX gains are approximately the same (nearly one) and OKN gain is markedly decreased in both directions.

Lesions of the visual motor pathways from the parieto-occipital cortex to the pons lead to impaired smooth pursuit and optokinetic slow components toward the side of the lesion.[86,87,92] The abnormal visual ocular control does not impair VOR responses but does alter visual-vestibular interaction. Typical responses to the four sinusoidal ro-

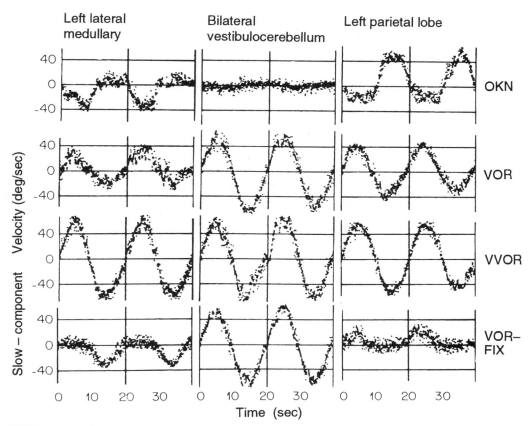

FIGURE 6–35. Plots of slow component velocity versus time from the four standard sinusoidal rotatory tests (0.05 Hz, peak velocity 60° per second in a variety of patients with CNS lesions. (From Baloh, RW, et al: Quantitative assessment of visual-vestibular interaction using sinusoidal rotatory stimuli. In Honrubia, V, and Brazier, MAB (eds): Nystagmus and Vertigo: Clinical Approaches to the Patient with Dizziness. UCLA Forum in Medical Sciences, No 24. Academic Press, New York, 1982, p 233, with permission.)

tatory test conditions in a patient with a deep parietal lobe lesion are shown in Figure 6–35 (*right*). OKN gain is normal to the right and markedly decreased to the left. VOR gain is normal in both directions, but the patient was unable to inhibit VOR slow components to the right with fixation (i.e., VOR-FIX gain is increased to the right). VVOR gain is slightly asymmetric, with lower gain to the left than to the right. As noted, in patients with minimal or absent sinusoidal OKN and smooth pursuit, sinusoidal VOR, VVOR and VOR-FIX responses are almost identical (Figure 6–35, *center*).

In summary, modern rotational testing examines the VOR as well as visual vestibular interaction. Lesions of the peripheral vestibular system typically impair only the VOR, whereas lesions of the CNS impair OKN and visual-vestibular interaction. The pattern of abnormal responses can help localize the lesions within central pathways. A summary of diagnostic possibilities offered by combined use of the visual-vestibular interaction battery is shown in Table 6–5.

TABLE 6–5 Summary of Diagnostic Implications of the Visuovestibular Interaction Test

Location of Lesion	OKN		VOR		VVOR		VOR-FIX	
	Gain[a]	Phase	Gain[a]	Phase	Gain[a]	Phase	Gain[a]	Phase[b]
Labyrinth or eighth nerve unilateral	Normal	Normal	Decreased contralaterally[c] acutely	Increased phase lead	Normal	Normal	Normal	—
Bilateral	Low normal	Normal	Decreased bilaterally	Increased phase lead	Low normal	Normal	Normal	—
Lateral medulla	Decreased bilaterally ipsilaterally > contralaterally	Normal	Asymmetric variable direction	Increased phase lead	Low normal	Normal	Increased bilaterally ipsilaterally > contralaterally	—
Bilateral vestibulo-cerebellum	Decreased bilaterally	Normal	Increased bilaterally	Normal	Normal	Increased phase lead	Increased bilaterally	—
Unilateral parietal lobe	Decreased ipsilaterally[c]	Normal	Normal	Normal	Decreased ipsilaterally[c]	Normal	Increased contralaterally	—

[a]Peak slow-phase eye velocity/peak stimulus velocity.
[b]Normal subjects completely inhibit the VOR at this frequency and peak velocity.
[c]Direction of slow-component eye movement.
Source: From Honrubia and Brazier,[118] p 231, with permission.

Subjective Vestibular Tests

Although simple in concept, the quantification of the sensation of self-motion, which is the most common problem of vestibular patients, has been a difficult task for clinicians. With vestibular stimulation, it is often difficult to recognize the beginning of motion and to differentiate purely vestibular-derived information from that obtained through visual, tactile, or proprioceptive stimuli. Indeed, because of these interactions, even normal humans experience a variety of illusions of motion which can lead to hazardous situations.

Of the vestibular system, the psychophysics of semicircular canals have been the most intensively studied. The canals are thought to operate like velocity sensors in the frequency range of head movements. For example, when subjects are stimulated with angular rotations, they qualitatively describe the sensation as "moving" to the left or to the right. The characteristics of these psychophysical phenomena follow the prediction of the pendulum model of vestibular function in that perception of motion corresponds to velocity of head motion in a manner similar to the slow velocity component of eye movement being associated with this stimulus. In accordance with this model, the threshold for the perception of motion is approximately 1° per second for all frequencies within the range of natural head movements (Fig. 6–36).[130]

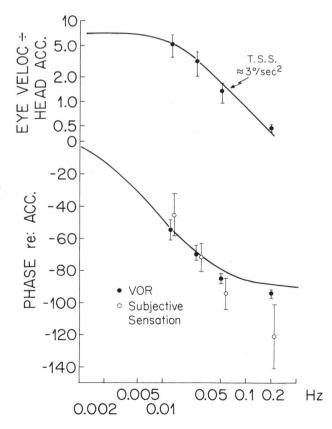

FIGURE 6–36. Summary of gain and phase measurements of VOR and of phase measurements of subjective sensation evaluations in normal subjects. Bars indicate 1 standard deviation around mean values. Abscissa indicates frequency of stimulus; ordinate indicates ratio of eye velocity to head acceleration (*top*) or phase of responses in relation to head acceleration (*bottom*). In the latter, all values are negative, indicating lag of reflex reactions to stimuli. Also indicated is the threshold for sensation in terms of acceleration for a sinusoidal stimulus of 0.05 Hz (about 3.0° per second). (From Honrubia, V, et al: Comparison of vestibular subjective sensation and nystagmus responses during computerized harmonic acceleration tests. Ann Otol Rhinol Laryngol 91:498, 1982, with permission.)

The evaluation of these psychophysical data is still in the experimental stage, but some important observations have been made in a recent study.[131–133] Using physiological sinusoidal stimulation of the HSCs, it was shown that subjects, while being rotated and asked to fixate on a visual target (VT) moving vertically, judge the velocity of the VT in a simple trigonometric interaction between the eye velocity of the vestibular compensatory eye movement (horizontally moving, slow component nystagmus in the dark) and the VT's velocity. The VT is no longer perceived as vertical but as if moving in a tilted angle. This occurs in spite of the fact that the subjects' eyes are fixating on the movable VT and reproduce perfectly its pure vertical trajectory (Fig. 6–37 and Fig. 6–38). That is, subjects experience the illusion that the VT's trajectory is the resulting vector between its velocity and the "normal" vestibular slow component velocity—

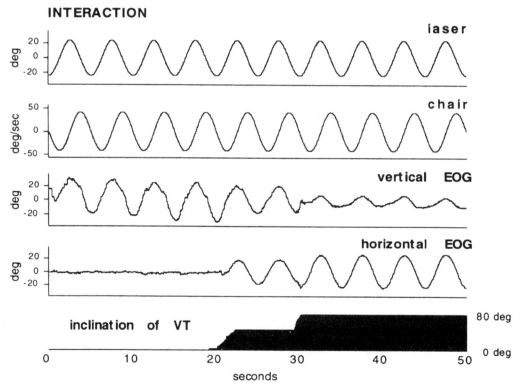

FIGURE 6–37. Interaction. This figure displays raw data from the horizontal vestibular and vertical visual interactive motor-psychophysical experiment. The first record shows the position of the laser as a function of time. The peak velocity is 30° per second and the frequency is 0.2 Hz. The third record shows the vertical electro-oculographic (EOG) signal. The fourth record is the corresponding horizontal EOG signal. The fifth record shows the angle of inclination from the vertical of the tracking laser. The changes in the visual target angle trajectory occur at the same time as the amplitude changes in the vertical and horizontal records. As the subject intends to rectify the motion of the tilted visual target toward a subjective vertical plane there is a diminution of the vertical EOG associated with a corresponding increase of the horizontal EOG. The earlier part of the horizontal EOG is flat as the eye moves strictly vertical, even though the subject believes it is tilted to the side. The final vertical illusion was approximately 80°. (From Honrubia, V, and Greenfield, A: A novel psychophysical illusion. Am J Otol 19(4):517, 1998, with permission.)

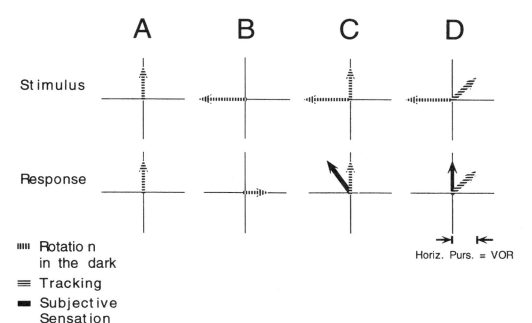

FIGURE 6–38. Schematic representation of stimulus-response expectations underlying experiments of visual-vestibular eye movements and subjective sensation interaction. (*A*) Laser tracking in the vertical direction only. (*B*) Horizontal vestibular stimulation only, with no targets for fixation. (*C*) Superposition of the first two cases. (*D*) Situation after inclination of the visual target trajectory so that it appears vertical to the subject. The magnitude of the horizontal component is indicated at "Horiz. Purs." It is expected that this component will be equal to the response in (*B*). Tracking stimuli and responses are indicated by arrows shaded with a horizontal pattern. Vestibular stimuli and responses are indicated by arrows shaded with a vertical pattern. Subjective responses are shown by solid arrows. (From Honrubia, V, and Greenfield, A: A novel psychophysical illusion. Am J Otol 19(4):516, 1998, with permission.)

without interaction. The illusion is corrected by tilting the VT by an angle whose magnitude is predicted by the magnitude of the vestibular slow component velocity.

The results of these experiments are consistent with the notion that the brain uses vestibular nerve inputs to determine the position of the head in relation to the earth coordinates. During unnoticeable vestibular stimulation, such as in these experiments, when the subjects are rotated in the dark and fixating on the moving light, the afferent vestibular nerve input must subconsciously change the brain internal reference center for orientation, creating an illusionary change in the moving light trajectory. In other words, the vestibular nerve input modulates the brain's estimation of self motion and position and as a consequence, the trajectory of an earth fixed reference—the vertically moving visual target—is erroneously interpreted as moving obliquely.

An interesting corollary of this observation is the thought that a similar mechanism operating in patients with spontaneous nystagmus will result in an illusion of motion of the environment while the patient is stationary, as is the case with most patients. The magnitude of the error should be related to the vestibular stimuli that will produce an equivalent velocity in the slow component eye movement. Furthermore, patients will also have difficulty judging the relative motion of objects around them. Although more research needs to be conducted in this area, it is obvious that the examiner should be acutely aware of and understand the disorientation experienced by patients.

REFERENCES

1. Baloh, RW, and Honrubia, V: In Plum, F, et al (eds): Clinical Neurophysiology of the Vestibular System, 2 ed. Contemporary Neurology Series. FA Davis, Philadelphia, 1990.
2. Honrubia, V: Contemporary vestibular function testing: Accomplishments and future perspectives. In Clinical Applications of Vestibular Science Symposium, 1994. University of California, Los Angeles: Otolaryngology—Head and Neck Surgery, 1994.
3. Honrubia, V, et al: Quantitative evaluation of dizziness characteristics and impact on quality of life. Am J Otol 17:595, 1996.
4. Fenn, WO, and Hursh, JB: Movements of the eyes when lids are closed. Am J Physiol 118:8, 1937.
5. Pousner, ER, and Lion, KS: Testing eye muscles. Electronics 23:96, 1950.
6. Coats, AC: Electronystamography. In Bradford, L (ed): Physiological Measures of the Audio-Vestibular System, Academic Press, New York, 1975, p 37.
7. Barber, HO, and Stockwell, CW: Manual of Electronystagmography. Mosby, St Louis, 1976.
8. Kamei, T, and Kornhuber, HH: Spontaneous and head shaking nystagmus in normals and in patients with central lesions. Can J Otolaryngol 3:372, 1974.
9. Barber, HO, and Wright, G: Positional nystagmus in normals. Adv Otorhinolaryngol 19:276, 1973.
10. Lin, J, et al: Direction-changing positional nystagmus: Incidence and meaning. Am J Otolaryngol 7:306, 1986.
11. Barry, W, and Melvill Jones, G: Influence of eye lid movement upon electro-oculographic recording of vertical eye movements. Aerospace Med 36:855, 1965.
12. Honrubia, V, et al: Computer analysis of induced vestibular nystagmus. Rotatory stimulation of normal cats. Ann Otol Rhinol Laryngol 3(suppl 3):7, 1971.
13. Baloh, RW, et al: On-line analysis of eye movements using a digital computer. Aviat Space Environ Med 51:563, 1980.
14. Leigh, RJ, and Zee, DS: The Neurology of Eye Movements. FA Davis, Philadelphia, 1983.
15. Lorente De No, R: Observations on nystagmus. Acta Otolaryngol (Stockh) 21:46, 1935.
16. Cogan, DG: Congenital nystagmus. Can J Ophthalmol 2:4, 1967.
17. Baloh, RW, et al: Periodic alternating nystagmus. Brain 99:11, 1976.
18. Davis, DG, and Smith, JL: Periodic alternating nystagmus. A report of eight cases. Am J Ophthalmol 72:757, 1971.
19. Baloh, RW, et al: Eye movements in patients with Wallenberg's syndrome. Ann N Y Acad Sci 374:600, 1981.
20. Baloh, RW, and Yee, RD: Spontaneous vertical nystagmus. Rev Neurol 145:527, 1989.
21. Halmagyi, GM, et al: Downbeating nystagmus. A review of 62 cases. Arch Neurol 40:777, 1983.
22. Fisher, A, et al: Primary position upbeating nystagmus. A variety of central positional nystagmus. Brain 106:949, 1983.
23. Aschoff, JC, et al: Acquired pendular nystagmus with oscillopsia in multiple sclerosis: A sign of cerebellar nuclei disease. J Neurol Neurosurg Psychiatr 37:570, 1974.
24. Baloh, RW, et al: Cerebellar-pontine angle tumors. Results of quantitative vestibulo-ocular testing. Arch Neurol 33:507, 1976.
25. Hood, JD: Further observations on the phenomenon of rebound nystagmus. Ann N Y Acad Sci 374:532, 1981.
26. Baloh, RW, et al: Internuclear ophthalmoplegia. II. Pursuit, optokinetic nystagmus, and vestibulo-ocular reflex. Arch Neurol 35:490, 1978.
27. Cogan, DG, et al: Unilateral internuclear ophthalmoplegia: Report of eight clinical cases and one post-mortem study. Arch Ophthalmol 44:783, 1950.
28. Spooner, JW, and Baloh, RW: Eye movement fatigue in myasthenia gravis. Neurology 29:29, 1979.
29. Barany, R: Neue Untersuchungsmethoden, die Beziehungen zwischen Vestibular-apparat, Kleinhirn, Grosshirn and Ruckenmark betreffend. Wien med Wchnschr 60:2033, 1910.
30. Jongkees, LBW: On positional nystagmus. Acta Otolaryngol (suppl)159:78, 1961.
31. Nylen, CO: Positional nystagmus. A review and future prospects. J Laryngol Otol 64:295, 1950.
32. Dix, M, and Hallpike, C: The pathology, symptomatology and diagnosis of certain common disorders of the vestibular system. Ann Otol Rhinol Laryngol 61:987, 1952.
33. Schuknecht, HF: Pathology of the Ear. Harvard Univ. Pr., Cambridge, MA, 1974.
34. Hall, SF, et al: The mechanics of benign paroxysmal vertigo. J Otolaryngol 8:151, 1979.
35. Parnes, LS, and McClure, JA: Posterior semicircular canal occlusion in the normal hearing ear. Otolaryngol Head Neck Surg 104:52, 1991.

36. Welling, D, et al: Particulate matter in the posterior semicircular canal. Laryngoscope 107:90, 1997.
37. Epley, JM: The canalith repositioning procedure: For treatment of benign paroxysmal positional vertigo. Otolaryngol Head Neck Surg 107:399, 1992.
38. Ito, M: The vestibulo-cerebellar relationships: Vestibulo-ocular reflex arc and flocculus. In Naunton, R.F. (ed): The vestibular system. Academic, New York, 1975.
39. Lorente De No, R: Anatomy of the eighth nerve: The central projection of the nerve endings of the internal ear. Laryngoscope 43:1, 1933.
40. Lorente De No, R: Vestibulo-ocular reflex arc. Arch Neurol Psychiatr 30:245, 1933.
41. McClure, JA: Horizontal canal BPV. J Otolaryngol 14:30, 1985.
42. Pagnini, P, et al: Benign paroxysmal vertigo of the horizontal canal. Orl J Otorhinolaryngol Relat Spec 51:161, 1989.
43. Baloh, RW, et al: Horizontal semicircular canal variant of benign positional vertigo. Neurology 43:2542, 1993.
44. Baloh, RW, et al: Persistent direction-changing positional nystagmus: Another variant of benign positional nystagmus? Neurology 45:1297, 1995.
45. Epley, JM: Positional vertigo related to semicircular canalithiasis. Otolaryngol Head Neck Surg 112:154, 1995.
46. Epley, J: Caveats in particle repositioning for treatment of canalithiasis (BPPV). Oper Tech Otolaryngol Head Neck Surg 8:68, 1997.
47. Baloh, RW, et al: Benign paroxysmal positional nystagmus. Am J Otolaryngol 1:1, 1979.
48. Honrubia, V, et al: Paroxysmal positional vertigo syndrome. Am J Otol 20:o–o, 1999.
49. Baloh, RW, et al: The mechanism of benign paroxysmal positional nystagmus. Adv Otorhinolaryngol 25:161, 1979.
50. Baloh, RW, et al: Benign positional vertigo: clinical and oculographic features in 240 cases. Neurology 37:371, 1987.
51. Grand, W: Positional nystagmus: An early sign in medulloblastoma. Neurology 21:1157, 1971.
52. Gregorius, FK, et al: Positional vertigo with cerebellar astrocytoma. Surg Neurol 6:283, 1976.
53. Cawthorn, T, and Hinchcliffe, R: Positional nystagmus of the central type as evidence of subtentorial metastases. Brain 84:415, 1961.
54. Barber, HO: Positional nystagmus: Testing and interpretation. Ann Otol Rhinol Laryngol 73:838, 1964.
55. Lau, CG, et al: A linear model for visual-vestibular interaction. Aviat Space Environ Med 49:880, 1978.
56. Honrubia, V, et al: Evaluation of rotatory vestibular tests in peripheral labyrinthine lesions. In Nystagmus and Vertigo: Clinical Approaches to the Patient with Dizziness. UCLA Forum in Medical Sciences. Academic, New York, 1982.
57. Henriksson, NG: The correlation between the speed of the eye in the slow phase of nystagmus and vestibular stimulus. Acta Otolaryngol (Stockh) 45:120, 1955.
58. Honrubia, V, et al: Vestibulo-ocular reflexes in peripheral labyrinthine lesions: II. Caloric testing. Am J Otolaryngol 5:93, 1984.
59. Sills, AW, et al: Caloric testing 2. results in normal subjects. Ann Otol Rhinol Laryngol Suppl 86(suppl 43):7, 1977.
60. Lisberger, SG, et al: Visual motion processing and sensory-motor integration for smooth pursuit eye movements. Annu Rev Neurosci 10:97, 1987.
61. Collewijn, H, and Tamminga, EP: Human smooth and saccadic eye movements during voluntary pursuit of different target motions on different backgrounds. J Physiol 351:217, 1984.
62. Baloh, RW, and Honrubia, V: Reaction time and accuracy of the saccadic eye movements of normal subjects in a moving-target task. Aviat Space Environ Med 47:1165, 1976.
63. Crane, TB, et al: Analysis of characteristic eye movement abnormalities in internuclear ophthalmoplegia. Arch Ophthalmol 101:206, 1983.
64. Meienberg, O, et al: Clinical and oculographic examinations of saccadic eye movements in the diagnosis of multiple sclerosis. Arch Neurol 43:438, 1986.
65. Metz, HS, et al: Ocular saccades in lateral rectus palsy. Arch Ophthalmol 84:453, 1970.
66. Solingen, LD, et al: Subclinical eye movement disorders in patients with multiple sclerosis. Neurology 27:614, 1977.
67. Yee, RD, et al: Rapid eye movements in myasthenia gravis. II. Electro-oculographic analysis. Arch Ophthalmol 94:1465, 1976.
68. Leigh, RJ, et al: Abnormal ocular motor control in Huntington's disease. Neurology 33:1268, 1983.
69. Troost, BT, and Daroff, RB: The ocular motor defects in progressive supranuclear palsy. Ann Neurol 2:397, 1977.
70. Baloh, RW, et al: Effect of alcohol and marijuana on eye movements. Aviat Space Environ Med 50:18, 1979.
71. Gentles, W, and Thomas, EL: Commentary. Effect of benzodiazepines upon saccadic eye movements in man. Clin Pharmacol Ther 12:563, 1971.
72. Wilkinson, IM, et al: Alcohol and human eye movement. Brain 97:785, 1974.
73. Zee, DS, et al: Ocular motor abnormalities in hereditary cerebellar ataxia. Brain 99:207, 1976.
74. Furman, JM, et al: Eye movements in Friedreich's ataxia. Arch Neurol 40:343, 1983.

75. DeJong, JD, and Jones, GM: Akinesia, hypokinesia, and bradykinesia in the oculomotor system of patients with Parkinson's disease. Exp Neurol 32:58, 1971.
76. White, OB, et al: Ocular motor deficits in Parkinson's disease. II. Control of the saccadic and smooth pursuit systems. Brain 106:571, 1983.
77. Sharpe, JA, et al: Control of the saccadic and smooth pursuit systems after cerebral hemidecortication. Brain 102:387, 1979.
78. Zee, DS, et al: Congenital ocular motor apraxia. Brain 100:581, 1977.
79. Baloh, RW, et al: Ataxia-telangiectasia. Quantitative analysis of eye movements in six cases. Neurology 28:1099, 1978.
80. Spooner, JW, et al: Effect of aging on eye tracking. Arch Neurol 37:575, 1980.
81. Zackon, DH, and Sharpe, JA: Smooth pursuit in senescence: Effects of target velocity and acceleration. Acta Otolaryngol 104:290, 1987.
82. Holzman, PS, et al: Smooth-pursuit eye movements, and diazepam, CPZ, and secobarbital. Psychopharmacologia 44:112, 1975.
83. Rashbass, C: The relationship between saccadic and smooth tracking eye movements. J Physiol 159:326, 1961.
84. Yee, RD, and Al, E: Pathophysiology of optokinetic nystagmus. In Nystagmus and Vertigo: Clinical Approaches to the Patient with Dizziness. UCLA Forum in Medical Sciences. New York, Academic, 1982.
85. Baloh, RW, et al: Vestibulo-ocular function in patients with cerebellar atrophy. Neurology 25:160, 1975.
86. Baloh, RW, et al: Optokinetic nystagmus and parietal lobe lesions. Ann Neurol 7:269, 1980.
87. Leigh, RJ, and Tusa, RJ: Disturbance of smooth pursuit caused by infarction of occipitoparietal cortex. Ann Neurol 17:185, 1985.
88. Zasorin, NL, et al: Influence of vestibulo-ocular reflex gain on human optokinetic responses. Exp Brain Res 51:271, 1983.
89. Honrubia, V, and Luxon, L: Optokinetic nystagmus with reference to the smooth-pursuit system. In Oosterveld, W (ed): Otoneurology, Wiley, Chichester, 1984, p 195.
90. Yee, RD, et al: Slow build-up of optokinetic nystagmus associated with downbeat nystagmus. Invest Ophthalmol Vis Sci 18:622, 1979.
91. Lafortune, S, et al: Human optokinetic after nystagmus. Acta Otolaryngol 101:183, 1986.
92. Baloh, RW, et al: Clinical abnormalities of optokinetic nystagmus. In Lennerstrand, G, and Zee, D (eds): Functional Basis of Ocular Motility Disorders. Pergamon, New York, 1982, p 311.
93. Schmaltz, G: The physical phenomena occurring in the semicircular canals during rotatory and thermic stimulation. Proc Roy Soc Med 25:359, 1932.
94. Paige, GD: Caloric responses after horizontal canal inactivation. Acta Otolaryngol 100:321, 1985.
95. Scherer, H, and Clarke, AH: The caloric vestibular reaction in space. Physiological considerations. Acta Otolaryngol 100:328, 1985.
96. Baertschi, AJ, et al: A theoretical and experimental determination of vestibular dynamics in caloric stimulation. Biol Cybern 20:175, 1975.
97. Zangemeister, WH, and Bock, O: The influence of pneumatization of mastoid bone on caloric nystagmus response. A clinical study and a mathematical model. Acta Otolaryngol 88:105, 1979.
98. Baloh, RW, et al: Caloric testing. 1. Effect of different conditions of ocular fixation. Ann Otol Rhinol Laryngol Suppl 86(suppl 43):1, 1977.
99. Takemori, S: Visual suppression test. Clin Otolaryngol 3:145, 1978.
100. Cogan, D: Neurologic significance of lateral conjugate deviation of the eyes on forced closure of the lids. Arch Ophthalmol 39:37, 1984.
101. Working Group on Evaluation of Tests for Vestibular Function, CoH, Bioacoustics, and Biomechanics: Evaluation of Tests for Vestibular Function. In Aviation, Space & Environmental Medicine. Alexandria, VA, Aerospace Medical Assoc., 1992.
102. Baloh, RW, et al: Caloric testing. 3. Patients with peripheral and central vestibular lesions. Ann Otol Rhinol Laryngol Suppl 86(suppl 43):24, 1977.
103. Elidan, J, et al: On the vertical caloric nystagmus. J Otolaryngol 14:287, 1985.
104. Norre, ME: Caloric vertical nystagmus: The vertical semicircular canal in caloric testing. J Otolaryngol 16:36, 1987.
105. Uemura, T, and Cohen, B: Effects of vestibular nuclei lesions on vestibulo-ocular reflexes and posture in monkeys. Acta Otolaryngol Suppl 315:1, 1973.
106. Furman, JM, and Baloh, RW: Otolith-ocular testing in human subjects. Ann N Y Acad Sci 656:431, 1992.
107. Barany, R: Physiologie und Pathologie des Bogengangsapparates beim Menschen. Deuticke, Vienna, 1907.
108. Montandon, A: A new technique for vestibular investigation. Acta Otolaryngol 39:594, 1954.
109. Sills, AW, et al: Algorithm for the multi-parameter analysis of nystagmus using a digital computer. Aviat Space Environ Med 46:934, 1975.
110. Baloh, RW, et al: Quantitative vestibular testing. Otolaryngol Head Neck Surg 92:145, 1984.
111. Honrubia, V, et al: Vestibulo-ocular reflexes in peripheral labyrinthine lesions: I. Unilateral dysfunction. Am J Otolaryngol 5:15, 1984.

112. Baloh, RW, et al: Impulsive and sinusoidal rotatory testing: A comparison with results of caloric testing. Laryngoscope 89:646, 1979.
113. Baloh, RW, et al: Changes in the human vestibulo-ocular reflex after loss of peripheral sensitivity. Ann Neurol 16:222, 1984.
114. Jenkins, HA, et al: Evaluation of multiple-frequency rotatory testing in patients with peripheral labyrinthine weakness. Am J Otolaryngol 3:182, 1982.
115. Honrubia, V, et al: Ewald's second law of labyrinthine function and the vestibulo-ocular reflex. In The Vestibular System: Function and Morphology. Springer-Verlag, Berlin, 1981.
116. Baloh, RW, et al: Ewald's second law re-evaluated. Acta Otolaryngol 83:475, 1977.
117. Wolfe, J, et al: Low-frequency harmonic acceleration in the evaluation of patients with peripheral labyrinthine disorders. In Nystagmus and Vertigo: Clinical Approaches to the Patient with Dizziness. UCLA Forum in Medical Sciences. New York, Academic, 1982.
118. Honrubia, V, et al: Ewald's second law of labyrinthine function and the vestibulo-ocular reflex. In Gualtierotti, T (ed): The Vestibular System: Function and Morphology. Springer-Verlag, Berlin, 1981, p 509.
119. Honrubia, V, et al: Vestibulo-ocular reflex changes following peripheral labyrinthine lesions. In Ruben, RW (ed): The Biology of Change in Otolaryngology, Proceedings of the Midwinter Meeting, Association for Research in Otolaryngology. Elsevier, Amsterdam, 1986, pp 155–170.
120. Baloh, RW, et al: Horizontal vestibulo-ocular reflex after acute peripheral lesions. Acta Otolaryngol Suppl 468:323, 1989.
121. Goldberg, J, and Fernandez, C: Physiology of peripheral neurons innervating semicircular canals of the squirrel monkey. III. Variations among units in their discharge properties. J Neurophysiol 34:676, 1971.
122. Thurston, SE, et al: Hyperactive vestibulo-ocular reflex in cerebellar degeneration: Pathogenesis and treatment. Neurology 37:53, 1987.
123. Honrubia, V, et al: The patterns of eye movements during physiologic vestibular nystagmus in man. Trans Am Acad Ophthalmol Otolaryngol 84:339, 1977.
124. Lau, CG, and Honrubia, V: Fast component threshold for vestibular nystagmus in the rabbit. J Comp Physiol 160:585, 1987.
125. Baloh, RW, et al: Eye movements in patients with absent voluntary horizontal gaze. Ann Neurol 17:283, 1985.
126. Baloh, RW, et al: Internuclear ophthalmoplegia. I. Saccades and dissociated nystagmus. Arch Neurol 35:484, 1978.
127. Waespe, W, and Henn, V: Gaze stabilization in the primate. The interaction of the vestibulo-ocular reflex, optokinetic nystagmus, and smooth pursuit. Rev Physiol Biochem Pharmacol 106:37, 1987.
128. Honrubia, V: Vestibular adaptation—Introduction. In Vestibular Adaptation Symposium. University of California, Los Angeles, 1996.
129. Hyden, D, et al: Human visuo-vestibular interaction as a basis for quantitative clinical diagnostics. Acta Otolaryngol 94:53, 1982.
130. Honrubia, V, et al: Comparison of vestibular subjective sensation and nystagmus responses during computerized harmonic acceleration tests. Ann Otol Rhinol Laryngol 91:493, 1982.
131. Honrubia, V, et al: Subjective sensation during interaction between horizontal vestibular and vertical pursuit stimulation. Ann N Y Acad Sci 781:407, 1996.
132. Honrubia, V, and Greenfield, A: A novel psychophysical illusion resulting from interaction between horizontal vestibular and vertical pursuit stimulation. Am J Otology 19:513, 1998.
133. Honrubia, V, et al: Optokinetic and vestibular interactions with smooth pursuit: Psychophysical responses. Acta Otolaryngol 112:163, 1992.

CHAPTER 7

Clinical Changes in Vestibular Function With Time After Unilateral Vestibular Loss

Ian S. Curthoys, PhD and G. Michael Halmagyi, MD

It has been known for a more than a century that acute total loss of a previously intact labyrinth, unilateral vestibular loss (or unilateral vestibular deafferentation [uVD]) invariably results in a stereotyped pattern of disruption of equilibrium in species as diverse as fish, amphibians, birds, rodents, monkey, and man. Although the loss is usually permanent, the sensory and motor disruption it causes is usually only temporary. The process of recovery from the neurologic effects of acute uVD is termed **vestibular compensation**.[1-8]

Unilateral vestibular loss is a common clinical event. It occurs as a result of disease, such as acute vestibular neuritis, or as a result of surgical treatment, such as unilateral labyrinthectomy or unilateral vestibular neurectomy. Although most patients recover well from uVD, some do not, and the cause of the poor compensation of those few patients is a question of great research interest. The aim of this chapter is to describe the pattern of onset and resolution of the sensory and motor components after uVD, and the pathophysiological basis of the uVD syndrome in humans.

CONSEQUENCES OF UNILATERAL VESTIBULAR LOSS IN HUMANS

Immediately after uVD, humans invariably experience intense dysequilibrium. This dysequilibrium has both sensory and motor components that can be further categorized as static or dynamic. **Static components** are those present when the person is at rest, whereas the **dynamic components** are those evident only during movement; that is during stimulation of the sole remaining labyrinth by angular or linear acceleration. Some of these perceptual abnormalities are temporary, whereas others appear to be permanent.

It is important to emphasize that the syndrome that develops following acute loss of a normal labyrinth is totally stereotyped in pattern and duration in each species. Some species recover within a few hours (goldfish),[9] whereas in other species recovery takes hours, days, or weeks. Certain behavioral components are invariably present and in any particular species; each component changes over time with a characteristic temporal profile.

To measure precisely the pattern and resolution of the uVD syndrome in humans, it is best to study the same patients before and after surgical deafferentation of one intact labyrinth. Although such cases and the facilities for studying them are few, some long-term quantitative data on the precise sensory and motor consequences of uVD in humans has recently become available.[10–12] In particular, some patients with Ménière's disease probably have normal or near normal labyrinthine function between attacks of vertigo and some of these patients have been studied before and after unilateral vestibular neurectomy.

Static Sensory Components

After surgical uVD, immediately on recovering from the anesthesia, patients experience two different false spatial sensations (i.e., illusions). Both occur at rest, and both resolve within 1 to 2 days. One is an illusion of angular motion in yaw and the other is an illusion of linear tilt in roll. The angular motion illusion is a false sense of angular rotation, either of self or of the world. With eyes closed, the illusion is of self-motion with the body turning about its long axis toward the uVD side. With eyes open, the illusion is of world-motion, now in the opposite direction. These false sensations of rotation are called vertigo. The linear tilt illusion is a false sense of body roll-tilt about the naso-occipital (or roll) axis, again toward the side of the uVD.

Both illusions are probably due to the asymmetry in resting neural activity between the two vestibular nuclei. This asymmetry occurs as a result of the sudden profound decrease in resting activity in the deafferented vestibular nucleus produced by the uVD.[13,14] These illusions occur because it seems that whenever the level of neural activity in one vestibular nucleus exceeds the level of activity in the other, the imbalance is interpreted by the brain as rotation or tilt toward the side generating the higher level of activity. Such an imbalance occurs during a real angular acceleration or a real linear tilt in roll, but also after uVD. The relatively higher level of neural activity in the medial vestibular nucleus (MVN) on the intact side, as compared to the level of activity on the lesioned side, is interpreted by the brain as rotation toward the intact side. Similarly the relatively higher level of resting neural activity in the lateral vestibular nucleus (LVN) of the intact side, is interpreted by the brain as roll-tilt toward the intact side. In both cases the imbalance of neural activity produced by unilateral loss is similar to the imbalance produced by natural stimulation.

Dynamic Sensory Components

Deficits in the perception of angular and linear acceleration stimulation have been found after uVD. Although both deficits improve with time after uVD, in some patients some deficit appears to be permanent.

ANGULAR ACCELERATION PERCEPTION

To evaluate the precision of yaw angular acceleration perception, subjects seated in a rotating chair were asked in a recent study to counter-rotate themselves following a passive rotation in the dark. Brookes et al[15] showed that normal subjects passively rotated through an angle of between 30° and 180° (at a velocity of 80° per second) can, when given control over chair rotation, return the chair precisely back to its starting position. Some chronic uVD patients consistently under-responded to rotations toward the uVD side whereas they were able to respond correctly to rotations toward the intact side. Other uVD patients were able to respond correctly to rotations to either side. These results indicate that perception of angular rotation toward the lesioned side is impaired following uVD, and that this impairment compensates with time in some patients.

LINEAR ACCELERATION PERCEPTION

A normal subject on earth is continuously stimulated by the linear acceleration of gravity. If the person is upright then the direction of the gravitational vector corresponds to the longitudinal axis of his body. If the person is tilted in his coronal (i.e., roll) plane, about his naso-occipital axis, then the angle between his body long axis and the gravitational linear acceleration vector is called the roll-tilt angle. In our terms, the person is said to be experiencing roll-tilt stimulation. Roll-tilt stimulation activates the linear acceleration sensors of the inner ear: the otolithic receptors in the utricle and the saccule of each labyrinth (see Chapter 8).

Another method of producing roll-tilt stimulation is centrifugation. If a subject, seated upright on a centrifuge with his interaural axis parallel to the centrifuge arm, is rotated at a constant angular velocity, he will be subject to a centrifugal linear acceleration (but no angular acceleration). For convenience we refer to centrifugal rather than to centripetal accelerations because the otolithic receptor hair cells are bent in the direction of the centrifugal acceleration. During constant velocity rotation the centrifugal linear acceleration and the gravitational linear acceleration will sum to produce a resultant gravitoinertial force. This resultant force is in the coronal plane and is directed away from the body long axis. It is also a roll-tilt stimulus. If the subject is now centrifuged in total darkness to exclude visual cues to verticality, he will experience an irresistible sensation of being tilted in the roll plane.

Roll-tilt perception is the subjective conscious sensation of body tilt produced by roll-tilt stimulation. If during centrifugation the subject views a luminous, rotatable bar attached to the centrifuge chair and aligned with his interaural axis, the bar will appear to him to be tilted (i.e., rolled) with his body, by the same amount as his body appears to have rolled. This tilt of the subjective visual horizontal with respect to the perceived gravitational horizontal during centrifugation is called the oculogravic "illusion."[16,17] A subject's ability to sense this roll-tilt stimulus during centrifugation can be accurately measured by requiring the subject to return the small visible bar so that it is aligned with respect to the perceived direction of the gravitational horizontal with respect to his interaural axis. The following example shows how this can be done.

Consider a subject sitting upright on a centrifuge, 1 meter from the rotation axis, with his left ear directed toward the rotation axis (Fig. 7–1). The centrifuge rotates at a constant velocity of 30 rpm (equal to 180° per second) in darkness. Because gravitational and linear acceleration are identical physical forces, the subject now cannot but

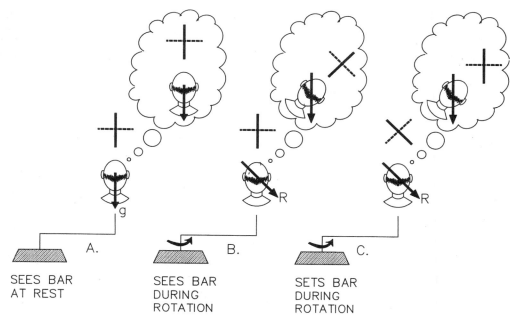

SEES BAR
AT REST

SEES BAR
DURING
ROTATION

SETS BAR
DURING
ROTATION

FIGURE 7–1. Measurement of linear acceleration perception using the oculogravic illusion. *(A)* With the centrifuge at rest in an otherwise darkened room, a normal subject *(shown from behind)*, seated with his interaural axis parallel to the long axis of the centrifuge arm and with his left ear towards the axis of rotation, views a dimly illuminated, gravitationally horizontal, rotatable bar shown here with interrupted lines. At rest he correctly perceives the bar as aligned not only with the gravitational horizontal, but also with his interaural axis. *(B)* When the centrifuge with its 1-meter arm turns at a constant velocity of 180° per second the gravito-inertial resultant force will be directed 45° from the gravitational vector, towards the subject's right labyrinth. In the otherwise darkened room the subject can now only assume that the resultant force is the gravitational force and therefore perceives that his own body long axis has rotated 45° to his right; he will sense a 45° roll-tilt to his right. The illuminated bar is, however, still physically aligned with his own interaural axis and not with the resultant force, so that he perceives the bar as also having rolled with him, 45° to the right. *(C)* When required to set the bar to the perceived gravitational horizontal, the subject does so by rotating the bar 45° to his left (i.e., counter clockwise) and so accurately aligns the bar normal to the resultant force. (From Dai, et al[10]).

regard the gravitoinertial resultant as his subjective gravitational vertical. Because the resultant is now directed from his left to his right, the only percept that will accord with his sensations is that he has been tilted onto his right side.

The angle of resultant linear acceleration is simple to calculate; in this case it is 45°. A normal subject will sense the direction of this resultant accurately, and will therefore perceive that his body has been roll-tilted 45° to his right. If he now views a dimly illuminated, rotatable light bar that is attached to the centrifuge chair, and is physically aligned parallel with his interaural axis (and therefore also normal to the gravitational vertical) it will appear that the bar has tilted with him to the right, also by 45°. He can now indicate the precise angle of perceived body tilt by rotating the bar to his left until it is set to where he perceives the gravitational horizontal to be. Normal subjects centrifuged in darkness can indicate their perception of roll-tilt accurately; they can set a light bar to within 5° of the gravitational horizontal on 95 percent of attempts. These observations show that roll-tilt perception can be accurately measured by nulling the oculogravic illusion and raise the possibility of using roll-tilt perception to measure otolith function clinically. Because roll-tilt perception partly depends on otolithic sensory input and normal subjects have accurate roll-tilt perception, it is possible to test otolith function clinically by means of the oculogravic illusion.

In a study of 30 patients before and after uVD,[10] we found that 1 week after operation all 30 patients showed a loss of sensitivity when given a roll-tilt stimulus toward their affected ear. They showed an asymmetry of roll-tilt perception in that they had a smaller oculogravic illusion for roll-tilt stimuli directed to their affected ear than they had before the operation (Fig. 7–2). This loss of sensitivity became increasingly evident with increasing roll-tilt stimulus angles. Furthermore, even when tested 6 months after uVD, these patients still showed a significant loss of sensitivity to linear accelerations that were medially directed with respect to the single functioning utricle (Fig. 7–3). Asymmetries of roll-tilt perception have been shown during simple roll-tilts to the left and right on a tilting chair.[18–20]

These results indicate that total uVD causes a deficit in roll-tilt perception of linear accelerations directed toward the lesioned side and, although this deficit compensates over time, this compensation is incomplete, and a small but detectable deficit in roll-tilt perception toward the lesioned side is a permanent legacy of uVD.

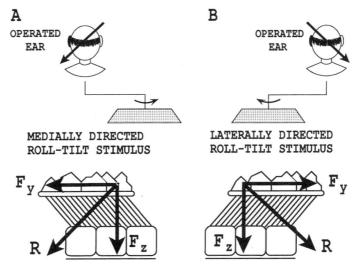

FIGURE 7–2. Medial versus lateral roll tilt stimulation following unilateral vestibular loss. Schematic representation of roll-tilt stimulation of the remaining intact right labyrinth of a patient who has had a left vestibular loss. The patient, viewed from behind, sits across the centrifuge arm so that his interaural axis is colinear with the centrifugal linear acceleration. If his intact right labyrinth is positioned away toward the rotation axis *(A)*, then its otoconial membrane will be displaced medially, toward the center of the head, and he is said to be subject to a medially-directed roll-tilt stimulus. If his intact right labyrinth is positioned away from the rotation axis *(B)*, its otoconial membrane will be displaced laterally, away from the center of the head, and he is said to be subject to a laterally-directed roll-tilt stimulus. The direction of the centrifugal acceleration indicates the direction of bending of the hair cells. The resultant *(R)* has two components: *Fy*, the roll-shear component which acts in the interaural axis, across the mean utricular plane, and *Fz* the component due to gravitational acceleration which acts as a compressive force in the body longitudinal axis. Fz is constant at 1g during centrifugation. (From Dai, et al[10]).

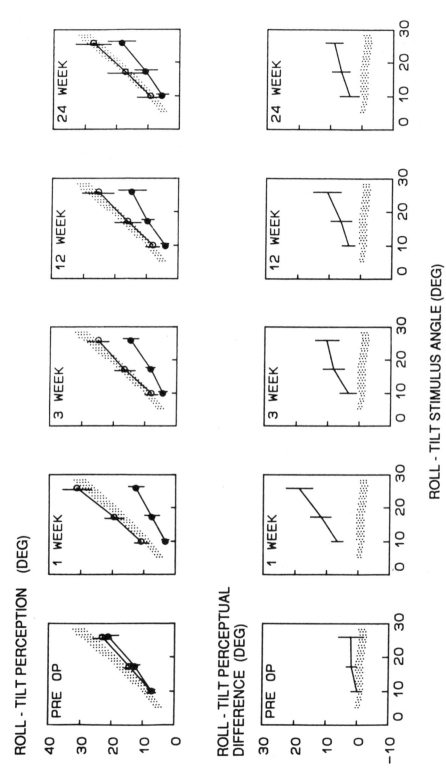

ROLL - TILT STIMULUS ANGLE (DEG)

FIGURE 7–3. Linear acceleration perception before and after unilateral vestibular loss. Summary of results of linear acceleration perception from 33 patients compared to 31 normal subjects. Linear acceleration perception from 33 patients compared to 31 normal subjects at 10°, 17°, and 26° roll-tilt stimulus angle, before and at various times from 1 to 24 weeks after unilateral vestibular loss. Shaded areas show two-tailed confidence intervals for normal subjects. (*Top row.*) Absolute values of perceived roll-tilt angle: open symbols show settings for linear accelerations directed towards the intact labyrinth (i.e., laterally directed roll-tilt stimulation); filled symbols show settings for linear accelerations directed toward the operated labyrinth (i.e., medially directed roll-tilt stimulation). The large interaural difference present 1 week after operation has decreased by 3 weeks but is still abnormal at all stimulus levels even 24 weeks after operation. (*Bottom row.*) Interaural differences in roll-tilt perception remain abnormally high, perhaps indefinitely, after unilateral vestibular loss. (From Dai, et al,[10]).

177

The clinical significance of these results is that oculogravic tests of roll-tilt perception may prove a useful means of detecting severe unilateral loss of dynamic otolith function and may provide a way of monitoring a sensory component of vestibular compensation. Others who have conducted careful tests of roll-tilt perception at a number of angles using a simple tilting chair also confirm the clinical value of such a perceptual test.[18]

Static Motor Components

The static motor components of the uVD syndrome all reflect a motor offset or bias towards the deafferented side. These components reflect both canal and otolithic imbalances.

SPONTANEOUS NYSTAGMUS

A spontaneous horizontal nystagmus is invariably present immediately after uVD. The slow phases are always directed toward the lesioned side. Movements that are clinically apparent are quick phases, and these are directed away from the lesioned side. An observer sees a horizontal eye movement pattern beating away from the lesioned ear. The essential characteristics of uVD nystagmus are the same as that of any other peripheral vestibular nystagmus: it is largely horizontal, unidirectional, and suppressed by visual fixation. Visual fixation suppression may be so effective that the nystagmus will only be apparent when visual fixation is completely excluded, emphasizing the need to check for nystagmus in the absence of visual fixation in all patients with suspected uVD (Fig. 7–4). Clinically, it is possible to exclude visual fixation by using Frenzel glasses or by using an ophthalmoscope to view the fundus of one eye while the other eye is covered.[21] The presence of nystagmus in the absence of visual fixation, combined with the absence of nystagmus in the presence of visual fixation, is definitive evidence that there is a peripheral vestibular lesion, on the side from which the quick phases are beating.

Typically the patient will have primary position (second degree) nystagmus even with visual fixation for the first day after uVD, and then first degree gaze-evoked nystagmus until the end of the first week. Even after a month there will still be a low-velocity (2° to 3° per second) first degree gaze-evoked nystagmus present only in the absence of visual fixation. This appears to be a permanent legacy of uVD.

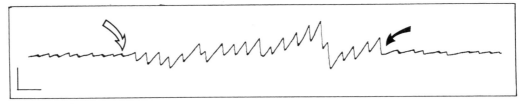

FIGURE 7–4. Peripheral vestibular nystagmus. Oculographic recording shows a left-beating primary-position nystagmus that is obvious only when visual fixation is removed *(open arrow)*, and is quickly suppressed again when visual fixation is permitted *(filled arrow)*. Peripheral vestibular nystagmus can be detected clinically by viewing the fundus of one eye while occluding the other. The patient had a right vestibular neurectomy the previous day. Upward deflections indicate rightward eye movements, downward deflections indicate leftward eye movements. Bar = 10° and 1 sec.

Recent studies suggest that spontaneous nystagmus is due to the loss of resting activity in type I secondary horizontal semicircular canal (HSCC) neurons in the medial vestibular nucleus on the same side as the lesion (called here the "ipsilesional" side). The intensity of the spontaneous nystagmus is held to be an accurate index of the relative resting rates of ipsilesional and contralesional type I HSCC canal neurons (see discussion of "Neural Activity in the Vestibular Nuclei during Vestibular Compensation").

Because the two vertical semicircular canals on one side are also deafferented by a uVD, it is surprising that the torsional component of unilateral nystagmus is so much less apparent than the horizontal component. In fact a prominent torsional component usually indicates that the lesion is in the vestibular nucleus rather than the labyrinth or vestibular nerve. There appears to be no entirely satisfactory explanation for these observations, probably because so few objective measurements of the three-dimensional components of spontaneous nystagmus component following uVD have been made.

OCULAR TILT REACTION

Following uVD there is a tonic ocular tilt reaction consisting of head tilt, conjugate eye torsion, and skew deviation, all directed to the lesioned side.[22] Although head tilt and skew deviation are usually very small, conjugate ipsilesional ocular torsion appears to be invariably present.[11,22–25] The direction of the torsion is always ipsilesional: the 12 o'clock meridians of both eyes are rotated toward the side of the uVD. The magnitude of the ocular torsion can be measured objectively by ocular fundus photography (Fig. 7–5). One week after uVD, there is up to 15° of ocular torsion (on average 9°); one month after uVD the ocular torsion has diminished to about half of the 1-week value. A small but statistically significant ocular torsion (2° to 3°) also appears to be a permanent legacy of uVD.

This change in ocular torsional position can be readily detected in perceptual tests, which show a bias in settings of the subjective visual vertical or horizontal toward the uVD side (see Chapter 8). A normal subject sitting upright in an otherwise totally darkened room can accurately align a dimly illuminated bar to within 2° of the gravitational vertical or horizontal. Thirty patients studied before and after uVD showed that, although their preoperative settings of the visible bar to the perceived gravitational horizontal were reasonably accurate, 1 week after operation they invariably set the bar so that it was tilted down on the side of the uVD, in some cases by up to 15°.[11] It must be emphasized that these patients reported that while seated upright they perceived themselves to be upright and they can set a nonvisual indicator (a somatosensory bar) to the perceived horizontal accurately. The settings of the visual bar correspond very closely to the size of the ocular torsion[11] and our more recent studies have confirmed the very close relationship between ocular torsional position and the visually perceived orientation of short lines.[26]

Although the setting of the visual bar returned toward the horizontal with time, it was still tilted by a mean of 4° 6 months or more after uVD. In all cases the magnitude of the tilting of the visual horizontal was closely correlated with the magnitude of the ocular torsion. It appears therefore that an ipsilesional tilting of the visual horizontal is a permanent legacy of uVD. This result has been confirmed by others.[18,27,28]

The clinical significance of these findings is that careful standardized measurement of the visual horizontal using a dim light bar in an otherwise totally darkened room gives valuable diagnostic information about vestibular (mainly otolithic) function[11,29] (see Chapter 8). A significant tilting of the visual horizontal indicates vestibu-

BEFORE RIGHT VESTIBULAR NEURECTOMY

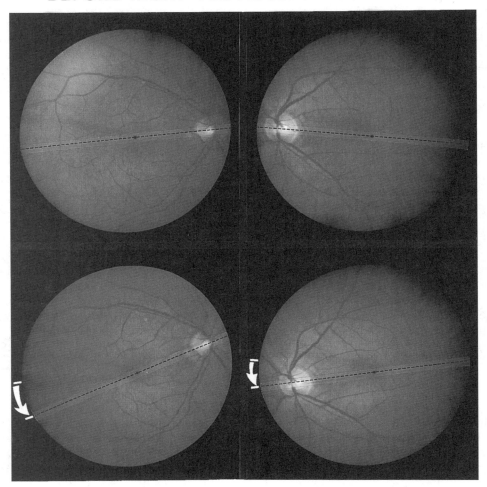

AFTER RIGHT VESTIBULAR NEURECTOMY

FIGURE 7–5. Fundus photographs of the left and right eye of a patient before *(top)* and 1 week after *(bottom)* right vestibular neurectomy. After operation there is tonic rightward torsion of the 12 o'clock meridian of each eye toward the patient's right side. The change in torsion angle measures 18° in the right eye and 16° in the left eye. When the patient was asked to set a luminous bar to the perceived visual horizontal in an otherwise darkened room he set the bar tilted toward his right side by 14.2° when viewing with the right eye and 15.1° when viewing with the left. (From Curthoys, et al[11]).

lar, probably otolithic, hypofunction on the side to which the patient tilts the bar. It is reasoned to be otolithic because semicircular canal activation or loss does not generate a tonically maintained eye position but rather a changing eye position (nystagmus). Although it appears that the tilting of the visual horizontal is due to ocular torsion, the mechanism of the ocular torsion itself is speculative. It is most likely similar to the mechanism of the spontaneous nystagmus that occurs after uVD and reflects decreased resting activity in otolithic secondary vestibular neurons in the ipsilesional vestibular nucleus, owing to loss of input from primary otolithic neurons.[30]

LATEROPULSION

Following uVD there is a position offset or "lateropulsion" of limb and body posture toward the operated side evident in the absence of visual fixation. Many clinical tests can be used to demonstrate this offset including the Barany past pointing test, the Fukuda vertical writing test, or the Unterberger stepping test. Although these are all positive in the first postoperative week, they return to normal after about a month.

POSTURAL DYSEQUILIBRIUM

Despite the apparent return to normal posture on clinical tests, posturographic tests using a standardized posture platform test often show a permanent deficit in postural equilibrium following uVD.[31] This deficit becomes evident if the movements of either the platform alone, or of the platform and the visual surround together, are referenced to the body sway. Static posturography on the other hand yields paradoxical results with those patients who were visually dependent before uVD becoming less so and vice versa.[32] The relationship of these posturographic abnormalities to other tests of vestibular function and to the overall clinical state after uVD is not yet clear. There are many unanswered questions. For example, is a permanent posturographic deficit after uVD simply the result of the UL, or does it imply a subclinical abnormality in the remaining labyrinth be detected before uVD? What is the relationship between an abnormal posturogram and symptomatic chronic vestibular insufficiency? These questions impact both the physical and surgical treatment of vestibular disorders, and these matters are addressed in detail in other chapters.

Dynamic Motor Components

HORIZONTAL VESTIBULO-OCULAR REFLEXES

The changes which occur in the horizontal vestibulo-ocular reflex (VOR) after uVD have been investigated in many species, including monkey and human. The results obtained depend on the stimulus used. In response to low-frequency (1 Hz) low-acceleration ($100°/sec^2$) symmetrical (i.e., sinusoidal) horizontal angular acceleration immediately after uVD, there is a severe and asymmetrical horizontal VOR (HVOR) deficit. The deficit persists for about a month in humans, and then improves so that by 1 year after uVD the HVOR (in response to this type of stimulus) is normal or near normal.[33–35] This improvement in the low-frequency, low-acceleration HVOR is commonly used as an index of vestibular compensation.

If angular accelerations in a natural range are used, a different result is obtained. In monkeys, immediately after uVD there is a profound deficit of both the ipsilesional and contralesional HVOR, but some recovery is already apparent by the second postoperative day. The VOR deficit is most apparent with the fastest head movements. In monkeys, Fetter and Zee[36] have shown, using a test stimulus consisting of constant $125°/sec^2$ angular acceleration stimulation lasting for 2 to 3 seconds, that 3 months after operation the ipsilesional HVOR still has a mean gain that is only 60% of normal and the contralesional HVOR has a gain that is 80% of normal. Using abrupt passive unpredictable head rotations with an angular acceleration up to 3000° per second, we have shown in humans that the ipsilesional HVOR gain up to 2 years after operation is on average still only 25% of normal[12,37,38] (Fig. 7–6 and Fig. 7–7). Some patients may

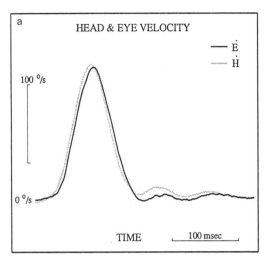
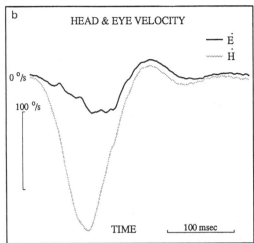

FIGURE 7–6. Single head impulses from a patient 3 years after unilateral vestibular neurectomy. Head velocity is shown in interrupted lines, eye velocity in continuous lines. Eye velocity more or less mirrors head velocity in response to the ampullopetal excitation produced by head rotation toward the intact side. In contrast eye velocity lags head velocity from the onset of head rotation in response to ampullofugal disfacilitation produced by head rotation toward the deafferented side. (From Halmagyi, et al[12]).

show some recovery of gain during this time, but the gain is always less than is physiologically adequate for stabilizing the retinal image during head movement. From this one can presume that the high-acceleration response of the HVOR is never restored to normal after uVD. It appears that dynamic equilibrium, just like static equilibrium, is permanently impaired by uVD.

Two signs of HVOR asymmetry can be detected clinically: head-shaking nystagmus[39] and the head-impulse sign.[40] Head-shaking nystagmus is horizontal nystagmus with quick phases directed toward the normal ear that appears for 3 to 10 seconds after 20 seconds or so of active horizontal head shaking. Like any other type of peripheral vestibular nystagmus, it is absent in the presence of visual fixation and present only in the absence of visual fixation. It is most readily observed using Frenzel glasses. Head-shaking nystagmus is a direct result of the inherent right-left sensory asymmetry of each horizontal semicircular canal (Ewald's second law), signaling to a brainstem neural network, which normally perseverates the peripheral vestibular input (the velocity storage integrator). Head-shaking nystagmus requires a properly functioning velocity storage integrator and can be absent after uVD.[41] The head-impulse sign consists of a compensatory saccade toward the intact ear during or immediately after a rapid passive unpredictable horizontal head rotation toward the affected ear. The sign is always positive in patients with severe unilateral loss of HSCC function. The head-impulse test also depends on Ewald's second law and the ability of rapid head impulses to drive the afferents of the single remaining HSCC to silence.

VERTICAL VESTIBULO-OCULAR REFLEXES

Normal subjects have a symmetric near-unity gain for their pitch VOR in response to 0.4 to 1.6 Hz active sinusoidal head oscillation both in upright and in onside posi-

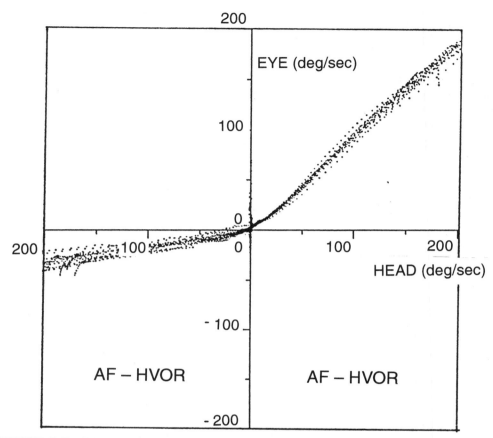

FIGURE 7–7. Horizontal eye velocity plotted as a function of horizontal head velocity for 20 horizontal head impulses in a patient who had undergone a left vestibular neurectomy 3 years previously. There is a profound HVOR deficit in response to head impulses directed toward the deafferented side—the ampullofugal (AF) HVOR. In contrast the HVOR in response to head impulses directed toward the intact side is normal—the ampullopetal (AP) HVOR. (From Halmagyi, et al[12]).

tions.[42] In response to high-acceleration passive head impulses in the upright position, normal subjects have a symmetrical pitch and roll VOR. The gain of the pitch VOR is close to 1, but the gain of the roll VOR is around 0.7. Following uVD there is a bidirectional pitch VOR deficit, and a unidirectional deficit for ipsilesional roll head rotations.[43–48]

DYNAMIC RESPONSES TO OTOLITHIC STIMULATION

During simple roll-tilt of the head, if the head is maintained in a rolled head position (e.g., rolled so that it is toward the left shoulder), the action of the linear acceleration of gravity on the inner ear is different to that with head vertical. The otolithic sensors in the inner labyrinth sense this linear acceleration and cause a reflexive response—a torsion or roll of both eyes, the visual axes in the direction opposite to the direction of the roll-tilt—called ocular counterrolling (OCR). OCR is one of the few accepted measures of otolith operation,[49,50] but it has been shown that uVD does not appear to produce consistent changes in the amplitude of OCR during roll-tilt towards the affected or to the intact ear. There have been few reports of comparable measurements of OCR before and after uVD.

Brief impulsive linear accelerations directed along an interaural axis also activate otolithic receptors and generate a horizontal eye velocity response (an otolith-ocular reflex). This response is equal in magnitude for accelerations directed to either side. There have been reports that there is a smaller response for linear accelerations directed to the intact ear than accelerations directed to the operated ear in post-uVD patients, but the response asymmetry declines within a few weeks.[51,52]

Summary of Changes in Vestibular Function With Time after Lesions

- *Angular rotation illusion:* maximum during first few hours, completely resolved by the third day after uVD.
- *Roll tilt illusion:* maximum during first few hours, completely resolved by third day.
- *Angular acceleration perception deficit:* maximum during first week; in some cases completely resolved at 1 year but in other cases deficit still present; data incomplete.
- *Linear acceleration perception deficit:* maximum during the first week; largely but incompletely resolved within 1 year.
- *Spontaneous nystagmus:* maximum during the first 2 days; improved at 1 week; largely but incompletely resolved within 1 year.
- *Ocular torsion:* maximum during the first week; largely but incompletely resolved within 1 year.
- *Lateropulsion:* maximum during the first 3 days; improved by 1 week; completely resolved within 1 year.
- *Postural dysequilibrium:* maximum during first week; incompletely resolved within 1 year.
- *Horizontal VOR deficit:* maximum during the first week; partial recovery at 1 month; near-complete recovery within 1 year in response to low acceleration stimulation; no significant recovery at all in response to high-acceleration stimulation.
- *Vertical VOR deficit:* persistent deficit at 1 year in response to high acceleration stimulation; data incomplete.
- *Ocular counterrolling:* no long-lasting asymmetry of ocular counterrolling during roll-tilt stimulation. Whether there is an asymmetry early after uVD remains to be established conclusively.

FACTORS INFLUENCING THE RESTORATION OF STATIC AND DYNAMIC EQUILIBRIUM

There is little reliable quantitative information regarding the effects of any physical or chemical interventions on the rate or extent of vestibular compensation in humans. The data that are available come from studies on cats, monkeys, and guinea pigs; much of it is incomplete, inconclusive, or contradictory (for a recent review see Smith and Curthoys,[4] Curthoys and Halmagyi,[5] Dieringer,[6] Vidal *et al.*[8] One reason for these contradictions could be that the large number of different inputs to the vestibular nuclei may all directly or indirectly affect the activity of vestibular nucleus neurons. It should be noted that in general the restoration of static equilibrium (i.e., static compensation) is remarkably robust; very little appears to hasten or hinder it. That robustness is in contrast to the restoration of dynamic equilibrium. Dynamic compensation, which appears to depend at least in part in intact visual, vestibular, and proprioceptive sensory inputs, is usually incomplete.

Visual Inputs

Studies in animals have shown that visual deprivation has no effect on the resolution of the static motor component, spontaneous nystagmus[53a,53b] but such deprivation impedes the recovery of roll head tilt,[54a] which is part of the ocular tilt reaction. Although bilateral occipital lobectomy has no effect on the resolution of spontaneous nystagmus, it does impede the recovery of the HVOR to low-acceleration stimulation.[53] Visual inputs do augment the diminished muscle responses to linear acceleration[54b] and the deficient righting reflexes[55] that occur after uVD. Visual motion deprivation delays recovery of locomotor equilibrium.[56]

Vestibular Inputs

There are only scant data on the effects of vestibular stimulation or deprivation on static or dynamic compensation. In frogs, otolithic stimulation hastens whereas otolithic deprivation delays static compensation of head tilt.[57] In cat low-frequency, combined visual-vestibular stimulation helps reverse the symmetrical deficit in HVOR gain, which occurs in response to low-frequency stimulation following uVD,[58] but has no effect on the asymmetry of the HVOR. There are no data on the effects of vestibular deprivation on vestibular compensation in mammals.

Proprioceptive Inputs

Cervical proprioceptive input could be important in static compensation because head restraint retards resolution of head tilt and spontaneous nystagmus.[59] Somatosensory proprioceptive deprivation appears to retard static compensation,[54b] whereas somatosensory proprioceptive stimulation appears to facilitate the restoration of dynamic postural equilibrium.[60] Acute spinal lesions can produce a temporary decompensation of static postural symptoms.[61,62]

Medications

The restoration of near-normal levels of spontaneous activity in the neurons of the ipsilesional vestibular nucleus in the absence of reinnervation could have a neurochemical basis. Investigations so far have not revealed any changes in glutamate, dopamine, norepinephrine, acetylcholine, histamine, or serotonin receptors, which could account for the restoration of spontaneous activity (for recent reviews see Smith and Darlington,[63] de Waele et al.[7] In several species treatment with an ACTH fragment accelerates static compensation.[64–67] In cat, amphetamine and trimethobenzamide may facilitate both static and dynamic compensation.[68b]

Lesions

Data on the effects of lesions of the cerebellum or its connections on vestibular compensation are contradictory. Whereas some cerebellar lesion studies[68a] show a marked delay in the resolution of spontaneous nystagmus, others[69] show no effect. Although bilateral occipital lobectomy has no effect on the resolution of spontaneous nystagmus, it does impede the recovery of the HVOR to low-acceleration stimulation.[53] Lesions of the brain stem[70] or transcerebellar vestibular commissures[71] do not impede static compensation, at least in mammals. This suggests that input from the contralesional (intact) vestibular nucleus is not essential for static compensation. Section of the brainstem commissures might, however, abolish the HVOR.[80]

It is important to note that in patients with fluctuating vestibulopathies such as Ménière's disease, attacks of vertigo are brief compared with the time required for compensation. In humans compensation takes 3 to 5 days to get under way and a month or more to achieve a functionally useful level. Vestibular compensation cannot help the patient with recurrent or paroxysmal vertigo; the process is too slow. Compensation does, however, help the patient to recover after a permanent uVD.

Chronic Vestibular Insufficiency Following Unilateral Vestibular Loss

Chronic vestibular insufficiency (CVI) is a clinical syndrome consisting of gait ataxia and oscillopsia. The gait ataxia is always most evident when visual and proprioceptive inputs are disrupted, for example, when the patient tries to walk on uneven ground in the dark. The oscillopsia is only evident during head movement, for example, when the patient walks or runs, or when he looks rapidly from side-to-side while driving or crossing a road.[72] CVI can be due to central or peripheral vestibular lesions. It invariably occurs in patients who have severe bilateral loss of vestibular function as evidenced by absent HVOR responses to rapid accelerations and to 0°C caloric stimulation. A common cause of severe bilateral loss of vestibular function is aminoglycoside ototoxicity.[73] Although the CVI may be asymptomatic in some patients with severe bilateral vestibular loss during the activities of daily living, the symptoms and abnormalities can always be demonstrated under certain provocative conditions such as rapid head movements and eye closure on a soft surface.

We have found that certain uVD patients also experience symptomatic CVI.[74] Considering that recent data shows permanent and in some cases severe deficits of horizontal and vertical VORs and postural equilibrium following uVD, this is not entirely surprising.[12,31,45–48] What is surprising is that most uVD patients do not experience symptoms of CVI, even though their VOR and posturographic results are apparently indistinguishable from the results of those patients who do. From a therapeutic viewpoint, it is important to determine what differences there are between patients who do and those who do not experience symptoms of CVI following uVD. Do the symptomatic uVD patients have a subtle defect in the contralesional sole functioning labyrinth, or do they have some defect in the compensation process? This question is under investigation.

The clear result from our research on uVDs over the last 12 years is that when passive head movements with angular accelerations in the natural range are used, uVD patients show long-lasting and probably permanent deficits of their horizontal, vertical and torsional VORs.[44-48] These deficits contrast sharply with the relative ease with which VOR gain can be changed in normal healthy subjects in response to apparently comparable challenges.[75,76] Many studies have shown how the gain of the horizontal VOR (measured in darkness) can be changed as a result of wearing magnifying or minifying lenses for even just a few hours. The VOR gain changes in a direction so as to compensate for this visually induced "challenge." Why, then, does this well-established adaptive plasticity of the VOR of normal healthy subjects not act to restore the gains of the horizontal vertical and torsional VORs of post u-VD patients to a symmetrical value of 1.0?

There are many factors that may prevent mechanisms of VOR adaptive plasticity from operating after uVD. In uVDs the entire vestibular afferent input from one side has been removed, whereas in normal subjects both labyrinths project information to the brainstem and any head movement results in stimulation of both labyrinths symmetrically. To achieve a stable retinal image after uVD, the VOR would have to generate different VOR gains for rotations to each side. VOR plasticity studies to date have required increased or decreased VOR for both directions of rotation. Unilateral vestibular loss disrupts central processing of vestibular information—the so-called velocity storage integrator—and this may disrupt the neural substrates responsible for VOR modification (see Wade et al.[77] for a recent review). Our recent measures have shown that after uVD the axis of eye rotation is not appropriate in that it is not parallel to the axis of head rotation.[45,46] The axis of eye rotation changes during head rotation with the result that the image must be smeared across the retina because of inadequate eye velocity and inappropriate (and changing) axis of eye rotation. Both eye velocity and axis deficits are larger for head rotations toward the lesioned side.

Our present hypothesis is that patients who compensate well for uVD most probably learn to use other responses to minimize the effect of the eye velocity and eye axis deficits. The result is that they probably do not experience the retinal smear resulting from their permanently inadequate VOR. One way appears to be by eliminating smear; a blink during the head movement will effectively prevent the retinal image from being smeared because during the blink there will be no retinal image. Our current measures have confirmed that during natural head movements blinks are common in normal healthy subjects. Experimental measures require subjects to keep their eyes open during gaze shifts; in other words, the measures require subjects to suppress their natural blink response. Patients with uVD may simply be using this natural response mechanism to block out the retinal smear to which their doubly inadequate VOR would otherwise expose them.

NEURAL ACTIVITY IN THE VESTIBULAR NUCLEI DURING VESTIBULAR COMPENSATION

To appreciate the mechanisms of the uVD syndrome and vestibular compensations it is useful to look at the changes in neural activity underlying these changes in behavior (for recent reviews see Goldberg and Fernandez,[78] Smith and Curthoys,[4] and Cirelli et al.[79]

Normal Medial Vestibular Nucleus Activity

Two types of HSCC-driven neurons have been found in the medial vestibular nuclei of monkeys, cats, and guinea pigs. Both types of vestibular nucleus neurons, like primary vestibular neurons, discharge spontaneously (at rest) at rates sometimes in excess of 80 impulses per second. The discharge rate of type I neurons increases when the head acceleration is ipsilateral and decreases when the head acceleration is contralateral. The reverse applies to type II neurons, which increase their discharge rate in response to contralateral head accelerations and decrease their discharge rate in response to ipsilateral head accelerations (Fig. 7–8). The reason that type I and type II neurons respond oppositely is that, whereas type I neurons are excited by ipsilateral HSCC primary afferent neurons and are inhibited by ipsilateral type II neurons, type II neurons themselves are excited by contralateral type I neurons via commissural pathways (see Fig. 7–8). Motor and sensory equilibrium requires equal resting activity of type I neurons in the two medial vestibular nuclei. Type I neurons drive the HVOR by excitatory projections to abducens motoneurons and interneurons in the contralateral abducens nucleus.

Ipsilesional Medial Vestibular Nucleus Activity

Immediately after uVD there are changes in the activity of both type I and type II neurons in the medial vestibular nucleus on the operated side.[14,81b,82b,83a,84a,85a] The resting activity of type I neurons is decreased whereas the resting activity of type II neurons is increased. The decrease in resting activity of type I neurons reflects the loss of excitatory drive by HSCC primary afferent neurons. The increase in resting activity of type II neurons may reflect increased excitatory drive by contralesional type I neurons, which have become disinhibited by the decrease in the activity of contralesional type II neurons, which are themselves normally excited by ipsilesional type I neurons (see Fig. 7–8). As well as showing a reduced resting discharge rate, immediately after uVD ipsilesional type I neurons show a decrease in sensitivity to angular acceleration. The sensitivity of type II neurons to angular acceleration remains unchanged. In the days and weeks that follow, a remarkable series of changes occur in the resting activity of ipsilesional medial vestibular nucleus neurons. The resting discharge rates of both type I and type II neurons is restored to normal even though the medial vestibular nucleus no longer receives any afferent drive from its labyrinth. Data so far, mainly from the guinea pig and the gerbil, have shown a limited restoration of sensitivity of type I neurons to angular accelerations. This restoration of resting activity in type I neurons could also underlie the recovery of humans from the disabling consequences of uVD and the restoration of normal static equilibrium.

Contralesional Medial Vestibular Nucleus Activity

Immediately after unilateral loss there is an increase in the resting activity of contralesional type I neurons without much change in their sensitivity.[13,82b,83a,84a,85a] There

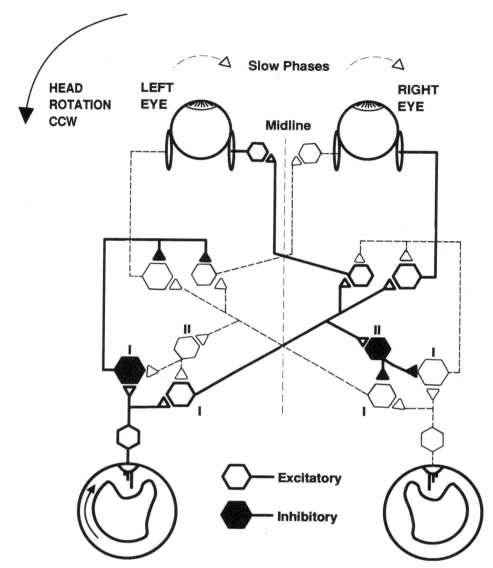

FIGURE 7–8. Schematic simplified representation of the responses in some of the identified connections of the normal HVOR pathways, in response to a counter-clockwise (i.e., leftward) head acceleration. Neurons from the left HSCC are shown in blue; neurons from the right HSCC are shown in yellow. Primary HSCC neurons, excitatory type I medial vestibular nucleus neurons, abducens motoneurons, abducens interneurons and medial rectus motoneurons are shown by open hexagonal symbols. Inhibitory type II medial vestibular nucleus neurons are shown by filled hexagonal symbols.

is also a decrease in the sensitivity of contralesional type II neurons without much change in resting activity. This increase in resting activity of type I neurons is due to decreased inhibition by type II neurons, which are themselves normally excited by ipsilesional type I neurons now silenced. In the following days and weeks, the resting activity of contralesional type I neurons is restored to normal and the resting activity of contralesional type II neurons increases to above normal. These changes in the resting activity of contralesional medial vestibular nucleus neurons occur despite the fact that the ipsilesional vestibular nucleus remains isolated from its labyrinth. However, the remarkable restoration of resting activity in ipsilesional type I neurons described above can account for the changes in activity of contralateral medial vestibular nucleus neurons. The restoration of contralesional type I resting activity to normal is presumably the result of the increased inhibition by contralesional type II neurons, now excited by the restored resting activity of ipsilesional type I neurons. Together with the decrease of contralesional type I resting activity to normal, there is a late decrease in contralesional type I sensitivity, whereas contralesional type II sensitivity remains low.

Normal Lateral Vestibular Nucleus Activity

Primary otolithic neurons project to secondary vestibular neurons mainly in the lateral (and descending) vestibular nuclei. The predominant response of lateral vestibular nucleus neurons is an increase in firing rate in response to ipsilateral tilts (i.e., laterally directed linear accelerations), the alpha response. The commissural connections between secondary otolithic neurons are poorly understood. Unlike the commissural connections of the HSCC secondary neurons in the medial vestibular nucleus, which are direct and functionally inhibitory, it appears that the commissural connections between the secondary otolithic neurons in the lateral vestibular nucleus are indirect and functionally excitatory. There are also interconnections between the lateral and medial vestibular nuclei and some medial vestibular nucleus neurons respond to both semicircular canal and otolithic stimulation. The changes that occur in the lateral vestibular nucleus after uVD vary between the rostroventral and dorsocaudal areas of the nucleus, which project to the cervicothoracic and lumbosacral segments of the spinal cord, respectively.

Ipsilesional Lateral Vestibular Nucleus Activity

There is a decrease in the proportion of roll-tilt responsive neurons in the rostroventral area, but not in the dorsocaudal area, as well as an overall decrease in the average resting activity of neurons.[81a] In contrast, there are increases in the number of position-sensitive neurons, in the tilt sensitivity of dorsocaudal neurons, and in the number of beta responses (increased firing with medially directed linear acceleration). With compensation there is little recovery in the resting activity of either alpha or beta neurons. The proportion of neurons in the rostroventral areas responsive to roll-tilt increases to normal whereas the sensitivity remains normal. The sensitivity of dorsocaudal neurons decreases to normal. The proportion of position sensitivity neurons and beta responses does not change.

Contralesional Lateral Vestibular Nucleus Activity

The proportion of roll-tilt–sensitive neurons is normal. The overall resting activity is slightly reduced. As in the ipsilesional lateral vestibular nucleus, there is an increase in position-sensitive neurons and beta responses, and a decrease in the roll-tilt sensitivity of neurons in the rostroventral areas. There are scanty data on the changes with compensation, but there appear to be few differences in the contralesional neuronal activity in normal and uncompensated cats.[82a]

SUMMARY

"Balance" is a common term used to describe the function of the vestibular system itself. Coincidentally, it also applies to the neural mechanism of vestibular operation. Unilateral loss or disease causes a massive disruption of this nicely balanced neural system and the behavioral symptoms are the manifestations of this imbalance. As the balance in neural activity between the two vestibular nuclei returns, behavioral symptoms, such as nystagmus, disappear. During this time there are significant anatomic changes occurring in the vestibular nuclei.[8,83b,84b,85b,86] Concurrently, other response mechanisms probably substitute for those compensatory responses permanently affected by the aberrant vestibular function. Neural equilibrium is disrupted by uVD in both the MVN and the LVN with consequences for static head and eye position, and for the dynamic response of both the canal and the otolithic systems to imposed stimuli. The major question still unanswered is the cause of the return of firing of neurons in the ipsilesional vestibular nucleus. The answer will likely be found in studies of the neurochemistry of the vestibular nuclei using detailed electrophysiology of the brain slice or isolated whole brain preparations.[87]

ACKNOWLEDGMENTS

This work was supported by the Australian National Health and Medical Research Council, the Garnett Passe and Rodney Williams Memorial Foundation, and by the RPA Hospital Neurology Department Trustees. We owe thanks to Ann Burgess for her meticulous proofreading of the manuscript.

REFERENCES

1. Schaefer, KP, and Meyer, DL: Compensation of vestibular lesions. In Kornhuber, HH (ed): Handbook of Sensory Physiology, Vol VI. Berlin, Springer Verlag, 1974, pp 463–490.
2. Precht, W: Recovery of some vestibuloocular and vestibulospinal functions following unilateral labyrinthectomy. Prog Brain Res 64:381, 1986.
3. Precht, W, and Dieringer, N: Neuronal events paralleling functional recovery (compensation) following peripheral vestibular lesions. Rev Oculomot Res 1:251, 1985.
4. Smith, PF, and Curthoys, IS: Mechanisms of recovery following unilateral labyrinthectomy: A review. Brain Res Rev 14:155, 1989.
5. Curthoys, IS, and Halmagyi, GM: Vestibular compensation: A review of the oculomotor, neural, and clinical consequences of unilateral vestibular loss. J Vestib Res 5:67, 1995.
6. Dieringer, N: "Vestibular compensation": Neural plasticity and its relations to functional recovery after labyrinthine lesions in frogs and other vertebrates. Prog in Neurobiol 46:97, 1995.
7. de Waele, C, et al: Neurochemistry of central vestibular pathways: A review. Brain Res Rev 20:24, 1995.
8. Vidal, PP, et al: Vestibular compensation revisited. Otolaryngol Head Neck Surg 119:34, 1998.
9. Weissenstein, L, et al: Vestibular compensation in the horizontal vestibulo-ocular reflex of the goldfish. Behav Brain Res 75:127, 1996.
10. Dai, MJ, et al: Linear acceleration perception in the roll plane before and after unilateral vestibular neurectomy. Exp Brain Res 77:315, 1989.
11. Curthoys, IS, et al: Human ocular torsional position before and after unilateral vestibular neurectomy. Exp Brain Res 85:218, 1991.

12. Halmagyi, GM, et al: The human horizontal vestibulo-ocular reflex in response to high-acceleration stimulation before and after unilateral vestibular neurectomy. Exp Brain Res 81:479, 1990.
13. Smith, PF, and Curthoys, IS: Neuronal activity in the contralateral medial vestibular nucleus of the guinea pig following unilateral labyrinthectomy. Brain Res 444:295, 1988.
14. Smith, PF, and Curthoys, IS: Neuronal activity in the ipsilateral medial vestibular nucleus of the guinea pig following unilateral labyrinthectomy. Brain Res 444:308, 1988.
15. Brookes, GB, et al: Sensing and controlling rotational orientation in normal subjects and patients with loss of labyrinthine function. Am J Otol 14:349, 1993.
16. Graybiel, A: The oculogravic illusion. AMA Arch Ophthalmol 48:605, 1952.
17. Graybiel, A, and Clark, B: Validity of the oculogravic illusion as a specific indicator of otolith function. Aerospace Med 36:1173, 1965.
18. Bergenius, J, et al: The subjective horizontal at different angles of roll-tilt in patients with unilateral vestibular impairment. Brain Res Bull 40:385, 1996.
19. Arshi, A, et al: Roll-tilt perception using a somatosensory bar task (abstract) Association for Research in Otolaryngology Meeting, St. Petersburg, Florida, February 5, 1998.
20. Tribukait, A, et al: The subjective visual horizontal for different body tilts in the roll plane—Characterization of normal subjects. Brain Res Bull 40:375, 1996.
21. Zee, DS: Ophthalmoscopy in the examination of patients with vestibular disorders. Ann Neurol 3:373, 1978.
22. Halmagyi, GM, et al: Ocular tilt reaction with peripheral vestibular lesion. Ann Neurol 6:80, 1979.
23. Wolfe, GI, et al: Ocular tilt reaction resulting from vestibuloacoustic nerve surgery. Neurosurg 32:417, 1993.
24. Vibert, D, et al: Ocular tilt reaction associated in sudden idiopathic unilateral peripheral cochleovestibular loss. J Otorhinol Relat Spec 57:310, 1995.
25. Safran, AB, et al: Skew deviation following vestibular neuritis. Am J Ophthalmol 118:238, 1994.
26. Wade, S, and Curthoys, IS: The effect of ocular torsional position on perception of the roll-tilt of visual stimuli. Vision Research 37:1071, 1997.
27. Vibert, D, et al: Diplopia from skew deviation in unilateral peripheral vestibular lesions. Acta Otolaryngol 116:170, 1996.
28. Tabak, S, et al: Deviation of the subjective vertical in long-standing unilateral vestibular loss. Acta Otolaryngol 117:1, 1997.
29. Friedmann, G: The judgement of the visual vertical and horizontal with peripheral and central vestibular lesions. Brain 93:313, 1970.
30. Pompeiano, O, et al: Central compensation of vestibular deficits. II. Influences of roll tilt on different-size lateral vestibular neurons after ipsilateral labyrinth deafferentation. J Neurophysiol 52:18, 1984.
31. Black, FO, et al: Effects of unilateral loss of vestibular function on the vestibulo-ocular reflex and postural control. Ann Otol Rhinol Laryngol 98:884, 1989.
32. Lacour, M, et al: Sensory strategies in human postural control before and after unilateral vestibular neurotomy. Exp Brain Res 115:300, 1997.
33. Jenkins, HA: Long-term adaptive changes of the vestibulo-ocular reflex in patients following acoustic neuroma surgery. Laryngoscope 95:1224, 1985.
34. Paige, GD: Nonlinearity and asymmetry in the human vestibulo-ocular reflex. Acta Otolaryngol (Stockh) 108:1, 1989.
35. Takahashi, M, et al: Recovery of vestibulo-ocular reflex and gaze disturbance in patients with unilateral loss of labyrinthine function. Ann Otol Rhinol Laryngol 93:170, 1984.
36. Fetter, M, and Zee, DS: Recovery from unilateral labyrinthectomy in rhesus monkey. J Neurophysiol 59:370, 1988.
37. Tabak, S, et al: Gain and delay of human vestibulo-ocular reflexes to oscillation and steps of the head by a reactive torque helmet. I. Normal subjects. Acta Otolaryngol. 117:785, 1997.
38. Tabak, S, et al: Gain and delay of human vestibulo-ocular reflexes to oscillation and steps of the head by a reactive torque helmet. II. Vestibular-deficient subjects. Acta Otolaryngol 117:796, 1997.
39. Hain, TC, et al: Head-shaking nystagmus in patients with unilateral peripheral vestibular lesions. Am J Otolaryngol 8:36, 1987.
40. Halmagyi, GM, and Curthoys, IS: A clinical sign of canal paresis. Arch Neurol 45:737, 1988.
41. Fetter, M, et al: Head-shaking nystagmus during vestibular compensation in humans and rhesus monkeys. Acta Otolaryngol (Stockh) 110:175, 1990.
42. Baloh, RW, and Demer, J: Gravity and the vertical vestibulo-ocular reflex. Exp Brain Res 83:427, 1991.
43. Allum, JH, et al: Long-term modifications of vertical and horizontal vestibulo-ocular reflex dynamics in man. I. After acute unilateral peripheral vestibular paralysis. Acta Otolaryngol (Stockh) 105:328, 1988.
44. Aw, ST, et al: Unilateral vestibular deafferentation causes permanent impairment of the human vestibulo-ocular reflex in the pitch plane. Exp Brain Res 102:121, 1994.
45. Aw, ST, et al: Three dimensional kinematics of the human vestibuloocular reflex response during high-acceleration head rotations after unilateral vestibular deafferentation and semicircular canal occlusion. J Neurophysiol 76:4009, 1996.
46. Aw, ST, et al: Three dimensional kinematics of the human vestibuloocular reflex response during high-acceleration head rotations: Speed gain and misalignment angle. J Neurophysiol 76:4021, 1996.

47. Aw, ST, et al: Compensation of the human vertical vestibulo-ocular reflex following occlusion of one vertical semicircular canal is incomplete. Exp Brain Res 103:471, 1995.
48. Cremer, PD, et al: Semicircular canal plane head impulses detect absent function of individual semicircular canals. Brain 121:699, 1998.
49. Diamond, SG, and Markham, CH: Binocular counterrolling in humans with unilateral labyrinthectomy and in normal controls. Ann NY Acad Sci 374:69, 1981.
50. Diamond, SG, and Markham, CH: Ocular counterrolling as an indicator of vestibular otolith function. Neurology 33:1460, 1983.
51. Bronstein, AM, et al: Compensatory otolithic slow phase eye movement responses to abrupt linear head motion in the lateral direction. Findings in patients with labyrinthine and neurological lesions. Acta Otolaryngol Suppl (Stockh) 481:42, 1991.
52. Lempert, T, et al: Effect of otolith dysfunction—impairment of visual acuity during linear head motion in labyrinthine defective subjects. Brain 120:1005, 1997.
53a. Fetter, M, et al: Effect of lack of vision and of occipital lobectomy upon recovery from unilateral labyrinthectomy in rhesus monkey. J Neurophysiol 59:394, 1988.
53b. Smith, PF, et al: The effect of visual deprivation on vestibular compensation in the guinea pig. Brain Res 364:195, 1986.
54a. Putkonen, PT, et al: Compensation of postural effects of hemilabyrinthectomy in the cat. A sensory substitution process? Exp Brain Res 28:249, 1977.
54b. Lacour, M, et al: Compensation of postural reactions to fall in the vestibular neurectomized monkey. Role of the remaining labyrinthine afferences. Exp Brain Res 37:563, 1979.
55. Igarashi, M, and Gutierrez, O: Analysis of righting reflex in cats with unilateral and bilateral labyrinthectomy. Otorhinolaryngology 445:279, 1983.
56. Xerri, C, and Zennou, Y: Sensory, functional and behavioural substitution processes in vestibular compensation. In Lacour, M, et al (eds): Vestibular Compensation: Facts, Theories and Clinical Perspectives. Paris, Elsevier, 1989, pp 35–58.
57. Flohr, H, et al: Concepts of vestibular compensation. In Flohr, H, and Precht, W (eds): Lesion-induced Neuronal Plasticity in Sensorimotor Systems. Berlin, Springer-Verlag, 1981.
58. Maioli, C, and Precht, W: On the role of vestibulo-ocular reflex plasticity in recovery after unilateral peripheral vestibular lesions. Exp Brain Res 59:267, 1985.
59. Pettorossi, VE, and Petrosini, L: Tonic cervical influences on eye nystagmus following labyrinthectomy: Immediate and plastic effects. Brain Res 324:11, 1984.
60. Igarashi, M: Physical exercise and the acceleration of vestibular compensation. In Lacour, M, et al (eds): Vestibular Compensation: Facts Theories and Clinical Perspectives. Elsevier, Paris, 1989 pp 131–144.
61. Jensen, DW: Reflex control of acute postural asymmetry and compensatory symmetry after a unilateral vestibular lesion. Neuroscience 4:1059, 1979.
62. Jensen, DW: Vestibular compensation: tonic spinal influence upon spontaneous descending vestibular nuclear activity. Neuroscience 4:1075, 1979.
63. Smith, PF, and Darlington, CL: Neurochemical mechanisms of recovery from peripheral vestibular lesions (vestibular compensation). Brain Res Review 16:117, 1991.
64. Flohr, H, and Luneburg, U: Influence of melanocortin fragments on vestibular compensation. In Lacour, M, et al (eds): Vestibular Compensation: Facts Theories and Clinical Perspectives. Elsevier, Paris, 1989. pp 161–174.
65. Gilchrist, DP, et al: Effects of flunarizine on ocular motor and postural compensation following peripheral vestibular deafferentation in the guinea pig. Pharmacol Biochem Behav 44:99, 1993.
66. Gilchrist, DP, et al: Evidence that short ACTH fragments enhance vestibular compensation via direct action on the ipsilateral vestibular nucleus. Neuroreport 7:1489, 1996.
67. Gilchrist, DP, et al: ACTH(4-10) accelerates ocular motor recovery in the guinea pig following vestibular deafferentation. Neurosci Lett 118:14, 1990.
68a. Courjon, JH, et al: The role of the flocculus in vestibular compensation after hemilabyrinthectomy. Brain Res 239:251, 1982.
68b. Peppard, SB: Effect of drug therapy on compensation from vestibular injury. Laryngoscope 96:878, 1986.
69. Haddad, GM, et al: Compensation of nystagmus after VIIIth nerve lesions in vestibulo-cerebellectomized cats. Brain Res 135:192, 1977.
70. Smith, PF, et al: Vestibular compensation without brainstem commissures in the guinea pig. Neurosci Lett 65:209, 1986.
71. Newlands, SD, and Perachio, AA: Effects of commisurotomy on vestibular compensation in the gerbil. Soc Neurosci Abstr 12:254, 1986.
72. Halmagyi, GM, and Henderson, CJ: Visual symptoms of vestibular disease. Aust N Z J Ophthalmol 16:177, 1988.
73. Halmagyi, GM, et al: Gentamicin vestibulotoxicity. Otolaryngol Head Neck Surg 111:571, 1994.
74. Halmagyi, GM: Vestibular insufficiency following unilateral vestibular deafferentation. Aust J Otolaryngol 1:510, 1994.
75. Berthoz, A, and Melvill Jones, G (eds): Adaptive Mechanisms in Gaze Control: Facts and Theories. Elsevier, Amsterdam, 1985.

76. Lisberger, SG: The neural basis for learning of simple motor skills. Science 242:728, 1988.
77. Wade, S, et al: Time constant of nystagmus slow phase velocity to yaw-axis rotation as a function of the severity of unilateral caloric paresis. Am J Otol 20, 1999.
78. Goldberg, JM, and Fernandez, C: The vestibular system. In: Handbook of Physiology. The Nervous System. Sensory Processes. Bethesda, MD, Physiological Society, 1981. pp 977–1022.
79. Cirelli, C, et al: *c-fos* Expression in the rat brain after unilateral labyrinthectomy and its relation to the uncompensated and compensated stages. Neuroscience 70:515, 1996.
80. Precht, W, et al: A mechanism of central compensation of vestibular function following hemilabyrinthectomy. J Neurophysiol 29:996, 1966.
81a. Xerri, C, et al: Central compensation of vestibular deficits. I. Response characteristics of lateral vestibular neurons to roll tilt after ipsilateral labyrinth deafferentation. J Neurophysiol 50:428, 1983.
81b. Markham, CH, et al: The contribution of the contralateral labyrinth to second order vestibular neuronal activity in the cat. Brain Res 138:99, 1977.
82a. Lacour, M, et al: Central compensation of vestibular deficits. III. Response characteristics of lateral vestibular neurons to roll tilt after contralateral labyrinth deafferentation. J Neurophysiol 54:988, 1985.
82b. Ris, L, et al: Neuronal activity in the ipsilateral vestibular nucleus following unilateral labyrinthectomy in the alert guinea pig. J Neurophysiol 74:2087, 1995.
83a. Ris, L, et al: Dissociations between behavioural recovery and restoration of vestibular activity in the unilabyrinthectomized guinea-pig. J Physiol 500:509, 1997.
83b. Gacek, RR, et al: Ultrastructural changes in vestibulo-ocular neurons following vestibular neurectomy in the cat. Ann Otol Rhinol Laryngol 97:42, 1988.
84a. Newlands, SD, and Perachio, AA: Compensation of horizontal canal related activity in the medial vestibular nucleus following unilateral labyrinth ablation in the decerebrate gerbil. I. Type I neurons. Exp Brain Res 82:359, 1990.
84b. Gacek, RR, et al: Ultrastructural changes in contralateral vestibulo-ocular neurons following vestibular neurectomy in the cat. Acta Otolaryngol Suppl (Stockh) 477:1, 1991.
85a. Newlands, SD, and Perachio, AA: Compensation of horizontal canal related activity in the medial vestibular nucleus following unilateral labyrinth ablation in the decerebrate gerbil. II. Type II neurons. Exp Brain Res 82:373, 1990.
85b. Gacek, RR, et al: Morphologic correlates of vestibular compensation in the cat. Acta Otolaryngol Suppl (Stockh) 462:1, 1989.
86. Gacek, RR, and Schoonmaker, JE: Morphologic changes in the vestibular nerves and nuclei after labyrinthectomy in the cat: a case for the neurotrophin hypothesis in vestibular compensation. Acta Otolaryngologica 117:244, 1997.
87. Vibert, N, et al: The vestibular system as a model of sensorimotor transformations. A combined in vivo and in vitro approach to study the cellular mechanisms of gaze and posture stabilization in mammals. Prog Neurobiol 51:243, 1997.

CHAPTER 8

Otolith Function Tests

G. Michael Halmagyi, MD
Ian S. Curthoys, PhD

The peripheral vestibular system is sensitive to both linear and angular accelerations: the semicircular canals sense angular acceleration while the otoliths, the saccule and the utricle, sense linear accelerations. Many different ways of testing otolith function have been proposed. These have included the measurement of horizontal, vertical, and torsional eye movements as well as psychophysical settings in response to linear accelerations produced on swings,[1] sleds,[2] centrifuges,[3] tilt-chairs,[4] and barbeque spits.[5] For an otolith function test to be clinically useful, it must be safe, practical, robust, and reproducible. The test also needs to be specific for, and sensitive to, otolith dysfunction, particularly unilateral otolith hypofunction. In our view, only two tests—the subjective visual horizontal and the vestibular evoked myogenic potentials—come near to fulfilling these requirements. Both have been regularly used in our clinical laboratories for several years, and what follows is in part a distillation of our own experience with these tests and of their scientific basis. Before considering these tests, however, some familiarity with the structure and function of the otoliths is necessary.

The balance organs in the inner ear—the vestibular sensory regions—are the gyros of the human body, and unnoticed they function continuously in an almost perfect fashion, providing the brain with information about head position and head movement. Until these organs fail no one really appreciates their significance in daily life, and anyone who has experienced an attack of vertigo will readily verify their importance. These biological gyros detect forces: the forces imposed by gravity and the forces generated when we move. They are constructed in such a way that different regions detect rotational forces and linear forces in any direction. The brain synthesizes the information from these separate force detectors to provide a global integrated summary of where we are and how we are moving. This realization is of clinical importance because it implies that disease affecting only one isolated region of the inner ear could have consequences for the overall integration of all of the vestibular sensory input. In this chapter, we deal only with the otoliths, the structures that sense linear forces, such as the force of gravity or the "straight line" acceleration experienced while accelerating at traffic lights.

OTOLITH STRUCTURE

The basic element of all vestibular transducers is the receptor hair cell, which is similar in both the angular and the linear force sensing systems (Fig. 8–1). The semicircular canals and the otoliths detect these two different forces not so much because of any differences in the intrinsic properties of the hair cells themselves but because of the way the structures that surround the hair cells are affected by the stimulating force. Each receptor cell has several, fine, hair-like *cilia* projecting from the cell body into a gelatinous overlying mass, the *otolithic membrane*. The longest cilium is called the *kinocilium;* it is located at one side of the receptor cell and has a specialized cross-sectional structure. The remaining cilia, the *stereocilia,* are of uniform cross-sectional structure and are arranged in a series of increasing height as they approach the kinocilium. Forces cause the otolithic membrane to slide so that the cilia of the receptor hair cells are bent.

Each labyrinth consists of endolymph-filled tubes and sacs containing receptor structures. The two specialized sacs are the *utricular sac* and the *saccular sac*. Contained within each of these sacs is a plate of specialized receptor hair cells and connective tissue, the *macula.* Each macula takes its name from the sac in which it is located, so that in each inner ear there is an utricular macula and a saccular macula. The terms *utricle* and *saccule* are often used to refer to the utricular and saccular maculae, although strictly speaking *utricle* and *saccule* refer to the membranous sacs that contain the maculae.

The two maculae have similar gross features. Embedded on the outer (free) surface of the otolithic membrane are dense crystals of calcium carbonate—the *otoconia.* On the inner surface of this membrane the cilia of the hair cells project into the membrane. The density of the otolithic membrane itself is similar to that of the surrounding endolymph 1.0 g/cm^3, but the density of the otoconia is almost 3 times greater, at 2.7 g/cm^3. These two receptor structures are together called the *otoliths* because their construction is similar and because both detect forces according to the same physical principle, namely that an imposed linear force displaces the relatively dense otoliths embedded in the otolithic membrane. The otolithic membrane then tends to slide across the surface of the macula, displacing the cilia of the receptor hair cells producing a change in hair cell resting membrane potential. The displacements of the otolithic membrane generated in this way by natural head movements in a 1-g environment are in the order of one micron.

The utricular and saccular maculae are almost perpendicular to one another. With the head erect the utricular macula is tilted by about 30° (open anterior) with respect to the horizontal plane of the head, whereas the saccular macula is almost vertical. These different orientations mean that the receptors on each macula will respond maximally to forces in different directions. The surface area of the human utricular and saccular maculae is only about 4.2 mm^2 and 2.2 mm^2 respectively. There are about 33,000 receptor hair cells in the utricular macula and about 19,000 in the saccular macula. As in other sensory systems, there is convergence of receptors to primary afferent nerves so that only about 6000 primary afferent nerve fibers supply the utricle and only about 4000 supply the saccule.

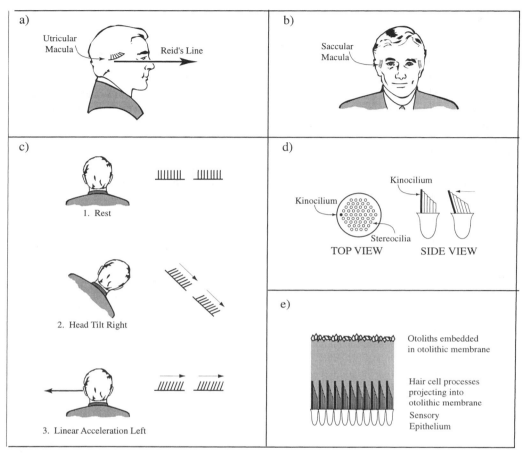

FIGURE 8–1. The structure and function of the otolithic system. (*A* and *B*) Schematic representation of the approximate orientation of the utricular and saccular maculae in the head. Reid's line is a standard reference line joining the center of the external ear and the lower edge of the bony orbit. (*C*) Three drawings show how different linear force stimuli affect the utricular receptor hair cells. The upper diagram (*1*) shows the back view of a person at rest with the cilia upright. Head tilts to the right cause the cilia to be deflected to the right (*2*); similarly a linear acceleration to the left (*arrow*) causes a deflection of the cilia to the right (*3*). (*D*) Schematic top-down view of a single receptor hair cell to show the polarization pattern. The kinocilium is located at one extreme of the upper surface of the cell. If the stereocilia are bent towards the kinocilium, as shown at the right, the receptor cell activity increases. (*E*) Schematic illustration of the organization of a macular surface. The crystals of calcium carbonate (the otoliths) are embedded in one side of the gelatinous otolithic membrane and the tips of the cilia project into the other side of this membrane. Forces cause the membrane to slide so that the cilia are bent thus stimulating the receptor cells.

NORMAL OTOLITH FUNCTION

Intracellular recordings from single isolated otolithic receptor hair cells subjected to controlled forces in precisely defined directions have shown that each receptor hair cell is polarized; that is it responds most strongly to forces in one direction and as the direction of the force deviates from that optimal direction, so the response of the receptor declines. This optimum direction is referred to as the cell's *polarization vector*. This physiological polarization corresponds to a morphological polarization in that receptor cells respond optimally when the imposed force shears the stereocilia towards the kinocilium. Receptor hair cells are arranged in a regular fashion across each macula so that the direction of the kinocilium of each cell shifts in direction by only a small amount relative to its neighbors with the result that there is a highly ordered arrangement of polarization vectors across each macula.

Primary afferent neurons synapse on a number of adjacent receptor hair cells so that some of the precision of tuning of the individual receptors is lost: afferent fibers respond to forces over a greater range of directions than do the individual receptors. Each afferent fiber exhibits a preference for forces in a particular direction, presumably reflecting the preferred orientation of the receptor hair cells on which the fiber synapses. For afferent fibers, just as for receptors, as the force direction deviates from the optimal direction, the fiber's firing frequency declines. Utricular afferents in general show a preference for forces directed across the plane of the macula, in other words, for laterally directed forces and similarly saccular afferents show a preference for forces directed vertically across the plane of the macula.

PRIMARY OTOLITHIC AFFERENTS

Recordings from primary otolithic afferent neurons in the vestibular nerve of experimental animals show a number of important characteristics (for a review see Goldberg & Fernandez[6]): (1) Primary otolithic afferents have a resting discharge rate. They fire at about 50 spikes per second even when there is no imposed force stimulus. (2) They have a *functional polarization vector.* This means that linear accelerations oriented in one particular direction will most effectively activate the afferent neuron. As the direction of the imposed force is deviated from this optimum direction, so the response of the afferent neuron declines. If the stimulus is directed exactly opposite to the preferred direction then the firing of the cell will be maximally suppressed. (3) They show a marked asymmetry in bidirectional sensitivity. This characteristic results in a larger increase in firing rate for forces in the excitatory direction than decrease in firing rate for the same magnitude of force in the opposite, disfacilitatory direction. (4) The spatial distribution of the directional preferences of all otolithic afferents is not uniform. In the squirrel monkey there is a directional preponderance so that more otolith afferents prefer ipsilaterally directed forces rather than contralaterally directed forces. There is 3:1 preponderance of ipsilateral force preferring utricular afferents whereas there is about a 1:1 distribution of up-and-down–force preferring saccular afferents. (5) At rest some otolithic afferents have a regular interspike interval whereas others show an irregular pattern of firing. The dynamic response characteristics of these two groups of neurons are quite different. Regular neurons show little adaptation to maintained forces, whereas the irregular neurons show a transient mode of responding: they fire vigorously during the change in the stimulus but adapt rapidly for a maintained stimulus. This means that even at the level of the afferent neurons leaving the macula, functional specialization has already taken place in that different aspects of the force stimulus are being signaled by these different parallel pathways.

Central Projections

Primary otolithic afferent neurons project to secondary vestibular neurons mainly in the lateral, medial, and descending vestibular nuclei. In some regions these otolithic projections show considerable overlap with the projections of horizontal semicircular canal afferents. The predominant response of lateral vestibular nucleus neurons is an increase in firing rate in response to ipsilateral tilts. Just as horizontal semicircular canal neurons in the medial vestibular nucleus are interconnected to the contralateral medial vestibular nucleus via commissural fibers, which play a major role in the neural operation of the system, so otolith-responsive neurons are interconnected to similar neurons in the opposite vestibular nucleus. However, the interconnections in the otolithic system are indirect and the functional mode of the bilateral interconnections is predominantly excitatory rather than inhibitory, as is the case of the horizontal semicircular canal system. Some cells in each vestibular nucleus can be activated both by semicircular canal and by otolithic stimulation. These convergent neurons integrate linear and angular acceleration input and thus help to maintain posture and equilibrium. The pathways from the otolithic regions of the vestibular nuclei to the ocular motor nuclei are poorly understood. Trochlear motoneurons can be disynaptically activated by electrical stimulation of the utricular nerve and increasing attention is being paid to two midbrain regions close to the oculomotor nuclei—the interstitial nucleus of Cajal and the rostral interstitial nucleus of the medial longitudinal fasciculus—which integrate inputs for torsional and vertical eye movement responses produced by otolithic stimulation. In particular it seems that the interstitial nucleus of Cajal has a major role in integrating otolithic input for coordinated eye and head responses to the linear forces detected by the otoliths. The neural substrate for the compensatory postural movements required by a linear acceleration are mediated by otolith-spinal projections—the lateral vestibulospinal tract arising in the lateral vestibular nucleus and the medial vestibulospinal tract arising in the medial vestibular nucleus.

Function of Otolithic Input

Electrical stimulation of the utricular nerve in the cat causes a distinct pattern of eye movement: a torsion of both eyes so that the upper poles of the eyes roll away from the side being stimulated.[7] Complementing that result are studies that have shown that unilateral section of the vestibular nerve causes a torsion of both eyes toward the operated side.[3,8] In natural movements the otoliths are activated and generate compensatory eye and postural responses. For example, tilting the head toward one shoulder causes the gravity vector to activate particular regions of the utricular and saccular maculae, and as a consequence the eyeball *torts* (or *rolls*) around the visual axis in a compensatory direction. At the same time, there is a complex pattern of activation of neck and trunk muscles acting to oppose this challenge to the equilibrium of the head.

The degree of this countertorsion or ocular *counter-rolling* is only about 10 percent of the head tilt, but it does depend on otolith function because subjects without otoliths do not show such counter-rolling.[4]

THE SUBJECTIVE VISUAL HORIZONTAL (OR VERTICAL): A TEST OF UTRICULAR FUNCTION

Physiological Background

A normal subject sitting upright in a totally darkened room can align a dimly illuminated bar to within 2° of the gravitational horizontal.[3] Studies of the ability of patients to do this, which we call setting the subjective visual horizontal (SVH), before and after total unilateral vestibular deafferentation (uVD) by either vestibular neurectomy or labyrinthectomy, yield interesting and important results.[8–11] Before uVD, the patients' settings are generally within the normal range; that is ±2° of the gravitational horizontal or vertical. After uVD, they invariably set the bar rotated toward the lesioned side, in some cases by up to 15°. They *set* the bar rotated toward the lesioned side because they *see* the gravitationally horizontal bar as being tilted toward the intact side. Although their settings of the bar return toward the true or gravitational horizontal with time, they are still tilted by a mean of 4°, 6 months or more after uVD. It appears, therefore, that a slight ipsilesional offset of the SVH is a permanent legacy of uVD. Furthermore, patients with acute unilateral peripheral vestibular lesions owing to diseases such as vestibular neuritis also set such a bar so that it is no longer aligned with the gravitational vector but is consistently tilted toward the side of the lesion.[12,13]

What could be the cause of this perceptual error? Is it an offset of the internal representation of the gravitational vertical as a result of the profound asymmetry in otolithic input to the vestibular nuclei that must occur after uVD? Arguing against this mechanism is the observation that despite the uVD, the patients do not feel that their own bodies are tilted; on the contrary, they feel themselves to be normally upright, even in the dark. In other words, although they rotate the bar toward the uVD side, it is not in order to null a perceived tilt of the bar with the body toward the intact side.

Another possible mechanism of the deviation of the SVH is a torsional deviation of the eyes as a part of the ocular-tilt reaction. The ocular-tilt reaction is a postural synkinesis consisting of head tilt, conjugate eye torsion, and hypotropia, all toward the same side. Some patients develop a florid temporary ipsilesional tonic ocular tilt reaction—including conjugate ocular torsion—after a unilateral peripheral vestibular lesion.[14] We therefore measured ocular torsional position as well as SVH before and after uVD.[8]

Following uVD, there is invariably an ipsilesional deviation of ocular torsion position: the 12 o'clock meridians of both eyes are invariably rotated toward the side of the uVD (Fig. 8–2). One week after uVD, there is up to 15° ipsilesional ocular torsion, and the magnitude of the ocular torsion closely correlates ($r = 0.95$) with the magnitude of the tilting of the SVH (Fig. 8–3). Furthermore, the torsional deviation gradually resolves, with a temporal pattern identical to that of deviation of the SVH. One month after uVD, both the ocular torsion and the tilting of the SVH are at half of the 1-week value. A slight but statistically significant ocular torsion (4° to 5°) appears to be a per-

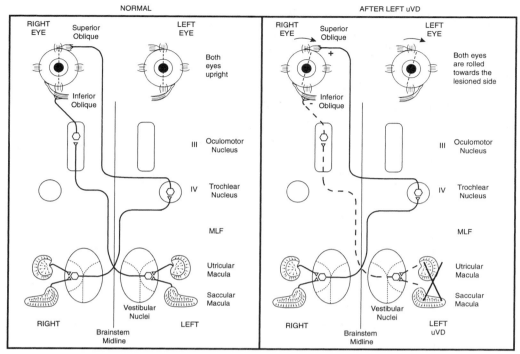

FIGURE 8–2. Explanation of the changes in torsional eye position after unilateral vestibular deafferentation (uVD). Normally second-order afferents from the vestibular nucleus send excitatory projections to the contralateral inferior oblique, and to the ipsilateral superior oblique, as well as the contralateral inferior rectus and ipsilateral superior rectus (not shown). Left uVD as shown here produces reduced tonic activity in the contralateral inferior oblique (and inferior rectus, not shown), so that the contralateral eye intorts, and reduced activity in the ipsilateral superior oblique (and superior oblique, not shown), so that the ipsilateral eye extorts. Through commissural disinhibition, one presumes that the left uVD increases tonic activity in the contralateral, right vestibular nucleus, and therefore increased tonic activity of the contralateral superior oblique, which also produces intorsion of the contralateral eye. (Figure by courtesy of Ms. Agatha Brizuela.)

manent legacy of uVD. Further support for the tight linkage between ocular torsional position and the SVH has come from related experiments in normals, which show that ocular torsion produces matching changes in perceived visual orientation.[15]

Although it appears that the offset of the SVH is due to ocular torsion, the mechanism of the ocular torsion itself is speculative. It could be similar to the mechanism of the spontaneous nystagmus that occurs after uVD and could reflect decreased resting activity in secondary vestibular neurons in the ipsilesional vestibular nucleus, owing to loss of input from primary vestibular neurons in those originating in the utricle. The evidence that tonic ocular torsion is utricular in origin depends in part on the argument that ocular torsion represents a tonic offset of the dynamic ocular counter-rolling mechanism (Fig. 8–4). It is generally accepted that dynamic counter-rolling is under utricular control.[4]

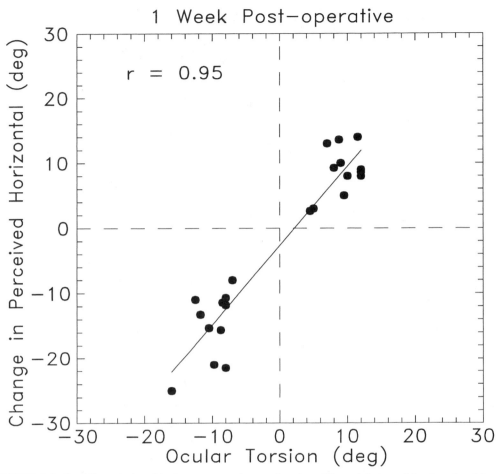

FIGURE 8–3. The relationship between ocular torsional position and the subjective visual horizontal. The average value 1 week after unilateral vestibular deafferentation of the change in ocular torsional position was calculated for each patient and correlated with that patient's average change in the visual horizontal. The correlation (0.95) is statistically significant. From Curthoys, et al[44] with permission.

Central Vestibular Lesions and Settings of the Subjective Visual Vertical

Patients with acute focal brainstem lesions commonly show a deviation of the subjective visual vertical (SVV) or SVH.[16, 17] Patients with lower brainstem lesions involving the vestibular nucleus set the SVV toward the side of the lesion, whereas patients with unilateral upper brainstem lesions involving the interstitial nucleus (of Cajal) and patients with unilateral cerebellar lesion involving the nodulus[18] set the SVV (or SVH) away from the side of the lesion. In most patients, there is also a deviation of the ocular torsional position (*cyclotorsion*) in the same direction as the deviation of the SVV. The relationship between the magnitude of the deviation of the SVV and of the ocular torsion

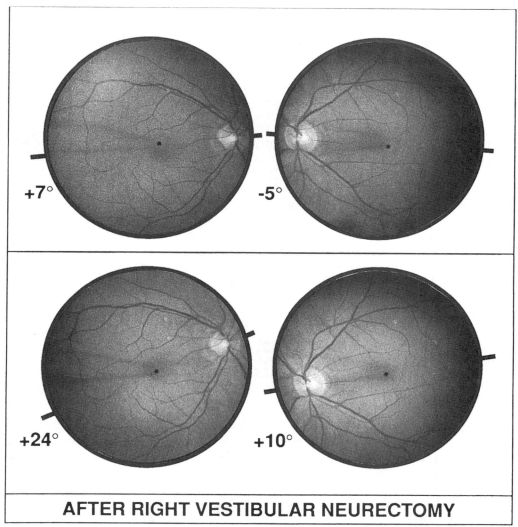

+7°

-5°

+24°

+10°

AFTER RIGHT VESTIBULAR NEURECTOMY

FIGURE 8–4. Ocular torsional position before and after uVD. Fundus photographs of the left and right eye of a patient before (*top row*) and one week after (*bottom row*) *right* vestibular neurectomy. After operation there is tonic rightward torsion of the 12 o'clock meridian of each eye toward the patient's *right* side. The torsion measures 17° in the right eye and 15° in the left eye. When the patient was asked to set a luminous bar to the perceived visual horizontal in an otherwise darkened room he set the bar tilted down on his right side by 14.2° when viewing with the right eye and 15.1° when viewing with the left.

is not as tight as with peripheral lesions, but is nonetheless present. There can be marked disparities between the amount of deviation of the SVV and of torsional deviation in the two eyes. For example, with lateral medullary infarcts, the excyclotorsion of the ipsilesional eye can be much larger than the incyclotorsion of the contralesional eye.

CLINICAL SIGNIFICANCE

The clinical significance of these findings is that careful, standardized measurement of the SVH or SVV, using a dim light-bar in an otherwise totally darkened room, can give valuable diagnostic information. A significant tilting of the SVV or the SVH indicates acute unilateral otolithic hypofunction of peripheral or central origin. It indicates either a lesion at the level of the end organ, vestibular nerve, or lower brainstem on the side to which the patient rotates the bar, or in the upper brainstem or caudal cerebellum on the side opposite to which the patient rotates the bar. Although the greater the deviation of the SVH or SVV is, the more acute as well as more extensive is the lesion, a small permanent deviation of the SVH-SVV might be a permanent legacy of central and of peripheral vestibular lesions.[8] The SVH test is insensitive to bilateral symmetrical impairment of otolith function since the deviation decreases as the patient compensates for the acute unilateral vestibular lesion (see Chapter 7).

VESTIBULAR-EVOKED MYOGENIC POTENTIALS: A TEST OF SACCULAR FUNCTION

Physiological Background

Brief (0.1 ms), loud (>95 dB), monaural clicks produce a large (60 to 300 mV), short latency (8 ms) inhibitory potential in the tonically contracting ipsilateral sternocleidomastoid muscle. The initial positive-negative potential has peaks at 13 (*p13*) and 23 ms (*n23*) and is abolished by selective vestibular neurectomy but not by profound sensorineural hearing loss; thus, even if the patient cannot hear the clicks there can nonetheless be normal *p13-n23* responses. Later components of the evoked response do not share the properties of the *p13-n23* potential and probably do not depend on vestibular afferents. Failure to distinguish between the early and late component waveforms could explain why earlier work along similar lines[19] was inconclusive.

For these reasons we have called the *p13-n23* response the *vestibular-evoked myogenic potential* (VEMP).[20] Unlike conventional evoked potentials such as brainstem auditory evoked potentials (BAEPs), which are generated by the synchronous discharge of nerve cells, the VEMP, while still an evoked potential, is generated by synchronous discharges of muscle cells or, rather, in groups of muscle cells innervated by a single motor neuron (i.e., a motor unit). This is why we call it a *myogenic* potential. Being a myogenic potential, the VEMP can be 500 to 1000 times larger than a brainstem potential (e.g., 200 microvolts versus less than 1 microvolt). Single motor unit recordings in the sternocleidomastoid muscle, which show a decreased firing rate synchronous with the surface VEMP, provide direct evidence of the myogenic origin of the potentials.[21]

When recording these potentials it is essential to remember that the amplitude of the VEMP is linearly related to the intensity of the click, and to the intensity of sternomastoid activation during the period of averaging, as measured by the mean rectified EMG. Therefore a conductive hearing loss abolishes the response simply by attenuating the intensity of the stimulus[22]; in such cases the VEMP can be elicited by a brisk tap to the forehead. Inadequate contraction of the sternomastoid muscles will also reduce the amplitude of the VEMP and failure to measure and control the intensity of muscle activation will produce spurious results.[22]

Several lines of evidence suggest that the VEMP arise from stimulation of the saccule (Fig. 8–5). Of all the vestibular end organs, the saccule is the most sensitive to sound.[23,24] It lies just under the stapes footplate in an ideal position to receive the full impact of a loud click delivered to the tympanic membrane.[25] Click-sensitive neurons in the vestibular nerve respond to tilts.[26,27] Most of these neurons originate in the saccular macula[26,28] and project to the lateral and descending vestibular nuclei as well as to other structures.[29,30]

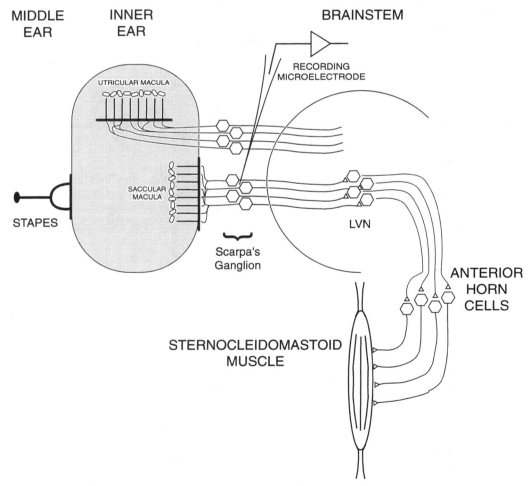

FIGURE 8–5. Explanation of the pathways for the click-evoked vestibular myogenic potential (VEMP). The loud click moves the stapes to activate receptors in the underlying saccular macula, which thereby causes via the vestibulospinal tract, disynaptic activation of ipsilateral C2 segment anterior horn cells supplying the sternomastoid muscle.

The VEMP measures vestibular function indirectly through a vestibulocollic reflex. Vestibulocollic reflexes are transmitted via the medial and lateral vestibulospinal tracts. The short latency of the onset of the VEMP suggests that it is mediated by a disynaptic pathway, projecting via the vestibulospinal tract. The responsible neural pathway must project ipsilaterally, as the *p13-n23* response is generated nearly exclusively by afferents arising from within the ipsilateral ear. The likely pathway is the ipsilateral medial vestibulospinal tract.[31]

Method

The technique for VEMP testing is simple and any equipment suitable for recording BAEPs will also be capable of recording VEMPs. Because the amplitude of the VEMP is linearly related to both the intensity of the click and the intensity of sternomastoid activation during the period of averaging, it is essential to ensure that the sound source is correctly calibrated and that the background level of rectified sternomastoid EMG activation is measured. The usual reason that VEMPs are absent or less than 50 microvolts in amplitude is either a conductive hearing loss or inadequate contraction of the sternomastoid muscles.

The VEMP test does not cause dizziness, and individual averages of 128 clicks can be completed in less than 3 minutes. Three superimposed averages usually give a clear result. The patient lies down for the test and activates the sternomastoid muscles for the averaging period by keeping her or his head raised from the pillow. The test cannot be done on uncooperative or unconscious patients, and is difficult for patients with painful neck problems to perform.

The function of one ear is best evaluated by comparing the amplitude of its VEMP with the amplitude of the VEMP from the other ear. Minor differences in latency occur commonly and might reflect differences in electrode placement over the muscle or differing muscle anatomy. Our own practice is to compare the amplitude of the responses generated by stimulation of each ear individually. For simple clinical screening, three runs of 128 averages with clicks of 100-dB intensity are sufficient. The peak-to-peak amplitudes can then be expressed relative to the level of background mean rectified EMG to create a ratio which largely removes the effect of differences in muscle activity. More accurate but more time-consuming correction can be made by making repeated observations with differing levels of tonic activation.[32] With this type of correction, we take asymmetries of greater than 2.5:1 as evidence of vestibular hypofunction on the side with the smaller potential. Uncorrected, amplitude asymmetries of up to 3:1 can occur in normals.

Clinical Applications

TULLIO EFFECT

Nystagmus produced by sound was first described, in pigeons, by Tullio. Loud sounds can sometimes produce nystagmus in humans. Patients who have nystagmus produced by loud sounds (the Tullio effect) complain of sound-induced oscillopsia rather than of sound-induced vertigo. They can have different underlying ear problems. Some appear to have a hypermobile stapes[33,34] whereas others appear to have a dehiscent superior semicircular canal.[35] Some have no other vestibular symptoms whereas others have vertigo and ataxia as well as sound-induced oscillopsia. The oscillopsia is due to vertical torsional nystagmus.[35,36] A characteristic abnormality in patients with the Tullio effect is a very large VEMP at an abnormally low threshold.[37] In normal subjects, the VEMP, just like the acoustic reflex, has a threshold. The VEMP threshold is normally about 85 to 90 dB NHL. In patients with the Tullio effect, the VEMP threshold is 10 to 20 dB lower than in normals and the VEMP amplitude at the usual 105 dB NHL stimulus level is huge (>500uV). If a VEMP can be consistently elicited at 70 dB NHL this probably indicates that the patient has the Tullio effect.

VESTIBULAR NEURITIS-NEUROLABYRINTHITIS AND BENIGN PAROXYSMAL POSITIONING VERTIGO

After an attack of vestibular neuritis about one patient in three develops posterior semicircular canal-type benign paroxysmal positioning vertigo (BPPV), usually within 3 months.[38] It is of some interest that patients who develop BPPV after vestibular neuritis have intact VEMPs, whereas those who do not have absent VEMPs. In other words, an intact VEMP seems to be a prerequisite for the development of post–vestibular-neuritis BPPV. The reason for this is probably that in those patients who develop post–vestibular-neuritis BPPV, only the superior vestibular nerve (innervating the anterior and lateral semicircular canals and the utricle) is involved. Because the inferior vestibular nerve innervates the posterior semicircular canal and the saccule, the presence of posterior canal BPPV and the preservation of the VEMP implies that the inferior vestibular nerve must have been spared. Support for this explanation comes from data that show preservation of posterior SCC vestibulo-ocular reflexes in some patients with vestibular neuritis.[39] (It should be recalled that clinical caloric tests measure only lateral semicircular canal function.)

ACOUSTIC NEUROMA

Although most patients with acoustic neuromas present with unilateral hearing loss, some present with vestibular ataxia. This is not entirely surprising; most "acoustic neuromas" actually arise not from the acoustic nerve but from one of the vestibular nerves, usually the inferior vestibular nerve.[40] Furthermore, pathologically they are not actually neuromas but schwannomas and should therefore be called "vestibular schwannomas" rather than acoustic neuromas. The VEMP, which is transmitted via the inferior vestibular nerve is abnormal—low amplitude or absent, in four out of five patients with acoustic neuroma.[41] Because the VEMP does not depend on cochlear or lateral semicircular canal function, it can be a valuable test in patients suspected of having an acoustic neuroma. This is because the VEMP test can be abnormal even if a BAEP test cannot be done because cochlear function is absent, and even if the caloric test of lateral semicircular canal function is normal.

MÉNIÈRE'S DISEASE

A recent study from Paris has found absent VEMPs from the affected ear in more than 50% of patients with Ménière's disease.[43] The loss of VEMP correlated with the low-frequency hearing loss but not with the loss of lateral SCC on caloric testing. Patients with absent VEMPs fared worse on condition 5 of the Equitest posturographic protocol, and these patients could be at greater risk of falls.

OTHER CONDITIONS

Initial experience with this technique suggests that the VEMP test can provide valuable information additional to that obtained by tests of lateral semicircular function such as caloric or rotational tests and by tests of utricular function such as the SVH test.[42] We have seen many patients with symptoms of unilateral or bilateral vestibulopathy (e.g. vertigo, ataxia) who have had normal tests of lateral semicircular canal function at a time the VEMP tests were unequivocally abnormal. The following is a typical example.

CASE STUDY

A 61-year-old, previously well male business executive developed sudden intense vertigo and nausea while driving home from work. He had to stop his car, vomited, and called for help. He was taken by ambulance to a hospital emergency room. On admission he was distressed by vertigo, retching, and vomiting. He was unable to stand. There was no spontaneous or positional nystagmus with or without visual fixation; the head impulse test was negative vertically as well as horizontally. A CT brain scan was normal. He was admitted to the hospital with the provisional diagnosis of cerebellar infarct. The following day he felt better and could now stand without support. At that time he noted that he could not hear in his left ear. Over the next 3 days his balance continued to improve but his hearing did not.

Investigations at that time revealed the following:

1. *Audiogram:* severe flat sensorineural hearing loss left ear; slight conductive loss right ear (Fig. 8–6A).
2. *Electronystagmogram:* minimal left beating gaze-evoked nystagmus in dark; normal caloric tests (Fig. 8–6B).
3. *Subjective visual horizontal:* more than 6° to the left (Fig. 8–6C).
4. *Vestibular-evoked myogenic potentials:* absent from left ear to clicks and to taps (Fig. 8–6D).

An MRI with contrast showed no abnormality in particular neither cerebellar infarction nor contrast enhancement of the inner ear.

Despite the absence of pain and vesicles he was given a tapering course of prednisone and zovirax on the chance that this was due to herpes zoster. His balance continued to improve but even 2 weeks later he still rotated to the left on the Unterberger (Fukuda) test and fell on the matted Romberg test. Within 1 month his hearing also improved but not quite back to normal, his subjective visual horizontal and his VEMPs both returned to normal.

COMMENT

This patient had acute neurolabyrinthitis affecting the cochlea, the saccule, and the utricle, but spared the semicircular canals. In some cases of acute neurolabyrinthitis, as in this one, the inner ear can recover most or all function. How-

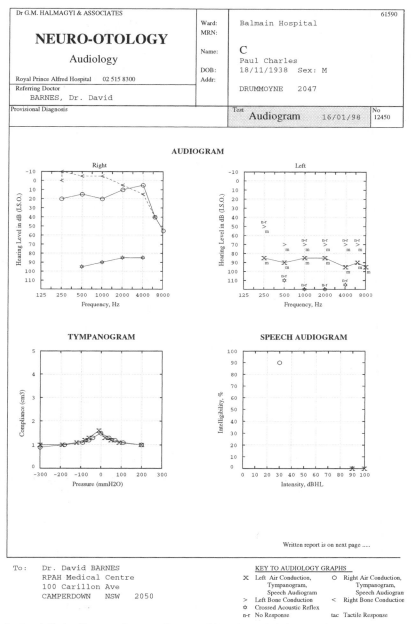

FIGURE 8–6. (*A*) Audiogram from a 61-year-old male with left neurolabyrinthitis. There is a severe sensorineural hearing loss on the left with absent acoustic reflexes and zero speech discrimination, all suggestive of a retrocochlear loss. On the right there is a slight conductive loss, asymptomatic and unrelated to the present problem.

(*Continues*)

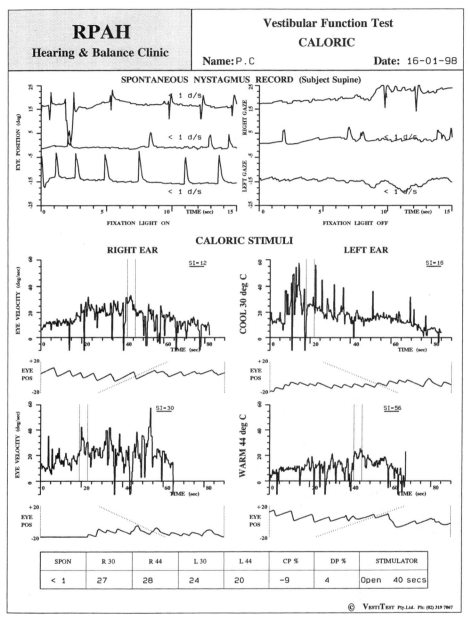

FIGURE 8–6. (Continued) (*B*) Electronystagmogram and caloric test from the same patient. There is minimal left beating gaze-evoked nystagmus in darkness (less than 1° per second slow-phase velocity). Bithermal caloric tests show symmetrical slow phase velocities from each ear. These findings indicate normal lateral semicircular canal function (see Halmagyi, et al[44]).

(Continues)

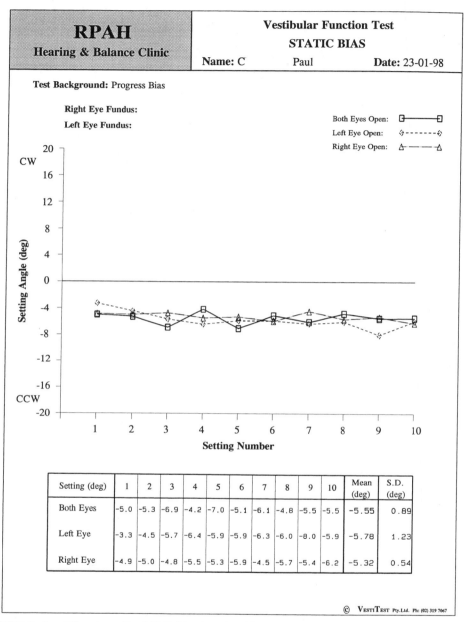

	RPAH Hearing & Balance Clinic	Vestibular Function Test STATIC BIAS
		Name: C Paul Date: 23-01-98

Test Background: Progress Bias

Right Eye Fundus:

Left Eye Fundus:

Both Eyes Open: ▭——————▭
Left Eye Open: ◇------◇
Right Eye Open: △————△

Setting (deg)	1	2	3	4	5	6	7	8	9	10	Mean (deg)	S.D. (deg)
Both Eyes	-5.0	-5.3	-6.9	-4.2	-7.0	-5.1	-6.1	-4.8	-5.5	-5.5	-5.55	0.89
Left Eye	-3.3	-4.5	-5.7	-6.4	-5.9	-5.9	-6.3	-6.0	-8.0	-5.9	-5.78	1.23
Right Eye	-4.9	-5.0	-4.8	-5.5	-5.3	-5.9	-4.5	-5.7	-5.4	-6.2	-5.32	0.54

© VestiTest Pty.Ltd. Ph: (02) 319 7067

FIGURE 8–6. (Continued) (*C*) Subjective visual horizontal (SVH) from the same patient. The patient makes ten settings of the SVH at his own speed. With each eye and then with both eyes open. There is a highly signficant offset of more than 5° to the left (the side of the hearing loss). Normal subjects can set the horizontal to within 2° of the gravitational horizontal.

(*Continues*)

Vestibular Evoked Myogenic Potentials

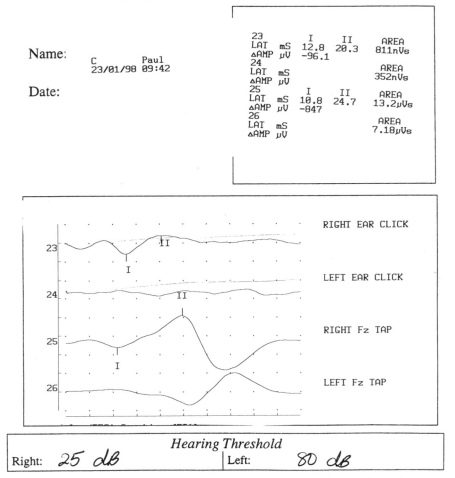

Name:

    C   Paul
    23/01/98 09:42

Date:

		I	II	AREA
23				
LAT	mS	12.8	20.3	811nVs
∆AMP	μV	-96.1		
24				
LAT	mS			AREA
∆AMP	μV			352nVs
25				
LAT	mS	10.8	24.7	AREA
∆AMP	μV	-847		13.2μVs
26				
LAT	mS			AREA
∆AMP	μV			7.18μVs

RIGHT EAR CLICK

LEFT EAR CLICK

RIGHT Fz TAP

LEFT Fz TAP

Hearing Threshold

Right: 25 dB | Left: 80 dB

FIGURE 8–6. (Continued) (*D*) Vestibular evoked myogenic potentials from the same patient. Channels 23 and 24 show the responses to 95 dB clicks; channels 25 and 26 show the response to forehead taps (Halmagyi, et al, 1995[21]). The responses are absent from the left. The absent tap responses show that the absent click reponses are not due to some conductive hearing loss in the left ear (that is being masked by the severe sensorineural loss), but due to loss of saccular function. The VEMP response to clicks has nothing to do with the audibility of the stimulus—it is present even if the click is not heard (see Colebatch, et al,[20]).

ever, even if the ear had not recovered (as would have been indicated by persistent loss of hearing and VEMP) the SVH would have returned to normal through central vestibular compensation (see Chapter 7).

SUMMARY

The SVH and the VEMP are simple, robust, reproducible, and specific tests of otolith dysfunction that can provide clinically useful diagnostic information in patients with vertigo and other balance disorders. Although they appear to have high specificity for otolith dysfunction, further clinical research will be required to establish their sensitivity.

ACKNOWLEDGMENTS

This work was supported by the National Health and Medical Research Council, the Garnet Passe and Rodney Williams Memorial Foundation and by the RPA Neurology Department Trustees.

REFERENCES

1. Baloh, RW, et al: Eye movements produced by linear accelerations on a swing. J Neurophysiol 60:2000, 1990.
2. Gianna, CC, et al: Eye movements induced by lateral acceleration steps. Exp Brain Res 114:124, 1997.
3. Dai, MJ, et al: Perception of linear acceleration before and after unilateral vestibular neurectomy. Exp Brain Res 77:315, 1989.
4. Diamond, SG, and Markham, CH: Ocular counterrrolling as an indicator of vestibular otolith function. Neurology 33:1460, 1983.
5. Furman, J, et al: Off vertical axis rotational responses in patients with peripheral vestibular lesions. Ann Otol Rhinol Laryngol 102:137, 1993.
6. Goldberg, JM, and Fernandez, C: The vestibular system. In Handbook of Physiology. The Nervous System III. Washington, American Physiologic Society, 1982, pp 977–1022.
7. Suzuki, J-I, Tokomasu, K, Goto, K: Eye movements from single utricular nerve stimulation in the cat. Acta Otolaryngol 68:350, 1969.
8. Curthoys, IS, et al: Human torsional ocular position before and after unilateral vestibular neurectomy. Exp Brain Res 85:218, 1991.
9. Boehmer, A, and Rickenmann, J: The subjective visual vertical as a clinical parameter of vestibular function in peripheral vestibular disease. J Vestib Res 5:35, 1995.
10. Bergenius, J, et al: The subjective horizontal at different angles of roll-tilt in patients with unilateral vestibular impairment. Brain Res Bull 40:385, 1996.
11. Tabak, S, et al: Deviation of the subjective vertical in long-standing unilateral vestibular loss. Acta Otolaryngol 117:1, 1997.
12. Friedmann, G: The influence of unilateral labyrinthectomy on orientation in space. Acta Otolaryngologica 71:289, 1971.
13. Vibert, D, et al: Evaluation clinique de la fonction otolithique par measure de la cyclotorsion oculaire et de la "skew deviation." Ann Otolaryngol (Paris) 110:87, 1993.
14. Halmagyi, GM, et al: Ocular tilt reaction due to peripheral vestibular lesion. Ann Neurol 6:80, 1979.
15. Wade, S, and Curthoys, IS: The effect of ocular torsional position on perception of the roll-tilt of visual stimuli. Vision Res 37:1071, 1997.
16. Dieterich, M, and Brandt, Th: Ocular torsion and tilt of the subjective visual vertical are sensitive brainstem signs. Ann Neurol 33:292, 1993.
17. Halmagyi, GM, et al: Tonic contraversive ocular tilt reaction with unilateral mesodiencephalic lesion. Neurology 40:1503, 1990.

18. Mossman, S, and Halmagyi, GM: Partial tonic ocular tilt reaction due to unilateral cerebellar lesion. Neurology 49:491, 1997.
19. Bickford, RG, et al: Nature of averaged evoked potentials to sound and other stimuli in man. Ann N Y Acad Sci 112:204, 1964.
20. Colebatch, JG, et al: Myogenic potentials generated by a click-evoked vestibulocollic reflex. J Neurol Neurosurg Psychiatr 57:190, 1994.
21. Halmagyi, GM, et al: Tapping the head activates the vestibular system: A new use for the clinical reflex hammer. Neurology 45:1927, 1995.
22. Ferber-Viart, C, Soulier, N, Duclaux, D, Dubreuil, C: Cochleovestibular afferent pathways of trapezius muscle responses to clicks in human. Acta Otolaryngol (Stockh) 118:6, 1998.
23. Young, ED, et al: Responses of squirrel monkey vestibular neurons to audio-frequency sound and head vibration. Acta Otolaryngol (Stockh) 84:352, 1977.
24. Didier, A, and Cazals, Y: Acoustic responses recorded from the saccular bundle on the eighth nerve of the guinea pig. Hearing Res 37:123, 1989.
25. Anson, BJ, and Donaldson, JA: Surgical anatomy of the Temporal Bone and Ear. Philadelphia, Saunders, 1973, p 285.
26. Murofushi, T, and Curthoys, IS: Physiological and anatomical study of click-sensitive primary vestibular afferents in the guinea-pig. Acta Otolaryngol (Stockh) 117:66, 1997.
27. Murofushi, T, et al: Responses of guinea pig primary vestibular neurons to clicks. Exp Brain Res 103:174, 1995.
28. McCue, MP, and Guinan, JJ: Sound-evoked activity in primary afferent neurons of the mammalian vestibular system. Am J Otol 18:355, 1997.
29. Murofushi, T, et al: Response of guinea pig vestibular nucleus neurons to clicks. Exp Brain Res 111:149, 1996.
30. Kevetter, GA, and Perachio, AA: Distribution of vestibular afferents that innervate the sacculus and posterior canal in the gerbil. J Comp Neurol 254:410, 1986.
31. Uchino, Y, et al: The sacculocollic reflex arc in cats. J Neurophysiol 77:3003, 1997.
32. Colebatch, JG, and Rothwell, JC: Vestibular-evoked EMG responses in human neck muscles. J Physiol 473:18P, 1993.
33. Deecke, L, et al: Tullio phenomenon with torsion of the eyes and subjective tilt of the visual surround. Ann N Y Acad Sci 374:650, 1981.
34. Dieterich, M, et al: Otolith function in man. Results from a case of otolith Tullio phenomenon. Brain 112:1377, 1989.
35. Minor, LB, Solomon, D, Zinreich, JS, Zee, DS: Tullio's phenomenon due to bone dehiscence of the superior semicircular canal. Arch Otolaryngol Head Neck Surg 124:249, 1998.
36. Rottach, KG, et al: Quantitative measurements of eye movements in a patient with Tullio phenomenon. J Vestib Res 6:255, 1996.
37. Colebatch, JG, et al: Click-evoked vestibular activation in the Tullio phenomenon. J Neurol Neurosurg Psychiatr 57:1538, 1994.
38. Büchele, W, and Brandt, T: Vestibular neuritis—horizontal semicircular canal paresis? Adv Otorhinolaryngol 42:157, 1988.
39. Fetter, M, and Dichgans, J: Vestibular neuritis spares the inferior division of the vestibular nerve. Brain 119:755, 1996.
40. Clemis, J, Balland, WJ, Baggot, PJ, Lyon, ST: Relative frequency of inferior vestibular schwannoma. Arch Otolaryngol 112:190, 1986.
41. Murofushi, T, et al: Vestibular evoked myogenic potentials in patients with acoustic neuromas. Arch Otolaryngol Head Neck Surg 124:509, 1998.
42. Heide, G et al: Click-evoked myogenic potentials in the differential diagnosis of vertigo. J Neurol Neurosurg Psychiat 66:787, 1999.
43. de Waele, C, Tran Ba Huy, P, Dirad, J-P, Freyys, G, Vidal, P-P: Saccular dysfunction in Ménière's disease. Amer J Otol 20:223, 1999.
44. Halmagyi, GM, et al: Testing the vestibulo-ocular reflex. In Alford, BR, et al (eds): Electrophysiologic Evaluation in Otolaryngology. Basel, Karger, 1997, pp 132–154.

CHAPTER 9

Audiological Assessment and Management

M. Cara Erskine, MEd
Hiroshi Shimizu, MD

AUDIOLOGICAL ASSESSMENT

The peripheral vestibular apparatus is connected to the cochlear duct, which holds the sensory organ of hearing. Pathological processes, therefore, can affect both the vestibular and cochlear organs, causing hearing impairment as well as dizziness. For example, the typical triad of Ménière's disease consists of episodic vertigo, fluctuating hearing loss, and tinnitus.[1] Labyrinthine fistula, ototoxicity, and acoustic neuroma are other examples that often present with both dizziness and hearing loss. Consequently, the audiological evaluation is required for early diagnosis in many cases of dizziness. The purpose of this chapter is to describe the:

1. Basic components of an audiological assessment as well as the more sophisticated measures of the auditory system used in diagnosis
2. Clinical application of the test results
3. Various methods used for auditory rehabilitation

Measurement of Behavioral Hearing Threshold

Hearing threshold is the faintest audible sound level and is expressed by the decibel (dB) notation. The decibel may be referred to as sound pressure level (SPL) or hearing level (HL). The unit used to describe the magnitude of the sound wave is called Pascal (Pa), and the weakest sound pressure audible to the human being at the frequency of 1000 Hertz (Hz) is 20 micro-Pascals (μPa). The decibel is not a fixed unit like the meter or gram, but an expression of a certain number of times greater than the reference level of 20 μPa. The decibel is defined as the logarithm of the ratio between a given sound pressure and the reference pressure. Namely,

$$dB\ SPL = 20 \log P1/P2$$

where P1 is sound pressure of a given sound, and P2 is the reference sound pressure (20 μPa). For example, a 20-dB SPL means a 10-fold increase (200 μPa) and a 60-dB SPL corresponds to a 1000-fold increase (20,000 μPa). Because the minimal audible SPL is different from frequency to frequency, the 0-dB dial reading on the audiometer was designed to present a pure tone of the minimal audible pressure under a given earphone regardless of frequency and is expressed in dB HL.

Hearing thresholds for pure tones are usually recorded on a graph called an *audiogram* (Fig. 9–1). Although the audible frequency range of young human ear is between 20 Hz and 20,000 Hz, hearing thresholds are measured mostly from 250 Hz to 8000 Hz for diagnostic objectives. The abscissa of the audiogram indicates dB HL and the ordinate indicates the frequencies for pure tones. Different symbols are used for the results obtained by *air conduction* (AC) and *bone conduction* (BC) with and without masking, in

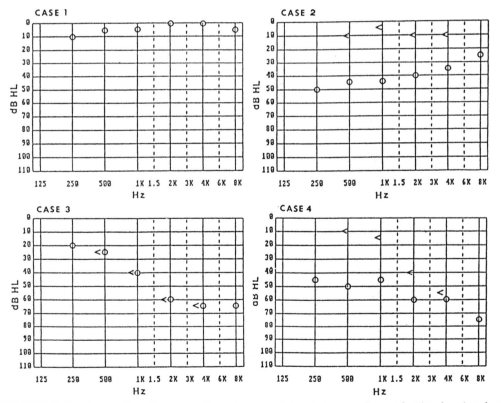

FIGURE 9–1. Types of audiograms. Case 1, normal hearing; case 2, conductive hearing loss; case 3, sensorineural hearing loss; case 4, mixed type hearing loss. ○ = air conduction, < = bone conduction.

sound field where pure tones are presented from the loudspeaker and for no response. Those symbols are usually shown on the audiogram form.

Because the behavioral hearing threshold depends on the patient's subjective response, the results are influenced by many factors such as attention, motivation, instruction, patient's physical condition, age, testing procedure, response criteria, and the audiologist's skill.

The AC threshold is measured by presenting pure tones either through the headphone or loudspeaker in the sound field. For BC testing, a BC oscillator is placed on the mastoid process behind the pinna. Because the sound reaches the cochlea directly, bypassing the external and middle ear conduction system, BC audiometry measures the function of the cochlea. The maximum BC threshold that can be measured is 65 dB to 70 dB HL.

Types of Hearing Loss

CONDUCTIVE HEARING LOSS

Conductive hearing loss is caused by a pathological condition that exists in the external ear canal or the middle ear. Case 2 in Figure 9–1 shows a typical audiogram of a conductive hearing loss characterized by elevated AC thresholds with a normal BC threshold. Audiograms showing significant gaps between AC and BC thresholds indicate the involvement of the external and/or middle ear. The main etiologies of conductive hearing loss include impact cerumen, foreign bodies in the external ear canals, acquired stenosis and closure of the external ear canal, disconnection of ossicular chain owing to injuries, otosclerosis, otitis media, cholesteatoma, barotrauma, genetic disorders, and neoplasms.

SENSORINEURAL HEARING LOSS

Hearing loss due to pathological conditions in the cochlea and/or the eighth nerve is called *sensorineural hearing loss*. The audiogram shows no gaps between AC and BC thresholds (case 3 in Fig. 9–1). The pathogenesis of sensorineural hearing loss includes injuries to the cochlea owing to temporal bone fracture, barotrauma, or noise, labyrinthitis, ototoxicity, Ménière's disease, aging process (presbyacusis), genetic process, some vascular and metabolic disorders, eighth-nerve Schwannoma, and meningioma in the cerebellopontine angle. Premature birth, hyperbilirubinemia, congenital infections (such as toxoplasmosis, syphilis, rubella, cytomegalovirus, and herpes), craniofacial anomalies, bacterial meningitis, hypoxia at birth, and prolonged mechanical ventilation are high risk factors for prelinguistic sensorineural hearing loss.

MIXED-TYPE HEARING LOSS

When both the external and/or middle ear and sensorineural system are involved, the audiogram reveals an elevation of BC thresholds but with AC-BC gaps as shown in Figure 9–1 (case 4). This type of loss is called *mixed-type hearing loss*. Mixed-type hearing loss can be seen in advanced otosclerosis, severe chronic otitis media, and some genetic hearing losses.

CLASSIFICATION OF HEARING LOSS

The degree of hearing loss is often expressed by *pure tone average* (PTA), which is the average hearing level of AC thresholds at 500 Hz, 1000 Hz, and 2000 Hz (Table 9–1). The frequency range between 500 Hz and 2000 Hz is referred to as the speech frequencies.

The classification shown in Table 9–1 may be adequate for adults who developed a hearing loss later in life, but is not necessarily appropriate for young children. For example, a loss of 30-dB PTA is classified as a mild hearing loss but is serious enough to cause a delay in speech and language development or difficulty understanding the teacher's speech in the classroom.[2]

Speech Audiometry

Ordinary speech audiometry typically consists of *speech reception threshold* (SRT) measurement and word recognition testing. The SRT is defined as the lowest level of speech at which the listener is able to repeat 50 percent of the two-syllable words (spondee) presented. If the patient is a young child, the SRT is sometimes estimated by presenting only familiar words to the child or letting the child identify pictures or toys on a tray. SRT measurement is essential to validate the reliability of PTA because the SRT should be within the 6-dB range of PTA. If no agreement is found between SRT and PTA, the reliability of the pure tone audiogram needs to be examined.

The *word recognition score* is expressed by the percentage of the *phonetically balanced* (PB) words that the listener can repeat correctly at a given level above the listener's SRT. By measuring the score at different speech intensity levels, starting from a low level and progressing to a high level, a word recognition score curve can be drawn (performance intensity function). The curve provides valuable information regarding the maximum score, called PB Max, and site of lesion. The PB Max is 88 to 100 percent and is usually obtained at 30 dB to 40 dB above SRT in normal listeners and patients with a conductive hearing loss. On the other hand, many patients with a cochlear hearing loss show PB Max at only 15 dB to 20 dB above the SRT with a score lower than normal. The PB Max is usually obtained at the most comfortable level (MCL) for speech. An abnormally narrowed range between the SRT and the MCL (dynamic range) is often referred to as *loudness recruitment*, which is one of the characteristics of cochlear sensorineural hearing loss. Patients with a precipitously downward sloping high-frequency hearing loss perform poorly in speech recognition testing because of

**TABLE 9–1. Classification
of Hearing Loss**

PTA (dB)	Classification
<15	Normal
16–25	Slight
26–40	Mild
41–55	Moderate
56–70	Moderately severe
71–90	Severe
>91	Profound

their inability to hear consonants. The PB Max, which is unproportionately poor for the degree of hearing loss and the configuration of audiogram, is often found in patients with a retrocochlear lesion, such as an acoustic neuroma and also in Ménière's disease. The speech recognition test is very important for differential diagnosis, assessment of the patient's communication ability, and evaluation for a hearing aid.

Acoustic Immittance Measurements

When a traveling sound wave reaches the tympanic membrane, a small portion of the sound energy is reflected at the tympanic membrane. The amount of reflection depends on the acoustic impedance (resistivity to the flow of acoustic energy) of the middle ear system. The middle ear analyzer is a device that measures a change in the acoustic impedance of the middle ear system by feeding the reflected sound received by a probe microphone to an impedance bridge. The measurement is called *acoustic immittance measurement* or *immittance audiometry,* and typically consists of *tympanometry* and *acoustic reflex measurement.*

Tympanometry measures a change in the compliance of the tympanic membrane and ossicular chain as a function of the air pressure in the external ear canal. When the air pressure in the external ear canal is matched to that in the middle ear, the compliance (mobility) of the tympanic membrane is highest. The testing results are depicted in a graph, referred to as a *tympanogram,* which reports the magnitude of acoustic transmission in terms of acoustic millimhos (mmhos) or as an equivalent volume of air in cubic centimeters or millimeters. The tympanogram is most commonly obtained with a single probe tone frequency of 226 Hz but multiple-frequency tympanometry (678 Hz or 1000 Hz in addition to 226 Hz) has been found to identify different types of ossicular chain disruptions.[3,4]

Five typical tympanograms are shown in Figure 9–2, and each type is associated with various middle ear disorders:

Type A: Normal middle ear air pressure and normal mobility of the tympanic membrane
Type As: Ossicular chain fixation, adhesive fixation, thickened or heavily scarred tympanic membrane, cholesteatoma, polyps, or granuloma
Type Ad: Ossicular chain discontinuity or flaccid tympanic membrane
Type B: Middle ear effusion, adhesive otitis media, tympanic membrane perforation, pressure-equalizing (PE) tube, impact cerumen, or artifact
Type C: Serous otitis media, or blocked eustachian tube

The acoustic reflex measurement has been used to identify site of lesion[5] or to identify and estimate hearing sensitivity.[6] The acoustic reflex occurs when the stapedius muscle contracts in response to a loud signal. A stimulus applied to either ear will cause muscles to contract binaurally. The reflex is tested at the point of maximum compliance of the middle ear and can be seen on the middle ear analyzer as a change in compliance. When an acoustic signal is presented continuously at 10 dB above the reflex threshold, the magnitude of the reflex is usually sustained for 10 seconds at 500 Hz and 1000 Hz. The measurement of the magnitude of reflex for the 10 seconds is called the *acoustic reflex decay test.* This test is primarily used to identify a lesion in the eighth nerve.

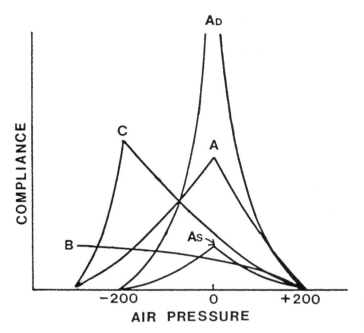

FIGURE 9–2. Types of tym-
panograms.

The acoustic reflex occurs at 70 dB to 100 dB HL in normal hearing individuals. However, the reflex is often seen at only 30 dB to 50 dB above hearing threshold in patients with a sensorineural hearing loss. The narrow range between the reflex threshold and the hearing threshold indicates a cochlear lesion. On the other hand, the patient with an acoustic tumor may show elevated acoustic reflex thresholds and also rapid reflex decay. The absence or elevation of reflex thresholds can be seen in stapes fixation as in otosclerosis, disarticulation of the middle ear ossicles, conductive hearing losses, and brain stem pathway disorders. The acoustic immittance measurements have also been used as a screening tool to identify middle ear disorders and hearing loss in young children.[7,8]

Auditory Brainstem Response Testing

By means of an average response computer, a series of time-locked electrical potentials evoked by acoustic stimuli can be recorded with a regular EEG electrode placed on the top of the head (vertex) or on the forehead below the hairline, and another electrode placed on each earlobe. The electrode on the earlobe ipsilateral to the ear stimulated is used as a reference electrode and the other as a ground electrode. The broad-band click-elicited auditory brainstem response (ABR) typically consists of a series of five or more evoked electrical potentials generated within the eighth nerve and the central auditory pathways of the brainstem (Fig. 9–3). At 70 dB nHL (70 dB above the mean value of click thresholds obtained from a group of normally hearing young adults), wave I occurs at around 1.6 ms after click onset and is followed by wave II at 2.8 ms, wave III at 3.8 ms, wave IV at 5.1 ms, and wave V at around 5.7 ms. Waves I and

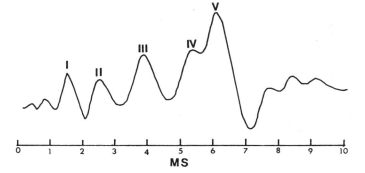

FIGURE 9–3. Basic morphology of auditory brainstem response (ABR). Wave I corresponds to the cochlea, acoustic N; wave II, acoustic N, cochlear Nu; wave III, superior olivary complex; wave IV, lateral lemniscus; wave V, inferior colliculus.

II arise primarily from the auditory nerve, but because of the complexity of the neuroanatomy of the auditory system in the brainstem, the later wave appears to be the summation of the electrical activity in more than one auditory source between the cochlear nucleus and inferior colliculus. The latency values get longer as the intensity is decreased, but the interwave interval is relatively[9] unaffected by the intensity of the acoustic signal.

Because the recording technique is noninvasive and the responses are highly sensitive and reproducible, ABR testing has become an important clinical tool in audiology, otology, and neurology.

CLINICAL APPLICATIONS OF AUDITORY BRAINSTEM RESPONSE TESTING

Estimation of Hearing Sensitivity

Assessment of hearing of difficult-to-test young children is crucial but requires special techniques. Brainstem response audiometry is a powerful tool for assessing the hearing of those children; it can be done in natural and sedated sleep. The click-elicited ABR estimates hearing sensitivity at 3000 Hz to 4000 Hz.[10–12] The morphology of the ABR with a conductive hearing loss is characterized by prolonged latency of each wave with normal or near-normal interwave intervals. The latency values are greatly influenced by the pathology of the cochlea and the configuration of audiogram. Sloping high-frequency cochlear hearing losses usually cause prolonged latencies without greatly affecting the wave I–V interval.[13] The prediction of hearing threshold in low and middle frequencies requires the use of tone bursts or more complex stimuli.[14]

An ABR can be obtained even in neonates (Fig. 9–4), and the effectiveness of neonatal hearing screening by means of ABR, particularly by automated ABR, in early identification of hearing impaired infants and early intervention has been well recognized.[15–18]

Identification of Lesions in the Auditory Nerve and Brainstem

The morphology, absolute latency, and interwave intervals of the ABR provide significant information regarding the condition of the VIIIth nerve and auditory pathway within the brainstem. Inconsistent morphology, abnormally prolonged latencies and/or interwave intervals, reversed wave I/V amplitude, and the absence of wave V, or the entire response, are indicative of lesions in the VIIIth nerve or the brainstem. The

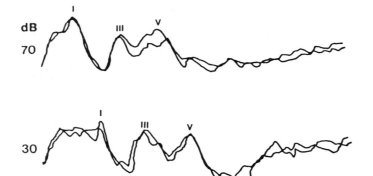

FIGURE 9–4. Auditory brainstem responses obtained from a 3-day-old baby.

abnormal ABR can be found in acoustic tumors (Fig. 9–5), brainstem tumors, demyelinating disorders such as multiple sclerosis and leukodystrophy, brain death, coma, head trauma, stroke or ischemia, hydrocephalus, sudden infant death syndrome, alcoholism, sleep apnea, and spastic dysphonia.[19,20] A general relationship between the level of the lesion and its effect on the ABR has been well recognized, but the abnormality of the ABR is not uniquely characteristic for a given pathology. For example, the complete absence of ABR can be seen in both acoustic tumor and multiple sclerosis.

Diagnostic and Prognostic Applications in Severe Head Injury in the Intensive Care Unit

ABR, often combined with somatosensory and visual evoked potentials, has been used for severely brain-damaged patients in the intensive care unit to monitor neurological status, localize the lesion, evaluate the effectiveness of medical and surgical treatment, determine brain death, or predict the patient's prognosis.[21] Because the patient is in critical condition, the interpretation of the evoked potential data requires careful considerations of the effects of various pharmacological agents, hypothermia, intracranial pressure, and arterial blood gases.

Intraoperative Monitoring

The recent development of electrophysiological and evoked potential monitoring during surgery has made a significant contribution in the improved intraoperative patient management and reduction of postoperative complications. Monitoring by ABR has proved useful for surgical procedures on the VIIIth nerve and brainstem, such as acoustic tumor resection, retrolabyrinthine vestibular nerve section, trigeminal nerve section, brainstem tumor resection, microvascular decompression of cranial nerves V or VII, and posterior fossa decompression.[22]

ELECTROCOCHLEOGRAPHY

Electrocochleography (ECoG) is the recording of acoustically evoked electrical potentials arising from the cochlea and the VIIIth nerve: *cochlear microphonic* (CM), *summation potential* (SP), and *whole action potential* (AP) of the VIIIth nerve.

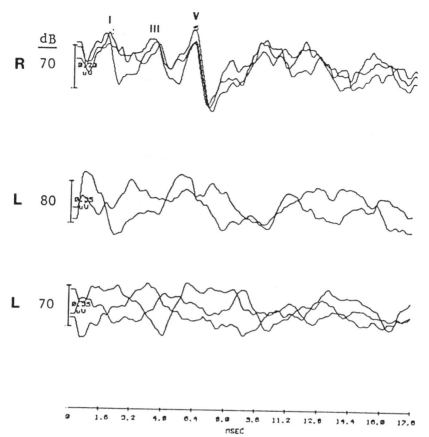

FIGURE 9–5. ABRs obtained from a 46-year-old patient who had a surgically confirmed acoustic neuroma on the left side. She had a moderate sensorineural hearing loss in the left ear. Repeated ABR on the left side at 70 dB and 80 dB nHL showed no discernible responses but clear responses were obtained when the right ear was stimulated.

The CM is an alternating current (AC) potential, which is generated by the hair cells. CM mimics the wave form of sound stimulation like the AC voltage from a microphone. For example, if a 1000-Hz pure tone is presented to the ear, the recorded CM is also a 1000-Hz sinusoidal wave and is maintained for the duration of the stimulation. However, the CM is not symmetrical about the baseline, indicating a shift of a direct current (DC). This shift of the baseline (DC shift) is called *SP.* It is not well known how the SP is generated, but it is believed to reflect the distortion in the hair cell transduction process. The whole VIIIth nerve AP is the summation of synchronized discharge from many auditory neurons. The wave I of the ABR represents the AP.

Those stimulus-related electrical potentials can be recorded with a needle electrode placed on the promontory through the tympanic membrane (TM) or by an electrode placed on the TM or the wall of the external ear canal near the TM. The shorter the distance between the electrode and cochlea, the larger is the amplitude of the potentials and the better is the signal-to-noise ratio. However, the TM or ear canal electrode (noninvert) is more popular than the transtympanic electrode in the United States because of its noninvasiveness. The invert electrode is preferably placed on Fz. The potentials can be elicited by either clicks or tone bursts at moderately high intensities. Because the CM mimics the wave form of the acoustic stimulus, it can be canceled out by adding the averaged CMs obtained with the stimuli of reversed polarities. When the CM is canceled out, the SP appears as step-like voltage during the stimulus period of tone bursts or on the leading edge of the AP waveform for clicks (Fig. 9–6). The AP is not affected by the polarity of the click.

CLINICAL APPLICATIONS

Attempts had been made to use ECoG to predict hearing threshold and identify the cite of lesion until ABR was accepted as being more sensitive and useful than ECoG.[24-27] Recently, ECoG has attained popularity in identifying and monitoring endolymphatic hydrops or Ménière's disease.[23,28–30] Normally, the amplitude of SP is very small compared with the AP amplitude. The range of SP/AP amplitude ratio is normally 10 to 50 percent, but exceeds 50 percent in many patients with Ménière's disease (see Fig. 9–6). Because Ménière's disease is characterized by episodic attacks of vertigo and fluctuating sensorineural hearing loss, whether or not ECoG is performed during the active stage of endolymphatic hydrops may alter the results. The "hit-rate" of ECoG seems to be poor with a mild or severe hearing loss in high frequencies.[31] Consequently, the absence of abnormally enlarged SP does not necessarily rule out Ménière's disease.

An enlargement of SP has also been found in both humans and experimental animals with perilymphatic fistula.[32] Perilymphatic fistula may result in secondary endolymphatic hydrops owing to a decrease in perilymph causing an enlarged SP. The

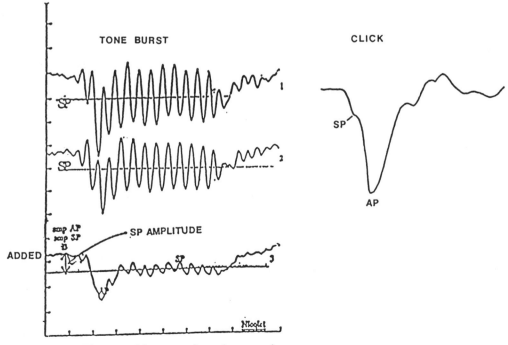

FIGURE 9–6. Electrocochleograms from the normal ear.

symptoms of perilymphatic fistula often mimic Ménière's syndrome. Another clinical application of ECoG has been to monitor the functional integrity of the VIIIth nerve and the auditory pathway in the brainstem during posterior fossa surgery.[33–36] One of the advantages of promontory ECoG with a transtympanic electrode is the significantly improved signal-to-noise ratio resulting from recording in the proximity of the VIIIth nerve.

Otoacoustic Emission

During the past decade, a dramatic change has evolved in our knowledge of the physiology of the cochlea by the discoveries of *otoacoustic emission*,[37] the *sharp basilar membrane tuning*,[38,39] and the *motility of the outer hair cells*.[40] We now know that the cochlea has both passive and active mechanisms, and that the cochlea emits sounds that can be recorded in the external ear canal. There are two types of otoacoustic emissions (OAEs). One is the OAE that can be recorded in the absence of acoustic stimulation and is called *spontaneous otoacoustic emission (SOAE)*. SOAEs are low intensity narrow band sounds which are present in 40 to 60 percent of healthy ears.

The other type of OAE is evoked by acoustic stimuli, called *evoked otoacoustic emission (EOAE)*. They can be elicited by clicks or tone pips (transiently evoked OAE:TEOAE), single, continuous pure tones (stimulus frequency OAE), and by two continuous pure tones separated by a prescribed frequency distance (distortion-product OAE). EOAEs can be detected in nearly all normal human ears.

To measure OAEs, a small probe tip, which contains a sensitive microphone and a sound source, is inserted into the external ear canal in a similar fashion used in acoustic immittance measurement. The emitted sound energy is amplified and fed into the computer-based dynamic signal analyzer. For details of the recording technique and to understand the wave forms of the OEAs, the reader is referred to Kemp et al.[41] Because of the objectivity of OAE measurement, noninvasiveness of the recording procedure, its frequency-specific nature, and the specificity for outer hair cells, the OAE has great potential to provide clinically significant information on cochlear function and pathology.[42–44] Because of the recent development of instrumentation, we can record OAEs from patients in clinical situations. However, the clinical application is still in the early stages of development. The most promising clinical application has been the use of transiently evoked OAEs (TEOAEs) for hearing screening of infants including neonates.[42,45–47] The ideal hearing screening for the difficult-to-test young infants requires that the test be fast, easy, noninvasive, highly sensitive, and low in false-positive and false-negative rates. The TEOAE are present in virtually all normal neonates[41,45,48,49] and are not present in adults with a mild hearing loss. The test time is reportedly only 12 minutes on the average, versus 26 minutes for ABR screening.[50] With these findings and miniaturization of the equipment, TEOAE and distortion product OAE (DPOAE) became powerful tools for newborn hearing screening.

MANAGEMENT OF HEARING IMPAIRMENT

Selection of the best amplification system for an individual must be based on thorough, individualized assessment of hearing function. The greatest potential benefits from a hearing aid are best achieved by those with moderate to severe hearing losses

(30 dB through 85 dB). Whereas most people with a hearing loss may benefit from an assistive listening device and/or hearing aid in selected situations, people with profound losses (no benefit from a hearing aid) may benefit from a cochlear implant. Clinicians generally agree that hearing-impaired people would benefit from aural rehabilitation, speech reading, and/or auditory training.

Hearing Aids

The function of a hearing aid is to amplify sound that will help the hearing-impaired utilize the residual hearing to the maximum. The first amplification system was the cupped ear, which gave an increase of about 10 dB in the high frequencies. Horns and speaking tubes were first used in the late 1800s as aids to hearing. The transistor hearing aids currently in use have greater flexibility, reduced size, and lower battery cost.

The electronic hearing aid is a miniature telephone with three basic parts: the microphone, which picks up the sound and converts it to an electrical signal; the amplifier, which increases the strength of the electrical signal; and the receiver, which converts the amplified sound back into acoustic energy.

TYPES OF HEARING AIDS

1. *Behind the ear* (BTE) (Fig. 9–7, center):   This hearing aid fits behind the pinna, is considered fairly rugged, is available in a wide variety of amplification configurations, and can be fit to the most severe hearing losses.
2. *In-the-ear/In-the-canal* (ITE/ITC):   These miniature hearing aids are custom-molded instruments. The electronic components are placed into the concha portion in the ITE (Fig. 9–7, left), and more deeply within the canal portion in the ITC (Fig. 9–7, right). The popularity of these hearing aids remains high in market share, 60% for ITE/ITC combined.[51]
3. *Completely-in-the-canal* (CIC):   This hearing aid is very small and fits deep in the ear canal. The main advantages lie in the invisibility, increased gain and output, and reduction of the occlusion effect and feedback.[52]

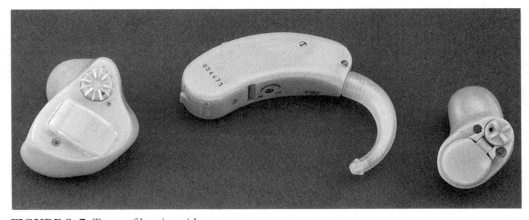

FIGURE 9–7. Types of hearing aids.

4. *Body hearing aid:* Up to 1955, this hearing aid was the only wearable one available but now accounts for less than 2 percent of the market. The body hearing aid usually is worn by people with a very profound hearing loss.

5. *Contralateral routing of sound* (CROS): A hearing aid shell is worn by each ear; one contains a hearing aid and the other a microphone emitter. The sound is picked up on the side with no usable hearing and routed to the better side by a radio frequency. This aid is helpful for people with profound unilateral hearing loss and near-normal hearing in the better ear, and helps users to understand speakers when they stand on the impaired side.

6. *Bilateral contralateral routing of sound* (BICROS): This system is the same as the CROS, but two microphones are connected to the same amplifier. BICROS is used when there is no hearing in one ear and a hearing loss in the other.

7. *Bone conduction hearing aid:* This hearing aid conducts the sound directly to the inner ear by bone vibration and bypasses the middle ear system. It is used when bone conduction is near normal or mildly depressed and the patient is unable to wear conventional hearing aids because of aural atresia or medical problems. This aid can be attached to a headband and placed tightly against the mastoid or it can be surgically implanted. The microphone and receiver are encased in a BTE device.

Hearing aids can be equipped with a telephone coil, which is an induction coil, to pick up electromagnetic signals directly from a telephone or a loop amplification system. Hearing aids are now available with a variety of circuits, such as automatic signal processing, digitally programmable hearing aids, truly digital sound processing, and K-AMP. These circuits help to improve their aided function in noise, the localization of sound, and when there is sensitivity to loud sounds.

If the patient has a bilateral hearing loss, the consensus has been to recommend two hearing aids to benefit from binaural hearing. Ross[53] reviewed 19 studies on monaural and binaural hearing aid use, and 15 of them showed binaural superiority. Users set the volume lower when wearing two hearing aids and were able to function better in noise. However, in a comparison trial of binaural and monaural hearing aid use, two hearing aids were preferred in everyday quiet situations but one aid was more effective in noise.[54]

Aural Rehabilitation

An aural rehabilitation program is always recommended as part of the hearing aid selection. Such a program is designed to help the individual integrate the use of the hearing aid with the proper adjustments in the environment to maximize their performance. Hearing aid users are taught how to manipulate background noise and select favorable seating. In addition, emphasis is placed on incorporating the auditory and visual modalities.[55] The goal of an aural rehabilitation program is to orient each person to their specific hearing aid and provide strategies for coping in all environments with the hearing aid.[56]

ASSISTIVE LISTENING DEVICES

Assistive listening devices (ALDs), are a significant adjunct to rehabilitation/habilitation process for the hearing impaired. "ALD" is broadly used to encompass the equipment designed to improve the communication ability of the hearing impaired population. The equipment primarily consists of: (1) ALD as in a loop amplifying system, hardware system, or infrared system; (2) assistive alerting device (AADs), such as bells and buzzers; (3) assistive signaling device (ASDs) referring to a signaling device, such as in flashing lights; and (4) telecommunication device for the disabled or TDDs and closed-captioning units for television.[57] These devices are needed because a hearing aid has limitations. Most individuals are dissatisfied with their hearing aid and few hearing aid users have no complaints. The ALDs bypass the background noise so that the signal goes directly from the speaker to the listener.

Aids can be categorized according to their commonality. This categorization includes:

1. *Hard wire devices*, in which the microphone is near the sound source and the signal is sent electronically to the ear of the listener. These devices include the Pocket Talker and a system called direct audio input which attaches directly to the hearing aid with a boot.
2. *Wireless listening systems* including the *loop system*, which is based on the principle of magnetic induction in which a signal from an amplifier is fed into a coil of wire that is placed around the room. The wire generates an audio frequency magnetic field, which is picked up by the telephone switch on the hearing aid.

Also included is the *infrared system*, in which sounds are picked up by a microphone and are transferred to an infrared beam emitted by a special light-emitting diode (LED). The listener wears a battery-operated infrared receiver with a volume control. These devices are popular in theaters, concert halls, and places of worship.

AADs are units that emit an alerting signal by converting a normal alerting sound to a low-frequency loud sound for the hearing impaired to hear. Smoke detectors, door bells, and telephones are some of the most frequently used units. ASDs transform the acoustic signal by transmitter to a visual or tactile sound. For example, a light can be activated when the door bell rings or a vibrating unit under the pillow can be attached to an alarm clock.

An informing device is a *telecommunication device* (TDD formerly TTY) for the severely hearing impaired and deaf, which allows them to communicate by telephone. This device allows for an acoustic coupler to convert the typed messages into sequences of tones. The signal is then converted into a readout enabling use of the phone lines. Closed-captioning television is a decoding device that provides readable messages for the hearing impaired and deaf.

ALDs and these other systems enrich the lives of the hearing impaired and the deaf, and allow for greater security and independence.[57,58]

Cochlear Implants

Cochlear implants are a viable choice for the profoundly hearing impaired population. They are appropriately fit only to those people who cannot achieve any benefit from a hearing aid. Cochlear implants produce a sensation of hearing by direct electrical stimulation of the acoustic nerve. This technique is not novel and was first reported by the Romans as a way to treat headache. The earliest report of direct electrical stimulation to the ear was reported in 1790 when Volta inserted metal rods into each ear and connected them to a circuit of 50 volts. He experienced the sense of a blow to the head.[59] It did not receive mention again until the 1900s. In 1957, Djourno and Eyries became the first group to stimulate the acoustic nerve of a deaf patient.[59]

Cochlear implants are implanted either outside the cochlea (round window, mastoid) and are referred to as extracochlear, or within the cochlea and called intracochlear. They are further defined by the number of channels: single or multi. The multichannel devices are the only ones that are being manufactured in the United States. They are reported to provide superior information over the single-channel units because they provide frequency-specific information about the signal.[60]

The main components of the cochlear implant (Fig. 9–8A) are: (1) the microphone, which sends an electrical equivalent of an acoustic stimulus to the signal processor; (2) the signal processor, which transforms the electrical input into the desired electrical stimuli; and (3) the surgically implanted system, in which the signal goes to one or more electrodes depending on the design of the device. The cochlear implant is now available as an ear-level device that is the same size as a behind-the-ear hearing aid (Fig. 9–8B).

More than 25,000 children and adults utilize multichannel devices worldwide, about 50 percent are able to understand some open-set information (no clues are provided to the patient).[61] Although outstanding results (e.g., being able to talk on the telephone) do occur, they are rare. Most patients, however, can carry on controlled conversations with visual cues.

The technology of the cochlear implant is continuing to improve as advances are made in coding strategies. The strategy can be manipulated depending on patient requirements. Under the current selection process, it cannot be predicted who will function well with the cochlear implant, but those who do best seem to be generally younger, motivated individuals who have good lip-reading skills and have only very recently lost their hearing.

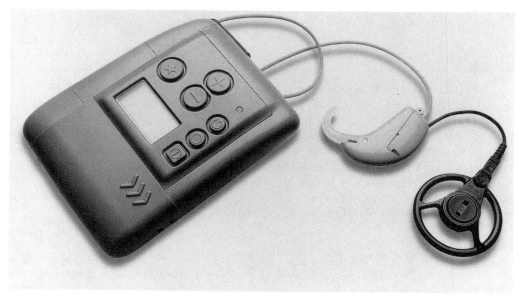

FIGURE 9–8A. A multichannel cochlear implant processor, microphone, and magnet coil (photograph courtesy of Cochlear Corporation).

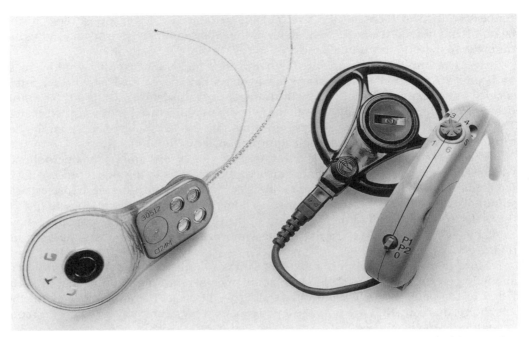

FIGURE 9–8B. Cochlear implant internal device electrode array and ear level cochlear implant (photograph courtesy of Cochlear Corporation).

The rehabilitation process is lengthy but vital to the success of the cochlear implant. The procedure involves tuning the speech processor by computer hook-up, orientation to the device, aural rehabilitation, and experiencing new environments while using the device.

Auditory Training

The concept of auditory training was originally noted in 1802 by Itard.[62] He began to systematically work on improving auditory skills in hearing-impaired children. The initial work usually begins with sound awareness tasks, gross sound discrimination, broad sound discrimination among simple speech patterns, and fine discrimination of speech. The concept is to maximize the use of residual hearing regardless of the degree of hearing loss. Controversy exists as to whether this approach is helpful, and reportedly there is little scientific evidence to support its value. There has been some small but statistically significant improvement noted in the area of speech recognition performance. The gains appear to be maintained over time.[63]

SPEECH READING/LIP READING

This skill is a multifactor process that involves how sounds look on the lips. Lip reading requires combining visual attention, situational and contextual cues, lighting, and distance from the speaker in order to achieve maximum benefit.[56] In the English language, about one-third of the sounds are visible on the lips; thus the combination of these factors is essential. Training in this skill is aimed at teaching systematic observation of visual symbols combined with optimal environmental factors and topic selection. The most common methods are: (1) synthetic (Nitchie), which uses materials in differing linguistic contexts (words to conversational speech); (2) analytic (Mueller-Walle, Jena), which works on isolated sounds and nonsense syllables which begins with visible sounds (/p/, /th/, /f/) and proceeds to low visibility sounds (/k/, /g/, /h/); and (3) eclectic (Kinzie), which combines both methods of using sounds in isolation and words in context.[62] Speech reading is considered an important component of the aural rehabilitation process, particularly for those individuals with significant hearing impairment.

Many newer approaches to aural rehabilitation have been introduced which include Alpiner's Progressive Approach (1993).[64] It is individually tailored to the patients' needs and looks at their goals and works with others within their social circle. Speech tracking, described by DeFilippo and Scott (1978),[65] which assesses the patient's ability to give information back verbatim as provided by the instructor. Another avenue is through laser video disc production, which can be operated by the patient and provide flexibility as the patient can work independently at home (1993).[66]

SUMMARY

The auditory and vestibular systems are often affected by the same disorders. Evaluation of auditory function in cases where dizziness is a complaint, therefore, contributes to the diagnosis of the patient's problem. This chapter has reviewed the numerous procedures for evaluating auditory function that can be incorporated into the total workup. Information obtained from tests about auditory function not only aids in diagnosis but is the basis for treatment and rehabilitation of the hearing loss itself.

REFERENCES

1. Pfaltz, CZ, and Matefi, L: Ménière's disease or syndrome? A critical review of diagnostic criteria. In Vosteen, KH, et al (eds): Ménière's Disease: Pathogenesis, Diagnosis and Treatment. Thieme-Stratton, New York, 1981, p 1.
2. Bess, FH, et al: Children with minimal sensorineural hearing loss: Prevalence, educational performance, and functional status. Ear Hear 19:339, 1998.
3. Lilly, DJ: Multiple frequency, multiple component tympanometry: New approaches to an old diagnostic problem. Ear Hearing 5:300, 1986.
4. Van Camp, KJ, and Vogeleer, M: Normative multi-frequency tympanometric data on otosclerosis. Scand Audiol 15:187, 1986.
5. Stach, BA, and Jerger, JF: Acoustic reflex patterns in peripheral and central auditory system disease. Semin Hearing 8:369, 1987.
6. Silman, S, et al: Prediction of hearing loss from the acoustic reflex threshold. In Silman, S (ed): The Acoustic Reflex Basic Principles and Clinical Application. Academic Press, New York, 1984, p 187.
7. Guidelines for screening for hearing impairment and middle ear disorders. American Speech, Language, and Hearing Association (suppl) 2:17, 1990.
8. Walters, RI, and Shimizu, H: Acoustic immittance screening of infants. Semin Hearing 11:177, 1990.
9. Coats, AC, and Martin, JL: Human auditory nerve action potentials and brainstem evoked responses. Arch Otolaryngol 103:605, 1977.
10. Jerger, J, and Mauldin, L: Prediction of sensorineural hearing level from the brain stem evoked response. Arch Otolaryngol 104:456, 1979.
11. McDonald, JM, and Shimizu, H: Frequency specificity of the auditory brain stem response. Am J Otolaryngol 2:36, 1989.

12. Shimizu, H: Some considerations on standardizing measurement and interpretation of brainstem response audiometry. In Starr, A, et al (eds): Sensory Evoked Potentials. Centro Ricerche e Studi Amplifon, Milan, Italy, 1984.
13. Bauch, CD, and Olsen, WO: The effect of 2000–4000 Hz hearing sensitivity on ABR results. Ear Hear 7:314, 1986.
14. Gorga, MP: Predicting auditory sensitivity from auditory brainstem response measurements. Semin Hear 20:29, 1999.
15. Hermann, BS, et al: Automated infant hearing screening using the ABR: Development and validation. Am J Audiol 4:6, 1995.
16. Stach, BA and Santilli, CL: Technology in newborn hearing screening. Semin Hearing 19:247, 1998.
17. Arehart, KH, et al: State of the States: The status of universal newborn hearing screening, assessment, and intervention systems in 16 States. Am J Audiol 7:101, 1998.
18. American Academy of Pediatrics: Newborn and infant hearing loss: Detection and intervention. Pediatrics 103:527, 1999.
19. Rowe, MJ: The brainstem auditory evoked response in neurological disorders: A review. Ear Hear 2:141, 1981.
20. Stockard, JJ, and Hecox, K: Brainstem auditory evoked potentials in sudden infant death syndrome (SIDS), "near-miss-SIDS," and infant apnea syndromes. Electroencephalogr Clin Neurophysiol 51:43, 1981.
21. Hall, JW, III and Tucker, DA: Sensory evoked responses in the intensive care unit. Ear Hear 7:220, 1986.
22. Edwards, BM and Kileny, PR: Audiologists in intraoperative neurophysiologic monitoring. Semin Hearing 19:87, 1998.
23. Coats, AC: The summating potential and Ménière's disease. Arch Otolaryngol 107:199, 1981.
24. Ruben, RJ, et al: Cochlear potentials in man. Laryngoscope 71:1141, 1961.
25. Cullen, JK, et al: Human acoustic nerve action potential recordings from the tympanic membrane without anesthesia. Acta Otolaryngol 4:15, 1972.
26. Sohmer, H, and Feinmesser, M: Electrocochleography in clinical-audiological diagnosis. Arch Otolaryngol 206:91, 1974.
27. Aran, JM: Contributions of electrocochleography to diagnosis in infancy. An eight year survey. In Gerber, SE and Mencher, GT (eds): Early Diagnosis of Hearing Loss. Grune & Stratton, New York, 1978, p 215.
28. Orchik, DJ, et al: Summating potential and action potential ratio in Ménière's disease before and after treatment. Am J Otol 19:478, 1998.
29. Levine, S, et al: Use of electrocochleography in the diagnosis of Ménière's disease. Laryngoscope 108:993, 1998.
30. Margolis, RH: Electrocochleography. Semin Hearing 20:45, 1999.
31. Coats, AC, et al: Auditory evoked potentials—The cochlear summating potential in detection of endolymphatic hydrops. Am J Otol 5:443, 1984.
32. Arenberg, IK, et al: ECoG results in perilymphatic fistula: Clinical and experimental studies. Otolaryngol Head Neck Surg 99:435, 1988.
33. Levine, RA, et al: Monitoring auditory evoked potentials during acoustic neuroma surgery: Insights into the mechanism of hearing loss. Ann Otol Rhinol Laryngol 93:116, 1984.
34. Ojemann, RG, et al: Use of intraoperative auditory evoked potentials to preserve hearing in unilateral acoustic neuroma removal. J Neurosurg 61:938, 1984.
35. Silverstein, H, et al: Simultaneous use of CO2 laser with continuous monitoring of eighth cranial nerve action potentials during acoustic neuroma surgery. Otolaryngol Head Neck Surg 92:80, 1984.
36. Silverstein, H, et al: Retrolabyrinthine vestibular neurectomy with simultaneous monitoring of eighth nerve and brainstem auditory evoked potentials. Otolaryngol Head Neck Surg 93:736, 1985.
37. Kemp, DT: Stimulated acoustic emission from within the human auditory system. J Acoust Soc Am 64:1386, 1978.
38. Khana, SM, and Leonard, DGB: Basilar membrane tuning in the cat cochlea. Science 215:305, 1982.
39. Sellick, PM, et al: Measurement of basilar membrane motion in the guinea pig using the Mossbauer technique. J Acoust Soc Am 72:131, 1982.
40. Brownell, WE: Observations on a motile response in isolated outer hair cells. In Webster, WR, and Aitken, LM (eds): Mechanisms of Hearing. Monash Univ. P. 1983, p 5.
41. Kemp, DT, et al: A guide to the effective use of otoacoustic emissions. Ear Hear 11:93, 1990.
42. Elberling, C, et al: Evoked acoustic emission: Clinical application. Acta Otolaryngolog (suppl) 421:77, 1985.
43. Ferber-Viart, C, et al: Is the presence of transient evoked otoacoustic emissions in ears with acoustic neuroma significant?
44. Robinette, MS: EOAE contributions in the evaluation of cochlear versus retrocochlear disorders. Semin Hearing 20:13, 1999.
45. Johnsen, NJ, et al: Evoked acoustic emissions from the human ear. IV. Final results in 100 neonates. Scand Audiol 17:27, 1988.
46. Bonfils, P, et al: Clinical significance of otoacoustic emission: A perspective. Ear Hear 11:155, 1990.
47. Stevens, JC, et al: Click evoked otoacoustic emissions in neonatal screening. Ear Hear 11:128, 1990.

48. Bonfils, P, et al: Evoked oto-acoustic emissions from adults and infants: Clinical applications. Acta Oto-laryngol 105:445, 1988.
49. Norton, SI, and Widen, JE: Evoked otoacoustic emissions in normal-hearing infants and children: Emerging data and issues. Ear Hear 11:121, 1990.
50. White, KR: The Rhode Island Project: Otoacoustic emissions and neonatal hearing screening. Presented at International Symposium on Otoacoustic Emissions, Kansas City, Missouri, May 9–11, 1991.
51. Strome, KE: A review of the 1997 hearing instrument market. Hearing Review 5:8, 1998.
52. Mueller, HG and Ebinger, KA: CIC hearing aids: Potential benefits and fitting strategies. Semin Hearing 17:61, 1996.
53. Ross, M: Binaural vs. monoaural hearing aid amplification for hearing impaired individuals. In Libby, ER (ed): Binaural Hearing and Amplification, vol 2. Zenetron, Chicago, 1980, p 1.
54. Schureurs, KK, and Olsen, WO: Comparison of monaural and binaural hearing aid use on a trial period basis. Ear Hear 6:198, 1985.
55. Tye-Murray, N: Foundations of Aural Rehabilitation. Singular Publishing Group, San Diego, 1998, pp 22–30.
56. Ross, M: Overview of aural rehabilitation. In Katz, J (ed): Handbook of Clinical Audiology. Williams & Wilkins, Baltimore, 1994, pp 592–594.
57. Pehringer, JL: Assistive devices: Technology to improve communication. Otolaryngol Clin North Am 22:143, 1989.
58. Vaughn, GR, et al: Assistive devices and systems (ALDS) enhance the lifestyles of hearing impaired persons. Am J Otology 9:101, 1988.
59. Luxford, WM, and Brackmann, DE: The history of cochlear implants. In Gray, RF (ed): Cochlear Implants. College-Hill, San Diego, 1985, p 1.
60. NIH Consensus Statement on Cochlear Implants in Adults and Children, V13, May 1995.
61. Osberger, MJ: Audiological rehabilitation with cochlear implants and tactile aids. American Speech, Language, and Hearing Association 32(4):38, 1990.
62. Ross, M: Overview of aural rehabilitation. In Katz, J (ed): Handbook of Clinical Audiology. Williams & Wilkins, Baltimore, 1994, pp 587–589.
63. Rubinstein, A, and Boothroyd, A: Effect of two approaches to auditory training on speech recognition by hearing impaired adults. Journal of Speech and Hearing Disorders 30:153, 1987.
64. Alpiner, JG, et al: Overview of rehabilitative audiology. In Alpiner, JG and McCarthy, PA (eds): Rehabilitative Audiology Children and Adults, ed 2. Williams & Wilkins, Baltimore, 1993, pp 13–14.
65. DeFilippo, CL and Scott, BL: A method for training and evaluating the reception of ongoing speech. J Acoust Soc Am 63:1186, 1978.
66. Alpiner, JG and Schow, RL: Rehabilitative evaluation of hearing impaired adults. In Alpiner, JG and McCarthy, PA (eds): Rehabilitative Audiology Children and Adults, ed 2. Williams & Wilkins, Baltimore, 1993, pp 245–250.

Medical Management

Pharmacological and Optical Methods of Treating Vestibular Disorders and Nystagmus

R. John Leigh, M.D.

Patients with vestibular disease may complain of vertigo, oscillopsia, or the visual consequences of nystagmus.[1] *Vertigo* consists of the illusion of turning and implies vestibular imbalance. *Oscillopsia* consists of illusory, to-and-fro, movements of the seen environment; when it occurs with head movements, it usually implies bilateral loss of vestibular function. Patients with spontaneous nystagmus, owing to vestibular or other processes, may also complain of oscillopsia when their heads are still. In this chapter, treatments for vertigo, oscillopsia, and the visual consequences of nystagmus will be reviewed, attempting to base therapies on known pathophysiology.

In trying to understand and treat the symptoms resulting from labyrinthine disorders, it is important to bear in mind the nature of the demands placed on the vestibular system *during natural activities, especially locomotion.* The purpose of the vestibulo-ocular reflex (VOR) is to maintain clear and stable vision during natural head movements. A major threat to clear vision is the head perturbations occurring during locomotion. This was first pointed out by the anonymous physician, J.C.,[2] who had lost vestibular function due to aminoglycosides: "During a walk I found too much motion in my visual picture of the surroundings to permit recognition of fine detail. I learned that I must stand still in order to read the lettering on a sign."

Figure 10–1 summarizes the peak velocities and predominant frequencies of head rotations measured in 20 normal subjects as they walked or ran in place. Note that although peak head velocity is generally below 150° per second, the predominant frequencies range from 0.5 Hz to 5 Hz.[3,4] The latter value is above the frequencies that vestibular physiologists have conventionally used to test patients with vestibular dis-

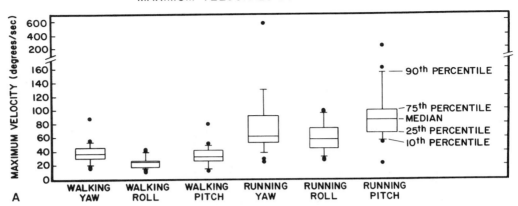

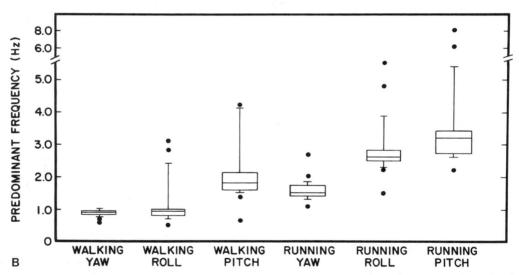

FIGURE 10–1. Summary of the ranges of (*A*) maximum velocity and (*B*) frequency of rotational head perturbations occurring during walking or running in place. Distribution of data from 20 normal subjects are displayed as Tukey box graphs, which show selected percentiles of the data. All values beyond the 10th and 90th percentiles are graphed individually as points. (From King, et al,[4] with permission.)

orders. Furthermore, in designing exercises to rehabilitate vestibular patients, strategies should be applied to use head movements that contain these sort of frequencies, which mainly result from transmitted heel-strike. Thus, in thinking about methods to improve vestibular symptoms, it is important to identify the functional goals for which the patient is aiming and so determine the physiological demands that will be made of the vestibular system to achieve it.

VERTIGO

Pathophysiology

As distinct from one's perception of self-motion during natural locomotion, vertigo is a distressing, illusory sensation of turning that is linked to impaired perception of a stationary environment. It is the mismatch between the actual multisensory inputs and the expected pattern of sensory stimulation with the head stationary that causes vertigo.[5] Whereas rotational vertigo connotes disturbance of the semicircular canals or their central projections, sensations of body tilt or impulsion (e.g., lateropulsion, levitation) imply otolithic disturbance.

Vertigo should be differentiated from other causes of "dizziness," such as presyncopal faintness, loss of stable balance, light-headedness, or psychological disorders (such as agoraphobia, acrophobia, or phobic vertigo syndrome).[6] Thus, accurate identification of symptoms is essential before starting therapies, although, in practice, diagnosis may be difficult.[7] Furthermore, even when patients do experience true vertigo, it may not be caused by organic disease. So, for example, certain individuals are prone to develop vertigo, unsteadiness, or malaise with motion, at height, and when assuming certain postures.[5]

Besides causing vertigo, sudden loss of tonic neural input from one labyrinth or vestibular nerve causes nystagmus and unsteadiness.[1,5] The nystagmus is typically mixed horizontal-torsional with slow phases directed toward the side of the lesion. The nystagmus is more marked on looking in the direction of the quick phases, a phenomenon known as Alexander's law.[1] Past-pointing to the side of the lesion reflects imbalance of vestibulospinal reactions.[5] Patients with rotational vertigo owing to acute, peripheral vestibular lesions are often uncertain as to the direction of their vertiginous illusions. This is because their vestibular sense indicates self-rotation in one direction, but their eye movements (slow phases of vestibular nystagmus) cause visual image movements that, when self-referred, connote self-rotation to the opposite side. It is therefore worthwhile to evaluate the vestibular sense alone by asking specifically about the perceived direction of self-rotation with the eyes closed, thus eliminating any possibly confounding visual stimuli. Although most patients with acute peripheral lesions recover within 1 or 2 months, some are left with recurrent vestibular symptoms and others develop benign paroxysmal positional vertigo.

Neuropharmacology of Vertigo and Nystagmus

Basic research has identified a number of neurotransmitters that appear to contribute to peripheral and central vestibular mechanisms (see Darlington and Smith,[8] Rascol et al,[9] and Dewaele et al[10] for reviews). The excitatory amino acid glutamate is likely to be the neurotransmitter at the vestibular hair cell to vestibular nerve afferent synapse, and also at the synapse between the vestibular nerve and medial vestibular nucleus (MVN). In both cases, it seems that kainate/AMPA (alpha-amino-3-hydroxy-5-methyl-4-isoxazole-proprionic acid) receptors are involved. Glutamate may also influence vestibular compensation acting on NMDA (*N*-methyl-D-aspartate) receptors. The neurotransmitter of the vestibular efferents, which project from brainstem to hair cells, is acetylcholine. Both MVN and lateral vestibular nucleus (LVN) neurons possess muscarinic and nicotinic acetylcholine receptors.

Within the vestibular nuclei, the inhibitory neurotransmitter gamma-aminobutyric acid (GABA) has been identified,[11] and $GABA_A$ receptors on MVN type I neurons may be the mechanisms of inhibition for projections from MVN type II neurons that receive commissural projections, and cerebellar Purkinje cells of the flocculus. A general principle concerning the *vestibular projections* is that inhibitory pathways to motoneurons mediating the vertical VOR use GABA, whereas the inhibitory pathways to motoneurons mediating the horizontal VOR utilize glycine.[12] Histamine, norepinephrine, dopamine, and serotonin also appear to exert effects on vestibular mechanisms. Thus, a large number of neurotransmitters and neuromodulators have been identified within vestibular and ocular motor structures, but the functional role of most of these molecules remains unclear.

One approach that has clarified the functional significance of these findings has been to study the behavioral effects of pharmacological inactivation by microinjection of agents that inactivate certain neurotransmitters. Straube et al[13] and Meetens et al[14] have measured the ocular motor deficits produced by microinjection of the weak GABA antagonist bicuculline and the strong GABA agonist muscimol into the vestibular and adjacent prepositus nuclei of monkeys and cats. Bicuculline induced nystagmus with increasing velocity waveforms that had horizontal and vertical components; the horizontal quick phases were directed ipsilaterally or contralaterally. On the other hand, muscimol caused loss of gaze-holding ("neural integrator") function that was evident as gaze-evoked nystagmus, with a shift in the "null" position away from primary position. These findings indicate that GABA is an important neurotransmitter for the vertical and horizontal VOR, and is also involved in the gaze-holding mechanism, which depends heavily on the medial vestibular and prepositus nuclei. Thus, the effects of these injections may represent varying combinations of vestibular imbalance and gaze-holding failure.

There is also evidence that control of the dynamic property of the VOR referred to as *velocity storage* (enhancement of vestibular time constant from that of the cupula to that of the VOR) by the nodulus and uvula is achieved by inhibitory pathways that use GABA.[15] Experimental lesions of the nodulus and uvula cause prolongation of velocity storage and periodic alternating nystagmus (PAN).[16] The $GABA_B$ agonist baclofen is able to abolish PAN owing to experimental or clinical lesions.[17]

Clinical evidence has also supported a role for nicotinic acetylcholinergic mechanisms in vertical eye movements that are probably mediated by the vestibular system. First, it has been shown that nicotine can produce upbeat nystagmus in normal subjects in darkness.[18] Second, intravenous physostigmine may increase the intensity of downbeat nystagmus.[19] Third, scopolamine suppresses downbeat nystagmus in some patients.[20]

Treatment

The general goals in treatment are to eliminate vertigo (illusion of motion) and accompanying neurovegetative symptoms (nausea, vomiting, anxiety), and to promote (or, at least, not hinder) the normal process of vestibular compensation. In certain cases, such as vertigo owing to migraine, it may be possible to treat the underlying cause. Usually, however, the treatment is symptomatic.

In *acute vertigo* owing to a peripheral vestibular lesion, functional recovery is the rule in the ensuing weeks. Recent evidence suggests that drugs that have a "sedative

TABLE 10–1. Some Commonly Used Vestibular Sedatives[1]

Drug	Class	Dosage	Comments	Precautions
Meclizine (Antivert)	Antihistamine Anticholinergic	Oral: 25 mg or 50 mg, qd or bid	Peak effects 8 hours after ingestion; less sedative	Asthma, glaucoma, prostate enlargement
Diphenhydramine (Benadryl)	Antihistamine Anticholinergic	Oral: 25–50 mg, q4–6h; IM: 10–50 mg	Mildly sedative	Asthma, glaucoma, prostate enlargement
Promethazine (Phenergan)	Antihistamine Anticholinergic Phenothiazine	Oral: 25 mg, q6h; Supp: 50 mg, q12h; IM: 25 mg, q12h	More sedative, more antiemetic	Asthma, glaucoma, prostate enlargement, epilepsy
Prochlorperazine (Compazine)	Antihistamine, Anticholinergic Phenothiazine	Oral: 5–10 mg q6h; Supp: 25 mg q12h; IM: 5–10 mg q6h	Sedative, antiemetic	Liver disease; in combination with CNS depressants or metoclopramide
Scopolamine (Transderm Scop)	Anticholinergic (nonselective muscarinic)	Transdermal patch, q3d Peak effect 4–8h after application	Less sedative, more antiemetic, suitable for motion sickness; Can cause confusion, mydriasis, "dependency"	Asthma, glaucoma, prostate enlargement
Droperidol (Inapsine)	Butyrophenone	IM or slow IV, 2.5–5.0 mg, q12h	Powerful antiemetic; sedative	Liver and kidney disease; Can cause hypotension and extrapyramidal side effects
Ondansetron (Zofran)	Serotonin 5-HT$_3$ receptor antagonist	Oral: 4–8 mg, tid; IV: 4 mg	Antiemetic, developed for patients receiving cancer chemotherapy; may be effective in controlling vertigo and nausea due to CNS disease (Rice and Ebers[28])	Headache; constipation

Abbreviations: IM, intramuscular; IV, intravenous; Supp, suppository.

241

effect" on the vestibular system should only be used for the first 24 hours.[21] Some drugs commonly used for treatment of vertigo, nausea, and vomiting are summarized in Table 10–1, and are discussed more fully in the reviews by Foster and Baloh,[22] and Rascol et al.[9] Most agents probably affect more than one neurotransmitter system and it has been suggested that, in intractable cases, a combination of different types of agent may be better than one alone.[23]

After the first 24 hours, drugs should be used sparingly and patients should be encouraged to get up and increase their activities; there is evidence that failure to do so will limit recovery.[21] During this period, a course of specific vestibular exercises may be indicated (see Chapter 14). Those patients who develop enduring vestibular symptoms may have an underlying central nervous system disorder, typically of the cerebellum,[24] and imaging studies are indicated. Other patients who complain of persistent symptoms may have either developed a phobic disorder,[6] or have the potential for secondary gain as a consequence of their injury.

Treatment of *recurrent vertigo* depends on the nature of the underlying disorder. For example, vertigo owing to migraine (including migraine without a headache) can usually be successfully managed medically (see Chapter 12). Recurrent vertigo owing to a perilymph fistula usually spontaneously recovers, although some patients require surgical repair (see Chapter 10).

On the other hand, vertigo owing to Ménière's disease is often difficult to manage, although a low-salt diet and diuretics help some patients.[25] Because the vestibular imbalance may be in a continuous state of flux, use of "vestibular sedatives" such as meclizine on a chronic basis is justified in some of these patients. Although systemic aminoglyoside administration, to abolish residual vestibular function, is now less commonly used in the treatment of Ménière's disease, injection of gentamicin into the middle ear had become a popular way to eliminate vertigo, especially when it arises from a deaf ear.[26,27]

Central neurological conditions, such as multiple sclerosis, vertebrobasilar ischemia, and posterior fossa mass lesions may cause severe, recurrent vertigo. When treatment of the underlying condition does not produce improvement, then "vestibular sedatives" are justified. Sometimes a combination of agents, such as anticholinergic (e.g., scopolamine) and an antidopaminergic agent (e.g., prochlorperazine) will bring more relief than a single agent.[23] Ondansetron, a serotonin 5HT-3 antagonist, has been reported to help some patients with vertigo owing to brainstem stroke.[28]

Benign paroxysmal positional vertigo is effectively treated in most cases by specific vestibular exercises or maneuvers (see Chapter 16)[29]; drugs are not indicated in this condition. A small percentage of patients do not improve with exercises and, for them, either surgical section of the nerve to, or plugging of, the posterior semicircular canal is effective.[30]

OSCILLOPSIA

Pathogenesis

Oscillopsia brought on or accentuated by head movement is usually of vestibular origin and reflects an inappropriate VOR gain or phase. Vision becomes blurred so that, for example, fine print on grocery items can only be read if the patient stands still in the store aisle. Oscillopsia is usually caused by excessive motion of images of sta-

---

BOX 10–1 Etiology of Oscillopsia[1]

Oscillopsia with head movements: Abnormal VOR

    Peripheral vestibular hypofunction
        Aminoglycoside toxicity
        Surgical section of eighth cranial nerve
        Congenital ear anomalies
        Hereditary vestibular areflexia
        Cisplatin therapy
        Idiopathic
    Central vestibular dysfunction
        Decreased VOR gain
        Increased VOR gain
        Abnormal VOR phase

Oscillopsia owing to nystagmus

    Acquired nystagmus (especially pendular, upbeat, downbeat, see-saw, or dissociated)
    Saccadic oscillations (psychogenic flutter/voluntary nystagmus, ocular flutter, microsaccadic flutter, and opsoclonus)
    Superior oblique myokymia (monocular oscillopsia)
    Congenital nystagmus (uncommon under natural illumination)

Central oscillopsia

    With cerebral disorders: seizures, occipital lobe infarction

---

tionary objects on the retina (Box 10–1). Excessive retinal slip not only causes oscillopsia, but also impairs vision. Oscillopsia with head movements may also occur as result of weakness of an extraocular muscle (e.g., abducens nerve palsy). Oscillopsia owing to nystagmus and other ocular oscillations occurs when the head is stationary.

An abnormal VOR may lead to oscillopsia during head movements in three ways: abnormal gain, abnormal phase shift between eye and head rotations, and a directional mismatch between the vectors of the head rotation and eye rotation. Disease of either the vestibular periphery or its central connections may be the cause (see Box 10–1).

Typically, oscillopsia is worse during locomotion but it may be noticed during chewing food and, in the most severe cases, it may occur due to transmitted cardiac pulsation.[2] In addition, visual acuity declines during head movements, and this can be easily demonstrated at the bedside by testing visual acuity first with the patient's head stationary, and then while rotating it side-to-side at 1 to 2 cycles per second.[1]

Oscillopsia may also occur with disorders of the central nervous system that change the gain or phase of the VOR. Thus, disease of the vestibulocerebellum may cause "vestibular hyperresponsiveness," particularly in the vertical plane. This occurs in patients with the Arnold-Chiari malformation,[1] and, occasionally, cerebellar patients are reported with increased gain of both the horizontal and vertical VOR.[31] In some patients with vestibulocerebellar dysfunction, the gain of the VOR is normal, but the phase relationship between head and eye movements is abnormal and causes retinal image slip.[32] Lesions of the medial longitudinal fasciculus (internuclear ophthalmoplegia in multiple sclerosis) may cause a low gain of the vertical VOR and produce oscillopsia with vertical head movements.[33]

Treatment

With time, compensation takes place in patients with oscillopsia owing to vestibular loss. A variety of factors, including potentiation of the cervico-ocular reflex, preprogramming of compensatory eye movements, and perceptual changes may account for this compensation.[2,34,35] Thus, drugs have little to offer. Exercises (see Chapter 13) and encouragement of the patient to resume activities such as walking are of key importance. Rarely, oscillopsia owing to a hyperactive VOR can be treated pharmacologically.[31] Paradoxically, patients who lack a VOR can read head-fixed visual displays during locomotion better than normal subjects can.[36] This is because clear vision of a head-fixed display requires that vestibular eye movements be suppressed or canceled. Because such patients have little or no VOR, it is easy to suppress vestibular eye movements. The practical application of this—in the future—might be development of head-fixed video displays of images obtained with cameras that can compensate for head perturbations.

NYSTAGMUS AND ITS VISUAL CONSEQUENCES

Pathogenesis

As indicated above, acquired nystagmus commonly causes impaired vision and oscillopsia—illusory movement of the environment. These symptoms, which are due to drift of images of stationary objects on the retina, interfere with reading and watching television, and the oscillopsia is often distressing to the patient. The relationship between retinal image velocity and visual acuity is a direct one: for higher spatial frequencies (which correspond to Snellen optotypes), image motion in excess of about 5° per second impairs vision.[37,38] On the other hand, the relationship between retinal image velocity and the development of oscillopsia is less consistent; the magnitude of oscillopsia is usually less than the magnitude of nystagmus. For example, in patients with downbeat nystagmus, oscillopsia is, on average, about one-third of the amplitude of the nystagmus.[39] This latter finding suggests that the brain compensates for the excessive retinal image motion and thus partly maintains visual constancy, although the mechanism is debated. Nevertheless, if retinal image drift, in patients with nystagmus, can be reduced below about 5° per second, then oscillopsia is usually abolished and vision is improved.[40]

Treatments

Some of the various drugs reported to suppress nystagmus are summarized in Box 10–2. *Gabapentin* has recently been shown to suppress or abolish acquired pendular nystagmus associated with multiple sclerosis or following brainstem stroke (oculopalatal tremor syndrome).[41] Acquired pendular nystagmus produces perhaps the most troubling visual disturbances of all forms of nystagmus, and most patients who take gabapentin will experience some relief (Fig. 10–2). However, not all such patients respond, and worsening of ataxia may be a troublesome side effect.

BOX 10–2   Treatments for Nystagmus and its Visual Consequences[1,17,41]

Drugs

  Gabapentin
  Baclofen
  Clonazepam
  Valproate
  Trihexyphenidyl
  Benztropine
  Scopolamine
  Isoniazid
  Carbamazepine
  Barbiturates
  Alcohol
  Acetazolamide
  Botulinum toxin

Optical devices

  Base-out prisms
  Other prism arrangements
  Spectacle lens-contact lens combination (for retinal image stabilization)

Invasive Procedures

  Operative treatment of Arnold-Chiari malformation
  Botulinum toxin

Baclofen is less effective in treating acquired pendular nystagmus than gabapentin (see Fig. 10–2) but, as discussed above, is usually effective in treating PAN.[17] Neither baclofen nor gabapentin are reliable treatments for downbeat nystagmus.[41] Other gabaergic agents, especially *clonazepam,* have been reported to be useful in the treatment of downbeat nystagmus.[17,42]

Anticholinergic agents may be effective in some patients with pendular or downbeat nystagmus. In one double-blind study, Barton et al[20] administered scopolamine, benztropine, and glycopyrrolate (a quaternary agent devoid of central nervous activity) intravenously. A single dose of scopolamine effectively reduced nystagmus and improved vision in all five patients with pendular nystagmus; benztropine was less effective, and glycopyrrolate had no significant effect. However, in a randomized, double-blind crossover trial of oral trihexyphenidyl and tridihexethyl chloride (a quaternary anticholinergic that does not cross the blood-brain barrier) only 1 out of 10 patients showed a decrease in nystagmus and an improvement of visual acuity with trihexyphenidyl.[43] Anticholinergic side effects included dry mouth, constipation, disturbed sleep, and tiredness. The discrepancy between these two studies could be explained by different subtypes of receptors antagonized or habituation to the drug effect after long-term oral use.

Other medications for nystagmus have not received such a systematic evaluation. However, *acetazolamide* is an effective treatment of the rare syndrome of familial periodic ataxia with nystagmus.[44] A recent open-label study reported that memantine, a glutamate antagonist not currently available in the United States, is effective in acquired pendular nystagmus.[45]

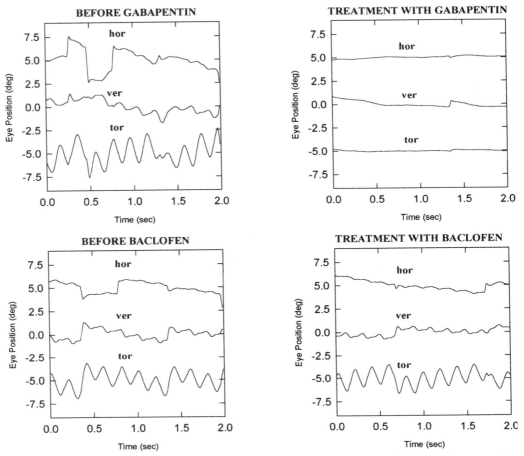

FIGURE 10–2. Representative data showing effects of gabapentin (*top*) or baclofen (*bottom*) of the nystagmus of the right eye of a 55-year-old woman with multiple sclerosis. The horizontal (hor) and torsional (tor) records have been offset from the vertical (ver) records, which is aligned about 0, for clarity of display; thus eye positions are relative rather than absolute. Upward deflections indicate rightward, upward or clockwise eye rotations, with respect to the patient. Gabapentin essentially abolished all components of this patient's nystagmus, whereas baclofen slightly reduced the vertical component. (From Averbuch-Heller, et al,[41] with permission.)

A number of optical devices have been suggested for treatment of nystagmus. One approach that often benefits patients whose nystagmus damps while viewing a near target is convergence prisms. An arrangement that is often effective is 7.00 diopter base-out prisms with −1.00 diopter spheres added to compensate for accommodation.[17,46] The spherical correction may not be needed in presbyopic individuals. Especially in some patients with congenital nystagmus, the improvement of visual acuity owing to nystagmus suppression when wearing base-out prisms may be sufficient for them to qualify for a driving license. Some patients with acquired nystagmus also benefit.[47] Occasionally, in patients in whose nystagmus is worse during near viewing, base-in prisms help.

Theoretically, it should be possible to use prisms to help patients whose nystagmus is quieter when the eyes are moved into a particular position in the orbit—the "null region." Thus, in patients with congenital nystagmus, there is usually some horizontal eye position in which nystagmus is minimized, and, in patients with downbeat nystagmus, the eyes may be quieter in upgaze. In practice, patients use headturns to bring their eyes to the quietest position, and only rarely are prisms that produce a conjugate shift helpful.

Another approach has been the development of an optical system to stabilize images on the retina during eye movements.[40,48,49] This system consists of a high-plus spectacle lens worn in combination with a high-minus contact lens (Fig. 10–3). Stabilization can be achieved if the power of the spectacle lens focuses the primary image close to the center of rotation of the eye. A contact lens is then required to extend back the focus onto the retina. Because the contact lens moves with the eye, it does not negate the effect of retinal image stabilization produced by the spectacle lens. With such a system it is possible to achieve up to about 90 percent stabilization of images on the retina. There are several limitations to the system, however. One is that it disables all eye movements (including the VOR and vergence), so that it is only useful while the patient is stationary and views monocularly. Another is that with the highest power components (contact lens of -58.00 diopters and spectacle lens of $+32$ diopters), the

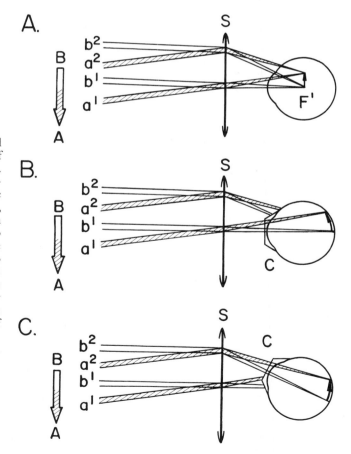

FIGURE 10–3. An optical method for stabilizing images of stationary objects upon the retina. (*A*) When viewing a distant object, AB, a convergent spectacle lens, S, will focus rays of light (b^1, b^2) from a point of interest B, on its focal point F^1, which is close to the center of rotation of the globe. Thus, if the eyeball were to rotate, light rays from point B would remain focused at the same point as in the eye. (*B*) A strongly divergent contact lens, C, extends back the focus from the center of the globe to the retina. (*C*) Because the contact lens moves with the eye, it does not negate the effect of retinal image stabilization produced by the spectacle lens, and rays of light from point B remain focused on the foveal region of the retina. (From Leigh, et al,[40] with permission.)

field of view is limited. Some patients with ataxia or tremor (such as those with multiple sclerosis) have difficulty inserting the contact lens. However, initial problems posed by rigid polymethyl methacrylate contact lenses have been overcome by development of gas-permeable or even soft contact lenses.[49] Most patients do not need the highest power components for oscillopsia to be abolished and vision to be useful. We have found that, in selected patients, the device may prove useful for limited periods of time, for example, if the patient wishes to watch a television program.

Invasive procedures such as the Kestenbaum operation, which effectively treats certain patients with congenital nystagmus, are of uncertain value in the treatment of acquired forms of nystagmus.[17] Neurosurgery does have a clear role in the therapy of the Arnold-Chiari syndrome; suboccipital decompression is reported to improve downbeat nystagmus and prevent progression of other neurological deficits.[50] Injection of botulinum toxin either into selected extraocular muscles or into the retrobulbar space will temporarily abolish or suppress nystagmus, but the side effects of ptosis and diplopia limit the therapeutic value, except in selected patients.[17,51,52]

SUMMARY

Disruption of the peripheral or central vestibular system often results in vertigo, oscillopsia, and nystagmus. Acute vertigo from peripheral vestibular lesions usually recovers spontaneously and vestibular suppressant medications, although appropriate during the first 24 hours, should be used sparingly after that initial period. The use of medications in recurrent vertigo is dependent on the specific disorder affecting the vestibular system. Oscillopsia owing to loss of the vestibular sense often improves spontaneously and medications do not aid recovery. Oscillopsia owing to nystagmus may be helped if gabapentin, baclofen, clonazepam, or acetazolamide can reduce the ocular oscillations. Several different optical devices have been developed as treatment for the visual consequences of nystagmus. No medications or optical devices can be applied uniformly to all patients; careful diagnosis of the problem must be made before any of these treatments is attempted.

ACKNOWLEDGMENTS

This work was supported by USPHS grant EY06717, the Department of Veterans Affairs, and the Evenor Armington Fund.

REFERENCES

1. Leigh, RJ, and Zee, DS: The Neurology of Eye Movements, ed 3. Oxford University Press, New York, 1999.
2. J.C.: Living without a balancing mechanism. N Engl J Med 246:458, 1952.
3. Das, VE, et al: Head perturbations during walking while viewing a head-fixed target. Aviat Space Environ Med 66:728, 1995.
4. King, OS, et al: Control of head stability and gaze during locomotion in normal subjects and patients with deficient vestibular function. In Berthoz, A, et al (eds): Second Symposium on Head-Neck Sensory-Motor System. Oxford Univ. Pr., New York, 1991.
5. Brandt, T: Vertigo: Its Multisensory Syndromes. Springer, New York, 1991.
6. Brandt, T: Phobic postural vertigo. Neurology 46:1515, 1996.

7. Nedzelski, JM, et al: Diagnoses in a dizziness unit. J Otolaryngol 15:101, 1986.
8. Darlington, CL, and Smith, PFS: What neurotransmitters are important in the vestibular system. In Baloh, RW, and Halmagyi, GM (eds): Disorders of the Vestibular System. Oxford Univ. Pr., New York, 1996, pp 140–144.
9. Rascol, O, et al: Antivertigo medications and drug-induced vertigo. Drugs 50:777, 1995.
10. Dewaele, C, et al: Neurochemistry of the central vestibular pathways. Brain Res Rev 20:24, 1995.
11. Spencer, RF, et al: The pathways and functions of GABA in the oculomotor system. In Mize, RR, et al (eds): Progress in Brain Research. Elsevier, New York, 1992, pp 307–331.
12. Spencer, RF, et al: Evidence for glycine as an inhibitory neurotransmitter of vestibular, reticular, and prepositus hypoglossi neurons that project to the cat abducens nucleus. J Neurosci 9:2718, 1989.
13. Straube, A, et al: Differential effects of bicuculline and muscimol microinjections into the vestibular nuclei on simian eye movements. Exp Brain Res 86:347, 1991.
14. Mettens, P, et al: Effect of muscimol microinjections into the prepositus hypoglossi and medial vestibular nuclei on cat eye movements. J Neurophysiol 72:785, 1994.
15. Cohen, B, et al: Baclofen and velocity storage: A model of the effects of the drug on the vestibulo-ocular reflex in the rhesus monkey. J Physiol (Lond) 393:703, 1987.
16. Waespe, W, et al: Dynamic modification of the vestibulo-ocular reflex by the nodulus and uvula. Science 228:199, 1985.
17. Leigh, RJ, et al: Treatment of abnormal eye movements that impair vision: Strategies based on current concepts of physiology and pharmacology. Ann Neurol 36:129, 1994.
18. Sibony, PA, et al: Nicotine and tobacco-induced nystagmus. Ann Neurol 28:198, 1990.
19. Dieterich, M, et al: The effects of baclofen and cholinergic drugs on upbeat and downbeat nystagmus. J Neurol Neurosurg Psychiatr 54:627, 1991.
20. Barton, JJS, et al: Muscarinic antagonists in the treatment of acquired pendular and downbeat nystagmus. A double-blind randomized trial of three intravenous drugs. Ann Neurol 35:319, 1994.
21. Zee, DS: Perspectives on the pharmacotherapy of vertigo. Arch Otolaryngol 111:609, 1985.
22. Foster, C, and Baloh, RW: Drug therapy for vertigo. In Baloh, RW, and Halmagyi, GM (eds): Disorders of the Vestibular System. Oxford Univ. Pr., New York, 1996, pp 541–550.
23. Peroutka, SJ, and Snyder, SH: Antiemetics: Neurotransmitter receptor binding predicts therapeutic actions. Lancet March 20th:658, 1982.
24. Rudge, R, and Chambers, BR: Physiological basis for enduring vestibular symptoms. J Neurol Neurosurg Psychiatr 45:126, 1982.
25. Andrews, JC, and Honrubia, V: Meniere's disease. In Baloh, RW, and Halmagyi, GM (eds): Disorders of the Vestibular System. Oxford Univ. Pr., New York, 1996, pp 300–317.
26. Nedzelski, J, et al: Intratympanic gentamycin installation as treatment of unilateral Meniere's disease: Update of an ongoing study. Am J Otol 14:278, 1993.
27. Murofushi, T, et al: Intratympanic gentamycin in Meniere's disease: Results of therapy. Am J Otol 18:52, 1997.
28. Rice, GP, and Ebers, GC: Ondansetron for intractable vertigo complicating acute brainstem disorders. Lancet 345:1182, 1995.
29. Brandt, T, et al: Therapy for benign paroxysmal positioning vertigo, revisited. Neurology 44:796, 1994.
30. Parnes, LS, and McClure, JA: Posterior semicircular canal occlusion for intractable benign paroxysmal positional vertigo. Ann Otol Rhinol Laryngol 99:330, 1990.
31. Thurston, SE, et al: Hyperactive vestibulo-ocular reflex in cerebellar degeneration: Pathogenesis and treatment. Neurology 37:53, 1987.
32. Gresty, MA, et al: Disorders of the vestibulo-ocular reflex producing oscillopsia and mechanisms compensating for loss of labyrinthine function. Brain 100:693, 1997.
33. Ranalli, PJ, and Sharpe, JA: Vertical vestibulo-ocular reflex, smooth pursuit and eye-head tracking dysfunction in internuclear ophthalmoplegia. Brain 111:1299, 1988.
34. Bronstein, AM, and Hood, JD: Oscillopsia of peripheral vestibular origin. Acta Otolaryngol (Stockh) 104:307, 1987.
35. Kasai, T, and Zee, DS: Eye-head coordination in labyrinthine-defective human beings. Brain Res 144:123, 1978.
36. Das, VE, et al: Measuring eye movements during locomotion. Filtering techniques for obtaining velocity signals from a video-based eye monitor. J Vestib Res 6:455, 1996.
37. Carpenter, RHS: The visual origins of ocular motility. In Cronly-Dillon, JR (ed): Vision and Visual Function, Vol 8. Eye Movements. MacMillan, London, 1991, pp 1–10.
38. Burr, DC, and Ross, J: Contrast sensitivity at high velocities. Vision Res 22:479, 1982.
39. Buchele, W, et al: Ataxia and oscillopsia in downbeat-nystagmus vertigo syndrome. Adv Oto-Rhino-Laryngol 30:2891, 1983.
40. Leigh, RJ, et al: Effects of retinal image stabilization on acquired nystagmus due to neurological disease. Neurology 38:122, 1988.
41. Averbuch-Heller, L, et al: A double-blind controlled study of gabapentin and baclofen as treatment for acquired nystagmus. Ann Neurol 41:818, 1997.
42. Currie, JN, and Matsuo, V: The use of clonazepam in the treatment of nystagmus-induced oscillopsia. Ophthalmology 93:924, 1986.

43. Leigh, RJ, et al: The effect of anticholinergic agents upon acquired nystagmus: A double-blind study of trihexyphenidyl and tridihexethyl chloride. Neurology 41:1737, 1991.
44. Zasorin, NL, et al: Acetazolamide-responsive episodic ataxia syndrome. Neurology 33:1212, 1983.
45. Starck, M, et al: Drug therapy for acquired pendular nystagmus in multiple sclerosis. J Neurol 244:9, 1997.
46. Dell'Osso, LF: Improving visual acuity in congenital nystagmus. In Smith, JL, and Glaser, JS (eds): Neuro-ophthalmology. Mosby, St. Louis, 1973, pp 98–106.
47. Lavin, PJM, et al: Downbeat nystagmus with a pseudocycloid waveform: Improvement with base-out prisms. Ann Neurol 13:621, 1983.
48. Rushton, D, and Cox, N: A new optical treatment for oscillopsia. J Neurol Neurosurg Psychiatr 50:411, 1987.
49. Yaniglos, SS, and Leigh, RJ: Refinement of an optical device that stabilizes vision in patients with nystagmus. Optometry Vision Sci 69:447, 1992.
50. Pedersen, RA, et al: Intermittent downbeat nystagmus and oscillopsia reversed by suboccipital craniectomy. Neurology 30:1239, 1980.
51. Leigh, RJ, et al: Effectiveness of botulinum toxin administered to abolish acquired nystagmus. Ann Neurol 32:633, 1992.
52. Tomsak, RL, et al: Unsatisfactory treatment of acquired nystagmus with retrobulbar botulinum toxin. Am J Ophthalmol 119:489, 1995.

CHAPTER 11

Surgical Management of Vestibular Disorders

Douglas E. Mattox, MD

The diagnosis of vestibular disorders is complicated by overlapping symptoms among the various disorders and the lack of pathognomonic diagnostic tests. At times, determining which inner ear is causing the symptoms may even be difficult. Most patients' symptoms can be managed with the medical and physical therapy measures described elsewhere in this book. However, surgical intervention may be appropriate when the symptoms have failed to respond to aggressive nonsurgical medical management.

With the exception of acoustic tumors, vestibular disorders are a matter of lifestyle and comfort, and are not life threatening. Therefore, the patient living with the symptoms must make the decision whether to proceed with surgery. The physician should discuss the likelihood of a successful outcome, as well as the nature of potential complications, and leave the ultimate decision up to the patient. In the author's experience, patients have a broad spectrum of responses to their symptoms of vertigo. Some patients want immediate intervention; others will consider surgery only when life becomes unbearable.

ACOUSTIC NEUROMAS (VESTIBULAR SCHWANNOMA)

Acoustic neuromas are nerve sheath tumors occurring in the internal auditory canal or cerebellopontine angle.[1] They are the third most common intracranial tumor and account for 8 to 10 percent of all intracranial tumors. Most patients with acoustic neuromas present with progressive unilateral sensorineural hearing loss. However, some patients first complain of vestibular symptoms or sudden hearing loss.[2]

An acoustic neuroma should be suspected in any patient with an unexplained unilateral sensorineural hearing loss, particularly if the patient has abnormal brainstem auditory responses or hypoactive (or absent) caloric responses. Magnetic resonance imaging (MRI) with gadolinium contrast has become the gold standard for the diagnosis of these tumors. Although there are rare instances of false-positive scans, usually owing to arachnoiditis, an enhancing mass in the cerebellopontine angle extending into the internal auditory meatus is almost always an acoustic neuroma.

Once the diagnosis is established, there are three therapeutic options: watchful waiting, radiosurgery, and surgical removal. *Watchful waiting* is indicated only for patients with very small intracanalicular tumors in which the diagnosis is inconclusive, and for patients who are elderly or in poor medical condition. Several recent series have reported the results of this approach. Wiet et al[3] found that 40 percent of 53 patients had continued growth of their tumors and required intervention over a mean follow-up of about 2 years. More frightening is an experience reported by Charabi et al.[4] In this series, 34 percent of 123 patients followed for a mean of 3.4 years required intervention for enlarging tumors and seven died of brainstem compression secondary to the tumor. Therefore, it may be concluded that there is a significant risk of tumor enlargement, and if a "wait-and-see" approach is taken, the importance of serial scans repeated at 6- to 12-month intervals must be emphasized to the patient.

Radiosurgery is a new modality, whose role in the treatment of acoustic neuromas is still being investigated.[5,6] A single treatment of high-dose irradiation is administered by stereotactically focusing multiple radiation sources on the tumor. Because the radiation beams come from many different angles, an extremely high radiation dose is delivered to the tumor where the beams intersect. With proper geometric planning, the surrounding neural and vascular structures are spared the high dose of radiation.

The initial results of radiosurgery are encouraging. Tumor control is achieved in 70 to 80 percent of patients, and the procedure has a low incidence of complications, especially facial paralysis.[5,6] The vascular supply to the cochlea is not spared, however, and approximately 60 percent of patients develop hearing loss.[5] This treatment is ideal for recurrent tumors and for patients whose medical problems make them a poor surgical risk. Radiosurgery is currently available in very few centers, but, no doubt, will develop wider use as availability of the devices increases.

Surgical removal of acoustic tumors has been the treatment of choice since described by Harvey Cushing in 1917.[7] Three basic approaches are used for removal of acoustic neuromas: (1) middle fossa craniotomy, (2) translabyrinthine approach, and (3) suboccipital craniotomy.[8,9] The choice of the approach is based on the size and location of the tumor and whether any attempt will be made to preserve hearing.[8,9]

Middle Cranial Fossa

The middle cranial fossa approach is used for tumors confined to the internal auditory canal in patients who have usable hearing (Fig. 11–1). A vertical incision is made in the scalp superior to the external auditory canal. The soft tissues are elevated from the bone and a 3 × 4-cm temporal craniotomy is performed. The dura and temporal lobe are elevated from the floor of the middle cranial fossa. The internal auditory canal is identified by drilling the bone overlying it. The facial nerve, mastoid air-cell system, and superior semicircular canal are important landmarks. The bone is thinned over the entire extent of the internal auditory canal, and then the dura of the canal is incised. Care is taken not to damage the facial nerve in the anterior superior quadrant of the internal auditory canal. The cochlear nerve is anterior inferior in the canal and safely out of harm's way.

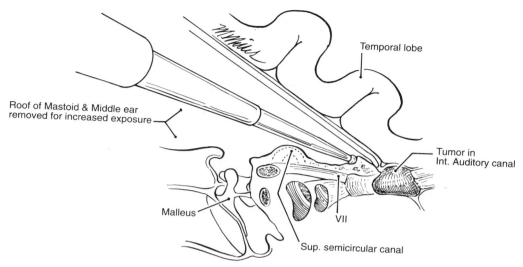

FIGURE 11–1. Middle fossa. This coronal section through the internal auditory canal and middle ear shows the exposure of the internal auditory canal through the middle fossa. A drill is shown passing through a small temporal craniotomy. The temporal lobe is elevated extradurally. The superior semicircular canal is identified and the internal auditory canal exposed by removing the bone over the auditory canal medial to the superior semicircular canal.

The advantage of the middle cranial fossa approach is that the inner ear and hearing are not destroyed in the approach. Care must be taken to avoid damaging the facial nerve because it is superficial in the dissection. Managing tumors that extend through the porus acusticus into the posterior fossa using the middle cranial fossa approach is very difficult. This procedure, therefore, is indicated only for tumors limited to the internal auditory canal.

Recovery after middle fossa craniotomy is prompt. Unless the patient has significant vestibular symptoms, he or she should be up and about the next day. Cerebrospinal fluid (CSF) leakage is unlikely, but the patient should be checked for both external leak and a leak down the eustachian tube into the nasopharynx after this approach and all other approaches described in this section.

Translabyrinthine Approach

The translabyrinthine approach is the procedure of choice for tumors up to 2.5 cm in diameter when hearing preservation is not a consideration (Fig. 11–2). The tumor is approached similar to a standard mastoidectomy. The cortical and pneumatized bone of the mastoid are drilled away to expose the sigmoid sinus, posterior fossa dura, and middle fossa dura. The facial nerve is protected by identifying it within its bony canal. A complete labyrinthectomy is performed to expose the internal auditory canal. Once the intracanalicular portion of the tumor is mobilized, the dura of the posterior fossa is incised, and the remainder of the tumor is removed.

Recovery after translabyrinthine removal of acoustic tumors is generally prompt and patients can be out of bed in 2 to 3 days. This rapid recovery is attributable to the lack of pressure or retraction of the cerebellum during the procedure. The disadvan-

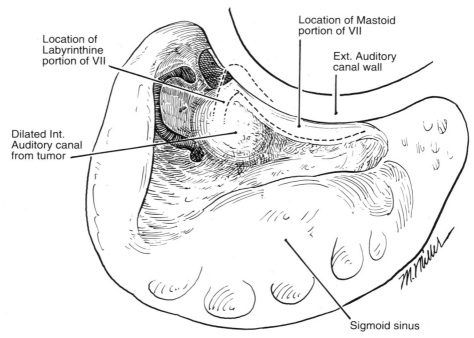

FIGURE 11–2. Translabyrinthine approach for removal of acoustic neuroma. A translabyrinthine approach to the internal auditory canal is shown in surgical position with anterior at the top and superior to the left of the drawing. The tumor is exposed after completion of a labyrinthectomy (see Fig. 11–5). The internal auditory canal has been dilated by the tumor. Removal of the last shell of bone over the tumor as well as the bone from the posterior fossa will allow complete tumor removal.

tage of the translabyrinthine approach is that hearing is automatically sacrificed. The exposure is excellent for small- and medium-sized tumors, but is inadequate for tumors larger than 2.5 cm in diameter and those that are adherent to the brainstem. The ideal case for translabyrinthine removal has a clear separation between the tumor and the brainstem on computed tomography (CT) or MRI.

Suboccipital Craniectomy

Suboccipital craniectomy gives the best exposure when the tumor is large or adherent to the brainstem (Fig. 11–3). In rare cases in which there is good hearing preoperatively, the suboccipital approach offers the possibility of preserving hearing. Maintenance of hearing requires the preservation of both the cochlear nerve and the fragile capillary blood supply of the inner ear. Hearing can be spared in a one-third to one-half of the patients in whom this approach is attempted.[10]

The suboccipital craniectomy differs from the translabyrinthine approach in that the angle of the approach is from behind rather than in front of the sigmoid sinus. The incision is placed 5 to 6 cm behind the ear and a 5-cm piece of the occipital skull is removed. This defect is reconstructed with prosthetic mesh at the end of the procedure.

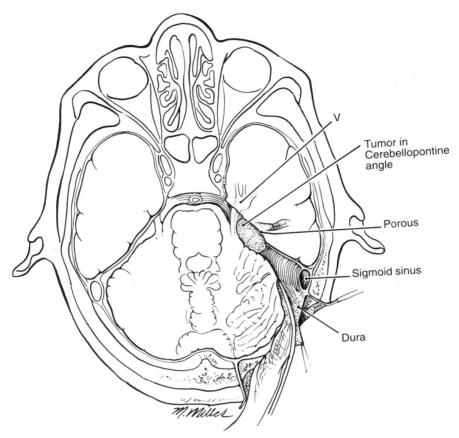

FIGURE 11–3. Suboccipital craniectomy. This axial section demonstrates a posterior fossa craniotomy behind the sigmoid sinus. The cerebellum drops away from the posterior surface of the temporal bone. The tumor is exposed in the cerebellopontine angle. The posterior lip of the internal auditory canal must be drilled away to remove the tumor extending into the canal.

The cerebellum lies between the craniotomy and the cerebellopontine angle; however, the surgery is performed in the lateral position, allowing the cerebellum to fall away by itself without additional retraction.

After the tumor is identified, the capsule of the tumor is incised and the central core of the tumor is removed with an ultrasonic aspirator or laser. After the tumor has been decompressed, the portion of the tumor within the internal auditory canal is removed by drilling away the posterior surface of the canal. The facial nerve is identified in the fundus of the internal auditory canal where its anatomy is constant. The tumor is mobilized from the brainstem and the seventh nerve is identified medial to the tumor.

Recovery time after a suboccipital craniotomy is slower than from the other two approaches because of the magnitude of the procedure, but patients are usually ready for discharge from the hospital within a week. Occasionally a patient will develop a postcraniotomy headache that requires long-term pain management.

Complications after acoustic neuroma surgery are relatively uncommon. Hearing loss always occurs in translabyrinthine procedures and is common after suboccipital removal of tumors greater than 1.5 centimeter. Transient facial paralysis is common with larger tumors. Permanent facial paralysis is seen in fewer than 5 percent of patients. CSF leaks can occur postoperatively, but are usually transient and rarely require secondary surgical correction.

MÉNIÈRE'S DISEASE

Although the underlying etiology of Ménière's disease is unknown, a consistent histopathological finding is hydrops (dilation) of the endolymphatic spaces.[11] The hydrops presumably results from a malfunction of the resorptive function of the endolymphatic sac. The classic constellation of symptoms includes fluctuating hearing loss, episodic vertigo, tinnitus, and a sensation of fullness in the ear.[12] These symptoms, however, do not necessarily develop simultaneously and many patients do not develop them all. Subcategories of Ménière's disease describe these other conditions; for instance, cochlear hydrops (fluctuating hearing loss alone) or vestibular hydrops (vestibular symptoms without hearing loss).[12]

In most patients, Ménière's disease is ultimately self-limited; over time the patient suffers deterioration of hearing and a gradual subsiding of the episodic dizzy spells. This evolution, however, may require 10 or 20 years. In the interim, the patient's lifestyle may be severely impaired.

Medical therapy of Ménière's disease rests on avoiding factors known to exacerbate the symptoms: stress, caffeine, alcohol, nicotine, and foods high in salt. Diuretics and vestibular suppressant drugs are usually prescribed. This regimen, known as the Furstenberg regimen, can adequately control the symptoms in up to three-quarters of patients.[13] A few patients, however, cannot be adequately managed by medical means alone and surgical intervention must be considered. The surgical procedures for Ménière's disease may be categorized as those designed to improve the function of the endolymphatic sac, and those that ablate the vestibular system, either with or without preservation of hearing.

Endolymphatic sac procedures attempt to reestablish the function of the sac as the resorptive organ for the endolymph of the inner ear by draining the excess endolymphatic sac into the mastoid cavity.[14] A standard postauricular mastoidectomy is performed and the sigmoid sinus, mastoid antrum and incus, facial nerve, and lateral and posterior semicircular canals are identified. The endolymphatic sac is found between the posterior surface of the temporal bone and the dura of the posterior fossa. The bone is thinned until the dura and the sac are identifiable through the last layer of bone. This bone is picked away to expose the dura and the overlying endolymphatic sac. The sac is opened and Silastic sheeting or another shunt device is inserted into the lumen of the endolymphatic sac and allowed to drape into the mastoid cavity. Care must be taken to open the endolymphatic sac without puncturing the underlying dura, which could result in a CSF leak. Any endolymph drained by the shunt is resorbed by the mucous membranes of the mastoid cavity.

It is almost an understatement to say that endolymphatic sac surgery is controversial. The fluid spaces involved are minuscule and the ability of mechanical means to improve function of the sac is doubtful. In a clinical trial, similar results were obtained with real and sham operations.[15] Nonetheless, the procedure controls the vertiginous attacks in one-half to two-thirds of patients, and has the advantage of relative ease and safety.

Although they are more complex procedures, control of vertigo is predictable and reliable in 90 to 95 percent of patients with either vestibular neurectomy or labyrinthectomy. These procedures should completely relieve the vertiginous attacks because vestibular input from that ear is completely eliminated. The loss of all vestibular function on one side can easily be compensated by an intact labyrinth on the opposite side.

When the hearing is worth preserving (the ability to detect speech, known as *speech reception threshold* is better than 60dB, and the ability to understand speech, or *discrimination score,* is better than 50 percent), a vestibular neurectomy through either the middle cranial fossa or retrolabyrinthine space is the procedure of choice.

The middle cranial fossa approach is the same as described above for acoustic tumors. Once the internal auditory canal has been identified and exposed, it can be opened and the superior and inferior of vestibular nerves divided.

The vestibular nerve can also be sectioned using either a retrolabyrinthine or retrosigmoid (suboccipital) approach (Fig. 11–4). In the retrolabyrinthine approach a complete mastoidectomy is performed as described for the endolymphatic sac procedure.[16] In addition, all of the bone medial to the sigmoid sinus is removed to expose the posterior fossa dura. The dura is opened to expose the cerebellopontine angle. The vestibular and auditory branches of the eighth nerve are directly in the field of view and the vestibular nerve is divided. A disadvantage of this approach is that the auditory and vestibular portions of the eighth nerve are fused as they exit the brainstem and may not have separated before they enter the internal auditory canal. Some surgeons have advocated a retrosigmoid approach to drill away the posterior lip of the internal audi-

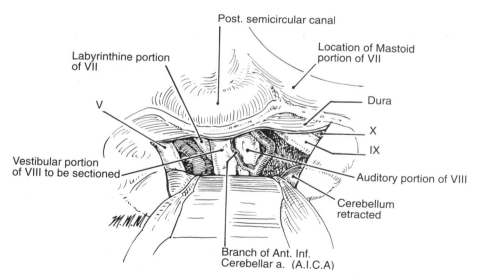

FIGURE 11–4. Retrolabyrinthine vestibular nerve section. This surgeon's view of a right ear in surgical position (anterior—*top;* superior—*left*) shows the exposure for a retrolabyrinthine nerve section. The cerebellopontine angle is exposed by removing the posterior surface of the temporal bone between the sigmoid sinus and the posterior semicircular canal. The dura is opened, and the seventh and eighth nerves are identified. The demarcation between the vestibular and auditory portions of the nerve is usually marked by a small branch of AICA. The vestibular portion of the eighth nerve (superior half) is divided.

tory canal. This procedure permits identification of the vestibular nerve after it has separated from the auditory nerve.[17]

If hearing preservation is not a goal, for example in cases of unilateral Ménière's disease with severely impaired hearing or discrimination, a labyrinthectomy is the most effective treatment. Labyrinthectomy can be performed either through the external auditory canal or through the mastoid (Fig. 11–5). In the transcanal approach, the tympanic membrane is elevated to expose the middle ear. The stapes is removed and the vestibule is opened between the oval and round windows. The saccule, utricle, and ampullae of the superior, lateral, and posterior semicircular canals are removed with an angled pick. Reaching the ampulla of the posterior semicircular canal is a blind maneuver and may leave neuroepithelium behind. For this reason, this author prefers the transmastoid approach. A standard mastoidectomy is performed and all three semicircular canals are identified. Each one in turn is drilled away and the neuroepithelium is identified under direct vision and removed. The three semicircular canals lead to the vestibule where once again the saccule and utricle are removed.

Recently there have been reports of attempts to selectively destroy the vestibular epithelium perfusing the lateral semicircular canal with streptomycin.[18] Although the initial reports were encouraging, subsequent multicenter studies have once again noted an unacceptably high incidence of sensorineural hearing loss.[19]

A less invasive procedure that has gained recent popularity is the use of intratympanic gentamicin to produce a chemical labyrinthectomy. Several protocols and dosing schedules have been reported, but in essence, a low dose of gentamicin is injected into the middle ear space, either directly through the tympanic membrane with topical anesthesia or through a myringotomy tube.[20,21] This procedure appears to produce good control of vertigo attacks, but poses significant risk to hearing.[22] It has the great advantage of being nonoperative, thus avoiding the risks of anesthesia and surgery, and the cost of hospitalization. However, even though it is a simple procedure, it must be taken with the same seriousness as any other destructive procedure on the labyrinth.

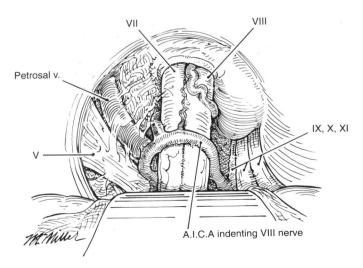

FIGURE 11–5. Labyrinthectomy. A transmastoid labyrinthectomy of the right ear (anterior—*top;* superior—*left*). The three semicircular canals have been identified, and the lateral and posterior canals have been partially opened. The canals will be completely removed, and the vestibule will be opened to remove all neuroepithelium.

In all the procedures described, the implicit belief is that the disease is unilateral, or if bilateral, the side producing the majority of symptoms can be determined. Surgical procedures, however, are seldom, if ever, indicated in patients who have active bilateral disease. These patients are extremely difficult to treat, but some hope can be offered with systemically administered streptomycin. Streptomycin is specifically toxic to the vestibular portion of the inner ear, and if given systemically will produce a bilateral chemical labyrinthectomy. Patients are given streptomycin, 1 g twice a day intramuscularly, until the vertigo subsides, usually in about 10 days. The patient is left the side effects of bilateral vestibular loss including difficulty walking in the dark and inability to keep the eyes fixed on a target during head movements (oscillopsia).[23]

POST-TRAUMATIC VERTIGO

Post-traumatic vertigo is managed in a manner identical to Ménière's disease with either a hearing-preserving or hearing-sacrificing form of vestibular ablation. Most authors, however, report less reliable control of recurrent attacks of dizziness.[24] The reasons for these results are unknown.

BENIGN PAROXYSMAL POSITIONAL VERTIGO

Unlike patients with Ménière's disease who develop spontaneous episodes of dizziness, those suffering from benign paroxysmal positional vertigo (BPPV) develop transient symptoms only when they assume certain positions.[12] The most common position is in a lateral or head-hanging position with the diseased ear undermost. The symptoms generally have a few seconds' latency before onset, develop in a crescendo-decrescendo pattern, demonstrate torsional nystagmus, and habituate on repeated trials. The site of the pathology is generally thought to be in the posterior semicircular canal. Schuknecht[11] has described debris on the cupula of the posterior semicircular canal, and he has given the condition the name "cupulolithiasis." The symptoms could arise from dislodged otoconia floating in the posterior semicircular canal as well as from those physically attached to the cupula.

BPPV is frequently a self-limiting condition that resolves regardless of what treatment is given.[12] A number of different physical therapy measures have been designed to dislodge the otoconia from the posterior semicircular canal. These measures are effective in the vast majority of patients (see Chapter 16).

Rarely, a patient has persistent symptoms despite physical therapy intervention and the passage of time. In these cases, two surgical procedures can be considered. The first is *singular neurectomy*—division of the branch of the vestibular nerve to the posterior semicircular canal.[25] This procedure is technically difficult and has been described by only a few centers. The singular nerve passes just medial to the round window niche before entering the ampulla of the posterior canal. The lip of the round window is drilled away, but the round window membrane must not be violated. Bone is removed posterior and inferior to the round window membrane with tiny diamond spurs to expose the singular canal. The canal is opened and the nerve avulsed.

Surgical blockade of the flow of endolymph in the posterior semicircular canal has been described recently.[26] In this procedure, the bony posterior semicircular canal is opened without violating the membranous labyrinth. Flow within the membranous labyrinth is blocked by occluding the bony and membranous canals with a bone plug. Reports from several centers confirm this is an effective and low-risk treatment for BPPV in those rare patients who fail to respond to particle-repositioning maneuvers.[27,28]

PERILYMPH FISTULA

Perilymph fistula is a direct communication between the inner ear and the middle ear, usually through the round or oval windows (Fig. 11–6).[29] Such leaks were initially described in association with barotrauma; however, spontaneous leaks are being described with increasing frequency. The symptoms of perilymph leak include hearing loss, usually sudden or episodic; vertigo associated with the hearing loss; and, more recently, patients have been described with generalized spatial disorientation and normal hearing. The diagnosis of perilymph fistula, and the indications and timing of surgery, are some of the most controversial subjects in the otological literature. To date

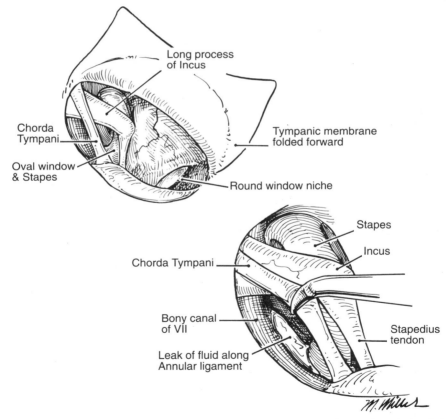

FIGURE 11–6. Perilymphatic fistula. A right middle ear exploration for perilymph fistula is shown in the surgical position (anterior—*top;* superior—*right*). The tympanic membrane has been reflected forward to expose the oval and round windows. Close inspection of the annular ligament of the oval window demonstrates a leak of perilymph. This will be closed with an autologous tissue graft.

there are no preoperative diagnostic tests that definitively confirm or exclude the presence of a perilymph fistula. Even upon surgical exploration there may be disagreements among observers as to the presence or absence of a fluid leak. Biochemical and fluorescent tracer studies as well as protein analyses are being developed as potential markers for the presence or absence of the perilymph fistula.[30]

The middle ear exploration for perilymph fistula is straightforward. The middle ear is approached through the external auditory canal and the tympanic membrane elevated. Both the oval and round windows are carefully observed for the repeated accumulation of fluid. The leak may become more obvious with a Valsalva maneuver (increased intrathoracic pressure against a closed glottis). The leak is repaired with autogenous tissue. Clinicians generally believe that the patient should remain on bedrest for some time after closure of perilymph fistula to allow the graft to heal in place.[29]

In most cases the patient feels better shortly after repair of a perilymph fistula. Patients with persistent symptoms present the physician with the difficult dilemma of deciding if the repair has failed or if the diagnosis was wrong in the first place.

VASCULAR LOOPS

Vascular loops are elongated or tortuous vessels (arteries or veins) within the intracranial cavity that are thought to press on nerve roots as they exit from the brainstem (Fig. 11–7). The first well-described vascular syndrome was hemifacial spasm, an uncontrollable twitching of one side of the face. This was found by Janetta et al[31] to be caused by an abnormal vessel pressing on the root-entry zone of the facial nerve. This concept has been expanded to include vestibular and auditory disorders.[32] The significance of these vascular loops is difficult to determine because the symptoms overlap other diagnostic categories, including Ménière's disease and perilymph fistula. Furthermore, tortuous vessels are common in the cerebellopontine angle of normal individuals, especially after middle age. Nonetheless, there are documented cases of vessels impinging on nerves causing abnormal stretching or displacement. It has been

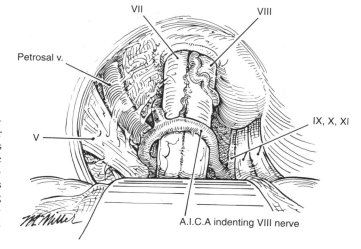

FIGURE 11–7. Retrolabyrinthine exposure of vascular compression. The exposure is the same as shown in Figure 11–4. The AICA is seen compressing the eighth nerve. This is treated by carefully elevating the vessel and interposing muscle or sponge material between the vessel and the nerve.

suggested that radiologic confirmation can be obtained with the combination of high-resolution CT with intravenous and air contrast.

Microvascular loop decompression is performed through a standard posterior craniectomy. The offending artery or vein is carefully dissected from the nerve and a small piece of muscle or teflon sponge is interposed to keep the vessel from pressing on the nerve.

SUMMARY

The development of surgical interventions for vertigo is a fascinating and challenging branch of neurotology. Unfortunately at the moment, most of the procedures used are ablative rather than restorative. Future developments in this field will be directed toward the rehabilitation and functional restoration of the diseased inner ear.

REFERENCES

1. Nager, GT: Acoustic neurinomas. Acta Otolaryngol (Stockh) 99:245, 1985.
2. Thomsen, J, et al: Acoustic neuromas: Progression of hearing impairment and function of the eighth cranial nerve. Am J Otol 5:20, 1983.
3. Wiet, RJ, et al: Conservative management of patients with small acoustic tumors. Laryngoscope 105:795, 1995.
4. Charabi, S, et al: Acoustic neuroma (vestibular schwannoma): Growth and surgical and nonsurgical consequences of the wait-and-see policy. Otolaryngol Head Neck Surg 113:5, 1995.
5. Yamamoto, M, and Noren, G: Stereotactic radiosurgery in acoustic neurinomas. No Shinkei Geka 18:1101, 1990.
6. Flickinger, JC, et al: Radiosurgery of acoustic neurinomas. Cancer 67:345, 1990.
7. Cushing, H: Tumors of the Nervus Acusticus and the Syndrome of the Cerebellopontine Angle. Saunders, Philadelphia, 1917.
8. Fisch, U, and Mattox, DE: Microsurgery of the Skull Base. Thieme, New York, 1988.
9. Brackmann, DE: A review of acoustic tumors: 1979–1982. Am J Otol 5:233, 1984.
10. Harner, SG, et al: Hearing preservation after removal of acoustic neurinoma. Laryngoscope 94:1431, 1984.
11. Schuknecht, HF: Pathology of the Ear. Harvard Univ. Pr., Cambridge, 1974.
12. Paparella, MM, et al: Ménière's disease and other labyrinthine diseases. In Paparella MM, et al (eds): Otolaryngology. Saunders, Philadelphia, 1991, p 1689.
13. Boles, R, et al: Conservative management of Ménière's disease: Furstenberg regimen revisited. Ann Otol 84:513, 1975.
14. Arenberg, IK: The fine points of valve implant surgery for hydrops: An update. Am J Otol 3:359, 1982.
15. Thomsen, J, et al: Placebo effect in surgery for Ménière's disease. Arch Otolaryngol 107:271, 1981.
16. Silverstein, H, and Norrell, H: Retrolabyrinthine vestibular neurectomy. Otolaryngol Head Neck Surg 90:778, 1982.
17. Silverstein, H, et al: Combined retrolab-retrosigmoid vestibular nerve neurectomy: An evolution in approach. Am J Otol 10:166, 1989.
18. Shea, JJ: Perfusion of the inner ear with streptomycin. Am J Otol 10:150, 1989.
19. Monsell, EM, and Shelton, C: Labyrinthectomy with streptomycin infusion for vertigo: Early results of a multicenter group. Am J Otol 13:416, 1992.
20. Nedzelski, JM, et al: Intratympanic gentamicin instilation as a treatment of unilateral Ménière's disease: Update of an ongoing study. Am J Otol 14:278, 1993.
21. Magnusson, H, and Padoanm, S: Delayed onset of ototoxic effects of gentamycin in treatment of Ménière's disease: Rationale for extremely low dose therapy. Acta Otolaryngol (Stockh) 111:671, 1991.
22. Toth, AA, and Parnes, LS: Intratympanic gentamicin therapy for Ménière's disease: Preliminary comparison of two regimens. J Otolaryngol 24:340, 1995.
23. Schuknecht, HF: Ablation therapy in the management of Ménière's disease. Acta Otolaryngol (Stockh) (suppl)132, 1975.
24. Kemink, JL, et al: Retrolabyrinthine vestibular nerve section: Efficacy in disorders other than Ménière's disease. Laryngoscope 101:523, 1991.
25. Gacek, RR: Singular neurectomy update. Ann Otol Rhinol Laryngol 91:469, 1982.

26. Parnes, LS, and McClure, JA: Posterior semicircular canal occlusion for intractable benign paroxysmal positional vertigo. Ann Otol Rhinol Laryngol 99:330, 1990.
27. Parnes, LS: Update on posterior canal occlusion for benign paroxysmal positional vertigo. Otolaryngol Clin North Am 29:333, 1996.
28. Zappia, JJ: Posterior semicircular canal occlusion for benign paroxysmal positional vertigo. Am J Otol 17:749, 1996.
29. Mattox, DE: Perilymph fistulas. In Cummings, CWC, et al (eds): Otolaryngology Head and Neck Surgery. Mosby, St Louis, 1986, p 3113.
30. Paugh, DR, et al: Identification of perilymph proteins by two-dimensional gel electrophoresis. Otolaryngol Head Neck Surg 104:517, 1991.
31. Janetta, PJ, et al: Etiology and definitive microsurgical treatment of hemifacial spasm. J Neurosurg 47:321, 1977.
32. Janetta, PJ: Neurovascular cross-compensation of the eighth cranial nerve in patients with vertigo and tinnitus. In Sammi, M, and Janetta, PJ (eds): The Cranial Nerves, Springer-Verlag, New York, 1981, p 552.

CHAPTER 12

Assessment and Management of Central Vestibular Disorders

Thomas Brandt, MD, FRCP
Marianne Dietrich, MD

Vestibular pathways run from the eighth nerve and the vestibular nuclei through ascending fibers, such as the ipsilateral or contralateral medial longitudinal fasciculus (MLF), the brachium conjunctivum, or the ventral tegmental tract to the ocular motor nuclei, the supranuclear integration centers in the rostral midbrain, and the vestibular thalamic subnuclei. From there they reach several cortex areas through the thalamic projection. Another relevant ascending projection reaches the cortex from vestibular nuclei via vestibular cerebellum structures, in particular the fastigial nucleus.

In the majority of cases, central vestibular vertigo syndromes are caused by dysfunction or a deficit of sensory input induced by a lesion. In a small proportion of cases, they are due to pathological excitation of various structures, extending from the peripheral vestibular organ to the vestibular cortex. Because peripheral vestibular disorders are always characterized by a combination of perceptual, ocular motor, and postural signs and symptoms, central vestibular disorders may manifest as "a complete syndrome" or with only single components. The ocular motor aspect, for example, predominates in the syndromes of upbeat or downbeat nystagmus. Lateral falls may occur without vertigo in vestibular thalamic lesions (thalamic astasia) or as lateropulsion in Wallenberg's syndrome.*

---

*Assessment and management of central vestibular disorders are largely adopted from a more detailed presentation in the book "Vertigo, Its Multisensory Syndromes."[1]

CLINICAL CLASSIFICATION OF CENTRAL VESTIBULAR DISORDERS

The "elementary" neuronal network of the vestibular system is the di- or trisynaptic vestibulo-ocular reflex (VOR). There is evidence for a useful clinical classification of central vestibular syndromes according to the three major planes of action of the VOR (Fig. 12–1): yaw, roll, and pitch.[2-4]

The plane-specific vestibular syndromes are determined by ocular motor, postural, and perceptual signs (Fig. 12–2):

- **Yaw plane signs** are horizontal nystagmus, past pointing, rotational and lateral body falls, horizontal deviation of perceived straight-ahead.

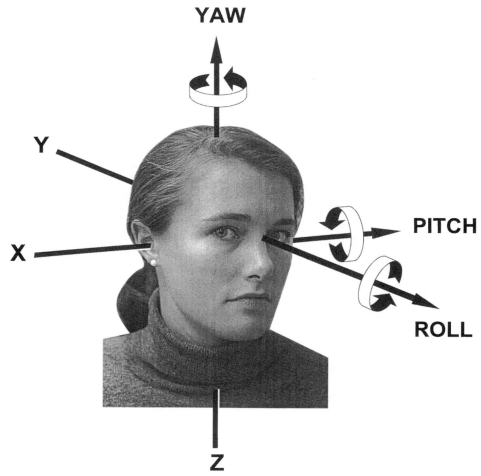

FIGURE 12–1. Schematic representation of the three major planes of action of the vestibulo-ocular reflex. Horizontal rotation about the vertical z axis = yaw; vertical rotation about the binaural y axis = pitch; vertical rotation about the x axis ("line of sight") = roll. Figure by courtesy of Alice Klinebase.

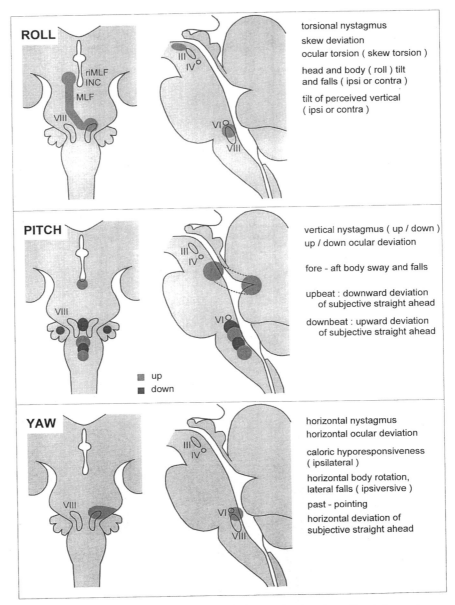

FIGURE 12–2. Topographic diagnosis of vestibular syndromes in roll, pitch, and yaw planes: schematic presentation of the distinct areas within the brainstem and vestibulocerebellum (frontal and sagittal views) in which a lesion induces a vestibulo-ocular tone imbalance in roll, pitch, or yaw plane. Typical ocular motor, postural, and perceptual signs are torsional, vertical (up/downbeat), or horizontal nystagmus. A tone imbalance in roll indicates unilateral "graviceptive" pathway lesions from the medial or superior vestibular nuclei (inducing ipsiversive signs), crossing midline to the contralateral MLF and the rostral integration centers for vertical and torsional eye movements, the INC and riMLF (inducing contraversive signs). A tone imbalance in pitch indicates paramedian bilateral brainstem lesions at pontomesencephalic or pontomedullary level, the brachium conjunctivum, or the flocculi. It is striking that pontomedullary lesions may induce either upbeat or downbeat nystagmus or transitions between the two, whereas binocular flocculus lesions result only in downbeat nystagmus and a pontomesencephalic lesion only in upbeat nystagmus. A tone imbalance in yaw indicates a unilateral pontomedullary lesion involving the medial and superior vestibular nucleus. This area overlaps with roll and pitch function of the VOR, which explains the frequency of mixed vestibular syndromes in more than one plane (riMLF = rostral interstitial nucleus of the medial longitudinal fasciculus, INC = interstitial nucleus of Cajal, III = oculomotor nucleus, IV = trochlear nucleus, VI = abducens nucleus, VIII = vestibular nucleus.)[25]

- **Roll plane signs** are torsional nystagmus, skew deviation, ocular torsion, tilts of head, body, and perceived vertical.
- **Pitch plane signs** are upbeat/downbeat nystagmus, forward/backward tilts and falls, vertical deviations of perceived straight-ahead.

The defined VOR syndromes allow for a precise topographic diagnosis of brainstem lesions as to their level and side (Fig. 12–3[3,4]).

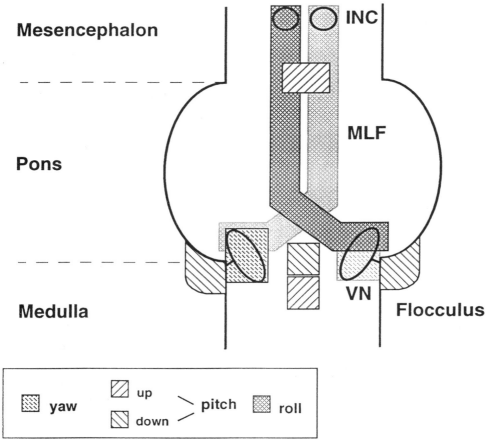

FIGURE 12–3. Vestibular syndromes in roll, pitch, and yaw planes: critical areas are schematically represented based on our current knowledge of vestibular and ocular motor structures and pathways, a lesion of which causes a vestibular tone imbalance in one of the three major planes of action. The mere clinical sign of a vertical, torsional, or horizontal nystagmus—if central-vestibular—allows a topographic diagnosis of the lesion, although the particular vestibular structures involved are still under discussion. Whereas a vestibular tone imbalance in the roll plane indicates unilateral brainstem lesions (a crossing in the pons), vertical nystagmus indicates bilateral lesions. Two separate causative loci are known for upbeat nystagmus: medullary or pontomesencephalic. Downbeat nystagmus indicates a bilateral paramedian lesion of the commissural fibers between the vestibular nuclei or a bilateral flocculus lesion. Horizontal nystagmus indicates unilateral pontomedullary lesions involving the vestibular nuclei. The differentiation of vestibular ocular motor signs according to the three major planes of action of the VOR and their mapping to distinct and separate areas in the brainstem are helpful for topographic diagnosis and for avoiding incorrect assignment of clinical signs to brainstem lesions identified with imaging techniques (INC = interstitial nucleus of Cajal, MLF = medial longitudinal fasciculus, VN = vestibular nucleus).[3]

TABLE 12–1 Central Vestibular Syndromes

Site	Syndrome	Mechanism/Etiology
Vestibular cortex (multisensory)	Vestibular epilepsy	Vestibular seizures are auras (simple or complex partial multisensory seizures)
	Volvular epilepsy	Sensorimotor "vestibular" rotatory seizures with walking in small circles
	Nonepileptic cortical vertigo	Rare rotatory vertigo in acute lesions of the parietoinsular vestibular cortex
	Spatial hemineglect (contraversive)	Multisensory horizontal deviation of spatial attention with (right) parietal or frontal cortex lesions
	Transient room-tilt illusions	Paroxysmal or transient mismatch of visual- and vestibular 3-D spatial coordinate maps in vestibular brainstem, parietal, or frontal cortex lesions
	Tilt of perceived vertical with body lateropulsion (mostly contraversive)	Vestibular tone imbalance in roll with acute lesions of the parietoinsular vestibular cortex
Thalamus	Thalamic astasia	Dorsolateral vestibular thalamic lesions
	Tilt of perceived vertical (ipsiversive or contraversive) with body lateropulsion	Vestibular tone imbalance in roll
Mesodiencephalic brainstem	Ocular tilt reaction (contraversive; ipsiversive if paroxysmal)	Vestibular tone imbalance in roll (integrator-OTR with INC lesions)
	Torsional nystagmus (ipsiversive or contraversive)	Ipsiversive in INC lesions
		Contraversive in riMLF lesions
Mesencephalic brainstem	Skew torsion (contraversive)	Vestibular tone imbalance in roll with MLF lesions
	Upbeat nystagmus	Vestibular tone imbalance in pitch in bilateral brachium conjunctivum lesions
Ponto-medullary brainstem	Tilt of perceived vertical, lateropulsion, ocular tilt reaction	Vestibular tone imbalance in roll with medial and/or superior vestibular nuclei lesions
	Pseudo "vestibular neuritis"	Lacunar infarction or MS plaque at the root entry zone of the eighth nerve
	Downbeat nystagmus	Vestibular tone imbalance in pitch
	Transient room-tilt illusion	Acute severe vestibular tone imbalance in roll or pitch
	Paroxysmal room-tilt illusion in MS	Transversally spreading ephaptic axonal activity
	Paroxysmal dysarthria/ataxia in MS	Transversally spreading ephaptic axonal activation
	Paroxysmal vertigo evoked by lateral gaze	Vestibular nuclei lesion?
Medulla	Upbeat nystagmus	Vestibular tone imbalance in pitch? (nucleus prepositus hypoglossi)
Vestibular cerebellum	Downbeat nystagmus	Vestibular tone imbalance in pitch caused by bilateral flocculus lesions (disinhibition)
	Positional downbeat nystagmus	Disinhibited otolith-canal interaction in nodulus lesions?
	Familial episodic ataxia (EA1 with myokymia and EA2 with vertigo)	EA1=autosomally dominant inherited potassium channelopathy; EA2=autosomally dominant inherited calcium channelopathy
	Encephalitis with predominant vertigo	Viral infection of cerebellum
	Epidemic vertigo	Viral infection of cerebellum

- A tone imbalance in yaw indicates lesions of the lateral medulla including the root entry zone of the eighth nerve and/or the vestibular nuclei.
- A tone imbalance in roll indicates unilateral lesions (ipsiversive at pontomedullary level, contraversive at pontomesencephalic level).
- A tone imbalance in pitch indicates bilateral (paramedian) lesions or bilateral dysfunction of the flocculus.

Some vestibular disorders are characterized by a simultaneously peripheral and central vestibular involvement. Examples are large acoustic neurinomas, infarctions of the anterior inferior cerebellar artery, head trauma, and syndromes induced by alcohol intoxication. Others may affect the vestibular nerve root in the brainstem, where the transition between the peripheral and central nervous system has been defined as the Redlich-Oberstein zone (lacunar infarction or focal demyelination in multiple sclerosis [MS] mimicking vestibular neuritis).

Cortical vestibular syndromes include vestibular seizures and lesional dysfunction with tilt of the perceived vertical, lateropulsion, and, rarely, rotational vertigo. There is no primary vestibular cortex, but the parietoinsular vestibular cortex[5] seems to act as a kind of main integration center. Dysfunction of this multisensory and sensorimotor cortex for spatial orientation and self-motion perception may be involved in spatial hemineglect and rare paroxysmal room-tilt illusions.

Most central vertigo syndromes have a specific locus (Table 12–1) but not a specific etiology. The etiology may, for example, be vascular, autoimmunologic, as in MS, inflammatory, neoplastic, toxic, or traumatic.

VESTIBULAR DISORDERS IN (FRONTAL) ROLL PLANE

The "graviceptive" input from the otoliths converges with that from the vertical semicircular canals at the level of the vestibular nuclei[6] and the ocular motor nuclei[7,8] to subserve static and dynamic vestibular function in pitch (up and down in the sagittal plane) and roll (lateral tilt in the frontal plane). In the "normal" position in the roll plane, the subjective visual vertical (SVV) is aligned with the gravitational vertical, and the axes of the eyes and the head are horizontal and directed straight ahead.

Signs and symptoms of a vestibular dysfunction in the roll plane can be derived from the deviations from normal function. A lesion-induced vestibular tone imbalance should result in a syndrome consisting of a perceptual tilt (SVV), vertical misalignment of the visual axes (skew deviation), ocular torsion (Fig. 12–4), or a complete ocular tilt reaction (OTR); the triad of head tilt, skew deviation, and ocular torsion.

There is convincing evidence that all the following signs and symptoms reflect vestibular dysfunction in the (frontal) roll plane:

- OTR
- Skew deviation (skew-torsion sign)
- Spontaneous torsional nystagmus
- Tonic ocular torsion (monocular or binocular), if not caused by infranuclear ocular motor disorders
- Tilt of perceived SVV (with binocular and monocular viewing)
- Body lateropulsion

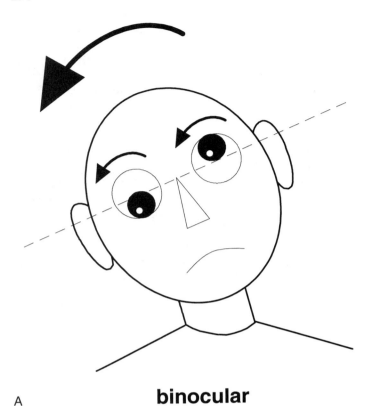

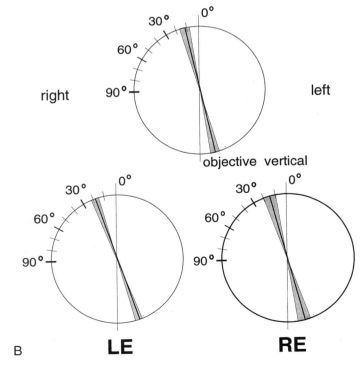

FIGURE 12–4. (A) Patient with OTR to the right with rightward head tilt, skew deviation (right eye undermost), and predominant ocular torsion (excyclotropia) of the undermost eye due to an acute Wallenberg's syndrome of the right medulla. (B) Perceptual tilts of SVV of about 12–18° under binocular and monocular (LE, RE) viewing conditions.

TABLE 12–2 Frequency of Subjective Visual Vertical Tilt, Skew Deviation, Ocular Torsion, and Ocular Tilt Reaction in Acute Unilateral Brainstem and Thalamic Infarctions

Lesion	Patients (*n*)	SVV Tilt (Percent)	Ocular Torsion (%)		Skew (Percent)	OTR (Percent)
			Monocular	Binocular		
Mesodiencephalic						
Paramedian thalamic	14	64	29[a]	43[a]	57	57
Posterolateral thalamic	17	65	13[b]	20[b]	0	0
Anterior polar thalamic	4	0	0	0	0	0
Mesencephalic	16	94	54	38	37.5	25
Pontomesencephalic	12	92	64	18	25	25
Pontine	34	91	47	33	26.5	12
Pontomedullary	13	100	60	20	23	7.7
Medullary (Wallenberg's syndrome)	36	94	27	55	44	33
Total	111	94	47	36	31	

[a]Additional third nerve palsy.
[b]Slight torsion of about 2.8°.
SVV = subjective visual vertical; OTR = ocular tilt reaction.

Ocular motor or postural tilts as well as misadjustments of SVV point in the same direction, either clockwise or counterclockwise (as seen from the viewpoint of the examiner). The direction of all tilts is reversed if pathological excitation of unilateral "graviceptive" pathways is the cause of vestibular tone imbalance in roll rather than a lesional input deficit. The combination of static and dynamic signs is not surprising if one considers the functional cooperation of otoliths and vertical semicircular canals owing to their neuronal convergence within "graviceptive" pathways. These signs and symptoms may be found in combination or as single components at all brainstem levels. A systematic study of 111 patients with acute unilateral brainstem infarctions revealed that pathological tilts of SVV (94 percent) and ocular torsion (83 percent) are the most sensitive signs.[9] Skew deviation was found in one-third and a complete OTR in one-fifth of these patients (Table 12–2).

Current clinical data support the following preliminary topographic diagnostic rules based on vestibular signs and symptoms in roll (Fig. 12–5[3,4]):

1. The fundamental pattern of eye-head tilt in roll—either complete OTR or skew torsion without head tilt—indicates a unilateral peripheral deficit of otolith and vertical canal input or a unilateral lesion of "graviceptive" brainstem pathways from the vestibular nuclei (crossing midline at lower pontine level) to the interstitial nucleus of Cajal (INC) in the rostral midbrain.
2. Tilts of SVV, resulting from peripheral or central vestibular lesions from the labyrinth to the vestibular cortex, are the most sensitive sign of a vestibular tone imbalance in roll.
3. All tilt effects—perceptual, ocular motor, and postural—are ipsiversive (ipsilateral eye lowermost) and owing to unilateral peripheral or pontomedullary lesions be-

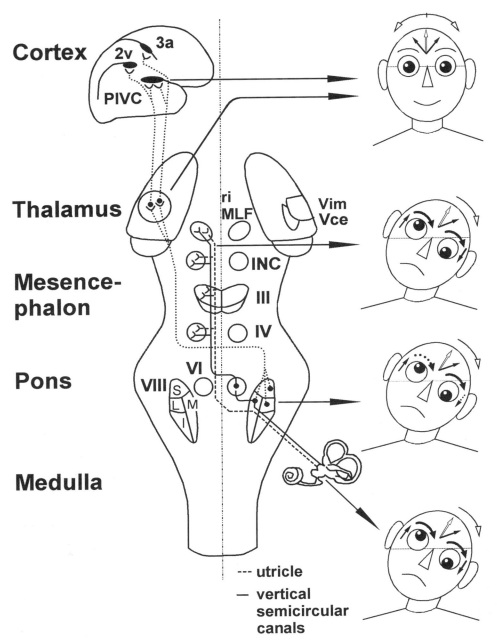

FIGURE 12–5. Vestibular syndromes in roll plane: Graviceptive pathways from otoliths and vertical semicircular canals mediating vestibular function in roll plane. The projections from the otoliths and the vertical semicircular canals to the ocular motor nuclei (trochlear nucleus IV, oculomotor nucleus III, abducens nucleus VI), the supranuclear centers of the INC, and the rostral interstitial nucleus of the MLF (riMLF) are shown. They subserve VOR in three planes. The VOR is part of a more complex vestibular reaction that also involves vestibulospinal connections via the medial and lateral vestibulospinal tracts for head and body posture control. Furthermore, connections to the assumed vestibular cortex (areas 2v and 3a and the parietoinsular vestibular cortex, PIVC) via the vestibular nuclei of the thalamus (Vim, Vce) are depicted. "Graviceptive" vestibular pathways for the roll plane cross at the pontine level. OTR (skew torsion, head tilt, and tilt of perceived vertical, SVV) is depicted schematically on the right in relation to the level of the lesion: ipsiversive OTR with peripheral and pontomedullary lesions; contraversive OTR with pontomesencephalic lesions. In vestibular thalamic lesions, the tilts of SVV may be contraversive or ipsiversive; in vestibular cortex lesions they are preferably contraversive. OTR is not induced by supratentorial lesions above the level of INC.[3]

low the crossing of the graviceptive pathways. They indicate involvement of the labyrinth, vestibular nerve, or medial and/or superior vestibular nuclei; the latter are mainly supplied by the vertebral artery.

4. All tilt effects in unilateral pontomesencephalic brainstem lesions are contraversive (contralateral eye lowermost) and indicate involvement of the MLF (paramedian arteries arising from basilar artery) or INC (paramedian superior mesencephalic arteries arising from the basilar artery).

5. OTR with unilateral (ponto)medullary lesions (vestibular nuclei) indicates the "ascending" (reflexive) type of a tone imbalance of the VOR in roll.

6. OTR owing to rostral midbrain lesions (INC) reflects the "descending" type of tone imbalance involving the neural integration center for eye-head coordination in roll.

7. Skew deviation is always combined with ocular torsion (skew-torsion sign). It manifests without head tilt if ascending pontomesencephalic "graviceptive" pathways are affected rostral to the downward branching of the vestibulospinal tract.

8. Unilateral lesions of ascending vestibular pathways rostral to the INC typically manifest with deviations of perceived vertical without concurrent eye-head tilt.

9. OTR in unilateral paramedian thalamic infarctions (paramedian thalamic arteries from basilar artery) indicates simultaneous ischemia of the paramedian rostral midbrain including the INC.

10. Unilateral lesions of the posterolateral thalamus can cause thalamic astasia and moderate ipsiversive or contraversive SVV tilts, thereby indicating involvement of the vestibular thalamic subnuclei (thalamogeniculate arteries).

11. Unilateral lesions of the parietoinsular vestibular cortex (PIVC) cause moderate, mostly contraversive SVV tilts (temporal branches of the middle cerebral artery or deep perforators) and "cortical lateropulsion."

12. An SVV tilt found with monocular but not with binocular viewing is typical for a trochlear or oculomotor palsy rather than a supranuclear "graviceptive" brainstem lesion.[10]

Tilt effects caused by paroxysmal activation of "graviceptive" pathways point in the opposite direction of those caused by lesional inhibition, such as unilateral infarction.[11-14] Thus, all clinical signs of vestibular dysfunction in roll can be helpful when determining not only the level but also the side of the brainstem lesion. If the level of damage is known from the clinical syndrome, the vestibular syndrome indicates the more severely affected side. Conversely, if the side of damage is clear from the clinical syndrome, the direction of OTR, skew deviation, and SVV tilt indicates the level on the brainstem.

Three types of vestibular disorders in roll can be thus described:[15]

1. "Ascending" VOR-OTR with pontomedullary lesions of the medial or superior vestibular nucleus or graviceptive pathways which subserve the VOR in the roll plane

2. Skew torsion without head tilt with unilateral lesions of the pontomesencephalic "graviceptive" pathways

3. "Descending" integrator-OTR with lesions of the rostral midbrain integration centers for eye-head coordination in the roll and pitch planes.

The "ascending, reflexive" type (lateral medulla) of OTR simply reflects a tone imbalance of the VOR, whereas the "descending integrator" type (rostral midbrain tegmentum) integrates signals of eye-head velocity with those of holding position and involves cortical control of the fundamental pattern of OTR during active locomotion. The (pontomesencephalic) "skew torsion" type results from lesions of ascending "graviceptive" pathways but does not cause head tilt, because vestibulospinal tracts are not involved. Unilateral infarctions of the brainstem cause dysfunction predominantly in the roll plane, less frequently in the yaw and pitch planes. Dysfunction in the pitch plane requires bilateral vestibular dysfunction.

Etiology

The two most common causes of tonic OTR are brainstem ischemia (especially Wallenberg's syndrome and unilateral paramedian thalamic plus rostral mesencephalic infarctions) and brainstem tumors.[11,16] We have also seen cases with unilateral thalamic hemorrhages, lower brainstem hemorrhages (cavernous angioma, lymphomas), after severe brainstem concussion, in MS, or associated with attacks of basilar migraine.

The paroxysmal OTR described in a patient with MS[13] may be a variant of the paroxysmal attacks assumed to arise from ephaptic spreading between adjacent demyelinated axons. We have observed repeated paroxysmal attacks of contraversive OTR with ipsiversive torsional nystagmus in the acute stage of Wallenberg's syndrome and in neurovascular cross-compression of the eighth nerve.

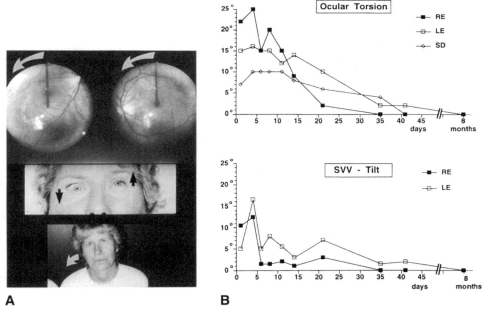

A   **B**

FIGURE 12–6. Patient with a left paramedian thalamic infarction presenting with a complete ocular tilt reaction (OTR) to the right. OTR consisted of contraversive head tilt of 20° (bottom); skew deviation of 10°, left eye over right eye; and ocular torsion of 15° to 20° (counterclockwise from the viewpoint of the observer). Natural course of ocular torsion, skew deviation (SD), and tilt of subjective visual vertical (SVV, in degrees) shows gradual recovery in 6 weeks. RE = right eye; LE = left eye.[17]

Natural Course and Management

The natural course and management of OTR depend on the etiology. OTR is usually transient; in cases of hemorrhage or infarction recovery occurs within a few days to weeks. However, it can be permanent, as we observed in a patient with severe brainstem concussion. Following unilateral brainstem infarctions, all features of OTR—postural, ocular motor, and perceptual—disappear naturally and gradually within 4 to 6 weeks or months (repeated measurements made in seven patients over a period of up to 1 to 3 years[17]) (Fig. 12–6). Repeated measurements of skew deviation, ocular torsion (OT), and tilts of SVV made during a single day showed consistent tilts.[9] Repeated measurements on subsequent days showed a gradual recovery, mostly within 30 days, both for OT and SVV (Fig. 12–7 and Fig. 12–8). Some patients, however, maintained a residual OT of a few degrees without a corresponding tilt of SVV for up to 2 years. Recovery is probably based on a functionally significant central compensation of a vestibular tone imbalance induced by a *unilateral* central lesion. The mechanisms underlying central compensation of central lesions may be similar to those of central compensation of peripheral vestibular lesions. Physical therapy may facilitate this central compensation, but this has not yet been proven in a prospective study.

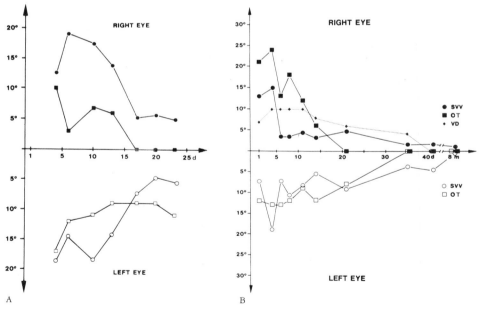

FIGURE 12–7. Two representative time courses of deviations of subjective visual vertical (SVV) and ocular torsion (OT) (separate for the left and right eyes) in a patient with Wallenberg's syndrome on the left (*A*) and a patient with unilateral lesion of the region of the interstitial nucleus of Cajal (INC) in the rostral midbrain tegmentum (*B*). Note the dissociated effects in the patient with Wallenberg's syndrome; OT and SVV deviated most in the ipsilateral left eye. Comparison of individual OT and SVV values in both patients shows varying dissociations of the net tilt. Both tend to normalize within 4 to 6 weeks, and fluctuations cannot be simply explained by methodological inaccuracy. VD = vertical divergence as skew deviation; d = days; m = months.[9]

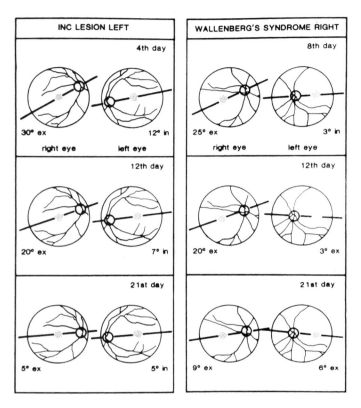

FIGURE 12–8. Schematic drawings from original fundus photographs made with the head upright, in a patient with a mesodiencephalic infarction on the left involving the region of the interstitial nucleus of Cajal (INC) (*left*) and a lateral medullary infarction on the right (*right*) in the acute stage (*top*) and 12 days and 21 days later, respectively (*bottom*). The anatomic structures involved were identified with MRI projections onto cytoarchitectonical sections of a stereotaxic brainstem atlas. Both binocular pathological ocular torsion (OT) in the mesodiencephalic lesion and the predominantly ipsilateral excyclotropia (ex) in the lateral medullary lesion exhibit spontaneous recovery to physiological excyclotropia of about 4° to 7°. After 21 days the patient with Wallenberg's syndrome showed a nearly normalized eye position (excyclotropia of 6° of the left eye and of 9° of the right eye), whereas the patient with the INC lesion on the left had a slight incyclotropia (in) of the left eye of 5°.[9]

Paroxysmal OTR in MS was treated effectively with carbamazepine[13]; baclofen had some therapeutic benefit in a patient with paroxysmal OTR and brainstem abscess.[14]

Thalamic and Cortical Astasia Associated with Subjective Visual Vertical Tilts

An association of SVV tilts with falls is also typical for posterolateral (vestibular subnuclei) thalamic lesions. Thalamic astasia[18] is a condition in which patients without paresis or sensory or cerebellar deficits are unable to maintain an unsupported, upright posture. Postural imbalance with a transient tendency to fall has been reported following therapeutic thalamotomy and thalamic hemorrhage.[19] According to our experience in some 30 patients with thalamic infarctions, the posterolateral type may cause contraversive or ipsiversive postural instability with SVV tilts, whereas the paramedian type (if it extends into the rostral midbrain) always causes contraversive falls.

Masdeu et al[20] have described astasia and gait failure with damage of the pontomesencephalic (locomotor) region. Although not discussed, it could also be explained in part by a vestibular tone imbalance in roll, especially since skew deviation was described as a feature of the syndrome.

Of 31 patients with cortical infarctions of the middle cerebral artery territory, 21 showed significant, mostly contraversive, pathological SVV tilts.[21] The overlapping area of these infarctions centered on the posterior insula, which is probably homologous to the parietoinsular vestibular cortex.[22,23] SVV tilts caused by vestibular cortex lesions may also be associated with (a compensatory) body lateropulsion. This explains the cortical phenomenon "pusher," which physical therapists readily recognize.

Torsional Nystagmus

The "graviceptive" input from the otoliths converges with that from the vertical semicircular canals to subserve static and dynamic vestibular function in roll. This combination of static and dynamic effects[24] is not surprising if one considers how these functions are corroborated. Our studies on OTR, lateropulsion, and SVV were concerned with static effects of vestibular dysfunction in roll.[3,25] These effects persist for days to weeks, during which time they spontaneously subside. In the acute stage of infarction, additional dynamic signs and symptoms occur, which consist of horizontal rotational vertigo and torsional nystagmus.[26,27] Fast phases of rotational nystagmus are contraversive in pontomedullary lesions, whereas the slow phases correspond in direction to the static deviation.

Several distinct and separate lesions (see Fig. 12–2) have been associated with torsional nystagmus, for example, lesions of the vestibular nuclei,[27,28] the lateral medulla,[26,29] in rare cases the MLF (as indicated by an association with internuclear ophthalmoplegia),[30,31] the INC, and the riMLF.[32–34] Fast phases of torsional nystagmus are

- Contraversive in pontomedullary lesions and
- Ipsiversive in paramedian pontine and mesencephalic (INC) lesions (rare exception: contraversive in riMLF lesion).

Jerk-waveform see-saw nystagmus (a torsional nystagmus with elevation of the intorting eye and depression of the extorting eye) is induced by an inactivation of the INC in the rostral midbrain and is also ipsiversive.[34]

The different locations of lesions causing different directions of torsional nystagmus first appear to be confusing. They can, however, be explained by the tonic torsional shift of eye position along the graviceptive pathways from the vestibular nuclei to the INC. A lesion of the (medial or superior) vestibular nucleus causes an ipsiversive tonic deviation (ipsiversive ocular torsion) with compensatory fast phases of the torsional nystagmus to the contralesional side. In view of the fact that the pathway within the MLF crosses to the contralateral side, an MLF lesion in the pontine and pontomesencephalic brainstem induces a tonic contraversive deviation and therefore a torsional nystagmus with the fast phases ipsilesional. The same is true for a lesion of the INC. The only exception to these directional rules for tone imbalance along the vestibular graviceptive pathways is the riMLF, a lesion of which causes a (possibly nonvestibular) ocular motor tone imbalance in the opposite direction.

VESTIBULAR DISORDERS IN (SAGITTAL) PITCH PLANE

A striking difference between vestibular tone imbalance in the roll and pitch planes is that roll dysfunction is caused by unilateral and pitch dysfunction by bilateral lesions of paired pathways in the brainstem or of the cerebellar flocculus.[4] This structural difference probably explains why a vestibular tone imbalance in pitch frequently occurs with various intoxications or metabolic disorders, which is unusual for tone imbalance in yaw or roll, unless as a functional decompensation of an earlier (compensated) tone imbalance. Downbeat and upbeat nystagmus are not merely ocular motor disorders, but central vestibular disorders that also affect orientation and balance. A tone imbalance in the pitch plane manifests as vertical upbeating or downbeating nystagmus, fore-aft head-and-body tilt, and deviation of the subjective straight-ahead toward the direction of the slow phase of the nystagmus.

Clinically, downbeat nystagmus occurs more frequently than upbeat nystagmus and is often permanent (as in Arnold-Chiari malformation), whereas upbeat nystagmus is usually a transient phenomenon. Lesional sites for upbeat nystagmus have been more precisely confirmed by clinical studies (bilateral lesions of the pontomesencephalic junction or the medulla) than those for downbeat nystagmus (bilateral pontomedullary lesions or bilateral flocculus dysfunction). In contrast, the pathomechanism of downbeat nystagmus appears to be clearer (tone imbalance of the VOR in pitch) than that of upbeat nystagmus, which can result from different pathomechanisms: a (perhaps vestibular) pontomesencephalic and a (perhaps nonvestibular) medullary one. Transitions between upbeat and downbeat nystagmus have been frequently described in paramedian pontomedullary lesions. Both types occur with paramedian plaques in MS, cerebellar degeneration, or drug intoxication. Whereas downbeat nystagmus is more typical for congenital craniocervical malformations (Arnold-Chiari malformation), upbeat nystagmus is more typical for MS, bilateral brainstem ischemia (basilar artery thrombosis), or brainstem tumors. Upbeat and downbeat nystagmus in the primary position of gaze may be the result of various intoxications (without structural lesion).

Downbeat nystagmus in the "primary" gaze position, or more particularly on lateral gaze, is often accompanied by oscillopsia and postural instability. This is a clearly defined and, depending on the lesional site, permanent association of symptoms, which often indicates structural lesions of the paramedian craniocervical junction.[35]

Downbeat nystagmus is present in darkness as well as with fixation; slow-phase velocity and amplitude increase on lateral gaze or with head extension or head movements in the sagittal (pitch) plane. Downbeat nystagmus may be present only on downward or lateral gaze. Slow-phase velocity is not consistently related to vertical gaze and, contrary to Alexander's law, may even be maximal on upward rather than downward gaze. Nystagmus is a jerk, usually with linear slow phases. It may exhibit changes of exponential velocity in slow phases, both increasing and decreasing.[36,37] Downbeat nystagmus may be episodic in Arnold-Chiari malformation[38] or paroxysmal.[28]

It has been reported that reversals from downbeat to upbeat nystagmus can be provoked by upward gaze deviation,[39] convergence,[40] or transitions from sitting to supine position.[41] Downbeat and upbeat nystagmus are the directional counterparts of a vestibular tone imbalance in the pitch plane. The close proximity of the areas causing either upbeat or downbeat nystagmus in the medulla agrees with the directional changes between the two. Reversals from upbeat to downbeat nystagmus have also been observed.[40,42,43]

Patients complain of a distressing illusory oscillation of the visual scene (oscillopsia) and postural imbalance. Both are obligatory but hitherto poorly studied symptoms of the syndrome. The retinal slip in downbeat nystagmus is misinterpreted as motion of the visual scene because the involuntary ocular movements that override fixation are not associated with an appropriate efference-copy signal. Oscillopsia is a permanent symptom, but the illusory motion is less than would be expected from the amplitude of the nystagmus; it increases with increasing amplitude; the mean ratio between the two is 0.37.[44]

Oscillopsia should be expected to cause an impairment of postural balance, because retinal image motion is a major cue for body stabilization. However, this kind of "visual ataxia" cannot simply account for the typical postural imbalance, which is a striking feature of the fore-aft body sway and includes a tendency to fall backward. This fore-aft postural instability can be interpreted to be a direction-specific vestibulospinal (or cerebellar) imbalance, because it can be observed when the eyes are closed. We believe that the objective measurable backward tilt represents a vestibulospinal compensation in the direction opposite to the perceived lesional "forward vertigo," which corresponds to downbeat nystagmus.[44,45] When the eyes are open, a measurable visual stabilization of body sway is preserved, but it does not sufficiently compensate for the visual ataxia. In downbeat nystagmus (more aptly termed "vestibular downbeat syndrome"), the patient's pathological postural sway with the eyes open depends on the direction of gaze; it increases with increasing amplitude of the nystagmus. Pathophysiologically, it is secondary to a combination of both vestibulospinal ataxia and reduced visual stabilization of posture owing to the nystagmus.

ETIOLOGY

The two most common causes of a downbeat nystagmus/vertigo syndrome are cerebellar ectopia (25 percent) (e.g., Arnold-Chiari malformation) and cerebellar degeneration (25 percent) (e.g., olivopontocerebellar degeneration). A further 10 to 20 percent of patients have a variety of conditions,[34,46] and in about 30 percent an unequivocal diagnosis of the cause cannot be established.

In cerebellar degeneration and drug-induced downbeat nystagmus, an asymmetric vestibulocerebellar disinhibition of the "Purkinje cell activity" on the vertical canal reflexes may be causative. Nutritional cerebellar syndromes owing to thiamine deficiency, in particular alcoholic cerebellar degeneration (see Box 12–1), not only cause a typical 3-Hz fore-aft oscillation of body sway[47] but also downbeating nystagmus.[46,48,49] Antiepileptic drugs, especially phenytoin[50] and carbamazepine,[51,52] can produce a reversible downbeat nystagmus with associated cerebellar signs, depending on the dosage of the drugs. Other causes include lithium toxicity,[46,53–55] felbamate intoxication,[56] or toluene abuse.[57] Severe magnesium depletion[58] and vitamin B_{12} deficiency[59] have been reported to result in downbeat nystagmus.

Other conditions associated with downbeat nystagmus are MS,[60] familial periodic ataxia, tumors of the posterior fossa, cerebellar degeneration,[61] paraneoplastic cerebellar degeneration,[62] infratentorial vascular diseases such as dolichoectasia of the vertebrobasilar artery,[63] hematomas, cavernomas, syringobulbia,[64] and encephalitis (Box 12–1).

Sometimes downbeat nystagmus is lithium induced in preexisting Arnold-Chiari malformation,[65] or caused as an intermittent syndrome by head tilt due to vertebral artery compression[66] or by a vermian arachnoid cyst with associated obstructive hy-

---

BOX 12–1 Downbeat Nystagmus (Vestibular Downbeat Syndrome)

Clinical syndrome

Downbeat nystagmus in the primary position of gaze (no suppression by fixation), increased on lateral gaze or head extension

Associated distressing oscillopsia and postural imbalance with a tendency to fall backward and vertical deviation of straight ahead

Saccadic downward pursuit

Transitions from downbeat to upbeat nystagmus possible

Incidence/age/sex

Depends on etiology, no obvious preference for sex, rare in children (congenital)

Pathomechanism

Tone imbalance of the vertical semicircular canal reflexes (pitch plane) modulated by otolithic input

Structural or functional lesions involve:

Either the floor of the fourth ventricle between the vestibular nuclei

Or vestibulocerebellar flocculus (intoxication, cerebellar degeneration)

Etiology

The two most common causes are cerebellar ectopia and cerebellar degeneration including alcoholic cerebellar degeneration

Other conditions: drugs (phenytoin, carbamazepine, lithium), MS, tumor, hematoma, vascular disease, encephalitis, magnesium depletion, vitamin B_{12} deficiency (see Table 12–1)

Course/prognosis

Frequently permanent when caused by structural lesions

Usually reversible when caused by intoxication or metabolic deficiency

Management

Depends on etiology (i.e., surgical decompression)

Medical treatment with baclofen, gabapentin (or clonazepam?)

Differential diagnosis

Acquired pendular nystagmus, gaze-evoked nystagmus, upbeat nystagmus, spasmus nutans (infants), vertical congenital nystagmus, ocular bobbing

---

drocephalus.[67] Downbeat nystagmus is rare in children. It may be hereditary congenital[68] as a persisting syndrome, or it may occur during infancy and resolve naturally.[69]

MANAGEMENT

Downbeat nystagmus owing to drugs, magnesium depletion, or vitamin B_{12} deficiency is usually reversible when the intoxication or the metabolic deficiency is reversed. Downbeat nystagmus owing to structural lesions in the posterior fossa is usually permanent, although a surgical suboccipital decompression in Arnold-Chiari malformation to relieve the compression of the herniating cerebellum against the caudal brainstem may lead to gradual improvement of some of the distressing symptoms.[70] Suboccipital craniotomy,[71] transoral removal of the odontoid process in the basilar impression,[72] of an osteophyt compressing the vertebral artery,[66] and surgical decompression of a syringomyelic cyst in the medulla,[67,73] were able to resolve the syndrome in individual patients. For one patient, base-out prisms were added to both spectacle lenses, because the convergence both dampened the nystagmus and decreased the oscillopsia.[36]

Target symptoms for symptomatic medical treatment are distressing oscillopsia and reduced visual acuity owing to the fixation nystagmus. Postural imbalance is less prominent and less distressing. It is our experience that baclofen suppresses downbeat as well as upbeat nystagmus and associated postural imbalance in some cases.[74] Baclofen appears to have a $GABA_B$-ergic effect with augmentation of the physiological inhibitory influence of the vestibulocerebellum on the vestibular nuclei. It was previously recommended for treatment of periodic alternating nystagmus.[75] Some more patients responded to gabapentin.[76] Muscarinic antagonists, in particular the anticholinergic drug scopolamine, reduced nystagmus in five patients with acquired pendular nystagmus and in two patients with downbeat nystagmus.[77] Benztropine was less effective. The $GABA_A$ agonist clonazepam (3 × 0.5 mg po daily) was used with some success to treat nystagmus and oscillopsia.[78,79] Physical balance training significantly improves postural instability in patients with a newly acquired downbeat nystagmus syndrome.[45] Box 12–1 summarizes the information given in this chapter about the downbeat nystagmus/vertigo syndrome.

Upbeat Nystagmus (Vestibular Upbeat Syndrome)

Upbeat nystagmus in the primary position of gaze with concomitant oscillopsia and postural instability is a pendant of downbeat nystagmus, and most probably reflects an imbalance of vertical VOR tone.[80] It has the same causes and involves central eye-head coordination in the pitch plane as mediated by pathways from the vertical semicircular canals and the otoliths. Because the manifestations are typically modulated by otolithic input arising from static head tilt, upbeat nystagmus is in a broader sense also a kind of positional nystagmus. As distinct from downbeat nystagmus, brainstem lesions are often found in patients with upbeat nystagmus. Two separate intra-axial brainstem lesions in the tegmentum of the pontomesencephalic junction and in the medulla near the perihypoglossal nuclei are likely to be responsible for this syndrome, but there is insufficient evidence to determine whether the cerebellar vermis is involved. Upbeat nystagmus indicates bilateral lesions of the pathways mediating VOR in pitch. However, not all forms of upbeat nystagmus must be vestibular. It can also arise from acquired asymmetries of the smooth pursuit or the gaze-holding neural integrator system.

ETIOLOGY

Upbeat nystagmus was observed in 26 of 17,900 patients examined at a neurotological clinic in Japan. The incidence rate was 0.145 percent.[81] The etiology of upbeat nystagmus is in general similar to that of downbeat nystagmus (Box 12–2). Malformation of the craniocervical junction and cerebellar degeneration seem to be less frequent than in downbeat nystagmus, whereas brainstem tumors and MS are more frequent. Upbeat nystagmus can be associated with bilateral vascular brainstem lesions (basilar thrombosis), hematoma, cavernoma, MS, encephalitis, abscess, or head injury. It has been repeatedly reported in alcoholic degeneration, especially in Wernicke's encephalopathy[40,82–84] or in single cases of Fisher's syndrome,[85] central diabetes insipidus,[86] Pelizaeus-Merzbacher disease,[87] and even associated with middle ear dis-

BOX 12–2   Upbeat Nystagmus (Vestibular Upbeat Syndrome)

Clinical syndrome

Upbeat nystagmus in the primary position of gaze (no suppression by fixation),
modulated by static head tilt
Associated distressing oscillopsia, postural imbalance, deviation of straight ahead
Saccadic upward pursuit
Transitions from upbeat to downbeat nystagmus possible

Incidence/Age/Sex

Depends on etiology, no obvious preference for sex, rare in children (congenital)

Pathomechanism

Tone imbalance of the vertical semicircular canal reflexes (pitch plane) modulated
by otolithic input
Structural or functional paramedian lesions involve:
Either pontomesencephalic junction (brachium conjunctivum? ventral tegmental
tract?)
Or medulla (perihypoglossal nuclei?)

Etiology

Brainstem tumors, infarction, hematoma, cavernoma, multiple sclerosis,
encephalitis, abscess, alcoholic degeneration (Wernicke's encephalopathy), drug
intoxication, nicotine (see Table 12.1)

Course/prognosis

Depending on etiology, gradual improvement by central compensation?
Usually reversible when caused by intoxication

Management

Medical treatment with baclofen (clonazepam?)
Physical exercise (eye movements and balance training)

Differential diagnosis

Acquired pendular nystagmus, gaze-evoked nystagmus, downbeat nystagmus,
spasmus nutans (infants), vertical congenital nystagmus, reversed ocular
bobbing

ease.[88] We have seen transient upbeat nystagmus associated with various intoxications, for example with antiepileptic drugs. Upbeat nystagmus can on rare occasions
be congenital.[89–92]

Neveling and Kruse[93] were the first to describe a tobacco-induced upbeat nystagmus, which Sibony et al,[94] investigated more thoroughly. This nicotine-induced nystagmus (after smoking one cigarette) can also be elicited by chewing nicotine gum.[95] It
obeys Alexander's law, but only occurs in darkness and is suppressed by visual fixation. It was reported to have a latency of 40 to 90 seconds, a duration of 10 to 20 minutes, and maximum slow-phase velocities at 2 to 3 minutes.[94] The degree of impairment in upward pursuit correlated with the intensity of nicotine-induced nystagmus
recorded in darkness.[96] Nicotinic receptors have been described in different parts of
the vestibular end organ,[97] the lateral and medial vestibular nucleus,[98] and in efferent
vestibular neurons.[99] It is not yet clear which structures are involved in nicotine-
induced upbeat nystagmus.

MANAGEMENT

Upbeat nystagmus may be associated with severe vertigo, ataxia, and nausea, particularly at first. Such patients may require vestibular sedatives (e.g., dimenhydrinate or scopolamine) as long as nausea lasts. Depending on the etiology, the natural history of this sign usually shows gradual improvement or disappears, in contrast to downbeat nystagmus, which is frequently permanent. Physical exercise involving fixation, eye movements, and postural balance will accelerate central compensation. Medical treatment is possible with baclofen (3 × 5 to 10 mg po daily), which has a beneficial effect on nystagmus amplitude, oscillopsia, and visual acuity in some patients (Fig. 12–9).[74] Cabamazepine was found to be effective in a single case of upbeat nystagmus due to multiple sclerosis.[100]

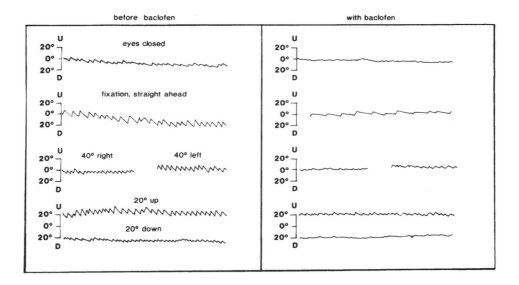

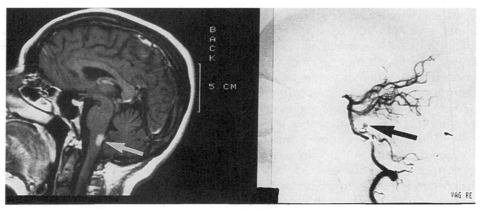

FIGURE 12–9. Partial suppression of upbeat nystagmus by medical treatment with baclofen in a patient suffering from a medullary metastasis. Vertical ENG recordings (*top*). MR scan and angiography of the vertebral artery (*bottom*).[74]

VESTIBULAR DISORDERS IN (HORIZONTAL) YAW PLANE

The clinical signs, both perceptual and motor, of a vestibular tone imbalance in the yaw plane include rotational vertigo, deviation of perceived straight-ahead, pastpointing, rotational and lateral body falls, and horizontal nystagmus.

Central vestibular syndromes manifesting purely in the yaw plane occur less frequently than those due to imbalance in the vertical pitch and roll planes for two reasons.[4] First, the area of a lesion that can cause a tone imbalance in yaw is comparatively small (root entry zone of the vestibular nerve, medial and superior vestibular nuclei, and the adjacent integration center for horizontal eye movements, the paramedian pontine reticular formation [PPRF]). In contrast, the area of a lesion that can cause vestibular tone imbalance in roll or pitch covers nearly the entire brainstem from the medulla to the rostral midbrain (see Fig. 12–2 and Fig. 12–3). The larger extent of the latter area is due to the greater separation of the vestibular nuclei and the ocular motor integration centers for vertical and torsional eye movements (riMLF and INC). Second, the area of a lesion that can theoretically cause a pure tone imbalance in the yaw plane adjoins and overlaps areas subserving vestibular function in roll and pitch (see Fig. 12–2 and Fig. 12–3). There is a multisensory convergence within the parallel neural network of the vestibular nuclei,[101] a lesion of which will cause mixed vestibular syndromes in more than one plane. A study of vestibular nuclei lesion in the monkey demonstrated a combined nystagmus: its horizontal component beat toward the contralateral side after rostral lesions and toward the ipsilateral side after caudal lesions.[102]

Some of the cases described as central variants of vestibular neuritis[103–107] caused by lesions of the medial vestibular subnucleus or the root entry zone of the vestibular nerve were probably not restricted to the yaw plane, because the case descriptions also contain signs and symptoms of VOR tone imbalance in other planes of action. There have been frequent reports that cerebellar infarctions owing to occlusion of the anterior inferior cerebellar artery (which may also supply the rostral vestibular nuclei) mimic vestibular neuritis.[103,108] The other main cause of confusion with disorders at the entry zone of the eighth nerve is multiple sclerosis.[45,105]

Hopf[104] has described two patients with symptoms and signs of vestibular neuritis, including horizontal semicircular canal paresis, who had in addition paresis of the masseter, temporal, and pterygoid muscles as well as impairment of the masseter reflex on the affected side. He argued that infarction of a small region ventrolateral to the floor of the fourth ventricle was causative, as structures serving both peripheral vestibular function and trigeminal motor function are present in this area. A demyelinating plaque in MS may mimic signs of vestibular neuritis, including caloric hyporesponsiveness if it is located at the root entry zone of the eighth nerve.[45] It is extremely important to carefully investigate ocular motor function in patients presenting with vestibular dysfunction which is apparently of peripheral origin; most central cases have some abnormalities incompatible with a peripheral disorder such as a contralateral gaze-evoked nystagmus or horizontal or vertical saccadic pursuit. The degree of horizontal canal paresis (as tested by caloric irrigation) is usually less severe (incomplete) than peripheral canal paresis. An MRI study demonstrated that canal paresis caused by brainstem lesions predominantly involved the medial and to a lesser extent the lateral vestibular nucleus as well as the proximal portion of the vestibular fascicle.[107]

Vestibular syndromes, when caused by unilateral pontomedullary lesions, frequently result in combined vestibular tone imbalance in more than one plane, such as a combination of torsional and horizontal nystagmus. This tone imbalance may manifest not only in spontaneous nystagmus but also in spontaneous or gaze-evoked ocular deviations. There may be an inappropriate horizontal ocular deviation during attempted vertical saccades (lateropulsion in Wallenberg's syndrome) or an inappropriate torsional deviation during attempted horizontal saccades ('torsipulsion').[26,109]

Sometimes the clinical manifestation of a particular ocular motor abnormality such as ocular tilt reaction allows one to identify the semicircular canal pathway affected (anterior or posterior). The different presentation of ocular tilt reaction in Wallenberg's syndrome with monocular dissociation of ocular torsion—either excyclotropia of the undermost eye or incyclotropia of the uppermost eye—indicates involvement of the posterior or the anterior semicircular canal pathways.[110] Lesions of the vestibular nuclei may also result in repetitive multidirectional paroxysmal nystagmus and vertigo, which have been reported to respond to treatment with carbamazepine.[38] The differential effects of a medullary lesion involving more than one VOR plane are not only reflected in the direction of eye movements but also in the preferred direction of increased body sway. Body sway histograms as measured by posturography are primarily diagonal in patients with Wallenberg's syndrome and moderate body lateropulsion (combination: roll and yaw), but primarily lateral in patients with severe body lateropulsion (roll greater than yaw).[110] This is also reflected by the close correlation between the tilt of perceived visual vertical and the severity of body lateropulsion, both indicators—perceptual and postural—of a vestibular imbalance in roll.[111]

VESTIBULAR CORTEX: LOCATIONS, FUNCTIONS, AND DISORDERS

The two major cortical functions of the vestibular system are spatial orientation and self-motion perception. These functions, however, are not specifically vestibular; they also rely on visual and somatosensory input. All three systems—vestibular, visual, and somatosensory—provide us with redundant information about the position and motion of our body relative to the external space. Although the vestibular cortex function is distributed among several multisensory areas in the parietal and temporal cortices, it is also integrated in a larger network for spatial attention and sensorimotor control of eye and body motion in space.

Animal studies have identified several distinct and separate areas of the parietal and temporal cortices which receive vestibular afferents, such as area 2v at the tip of the intraparietal sulcus,[112–114] area 3aV (neck, trunk, and vestibular region of area 3a) in the central sulcus,[115] PIVC at the posterior end of the insula,[22,23] and area 7 in the inferior parietal lobule.[116] Not only do these areas receive bilateral vestibular input from the vestibular nuclei, but they in turn directly project down to the vestibular nuclei.[5,117,118] Thus, corticofugal feedback may modulate vestibular brainstem function.

Our knowledge about vestibular cortex function in humans is less precise. It is derived mainly from stimulation experiments reported anecdotally in the older literature and from recent brain activation studies with PET[119] and fMRI.[120,121] It is not always possible to extrapolate from monkey species to human cortex, as Andersen and Gnadt[122] demonstrated for Brodmann's area 7 in rhesus monkey and humans. Area 2v corresponds best to the vestibular cortex as described by Foerster.[123] The PIVC corresponds best to a region from which Penfield and Jasper[124] were able to induce vestibular sensations by electrical stimulation with a depth electrode within the sylvian fissure, medial to the primary acoustic cortex.

The Parietoinsular Vestibular Cortex

In view of the strong interconnections between PIVC and other vestibular cortex areas (mainly 3aV and 2v) as well as the vestibular brainstem nuclei, Guldin and Grüsser[5] postulate that it is the core region within the vestibular cortical system in the monkey. About 50 percent of the neurons in this region respond to vestibular stimulation in addition to somatosensory, optokinetic, or visual stimulation. This area is involved not only in the processing of vestibular, somatosensory, and visual information, which is generated whenever the position of the body changes in relation to the extrapersonal space,[5] but also when stationary human subjects perform optokinetic nystagmus.[120,121]

Multimodal Sensorimotor Vestibular Cortex Function and Dysfunction

The vestibular, visual, and somatosensory systems cooperate to determine our internal representation of space and subjective body orientation in unique three dimensional coordinates, which are either egocentric (body-centered) or exocentric (world-centered). This is not a trivial process; two of the sensory systems are anchored in the head, which moves relative to the trunk. Retinal coordinates—dependent as they are on gaze and head position—and head-fixed labyrinthine coordinates would require continuous updating of the particular eye and head positions in order to deliver reliable input for adequate ocular motor and motor exploration of space. Nature seems to have solved this impossible sensorimotor control of a multilink and multiaxis system by multisensory coding of space in either common egocentric or exocentric rather than retinotopic or head-centered coordinates. This has been demonstrated for posterior parietal neurons.[125,126] Spatial information in nonretinal coordinates allows us to determine body position relative to visual space, which is a necessary prerequisite for accurate motor response. To obtain such a frame of reference, information coded in coordinates of the peripheral sensory organs (retina, otoliths, semicircular canals, and proprioceptors such as muscle spindles) must be transformed and integrated.[127] This function is most probably subserved by the posterior parietal cortex, a lesion of which produces a visuospatial hemineglect. Karnath et al[128,129] argued that neglect in brain-damaged patients is caused by a disturbance of the central transformation process that converts the sensory input coordinates from the periphery into an egocentric, body-centered coordinate system. The importance of the vestibular input for spatial orientation and the continuous updating of our internal representation of space becomes evident by the deficient spatial memory in microgravity during spacecraft missions. Large errors are made during prolonged microgravity when pointing at memorized targets, and it is the lack of knowledge of target position, not limb position, that is causative.[130]

In patients, an inappropriate vestibular input owing to peripheral or central dysfunction can cause paroxysmal "room-tilt illusions," the result of a mismatch of the two three-dimensional visual and vestibular coordinate maps. Furthermore, a plane- and direction-specific tilt of static spatial orientation occurs in disorders of the VOR, such as downbeat and upbeat nystagmus. Adjustments of subjective straight ahead exhibit an upward shift in downbeat nystagmus and a downward shift in upbeat nystagmus.[80] Here the tilt of perceived straight-ahead is elicited by the asymmetric vestibular tone in the pitch plane in the brainstem, which reaches the cortex by ascending projections. Vestibular syndromes caused only by cortical lesions have not yet been well defined. Static cortical spatial disorientation may occur as

- Paroxysmal room-tilt illusion in parietal or frontal lobe lesions
- Contralateral spatial hemineglect in inferior parietal or frontal lobe lesions
- Vertical neglect below the horizontal meridian in bilateral parieto-occipital lesions
- Tilts of perceived vertical (mostly contraversive) and body lateropulsion in unilateral PIVC lesions

Dynamic cortical spatial disorientation with apparent motion or rotational vertigo may occur

- In vestibular epilepsy with temporoparietal foci
- Rarely as a transient vertigo in acute lesions of the vestibular cortex

Spatial Hemineglect, a Cortical Vestibular Syndrome?

Spatial hemineglect impairs focal attention toward space on the contralesional side. It is most often induced by acute brain damage of the inferior parietal lobule of the right hemisphere[131] and occurs less frequently with acute right or left lesions of the frontal premotor cortex.[132] A recent report described a patient who had sequential strokes in both hemispheres. After suffering a right-sided parietal infarct, he had a severe unilateral spatial neglect, which abruptly disappeared following a second left-sided frontal infarct.[133] Other studies have described single patients with bilateral inferior parietal lobe lesions, which manifested in vertical neglect of the lower half-space below the horizontal meridian.[134,135] Mesulam[136] hypothesized that there is a cortical network for directed attention, in which the inferior parietal lobule modulates the shift of attention within extrapersonal space and the dorsolateral frontal area is responsible for generating exploratory motor behavior. A unilateral lesion leads to an imbalance of the bilateral tone and subsequently horizontal displacement of the sagittal midplane and subjective body orientation toward the lesioned side.

Studies showing that vestibular (caloric) stimulation significantly improved spatial functioning have demonstrated the important role of the vestibular system in neglect.[137,138] When vestibular stimulation was combined with neck muscle vibration, the horizontal deviation combined linearly, adding or neutralizing the effects observed during application of both types of stimulation.[127] This study also showed that the neglect patients displaced subjective body orientation ipsilesionally, which does not result from a disturbed primary perception or disturbed transmission of the vestibular or proprioceptive input from the periphery. Karnath et al[128,129] argued that the transformation process converting the sensory input coordinates from the periphery into egocentric (body-centered) coordinates is the critical mechanism that leads to hemineglect. This process must involve multisensory integration and motor behavior including eye and hand movements as well as walking trajectory.[139] Spatial hemineglect also includes the back space of the body.[140]

The concept of critical cortical areas involved in the control of spatial attention was derived from the study of patients with circumscribed lesions. Recent PET studies that visualize the activated neural system underlying visuospatial attention give further support for this view. Specifically, neocortical activations were observed in the right anterior cingulate gyrus, the intraparietal sulcus of the right posterior parietal cortex, and the mesial and lateral premotor cortices.[141]

Paroxysmal Room-Tilt Illusion

Room-tilt illusions are transient upside-down vision or apparent 90° tilts of the visual scene. In central vestibular disorders they can be induced by either acute vestibulocerebellar brainstem lesions or cortical dysfunction. The two causative cortical regions are the parieto-occipital area[142–144] and rarely the frontal lobe.[145] A lesion in these regions can also cause spatial hemineglect. Solms et al[145] have carefully reviewed 21 previously reported cases of transient upside-down vision and described the striking similarities.

Tiliket et al[146] reported that a sudden 90° room-tilt illusion could be elicited in three patients with unilateral brainstem lesions following vestibular stimulation by off-vertical rotary chair rotation. Furthermore, patients with peripheral bilateral vestibular failure may report transient room-tilt illusions on awakening in the morning. Our latter observation (unpublished) may be comparable to the reports of astronauts about occasional upside-down vision in microgravity.[147] We believe that room-tilt illusions are transient mismatches of the cortical visual and the vestibular three-dimensional coordinate maps that occur in 90° or 180° steps as the erroneous result of the attempted cortical match.[148] They should not be confused with the frequent tilts of subjective visual vertical, as they occur with unilateral peripheral vestibular brainstem, thalamus, or insular cortex lesions. The matching of two separate sensory three-dimensional coordinate maps must be plastic in order to compensate for visual-vestibular tone imbalances and/or to adapt to unusual environments (microgravity). The plasticity of this visual-vestibular interaction has been best demonstrated when wearing reversing prisms.[149]

Vestibular Epilepsy

Vestibular epilepsy (vestibular seizures or auras) is a rare cortical vertigo syndrome secondary to focal epileptic discharges in either the temporal lobe or the parietal association cortex[123,124,150]; multiple areas of both receive bilateral vestibular projections from the ipsilateral thalamus.

If vestibular seizures arise from different areas, the sensorimotor symptomatology may differ as regards apparent rotation or tilt,[151] with or without associated eye, head, and body deviation or epileptic nystagmus. Clinical data on the directions of apparent self-motion or surround-motion are mostly incomplete and imprecise. If the description is exact, as in rotatory seizures ("volvular epilepsy"), then the topographic localization of the underlying pathology is too inexact to permit its allocation to known vestibular areas.

An acute unilateral functional deficit of the vestibular cortex (e.g., in medial cerebral artery infarction) rarely manifests with vertigo,[152] unlike lesions in the vestibular area of the brainstem. It is not the functional loss but the focal discharge that causes central vertigo. This has been repeatedly demonstrated by stimulation experiments. Electrical stimulation of the human thalamus during stereotactic neurosurgical procedures induced sensations of movement in space, most frequently described as horizontal or vertical rotation or sensations of falling or rising.[153] These sensations were similar to those induced by stimulation of the vestibular cortex.[123,124]

Vertigo has long been considered a manifestation of epileptic auras.[154,155] Most information on auras (vestibular epilepsy), including case descriptions, comes from older textbooks, for example Bumke and Foerster[156] or Penfield and Jasper,[124] or review articles.[157,158] Original studies are relatively rare[159–162] in contrast to studies of the less important phenomenon of vestibulogenic epilepsy.

Knowledge of vestibular epilepsy has not advanced very much in the last 40 years because of the lack of pathophysiological data. The limited clinical data that exist consist of patients' descriptions, EEG recordings, and correlations of vestibular symptoms with the results of brain imaging techniques or surgical findings. Furthermore, the syndrome of vestibular epilepsy is not always well defined. Vertigo and dizziness in the sense of "lightheadedness" are often described by patients as part of the aura in complex partial seizures with temporal or extratemporal foci.[163] Most patients with (simple partial) vestibular seizures also have complex partial seizures or generalized tonic-clonic seizures.[162] Vestibular seizures must be distinguished from versive seizures that manifest with contralateral rotation of head and eye. The latter are typically associated with either motor cortex foci or are the result of seizure spread from the temporal lobes.

Epileptic nystagmus usually beats contraversive to the seizure focus and may be of vestibular, visual (optokinetic), or cortical ocular motor origin.[164]

MANAGEMENT

Vestibular seizures respond to antiepileptics. First-line drugs are carbamazepine or phenytoin; second-line drugs are gabapentine, sodium valproate, and lamotrigine.[165] If necessary and possible, surgical procedures may be considered.[166]

Paroxysmal Central Vertigo

Nonepileptic paroxysmal vertigo or other vestibular syndromes may result from pathological excitation of various vestibular structures.[167] Most of them occur in multiple sclerosis, but others may be associated with a brainstem abscess (paroxysmal ocular tilt reaction[14]) or an arteriovenous malformation with previous bleeding (repetitive paroxysmal nystagmus and vertigo[28]).

Different manifestations of paroxysmal vestibular syndromes of the brainstem have been described in MS:

- Paroxysmal dysarthria, ataxia, and vertigo[168]
- Paroxysmal ocular tilt reaction[13]
- Paroxysmal room-tilt illusion[169]

Paroxysmal dysarthria, vertigo, and ataxia, as described by Andermann et al,[168] are well known. They are probably one of the most common manifestations of paroxysmal attacks in MS.[170] The mechanism of these attacks has been suggested to be a transversely spreading ephaptic activation of adjacent axons within a partially demyelinated lesion in fiber tracts of the pontine tegmentum involving the brachium conjunctivum.[171] The attacks may be the initial symptom of MS. They last from a few seconds to a few minutes, and their frequency varies from a few per month to 200 per day. Sometimes they are provoked by hyperventilation or when rising. The character of the vertigo is rarely rotatory but more typically a kind of missing postural coordination, with ataxia and broad-based gait often associated with nystagmus or internuclear ophthalmoplegia.

Carbamazepine is a very effective treatment that in most cases results in the complete disappearance of the attacks[170,171] even in low dosages (200 to 400 mg/d). If untreated, they can continue for months or years. If carbamazepine eliminates the paroxysms for a period of weeks or months, the attempt should be made to discontinue the medication. Most patients will then remain free of paroxysms without antiepileptics.

Familial vertigo responds to azetazolamide. It includes a variety of autosomally dominant episodic ataxias,[172,173] which have recently been identified as channelopathies.

PAROXYSMAL VERTIGO EVOKED BY LATERAL GAZE

In the absence of vestibular stimulation, prolonged lateral eye deviation to the extreme left position for 5 to 20 seconds induced intense attacks of nystagmus and rotational vertigo with postural imbalance lasting from 50 to 90 seconds in rare patients with strokes in the vertebrobasilar territory, including the vestibular nuclei.[174]

Attempted convergence may evoke congenital and acquired forms of nystagmus,[175,176] or change upbeat nystagmus to downbeat nystagmus.[40] Sogg and Hoyt[90] described a family with attacks of vertical nystagmus, lasting from 20 to 90 minutes, which could be elicited by maintaining upward gaze. These attacks were, however, not accompanied by vertigo. Thurston et al[177] described a patient with periodically occurring conjugate eye and head turning, followed by nystagmus lasting for about 2 minutes, which was associated with focal seizure activity in the EEG.

CENTRAL VESTIBULAR FALLS WITHOUT VERTIGO

There are a few instances of what is probably central vestibular dysfunction. In such cases, patients without paresis or sensory or cerebellar deficits are unable to maintain an unsupported upright stance. They do not, however, complain of vertigo. Their conditions include thalamic astasia, lateropulsion in Wallenberg's syndrome or in PIVC lesions, and ocular-tilt reaction in pontomedullary or rostral midbrain lesions.

THALAMIC ASTASIA

Postural imbalance with a transient tendency to fall has been noted following therapeutic thalamotomy.[178-180] It has been attributed to muscle hypotonia or neglect and has also been observed after thalamic infarctions[181] and hemorrhages.[19,182] Masdeu and Gorelick[18] described 15 patients with "thalamic astasia," in the absence of motor weakness, sensory loss or cerebellar signs, due to lesions of different causes, all primarily involving superoposterolateral portions of the thalamus but sparing the rubral region. "Typically, when asked to sit up, rather than using the axial muscles, these patients would grasp the side rail of the bed with the unaffected hand or with both hands to pull themselves up." Thalamic astasia is transient and lasts for days or weeks, with the dorsothalamic region being the critical locus. Since posterolateral thalamic infarctions cause tilts of the perceived vertical that are either ipsiversive or contraversive,[17] thalamic astasia and tilts of perceived vertical may both reflect a vestibular tone imbalance. Furthermore, what Masdeu et al[20] described as astasia and gait failure with damage of the pontomesencephalic locomotor region involving the right pontine peduncle area may be associated with vestibular dysfunction in roll. Their patient presented with a contraversive skew deviation of 10°.

Thalamic hemiataxia differs from thalamic astasia and rarely occurs in isolation; it is usually associated with hemisensory loss without hemiparesis[183] or hemisensory loss and hemiparesis.[184] The lesions involve the ventral lateral nucleus of the thalamus and the adjacent posterior limb of the internal capsule and the mid-to-posterior thalamus containing the dentatorubrothalamic and ascending pathways.[183,184]

LATEROPULSION IN WALLENBERG'S SYNDROME

Lateropulsion of the body is a well-known transient feature of dorsolateral medullary infarction. These patients have irresistible, ipsiversive falls but generally no subjective vertigo. Different brainstem lesions from midbrain to medulla cause ipsiversive deviation of the subjective vertical.[9,110,185] Transient ocular-tilt reaction and ipsiversive deviations of SVV, which indicate a pathological shift in the internal representation of the gravitational vector, are typically found in Wallenberg's syndrome.[16,110] We hypothesized that the subjective vertigo is missing in these patients (despite a striking tendency to fall sideways), because individual multisensory postural regulation is adjusted to the deviated vertical. Lateropulsion then represents postural compensation of an apparent body tilt contraversive to the lesioned side. Despite the resulting postural imbalance and the conflicting true vertical, the body is continuously adjusted toward what the central nervous system erroneously computes as vertical.[16,110] This could explain why patients fall without vertigo or warning signals from the multisensory spatial orientation system. Lateropulsion without hemiparesis also occurs in cortical lesions. These patients with infarctions of the middle cerebral artery territory are well known to physiotherapists, who call such patients "pushers." It has been demonstrated that acute lesions of the PIVC cause contraversive tilts of the perceived visual vertical,[21] which makes it most likely that the cortical lateropulsion is also due to a vestibular tone imbalance in the roll plane.

Both lateropulsion in dorsolateral medullary lesions and in posterior insular lesions exhibit spontaneous recovery within days to weeks.[110] This process might be facilitated by physical therapy.

DROP ATTACKS

Sheldon[186,187] originally described drop attacks, which also represent falls without concurrent vertigo due to reflex-like hypotonia of antigravity muscles. The associated etiology is unknown in 69 percent of cases, cardiac in 12 percent, cerebrovascular insufficiency in 8 percent, combined cardiac and cerebrovascular disease in 7 percent, seizures in 5 percent, psychogenic in 1 percent, and vestibular following late Ménière's disease in only 3 percent of patients.[188] Patients with drop attacks have a surprisingly good long-term prognosis. **Hyperexplexia,** the sudden loss of postural tone evoked by startling stimuli, was exacerbated by superimposed posterior thalamic infarction.[189]

SUMMARY

Central vestibular syndromes are characterized by ocular motor, postural, and perceptual signs. They can be classified according to the three major planes of action of the VOR: yaw, roll, and pitch. A tone imbalance in yaw is characterized by horizontal nystagmus, past-pointing, rotational and lateral body falls, and deviation of the perceived straight-ahead. A tone imbalance in roll is defined by torsional nystagmus, skew deviation, ocular torsion, tilts of head, body, and the perceived vertical. Finally, a tone imbalance in pitch is characterized by upbeat or downbeat nystagmus, fore-aft tilts and falls, and vertical deviation of the perceived straight ahead. The thus defined syndromes allow for a precise topographic diagnosis as regards their level and side. Most signs and symptoms of central vestibular disorders resolve spontaneously within weeks to months owing to either recovery of the lesion or central compensation and substitution. The predominantly benign course of these syndromes may be facilitated by physical and drug therapy.

ACKNOWLEDGMENT

The authors wish to thank Ms. J. Benson for copyediting the manuscript.

REFERENCES

1. Brandt, Th: Vertigo, Its Multisensory Syndromes, ed 2. Springer-Verlag, London, 1999.
2. Brandt, Th: Man in motion. Historical and clinical aspects of vestibular function. Brain 114:2159, 1991.
3. Brandt, T, and Dieterich, M: Vestibular syndromes in the roll plane: topographic diagnosis from brainstem to cortex. Ann Neurol 36:337, 1994.
4. Brandt, T, and Dieterich, M: Central vestibular syndromes in the roll, pitch, and yaw planes: Topographic diagnosis of brainstem disorders. Neuro-ophthalmology 15:291, 1995.
5. Guldin, W, and Grüsser, O-J: The anatomy of the vestibular cortices of primates. In Collard M, et al (eds): Le Cortex Vestibulaire. Ipsen, Boulogne, 1996, p 17.
6. Angelaki, DE, et al: Two-dimensional spatio-temporal coding of linear acceleration in vestibular nuclei neurons. J Neurosci 13:1403, 1993.
7. Baker, R, et al: Synaptic connections to trochlear motoneurons determined by individual vestibular nerve branch stimulation in the cat. Brain Res 64:402, 1973.
8. Schwindt, PC, et al: Short latency utricular and canal input to ipsilateral abducens motoneurons. Brain Res 60:259, 1973.
9. Dieterich, M, and Brandt, Th: Ocular torsion and tilt of subjective visual vertical are sensitive brainstem signs. Ann Neurol 33:292, 1993.
10. Dieterich, M, and Brandt, Th: Ocular torsion and perceived vertical in oculomotor, trochlear and abducens nerve palsies. Brain 116:1095, 1993.
11. Halmagyi, GM, et al: Tonic contraversive ocular tilt reaction due to unilateral meso-diencephalic lesion. Neurology 40:1503, 1990.
12. Lueck, CJ, et al: A case of ocular tilt reaction and torsional nystagmus due to direct stimulation of the midbrain in man. Brain 114:2069, 1991.
13. Rabinovitch, HE, et al: The ocular tilt reaction. A paroxysmal dyskinesia associated with elliptical nystagmus. Arch Ophthalmol 95:1395, 1977.

14. Hedges, TR, and Hoyt, WF: Ocular tilt reaction due to an upper brainstem lesion: Paroxysmal skew deviation, torsion, and oscillation of the eyes with head tilt. Ann Neurol 11:537, 1982.
15. Brandt, T, and Dieterich, M: Two types of ocular tilt reaction: the "ascending" pontomedullary VOR-OTR and the "descending" mesencephalic integrator-OTR. Neuro-ophthalmology 19:83, 1998.
16. Brandt, Th, and Dieterich, M: Pathological eye-head coordination in roll: Tonic ocular tilt reaction in mesencephalic and medullary lesions. Brain 110:649, 1987.
17. Dieterich, M, and Brandt, Th: Thalamic infarctions: Differential effects on vestibular function in the roll plane (35 patients). Neurology 43:1732, 1993.
18. Masdeu, JC, and Gorelick, PB: Thalamic astasia: Inability to stand after unilateral thalamic lesions. Ann Neurol 23:596, 1988.
19. Verma, AK, and Maheshwari, MC: Hyperesthetic-ataxic-hemiparesis in thalamic hemorrhage. Stroke 17:49, 1986.
20. Masdeu, JC, et al: Astasia and gait failure with damage of the pontomesencephalic locomotor region. Ann Neurol 35:619, 1994.
21. Brandt, Th, et al: Vestibular cortex lesions affect perception of verticality. Ann Neurol 35:528, 1994.
22. Grüsser, O-J, et al: Localization and responses of neurons in the parieto-insular vestibular cortex of awake monkeys (Macaca fascicularis). J Physiol 430:537, 1990.
23. Grüsser, O-J, et al: Vestibular neurons in the parieto-insular cortex of monkeys (Macaca fascicularis): Visual and neck receptor responses. J Physiol 430:559, 1990.
24. Merfeld, DM, et al: The dynamic contributions of the otolith organs to human ocular torsion. Exp Brain Res 110:315, 1996.
25. Brandt, Th, and Dieterich, M: Central vestibular disorders in roll, pitch and yaw planes: Topographic diagnosis of brainstem disorders. Neuro-ophthalmology 15:291, 1995.
26. Morrow, MJ, and Sharpe, A: Torsional nystagmus in the lateral medullary syndrome. Ann Neurol 24:390, 1988.
27. Lopez, L, et al: Torsional nystagmus: A neuro-otological and MRI study of 35 cases. Brain 115:1107, 1992.
28. Lawden, MC, et al: Repetitive paroxysmal nystagmus and vertigo. Neurology 45:276, 1995.
29. Büttner, U, et al: The localizing value of nystagmus in brainstem disorders. Neuro-ophthalmol 15:283, 1995.
30. Dehaene, I, et al: Unilateral internuclear ophthalmoplegia and ipsiversive torsional nystagmus. J Neurol 243:461, 1996.
31. Noseworthy, JH, et al: Torsional nystagmus: Quantitative features and possible pathogenesis. Neurology 38:992, 1988.
32. Helmchen, C, et al: Contralesionally beating torsional nystagmus in a unilateral rostral midbrain lesion. Neurology 47:482, 1996.
33. Henn, V: Pathophysiology of rapid eye movements in the horizontal, vertical and torsional directions. In Büttner, U, and Brandt, Th (eds): Ocular Motor Disorders of the Brain Stem. Baillière Tindall, London, 1992, p 373.
34. Halmagyi, GM, et al: Jerk-waveform see-saw nystagmus due to unilateral meso-diencephalic lesion. Brain 117:789, 1994.
35. Cogan, DG: Downbeat nystagmus. Arch Ophthalmol 80:757, 1968.
36. Abel, LA, et al: Variable waveforms in downbeat nystagmus imply short-term gain changes. Ann Neurol 13:616, 1983.
37. Lavin, PJM, et al: Downbeat nystagmus with a pseudocycloid waveform: Improvement with base-out prisms. Ann Neurol 13:621, 1983.
38. Yee, RD, et al: Episodic vertical oscillopsia and downbeat nystagmus in a Chiari malformation. Arch Ophthalmol 102:723, 1983.
39. Baloh, RW, and Spooner, JW: Downbeat nystagmus: A type of central vestibular nystagmus. Neurology 31:304, 1981.
40. Cox, TA, et al: Upbeat nystagmus changing to downbeat nystagmus with convergence. Neurology 31:891, 1981.
41. Crevits, L, and Reynaert, C: Posture dependent direction reversal of spontaneous vertical nystagmus. Neuro-ophthalmology 11:285, 1991.
42. Rousseaux, M, et al: Upbeat and downbeat nystagmus occurring successively in a patient with posterior medullary hemorrhage. J Neurol Neurosurg Psychiatr 54:367, 1991.
43. Sakuma, A, et al: Primary position upbeat nystagmus with special reference to alteration to downbeat nystagmus. Acta Otolaryngol (Stockh) (suppl) 522:43, 1996.
44. Büchele, W, et al: Ataxia and oscillopsia in downbeat nystagmus/vertigo syndrome. Adv Oto-Rhino-Laryngol 30:291, 1983.
45. Brandt, Th, et al: Postural abnormalities in central vestibular brainstem lesions. In Bles, W, and Brandt, Th (eds): Disorders of Posture and Gait. Elsevier, Amsterdam, 1986, p 141.
46. Halmagyi, M, et al: Downbeating nystagmus, a review of 62 cases. Arch Neurol 40:777, 1983.
47. Dichgans, J, et al: Postural sway in normals and atactic patients: Analysis of the stabilizing and destabilizing effects of vision. Aggressologie 17:15, 1976.
48. Costin, JA, et al: Alcoholic downbeat nystagmus. Ann Ophthalmol 12:1127, 1980.

49. Zasorin, NL, and Baloh, RW: Downbeat nystagmus with alcoholic cerebellar degeneration. Arch Neurol 41:1301, 1984.
50. Alpert, JN: Downbeat nystagmus due to anticonvulsant toxicity. Ann Neurol 4:471, 1978.
51. Sullivan Jr, JD, et al: Acute carbamazepine toxicity resulting from overdose. Neurology 31:621, 1981.
52. Wheeler, SD, et al: Drug-induced downbeat nystagmus. Ann Neurol 12:227, 1982.
53. Halmagyi, GM, et al: Lithium-induced downbeat nystagmus. Am J Ophthalmol 107:664, 1989.
54. Coppeto, JR, et al: Downbeat nystagmus: Long-term therapy with moderate-dose lithium carbonate. Arch Neurol 40:754, 1983.
55. Corbett, JJ, et al: Downbeating nystagmus and other ocular motor defects caused by lithium toxicity. Neurology 39:481, 1989.
56. Hwang, TL, et al: Reversible downbeat nystagmus and ataxia in febamate intoxication. Neurology 45:846, 1995.
57. Malm, G, and Lyiug-Tunell, U: Cerebellar dysfunction related to toluene sniffing. Acta Neurol Scand 62:188, 1980.
58. Saul, RF, and Selhorst, JB: Downbeat nystagmus with magnesium depletion. Arch Neurol 38:650, 1981.
59. Mayfrank, L, and Thoden, U: Downbeat nystagmus indicates cerebellar or brainstem lesions in vitamin B_{12} deficiency. J Neurol 233:145, 1986.
60. Bronstein, AM, et al: Down beating nystagmus: Magnetic resonance imaging and neuro-otological findings. J Neurol Sci 81:173, 1987.
61. Baloh, RW, and Yee, RD: Spontaneous vertical nystagmus. Rev Neurol Paris 145:527, 1989.
62. Hammack, H, et al: Paraneoplastic cerebellar degeneration. II. Clinical and immunologic findings in 21 patients with Hodgkin's disease. Neurology 42:1983, 1992.
63. Jacobson, DM, and Corbett, JJ: Downbeat nystagmus associated with dolichoectasia of the vertebrobasilar artery. Arch Neurol 46:1005, 1989.
64. Bertholon, P, et al: Syringomyélobulbie posttraumatique et nystagmus vertical inférieur. Rev Neurol 149:355, 1993.
65. Monteiro, ML, and Sampaio, CM: Lithium-induced downbeat nystagmus in a patient with Arnold-Chiari malformation. Am J Ophthalmol 116:648, 1993.
66. Rosengart, A, et al: Intermittent downbeat nystagmus due to vertebral artery compression. Neurology 43:216, 1993.
67. Chan, T, et al: Intermittent downbeat nystagmus secondary to vermian arachnoid cyst with associated obstructive hydrocephalus. J Clin Neuroophthalmol 11:293, 1991.
68. Bixenman, WW: Congenital hereditary downbeat nystagmus. Can J Ophthalmol 18:344, 1983.
69. Weissman, BM, et al: Downbeat nystagmus in an infant: Spontaneous resolution during infancy. Neuro Ophthalmol 8:317, 1988.
70. Spooner, JW, and Baloh, RW: Arnold-Chiari malformation: Improvement in eye movements after surgical treatment. Brain 104:51, 1981.
71. Pedersen, RA, et al: Intermittent downbeat nystagmus and oscillopsia reversed by suboccipital craniectomy. Neurology 30:1239, 1980.
72. Senelick, RC: Total alleviation of downbeat nystagmus in basilar impression by transoral removal of the odontoid process. J Clin Neuroophthalmol 1:265, 1981.
73. Pinel, JF, et al: Downbeat nystagmus: Case report with magnetic resonance imaging and surgical treatment. Neurosurgery 21:736, 1987.
74. Dieterich, M, et al: The effects of baclofen and cholinergic drugs on upbeat and downbeat nystagmus. J Neurol Neurosurg Psychiatr 54:627, 1991.
75. Halmagyi, GM, et al: Treatment of periodic alternating nystagmus. Ann Neurol 8:609, 1980.
76. Auerbuch-Heller, L, et al: A double-blind controlled study of gabapentin and baclofen as treatment for acquired nystagmus. Ann Neurol 41:818, 1997.
77. Barton, JJ, et al: Muscarinic antagonists in the treatment of acquired pendular and downbeat nystagmus: A double-blind study, randomized trial of three intravenous drugs. Ann Neurol 35:319, 1994.
78. Chambers, BR, et al: Case of downbeat nystagmus influenced by otolith stimulation. Ann Neurol 13:204, 1983.
79. Currie, J, and Matsuo, V: The use of clonazepam in the treatment of nystagmus induced oscillopsia. Ophthalmology 93:924, 1986.
80. Dieterich, M, et al: Direction-specific impairment of motion perception and spatial orientation in downbeat and upbeat nystagmus in humans. Neurosci Lett 245:29, 1998.
81. Tokumasu, K, et al: Upbeat nystagmus in primary eye position. Acta Otolaryngol (Stockh) (suppl) 481:366, 1991.
82. Bender, MB, and Gormen, WF: Vertical nystagmus on direct forward gaze with vertical oscillopsia. Am J Ophthalmol 32:967, 1949.
83. Schmidt, D: Über die Bedeutung der Augensymptome zur Diagnostik der Wernicke Encephalopathie. Klin Mbl Augenheilk 161:36, 1972.
84. Zumstein, HR, and Meienberg, O: Upbeat nystagmus and visual system disorder in Wernicke's encephalopathy due to starvation. Neuro-Ophthalmology 2:157, 1982.

85. Yamazaki, K, et al: A case of Fisher's syndrome with upbeat nystagmus. Rinsho-Shinkeigaku 34:489, 1994.
86. Fujikane, M, et al: Central diabetes insipidus complicated with upbeat nystagmus and cerebellar ataxia. Rinsho-Shinkeigaku 32:68, 1992.
87. Trobe, JD, et al: Nystagmus of Pelizaeus-Merzbacher disease. A magnetic search-coil study. Arch Neurol 48:87, 1991.
88. Gresty, MA, et al: Primary position upbeating nystagmus associated with middle ear disease. Neuro-Ophthalmology 8:321, 1988.
89. Forsythe, WI: Congenital hereditary vertical nystagmus. J Neurol Neurosurg Psychiatr 18:196, 1955.
90. Sogg, RL, and Hoyt, WF: Intermittent vertical nystagmus in a father and son. Arch Ophthalmol 68:515, 1962.
91. Shibasaki, H, et al: Suppression of congenital nystagmus. J Neurol Neurosurg Psychiatr 41:1078, 1978.
92. Hoyt, CS, and Gelbert, SS: Vertical nystagmus in infants with congenital ocular abnormalities. Ophthalm Paediat Genet (Amsterdam) 4:155, 1984.
93. Neveling, R, and Kruse, KE: Über Nicotinnystagmus. Arch Ohr Heilk Z Hals Heilk 177:427, 1961.
94. Sibony, PA, et al: Tobacco-induced primary position upbeat nystagmus. Ann Neurol 21:53, 1987.
95. Sibony, PA, et al: Nicotine and tobacco-induced nystagmus. Ann Neurol 28:198, 1990.
96. Sibony, PA, et al: The effects of tobacco smoking on smooth pursuit eye movements. Ann Neurol 23:238, 1988.
97. Hiel, H, et al: Expression of nicotinic acetylcholine receptor mRNA in the adult rat peripheral vestibular system. Brain Res 738:347, 1996.
98. Phelan, KD, and Gallagher, JP: Direct muscarinic and nicotinic receptor-mediated excitation of rat medial vestibular nucleus neurons in vitro. Synapse 10:349, 1992.
99. Ishiyama, A, et al: Distribution of efferent cholinergic terminals and alpha-bungarotoxin binding to putative nicotinic acetylcholine receptors in the human vestibular end-organs. Laryngoscope 105:1167, 1995.
100. Iwata, A, et al: Primary position upbeat nystagmus reversed with carbamazepine. Eur J Neurol 3:260, 1996.
101. Leigh, RJ, and Brandt, Th: A re-evaluation of the vestibulo-ocular reflex: New ideas of its purpose, properties, neural substrate, and disorders. Neurology 43:1288, 1993.
102. Uemura, T, and Cohen, B: Effects of vestibular nuclei lesions on vestibulo-ocular reflexes and posture in monkeys. Acta Otolaryngol (Stockh) (suppl) 315:1, 1973.
103. Kömpf, D: Der benigne pseudovestibuläre Kleinhirninsult. Nervenarzt 57:163, 1986.
104. Hopf, HC: Vertigo and masseter paresis. A new brainstem syndrome. J Neurol 235:42, 1987.
105. Dieterich, M, and Büchele, W: MRI findings in lesions at the entry zone of the eighth nerve. Acta Otolaryngol (Stockh) (suppl) 468:385, 1989.
106. Disher, MJ, et al: Evaluation of acute vertigo: Unusual lesions imitating vestibular neuritis. Am J Otol 12:227, 1991.
107. Francis, DA, et al: The site of brainstem lesions causing semicircular canal paresis: An MRI study. J Neurol Neurosurg Psychiatr 55:446, 1992.
108. Amarenco, P, et al: Infarctus pontin inférolatéral: deux aspects cliniques. Rev Neurol (Paris) 146:433, 1990.
109. FitzGibbon, EJ, et al: Torsional nystagmus during vertical pursuit. Neuro-ophthalmology 16:79, 1996.
110. Dieterich, M, and Brandt, Th: Wallenberg's syndrome lateropulsion: Lateropulsion, cyclorotation and subjective visual vertical in 36 patients. Ann Neurol 31:399, 1992.
111. Brandt, Th, and Dieterich, M: Vestibular falls. J Vestib Res 3:3, 1993.
112. Schwarz, DWF, and Fredrickson, JM: Rhesus monkey vestibular cortex: A biomodal primary projection field. Science 172:280, 1971.
113. Fredrickson, JM, et al: Vestibular nerve projection to the cerebral cortex of the rhesus monkey. Exp Brain Res 2:318, 1966.
114. Büttner, U, and Buettner, UW: Parietal cortex area 2 V neuronal activity in the alert monkey during natural vestibular and optokinetic stimulation. Brain Res 153:392, 1978.
115. Ödkvist, LM, et al: Projection of the vestibular nerve to the area 3a arm field in the squirrel monkey (Saimiri sciureus). Exp Brain Res 21:97, 1974.
116. Faugier-Grimaud, S, and Ventre, J: Anatomic connections of inferior parietal cortex (area 7) with subcortical structures related to vestibulo-ocular function in a monkey (Macaca fascicularis). J Comp Neurol 280:1, 1989.
117. Abkarian, S, et al: Corticofugal connections between the cerebral cortex and brainstem vestibular nuclei in the macaque monkey. J Comp Neurol 339:421, 1994.
118. Jeannerod, M: Vestibular cortex. A network from directional coding of behavior. In Collard, M, et al (eds): Le Cortex Vestibulaire. Ipsen, Boulogne, 1996, p 5.
119. Bottini, G, et al: Identification of the central vestibular projections in man: A positron emission tomography activation study. Exp Brain Res 99:164, 1994.
120. Dieterich, M, et al: Horizontal or vertical optokinetic stimulation activates visual motion-sensitive, ocu-

lar motor, and vestibular cortex areas with right hemispheric dominance: An fMRI study. Brain 121:1479, 1998.

121. Bucher, SF, et al: Sensorimotor cerebral activation during optokinetic nystagmus: An fMRI study. Neurology 49:1370, 1997.

122. Andersen, RA, and Gnadt, JW: Posterior parietal cortex. In Wurtz, RH, and Goldberg, ME (eds): Reviews in Oculomotor Research. Vol 3, The Neurobiology of Saccadic Eye Movements. Elsevier, Amsterdam, 1989, p 315.

123. Foerster, O: Sensible Kortikale Felder. In Bumke, O, and Foerster, O (eds): Handbuch der Neurologie, Vol VI. Springer, Berlin, 1936, p 358.

124. Penfield, W, and Jasper, H: Epilepsy and the functional anatomy of the human brain. Little Brown, Boston, 1954.

125. Andersen, RA, et al: Encoding of spatial location by posterior parietal neurons. Science 230:456, 1985.

126. Galletti, C, et al: Parietal neurons encoding spatial orientations in craniotopic coordinates. Exp Brain Res 96:221, 1993.

127. Karnath, H-O: Subjective body orientation in neglect and the interactive contribution of neck muscle proprioception and vestibular stimulation. Brain 117:1001, 1994.

128. Karnath, H-O, et al: Trunk orientation as the determining factor of the "contralateral" deficit in the neglect syndrome and as the physical anchor of the internal representation of body orientation in space. Brain 114:1997, 1991.

129. Karnath, H-O, et al: Decrease of contralateral neglect by neck muscle vibration and spatial orientation of trunk midline. Brain 116:383, 1993.

130. Watt, DGD: Pointing at memorized targets during prolonged microgravity. Aviat Space Environ Med 68:99, 1997.

131. Vallar, G, and Perani, D: The anatomy of unilateral neglect after right hemisphere stroke lesions: A clinical CT correlation study in man. Neuropsychologia 24:609, 1986.

132. Husain, M, and Kennard, C: Visual neglect associated with frontal lobe infarction. J Neurol 243:652, 1996.

133. Vuilleumier, P, et al: Unilateral spatial neglect recovery after sequential strokes. Neurology 19:184, 1996.

134. Rapcsak, SZ, et al: Altitudinal neglect. Neurology 38:277, 1988.

135. Shelton, PA, et al: Peripersonal and vertical neglect. Brain 113:191, 1990.

136. Mesulam, M-M: A cortical network for directed attention and unilateral neglect. Ann Neurol 10:309, 1981.

137. Cappa, S, et al: Remission of hemineglect and anosognosia during vestibular stimulation. Neuropsychologia 25:775, 1987.

138. Vallar, G, et al: Exploring somatosensory hemineglect by vestibular stimulation. Brain 116:71, 1993.

139. Robertson, IH, et al: Walking trajectory and hand movements in unilateral left neglect: A vestibular hypothesis. Neuropsychologia 32:1495, 1994.

140. Vallar, G, et al: Spatial hemineglect in back space. Brain 118:467, 1995.

141. Nobre, AC, et al: Functional localization of the system for visuospatial attention using positron emission tomography. Brain 120:515, 1997.

142. Gerstmann, J: Über eine eigenartige Orientierungsströrung im Raum bei zerebraler Erkrankung. Wien medizin Wochenschr 76:817, 1926.

143. Halpern, F: Kasuistischer Beitrag zur Frage des Verkehrtsehens. Z gesamt Neurol Psychiatr 126:246, 1930.

144. Klopp, H: Über Umgekehrt- und Verkehrtsehen. Deutsch Zeitschr Nervenheilk 165:231, 1951.

145. Solms, M, et al: Inverted vision after frontal lobe disease. Cortex 24:499, 1988.

146. Tiliket, C, et al: Room tilt illusion. A central otolith dysfunction. Arch Neurol 53:1259, 1996.

147. Glasauer, S, and Mittelstaedt, H: Determinants of orientation in microgravity. Acta Astronautica 27:1, 1992.

148. Brandt, Th: The cortical matching of visual and vestibular 3-D coordinate maps. Ann Neurol 42:983, 1997.

149. Kohler, I: Die Methode des Brillenversuches in der Wahrnehmungspsychologie mit Bemerkungen zur Lehre der Adaptation. Z Exp Angew Psychol 3:381, 1956.

150. Schneider, RC, et al: Vertigo and rotational movement in cortical and subcortical lesions. J Neurol Sci 6:493, 1968.

151. Smith, BH: Vestibular disturbance in epilepsy. Neurology 10:465, 1960.

152. Brandt, Th, et al: Rotational vertigo in embolic stroke of the vestibular and auditory cortices. Neurology 45:42, 1995.

153. Hawrylyshyn, PA, et al: Vestibulothalamic projections in man—A sixth primary sensory pathway. J Neurophysiol 41:394, 1978.

154. Jackson, H: Diagnosis of epilepsy. Med Times Gazette 1:29, 1879.

155. Gowers, WR: The Borderlands of Epilepsy. Churchill, London, 1907.

156. Bumke, O, and Foerster, O (eds): Handbuch der Neurologie, Vol VI. Springer, Berlin, 1936.

157. Penfield, WG, and Kristiansen, K: Epileptic Seizure Patterns. Thomas, Springfield, 1951.

158. Karbowski, K: Schwindel und Epilepsie. Therapeut Umschau 41:705, 1984.

159. Riser, M, et al: A propos de 14 cas d'epilepsie giratoire. Rev Neurol 85:245, 1951.
160. Pedersen, E, and Jepson, O: Epileptic vertigo. Acta Psychiatr Neurol Scand (suppl) 108:301, 1956.
161. Hughes, MR, and Drachman, DA: Dizziness, epilepsy and EEG. J Nerve Ment Dis 38:431, 1977.
162. Kogeorgos, J, et al: Epileptic dizziness. Brit Med J 282:687, 1981.
163. Fried, I, et al: The anatomy of epileptic auras: Focal pathology and surgical outcome. J Neurosurg 83:60, 1995.
164. Kaplan, PW, and Tusa, RJ: Neurophysiologic and clinical correlations of epileptic nystagmus. Neurology 43:2508, 1993.
165. Schmidt, D, and Shorvon, S: The epilepsies. In Brandt, Th, et al (eds): Neurological Disorders: Course and Treatment. Academic, San Diego, 1996, p 159.
166. Noachtar, S, et al: Surgical therapy of epilepsy. In Brandt, Th, et al (eds): Neurological Disorders: Course and Treatment. Academic, San Diego, 1996, p 183.
167. Brandt, Th, and Dieterich, M: Vestibular paroxysmia (Disabling positional vertigo). Neuro-ophthalmology 14:359, 1994.
168. Andermann, F, et al: Paroxysmal dysarthria and ataxia in multiple sclerosis. Neurology (Minneap) 9:211, 1959.
169. Dogulu, CF, and Kansu, T: Upside-down reversal of vision in multiple sclerosis. J Neurol 244:461, 1997.
170. Espir, MLE, and Millac, P: Treatment of paroxysmal disorders in multiple sclerosis with carbamazepine (Tegretol). J Neurol Neurosurg Psychiatr 33:528, 1970.
171. Osterman, PO, and Westerberg, CE: Paroxysmal attacks in multiple sclerosis. Brain 98:189, 1975.
172. Griggs, RC, and Nutt, JG: Episodic ataxias as channelopathies. Ann Neurol 37:285, 1995.
173. Brandt, Th, and Strupp, M: Familial episodic ataxias. EA-1 and EA-2. Audiol Neurootol 2:273, 1997.
174. Büttner, U, et al: Paroxysmal spontaneous nystagmus and vertigo evoked by lateral eye position. Neurology 37:1553, 1987.
175. Sharpe, JA, et al: Convergence-evoked nystagmus. Congenital and acquired forms. Arch Neurol 32:191, 1975.
176. Oliva, A, and Rosenberg, ML: Convergence-evoked nystagmus. Neurology 40:161, 1990.
177. Thurston, STE, et al: Epileptic gaze deviation and nystagmus. Neurology 35:1518, 1985.
178. Hassler, R: Thalamic regulation of muscle tone and the speed of movement. In Purpura, DP, and Yahr, MD (eds): The Thalamus. Columbia Univ. Pr., New York, 1966, p 419.
179. Zoll, JG: Transient anosognosia associated with thalamotomy: Is it caused by proprioceptive loss? Confin Neurol 31:48, 1969.
180. Velasco, F, and Velasco, M: A reticulothalamic system mediating proprioceptive attention and tremor in man. Neurosurgery 4:30, 1979.
181. Cambier, J, et al: Lésions du thalamus droit avec syndrome de l'hemisphere mineur. Discussion du concept de négligence thalamique. Rev Neurol (Paris) 136:105, 1980.
182. Jenkyn, LR, et al: Language dysfunction, somesthetic hemi-inattention, and thalamic hemorrhage in the dominant hemisphere. Neurology 31:1202, 1981.
183. Solomon, DH, et al: The thalamic ataxia syndrome. Neurology 44:810, 1994.
184. Melo, TP, et al: Thalamic ataxia. J Neurol 239:331, 1992.
185. Friedmann, G: The judgement of the visual vertical and horizontal with peripheral and central vestibular lesions. Brain 93:313, 1970.
186. Sheldon, JH: The social medicine of old age: Report of an enquiry in Wolverhampton. Oxford Univ. Pr., London, 1948.
187. Sheldon, JH: On the natural history of falls in old age. Br Med J Clin Res 2:1685, 1960.
188. Meissner, I, et al: The natural history of drop attacks. Neurology 36:1029, 1986.
189. Fariello, RG, et al: Hyperekplexia exacerbated by occlusion of posterior thalamic arteries. Arch Neurol 40:244, 1983.

CHAPTER 13

Diagnosis and Management of Neuro-Otological Disorders Due to Migraine

Ronald J. Tusa, MD, PhD

Migraine is a common cause of episodic vertigo and dysequilibrium in children and adults. In practices treating patients with headaches, 27 to 33 percent of patients out of a population of 700 patients with migraine report episodic vertigo.[1,2] Thirty-six percent of these patients experience vertigo during their headache-free period; the others experience vertigo either just before or during a headache. The occurrence of vertigo during the headache period is much higher in patients with migraine headaches with aura (classic migraine) as opposed to migraine without aura (common migraine) (Kuritzky et al, 1981). In this chapter, the incidence of migraine, current classification and criteria used for diagnosing migraine, neuro-otological syndromes, and genetics related to migraine, and the management of migraine will be described.

INCIDENCE

Migraine is an extremely prevalent disorder. An epidemiologic study involving over 20,000 individuals between 12 and 80 years of age found that 17.6 percent of all adult females, 5.7 percent of all adult males, and 4 percent of all children had one or more migraine headaches per year.[3] This study used the diagnostic criteria recommended by the International Headache Society[4] (IHS), which will be described later. Of those individuals with migraine, approximately 18 percent experienced one or more attacks per month. In both males and females, the prevalence of migraine was highest between the ages of 35 and 45 years. The type and severity of migraine often varies within the same individual. Migraine with or without aura frequently begins between

12 and 30 years of age. After the age of 50, migraine is much less common, and it frequently presents as migraine aura without headache.[5]

CLASSIFICATION AND CRITERIA FOR DIAGNOSIS

Migraine disorders are usually subdivided into several types. To help standardize terminology and diagnostic criteria, a classification system for headaches was developed by the IHS.[4] This classification was based on 2 years of discussion among 100 individuals with representatives from seven countries. The classification and criteria for headaches pertinent to neuro-otological disorders is summarized in Box 13–1. The general features of the relevant types of migraine are discussed briefly; the features of specific neurotological disorders are discussed in greater detail.

BOX 13–1   IHS Classification of Headache

1.1   Migraine without aura (replaces common migraine).
  A. At least 5 attacks fulfilling criteria B–D.
  B. Headache attacks lasting 4 to 72 hours untreated. In children <15 years, attack may last 2 to 48 hours.
  C. Headache has at least two of the following characteristics:
    1. Unilateral location.
    2. Pulsating quality.
    3. Moderate or severe intensity that inhibits or prohibits daily activities.
    4. Aggravation by walking stairs or similar routine physical activity.
  D. During headache at least one of the following:
    1. Nausea and/or vomiting.
    2. Photophobia and phonophobia.
  E. At least one of the following.
    1. History and physical examinations do not suggest another disorder.
    2. History and physical examinations do suggest such disorder, but it is ruled out by appropriate investigations (e.g., MRI or CT scan of the head).

1.2   Migraine with aura (replaces classic migraine).
  A. At least 2 attacks fulfilling B:
  B. At least 3 of the following:
    1. One or more reversible aura symptoms indicating focal CNS dysfunction.
    2. At least one aura symptom develops gradually over more than 4 minutes, or 2 or more symptoms occur in succession.
    3. No aura symptom lasts more than 60 minutes unless more than one aura symptom is present.
    4. Headache occurs either before, during, or up to 60 minutes after aura is completed.
  C. Same as E above in criteria 1.1.

1.2.2   Migraine with prolonged aura (replaces complicated migraine).
  Fulfills criteria for 1.2, but at least one symptom lasts more than 60 minutes and less than 7 days.

(Continued)

BOX 13–1   *(Continued)*

1.2.4 Basilar migraine (replaces basilar artery migraine).

Fulfills criteria for 1.2, but two or more aura symptoms of the following types: Vertigo, tinnitus, decreased hearing, ataxia, visual symptoms in both hemifields of both eyes, dysarthria, double vision, bilateral paresthesia, bilateral paresis, decreased level of consciousness.

1.2.5 Migraine aura without headache (replaces migraine equivalent or acephalgic migraine). Fulfills criteria for 1.2 but no headache.

1.5   Childhood periodic syndromes that may be precursors to or associated with migraine.

1.5.1 Benign paroxysmal vertigo of childhood.
   A. Brief, sporadic episodes of disequilibrium, anxiety, and often nystagmus or vomiting.
   B. Normal neurological examination.
   C. Normal electroencephalogram.

1.6.2 Migrainous infarction (replaces complicated migraine).
   A. Patient has previously fulfilled criteria for 1.2.
   B. The present attack is typical of previous attacks, but neurological deficits are not completely reversible within 7 days and/or neuroimaging demonstrates ischemic infarction in relevant area.
   C. Other causes of infarction ruled out by appropriate investigations.

Adapted from Headache Classification Committee of the International Headache Society.[4]

Migraine without Aura

Migraine without aura, which replaces "common migraine," consists of periodic headaches that are usually throbbing and unilateral, exacerbated by activity, and associated with nausea, photophobia, and phonophobia. These headaches are frequently referred to as "sick" headaches (because of the nausea) or "sinus" headaches (because of their location). Patients usually prefer to lie down in a quiet, dark room during the headache and feel better after sleep. A family history for migraine can usually be obtained in the immediate family.

Migraine with Aura

Migraine with aura, which replaces "classic migraine," is associated with transient neurological symptoms consisting of sensory, motor, or cognitive disorders. These neurological disorders usually precede the headache, but may develop during or following the headache. The neurological disorder usually lasts 5 to 20 minutes, but can last as long as 1 hour. There are three relevant subtypes. The first is *migraine with prolonged aura,* in which neurological symptoms can last up to 7 days. The second is called *basilar migraine,* which replaces "basilar artery migraine," and presents with symptoms in the distribution of the basilar artery including vertigo, tinnitus, decreased hearing, and ataxia. The third is called *migraine aura without headache,* which replaces "migraine-equivalent spells" or "acephalgic migraine." This presents with the neurological disorders found in migraine with aura except there is no headache.

Childhood Periodic Syndromes

Childhood periodic syndromes may be precursors of or associated with migraine. The most important subtype is *benign paroxysmal vertigo of childhood,* which consists of spells of dysequilibrium and vertigo in children. These may or may not be associated with headache.

Migrainous Infarction

Migrainous infarction, which replaces "complicated migraine," is a migraine with aura associated with an infarct. The infarct can either be documented by neuroimaging or by an aura that does not resolve within 7 days.

The IHS classification was a mammoth undertaking, although it is still considered preliminary and subject to revision. The classification was primarily developed for research purposes and, therefore, diagnostic criteria were made very specific. Some members on the committee disagree with some of the criteria, such as excluding the bilateral nature of pain in some individuals with migraine.[6] A second edition to the classification has yet to be published.

NEURO-OTOLOGICAL SYNDROMES

A number of different neuro-otological syndromes have been described with migraine (Box 13–2). These disorders can be divided into those that are due to migraine and those that are associated with migraine.

BOX 13–2   Neuro-otological Disorders

Neuro-otological disorders due to migraine
1. Paroxysmal torticollis of infancy
2. Benign paroxysmal vertigo of childhood
3. Basilar migraine
4. Benign recurrent vertigo of adults
5. Migrainous infarct resulting in vertigo

Neuro-otological disorders associated with migraine
1. Motion sickness
2. Meniere's Disease
3. Benign paroxysmal positional vertigo

Disorders Due to Migraine

CHILDHOOD PERIODIC SYNDROMES

There are two neuro-otological disorders in children due to migraine. (1) *Benign paroxysmal vertigo of childhood* (IHS classification 1.5.1), which was first described by Basser.[7] This disorder consists of spells of vertigo and dysequilibrium without hearing loss or tinnitus.[8–12] The majority occurs between 1 and 4 years of age, but can occur anytime during the first decade. Vertigo and dysequilibrium typically last for minutes, but can last up to several hours. Patients may experience visual disturbance, flushing, nausea, and vomiting. In the majority cases, audiograms and caloric tests are normal. These patients also have normal physical examinations and normal EEGs. Initially, headache is usually not a major feature of these spells. Many of these patients eventually develop migraine with aura and there is frequently a positive family history for migraine. The differential diagnosis includes Ménière's disease, vestibular epilepsy, perilymphatic fistula, posterior fossa tumors, and psychogenic disorders. (2) *Paroxysmal torticollis of infancy* was not specifically classified by the IHS, but may fit into the same classification as benign paroxysmal vertigo of childhood; these disorders frequently occur in the same patient.[11] This disorder was first described by Snyder,[13] and has now been reported by a number of individuals.[14–16] Paroxysmal torticollis of infancy consists of spells of head tilt and rotation without vertigo, hearing loss, or tinnitus. These usually occur in the first 5 years of life and typically last between 10 minutes and several days. They may be associated with nausea, vomiting, pallor, agitation, and ataxia. In the majority of cases, audiograms and caloric tests are normal between the spells. This syndrome is believed to be due to migraine auras without headache. Some individuals complain of headache when they become older. The differential diagnosis includes posterior fossa tumors and torticollis.

BASILAR MIGRAINE

Basilar migraine (IHS classification 1.2.4) was first described by Bickerstaff,[17] and has been subsequently reported by a number of individuals.[18,19] This disorder consists of two or more neurological problems (vertigo, tinnitus, decreased hearing, ataxia, dysarthria, visual symptoms in both hemifields of both eyes, diplopia, bilateral paresthesia or paresis, decreased level of consciousness) followed by a throbbing headache. The majority of these occurs before 20 years of age, but can occur up until age 60. Vertigo typically lasts between 5 minutes and 1 hour. In the majority of cases, audiograms are normal. Many of these patients eventually develop more typical migraine headaches with aura, and there is frequently a positive family history for migraine. Transient ischemic attacks (TIAs) need to be considered before basilar migraine is diagnosed. TIAs within the vertebral-basilar circulatory system (vertebrobasilar insufficiency) may cause the same symptoms as basilar migraine, although TIAs usually last less than a few minutes.[20]

BENIGN RECURRENT VERTIGO IN ADULTS

This disorder was not formally classified by the IHS. Based on the symptoms, it may either be referred to as basilar migraine (1.2.4), or migraine aura without headache (1.2.5). This was first described by Slater,[21] and is the most common neurotological syndrome caused by migraine. This disorder consists of spells of vertigo, occasionally with tinnitus but without hearing loss.[22,23] In some individuals, jerk nystagmus may occur during the spell (see Case Study 1). Vertigo typically lasts between minutes and hours; the majority last less than 1 hour, and may occur with or without headache. The spells usually occur between the ages of 20 and 60. Peripheral and central vestibular deficits diagnosed by caloric and spontaneous eye movements during electronystagmography have been reported to occur in 5 to 80 percent of individuals with migraine in their headache-free period.[24a,b,25] This variation in abnormality may be due to a difference in criteria used for diagnosing vestibular deficits.[24] In the majority of cases, audiograms and caloric studies are normal. In this author's opinion, concomitant Ménière's disease was not always excluded in all cases. Therefore, it is not clear that permanent vestibular deficits can occur in migraine disease. Some individuals develop exercise-induced spells from a variety of physical activity including sit-ups, heavy lifting, intercourse, and strenuous aerobic exercises[26] (see Case Study 2). One needs to rule out Ménière's disease, benign paroxysmal positional vertigo, TIAs, vestibular epilepsy, and perilymphatic fistula before making a diagnosis of migraine-induced vertigo.

MIGRAINOUS INFARCTION

Migrainous infarction (IHS classification 1.6.2) is a migraine with aura associated with an infarct.[27–29] These strokes can be very focal, such as a small retinal stroke or infarct within portions of the optic nerve.[30,31] Whether similar focal infarcts can involve the labyrinth and eighth nerve is unclear. Sudden hearing loss owing to migrainous infarction of the labyrinth is quite rare.[32] Hearing loss, ear fullness, vertigo, and dysequilibrium due to a migrainous infarct in the territory of the anterior-inferior cerebellar artery also has been described,[33] as have vertigo and dysequilibrium due to migrainous infarct in the dorsal lateral medulla.[34]

Disorders Associated with Migraine

MOTION SICKNESS

Episodic dizziness, tiredness, pallor, diaphoresis, salivation, nausea and occasional vomiting induced by passive locomotion (e.g., riding in a car) or motion of the visual surround while standing still (e.g., viewing a rotating optokinetic stimulus or large screen motion picture) characterize motion sickness. Motion sickness is partially due to a visual-vestibular conflict or mismatch.[35] Twenty-six to sixty percent of patients with migraine have a history of severe motion sickness compared to 8 to 24 percent of the normal population.[1,36,37] The cause for this relation is not clear.

MÉNIÈRE'S DISEASE

There is a great deal of confusion between migraine aura without headache and vestibular hydrops (vestibular Ménière's disease).[38,39] Both can present with transient vertigo, ear fullness, or occasional tinnitus, but without any decrease in hearing. A history of headaches associated with the spells of vertigo may help to distinguish these two syndromes, but occasionally the diagnosis is only made following the patient's response to a therapeutic trial (see Case Study 3). Patients with well-documented Ménière's disease may later develop migraine aura without headache. Therefore, they may initially do well with treatment for Ménière's disease and then appear to fail to respond to treatment when in fact they have developed spells of vertigo due to migraine aura without headache (see Case Study 4). Kayan and Hood[1] and Hinchcliffe[40] noted a higher than expected incidence of both migraine and Ménière's disease in the same individual. Whether there is a causal link between these two disorders is unclear.

BENIGN PAROXYSMAL POSITIONAL VERTIGO

Benign paroxysmal positional vertigo (BPPV) and migraine in the same individual are reported frequently[1,41]; however the causal relationship remains obscure. We have occasionally seen patients who had a normal examination, but then developed BPPV following a migraine headache (see Case Study 5). This has also been reported to occur in children (8 to 12 years of age) following migraine.[42] This report was remarkable; BPPV is very rare in children and their cases were within one family. Whether BPPV following migraine is due to migrainous infarction in the distribution of the superior vestibular artery is still unclear.

PATHOPHYSIOLOGY

Neurochemical Mechanism

According to the neurogenic hypothesis, the aura of migraine is due to an area of neuronal dysfunction similar to a wave of spreading depression.[43] This neuronal dysfunction may be mediated by neurons containing serotonin (5-HT) within the trigeminal nucleus.[44] 5-HT is an intracranial vasoconstrictor; it rises during the migraine aura and falls during the headache. Platelet 5-HT levels drop rapidly during the onset of migraine. Through autoregulation, blood flow is reduced to this area of neuronal dysfunction. Thus, according to this hypothesis, the vascular changes of migraine are epiphenomena secondary to an underlying neurogenic mechanism. Dopamine receptors may also play a role in certain symptoms of migraine including yawning, drowsiness, irritability, nausea, vomiting, gastric paresis, and hypotension.[45]

Based on this hypothesis, treatment of migraine includes elimination of tyramine from the diet and the use of drugs that change vascular tone or alter serotonin and prostaglandin. There are a number of serotonin receptors, but 5-HT_1 may be the most involved. Agonists of these receptors block neuropeptide release and alter neurotransmission in trigeminovascular neurons.[46] These agonists are the most effective drugs in aborting migraine.

Genetics

The discovery of the genetic cause of certain types of migraine is one of the most promising breakthroughs in understanding and potentially treating this disorder. Familial hemiplegic migraine is an autosomal dominant disorder. In 50 percent of all families, this disorder is mapped to chromosome 19p13 in the gene called the CACNA1A (formerly called CACNL1A4[47]). This gene codes for a subunit of the P/Q

TABLE 13–1 CACNA1A Gene Defects that Cause AD Disorders

Gene Defect	Syndrome	Symptoms and Signs
Point mutation	Familial hemiplegic migraine	Episodic hemiparesis for up to 60 minutes followed by headache. GEN and DBN may persist after spells.
Point mutation	Episodic ataxia-2	Episodic ataxia and vertigo, GEN, DBN, decreased VOR cancel, decreased pursuit, normal VOR
CAG repeats	SCA 6	Progressive ataxia, GEN, DBN, decreased VOR cancel, decreased pursuit, normal VOR

Abbreviations: DBN, downbeat nystagmus; GEN, gaze-evoked nystagmus; VOR, vestibulo-ocular reflex.

voltage-gated neuronal calcium channel.[48] This same chromosome locus may be involved also in other forms of migraine aura.[49] Defects involving this gene are involved with other autosomal dominant disorders that have neurotologic symptoms (Table 13–1). The symptoms of these disorders overlap extensively.[50] Only 50 percent of families with familial hemiplegic migraine map to chromosome 19p13. Other families with this disorder map to chromosome 1 (1q21-q21).[51] Other chromosome defects are likely to be found in the future.

MANAGEMENT

Vertigo and dysequilibrium secondary to migraine usually respond to the same type of treatment as that used for migraine headaches. Migraine is triggered by a number of factors including stress, anxiety, hypoglycemia, fluctuating estrogen, certain foods, and smoking.[51–53] Treatment of migraine can be divided into (1) the reduction of risk factors, (2) abortive medical therapy, and (3) prophylactic medical therapy.

Reduction of Risk Factors

In my practice, all patients with migraine are given a management schedule to follow, which is explained at the time of their first visit (Box 13–3). I point out that there are several triggers for migraine, which are avoided by following the schedule.

STRESS

All patients are started on an aerobic exercise program to help reduce stress. This program is gradually increased until the individual is exercising 3 to 5 times per week for at least 30 minutes at the end of the day (jogging, swimming, fast walk, racquetball, tennis, etc). Several good aerobic exercise programs can be found in a paperback book by Cooper.[54] If patients are reluctant or unable to participate in an exercise program, other stress reduction programs can be very helpful. These include biofeedback and relaxation programs, which have been shown to significantly reduce the frequency of recurrent migraine disorders in clinical trials.[54a,b] Patients are urged to avoid hypoglycemia by eating something at least every 8 hours. Many individuals skip breakfast; the need to eat breakfast at the same time each morning, including weekends, is empha-

---

BOX 13–3   Schedule to Treat Migraine Disorders

1. Reduction of Stress
   a. Aerobic exercise at end of day (3 to 4 times/week). Get heart rate above 100 and sustain it for at least 20 minutes.
   b. Eat something at least every 8 hours to avoid hypoglycemia. Eat breakfast at same time each morning (breakfast on weekends should be at the same time as on weekdays).
   c. maintain a regular sleep schedule.
2. Do not smoke or chew any products that contain nicotine.
3. Avoid exogenous estrogen (oral contraceptives, estrogen replacement).
4. Follow diet.
5. Keep a diary.
   a. Note time and date of all headaches and/or spells that interfere with daily routine.
   b. Write down any foods that you had that are listed on the other side of this sheet during the 24 hours prior to the headache and/or spell.
   c. Bring diary in with you on your next visit!
6. Medications

---

sized. Finally, maintenance of a regular sleep schedule (going to bed and getting up at the same time each day) is strongly recommended.

NICOTINE

Patients who smoke cigarettes are urged to stop smoking.

ESTROGEN

If patients are taking estrogen supplements (other than vaginal creams), work with their gynecologist to either eliminate the supplement or reduce the estrogen to the lowest level possible for a 3-month trial.

DIET

All patients are placed on a diet schedule, which is given to them in written form (Table 13–2). This diet eliminates foods containing high levels of tyramine and other substances known to exacerbate migraine.[52a,b,55] Some of these foods cause migraine almost immediately (red wine, MSG); most cause migraine the next day (chocolate, nuts, cheese). Aspartame, found in Nutrasweet, can also provoke migraine.[56]

DIARY

Finally, all patients are asked to keep a careful diary, noting the time and date of all spells or headaches that interrupt their daily activities. They are asked to write down any foods from the list of "foods to avoid" (see Table 13–2) that they had during 24 hours prior to the headache or spell. This forces the individual to become more aware of the association of diet with migraine and potentially identifies certain foods they should avoid.

TABLE 13-2 Diet for Migraine Patients

	Foods Allowed	Foods to Avoid
Beverages	Decaffeinated coffee, fruit juice, club soda, noncola soda. Limit caffeine sources to 2 cups/d (coffee, tea, cola).	Chocolate, cocoa, certain alcoholic beverages (red wine, port, sherry, scotch, bourbon, gin). Excessive Nutrasweet (no more than 24 oz/d of diet drink).
Meats, fish, and poultry	Fresh or frozen turkey, chicken, fish, beef, lamb, veal, pork. Limit eggs to 3/week. Tuna or tuna salad.	Aged, canned, cured, or processed meats including ham or game, pickled herring, salad and dried fish; chicken liver, bologna; fermented sausage; any food prepared with meat tenderizer, soy sauce, or brewer's yeast; any food containing nitrates or tyramine (smoked meats including bacon, sausage, ham, salami, pepperoni, hot dogs).
Dairy products	Milk: Homogenized, 2% or skim. Cheese: American, cottage, farmer, ricotta, cream, Canadian, processed cheese slice. Yogurt (limit 1/2 cup/d)	Buttermilk, sour cream, chocolate milk. Cheese: Stilton, bleu, cheddar, mozzarella, cheese spread, Roquefort, provolone, gruyere, muenster, feta, parmesan, emmenthal, brie, brick,. camembert types, cheddar, gouda, romano
Breads, cereals	Commercial bread, English muffins, melba toast crackers, bagels. All hot and dry cereals.	Hot fresh homemade yeast bread, bread or crackers containing cheese. Fresh yeast coffee cake, doughnuts, sourdough bread. Any product containing chocolate or nuts.
Potato or substitute	White potato, sweet potato, rice, macaroni, spaghetti, noodles.	None.
Vegetables	Any except those to avoid.	Beans such as pole, broad, lima, Italian, fava, navy, pinto, garbanzo. Snow peas, pea pods, sauerkraut, onions (except for flavoring), olives, pickles.
Fruit	Any except those to avoid; limit citrus fruits to 1/2 cup/d (1 orange); limit banana to 1/2 per day	Avocados, figs, raisins, papaya, passion fruit, red plums.
Soups	Cream soups made from foods allowed in diet, homemade broth.	Canned soup, soup or bouillon cubes, soup base with yeast or MSG (read labels).
Desserts	Any cake, cookies without chocolate, nuts, or yeast. Any pudding or ice cream without chocolate or nuts. Flavored gelatin.	Any product containing chocolate including ice cream, pudding, cookies, cake or pies. Mincemeat pie.
Sweets	Sugar, jelly, jam, honey, hard candy.	Chocolate candy or syrup, carob.
Miscellaneous	Salt in moderation, lemon juice, butter or margarine, cooking oil, whipped cream, white vinegar, commercial salad dressings.	Pizza, cheese sauce, MSG in excessive amounts (including Chinese food and Accent), meat tenderizer, seasoned salt, yeast, yeast extract. Mixed dishes (including macaroni and cheese, beef stroganoff, cheese blintzes, lasagna, frozen TV dinners). Chocolate, nuts (including peanut butter). All nonwhite vinegars. Anything fermented, pickled or marinated.

Modified from Diamond[54] and Shulman et al.[55]

Medications

ABORTIVE MEDICAL THERAPY

The drugs used to abort attacks of migraine include aspirin, ibuprofen, isomethep-tene mucate (Midrin), ergotamine, dihydroergotamine, and 5-HT agonists (seroto-nin).[57] There are several types of serotonin receptors. It has been postulated that the abortive drugs are 5-HT$_1$ agonists, whereas the prophylactic drugs are 5-HT$_2$ antago-nists.[58] Table 13–3 lists the serotonin receptor medications and their uses. Sumatriptan is a potent agonist of the 5-HT$_1$ receptor but does not cross the blood-brain barrier well. Consequently, a host of other drugs are now coming onto the market with similar re-ceptor agonists including eletriptan, naratriptan, rizatriptan, and zolmitriptan. Dihy-droergotamine is also effective with 5-HT$_1$ agonism. These drugs are primarily de-signed to abort headache. They have not been found to be effective in aborting migraine auras to date. In fact, subcutaneous sumatriptan is totally ineffective when given during the aura.[59] There are also now a host of selective serotonin 5-HT$_3$ receptor antagonists that prevent nausea and vomiting (see Table 13–3). These drugs, plus dexamethasone, are the most effective regimen for prevention of acute vomiting caused by cancer chemotherapy. They have been found to be effective in other causes of severe nausea and vomiting including central vertigo,[60] but they have not yet been approved for these conditions. They are expensive and should not be used beyond a 24-hour period.

PROPHYLACTIC MEDICAL THERAPY

When migraine occurs several times a month, prophylactic daily medical therapy designed to prevent migraine should be used. There are a variety of drugs used in this capacity including beta-blockers, amitriptyline, calcium-channel blockers, lithium car-bonate, aspirin, and ibuprofen.[57] All of these drugs have been found to be effective in reducing the frequency and severity of headache with or without aura. These drugs have also been found to be useful in preventing migraine-associated dizziness.[61,62] Daily valproate recently has been found to be effective in preventing migraine head-aches[63] and has been approved for prophylactic treatment of migraine. To what extent this drug stops vertigo due to migraine is not known. With the exception of aspirin, ibuprofen, and valproate, the mode of action of these prophylactic drugs may be via their antagonist effect on 5-HT$_2$ receptors.[58]

Based on personal observations, this author has found that propranolol is quite ef-fective in preventing auras, including vertigo; therefore, it is the first drug used to treat patients with frequent migraine auras. Contraindications include congestive heart dis-ease, cardiac block, asthma, diabetes, and orthostatic hypotension. Patients start on 40-mg tablets, 1/2 tablet bid and increase this drug in 20-mg increments every 3 to 7 days, depending on patient tolerance of the drug. The effective dose is usually 80 to 200 mg/d. As this drug is increased, heart rate and blood pressure are monitored. Once the therapeutic dose is found, long-acting propranolol (80- to 120-mg capsules) may be prescribed. If they remain relatively symptom free for a few months, the medication is tapered every 1 to 2 weeks to the lowest effective dose.

Finally, acetazolamide (Diamox) 250 mg bid has been shown to decrease spells in patients with episodic ataxia-2. It may also be helpful in patients with familial hemi-plegic migraine[64] and those with familial migraine with vertigo.[65]

TABLE 13–3 Serotonin (5-HT) Receptor Drugs

Receptor	Chemical (Trade Name)	Dose	Indications	Side Effects
5-HT$_1$ agonists	Sumatriptan (Imitrex)	6 mg SQ, 25–100 mg PO or 20 mg nasal spray	Abortive therapy for migraine	Flushing, chest discomfort
	Zolmitriptan (Zomig)	2.5 mg PO	Abortive therapy for migraine	Flushing, chest discomfort
	Naratriptan	2.5 mg PO	Abortive therapy for migraine	Flushing, chest discomfort
	Eletriptan		Abortive therapy for migraine	Flushing, chest discomfort
	Rizatriptan		Abortive therapy for migraine	Flushing, chest discomfort
5-HT$_3$ antagonists	Ondansetron (Zofran)	8 mg PO × 2; 32 mg IV	Prevention of severe nausea and vomiting from chemotherapy	Mild headache and dizziness
	Dolasetron (Anzemet)	100 mg PO; 1.8 mg/kg IV	Prevention of severe nausea and vomiting from chemotherapy	Mild headache and dizziness
	Granisetron (Kytril)	2 mg PO; 10 μg/kg IV	Prevention of severe nausea and vomiting from chemotherapy	Mild headache and dizziness

CASE EXAMPLES

CASE STUDY 1

A 46-year-old owner of a blacktop paving company is referred for spells of vertigo, nausea, vomiting, oscillopsia, and diaphoresis for past 2 years, each lasting approximately 30 minutes. He had sustained tinnitus and hearing loss on the right side, which did not fluctuate with his spells of vertigo. In addition, he had a life-long history of sinus pressure discomfort in the forehead, eyes, and behind the nose, for which he took a decongestant. His last sinus discomfort was 3 years ago. In addition, he has recently had episodic flashes of light lasting 10 to 15 minutes. He has a history of hypertension and angina, but a normal EKG and coronary angiography. In the last 2 months, the frequency of his spells of vertigo increased to 1 per week and the last few spells were associated with left arm paresthesia and dysarthria. One spell was witnessed and the patient was found to have a sustained left-beating nystagmus for 20 minutes.

Comment

Migraine and Ménière's disease can be frequently difficult to distinguish. An important feature in this patient's history that points to migraine is that his tinnitus and hearing loss did not fluctuate with his spells. This feature applies only to patients that have sufficient hearing to notice fluctuation. Sinus headaches and migraine are also frequently confused; both can be located in the same area of the face and head. Episodic flashes of light are a helpful tip pointing to migraine aura. Basilar artery migraine is suggested by the other signs and symptoms during the spell, including paresthesias, dysarthria, and left-beating nystagmus.

Management and Outcome

A diagnosis of basilar artery stroke was considered. A four-vessel cerebral arteriogram was normal, as was an MRI of the head with contrast. In summary, this patient was thought to be having impending brainstem stroke with possible ischemia to the right brainstem resulting in vertigo, left-beating nystagmus, and left arm paresthesia. Of interest was that he also had angina with normal coronary arteries. He had a remote history of "sinus headaches" and recently has been experiencing scintillating scotomas. A diagnosis of basilar artery migraine (IHS classification 1.2.4) was made and his spells of vertigo stopped after he was placed on a diet and propranolol.

CASE STUDY 2

A 28-year-old real estate developer is referred for thirty 5 to 10 minute spells of dysequilibrium, vertigo, 15° tilt of world, and diplopia (vertical and horizontal) over the past 5 years. Many of these spells occurred during a variety of physical activities including running, weight lifting, intercourse, and strenuous aerobic exercises (rowing machine, stair-climber, and stationary bicycle).

Comment

Because of the exercise-induced nature of these spells, they were believed to be due to a perilymphatic fistula and surgery was initially recommended. Features more characteristic of migraine included the development of a dull soreness over his left occiput following each spell, the association of certain foods with spells (Chinese food, ice cream, cream cheese), and the frequent omission of breakfast. Migraine can be caused by exercise. Other features not consistent with a perilymphatic fistula were a normal audiogram and no history of barotrauma, ear surgery, or ear infection.

Management and Outcome

A diagnosis of basilar migraine (IHS classification 1.2.4) was made. These spells stopped after he was placed on the antimigraine schedule listed in Table 13–3.

CASE STUDY 3

A 47-year-old medical transcriptionist is referred for a 10-year history of spells of nausea, dysequilibrium, and occasional vomiting and ear fullness without hearing loss or tinnitus. Her audiogram was normal. She was diagnosed with probable Ménière's disease and treated with chlorothiazide (Diuril), dimenhydrinate (Dramamine), and no caffeine or nicotine. Because she continued to have bad attacks, she was then treated with scopolamine patches. She then began to develop headaches (usually left frontal), and ear pressure with some of the spells, worse in the summer. She had a history of severe headache with her menses since the age of 30. She had a normal caloric, CT scan of the head, and rotary chair test.

Comment

This is another case that illustrates the difficulty in distinguishing migraine from Ménière's disease. This patient started off with spells without headache. Because of a lack of headaches, she did not initially satisfy the criteria for migraine. Although rare, vestibular hydrops without hearing loss can occur. This entity usually eventually also affects hearing. Vestibular hydrops versus migraine aura without headache can present with identical symptoms. Until the diagnosis is secured, both entities are treated. Headaches eventually occurred.

Management and Outcome

She was diagnosed with migraine with aura (IHS classification 1.1) and migraine aura without headache (IHS classification 1.2.5). She was placed on an antimigraine schedule and treated with isometheptene at the onset of the spell, which did not help. She was then placed on an increasing dose of amitriptyline and eventually reached a dose of 50 mg each night. For the next year she continued to get a headache a few days before her menses, but no dizzy spells. Because of the complaint of difficulty getting up in the morning and a dry mouth, the amitriptyline was tapered and she was placed on an increasing dose of propranolol. She has had no headaches or spells of vertigo for the past 9 months.

CASE STUDY 4

A 35-year-old biochemist is referred for spells of vertigo, nausea, and vomiting lasting for less than 1 hour during the past year. As a teenager, she recalled having occasional bad "sinus headaches." Between the ages of 22 and 32 she had spells of vertigo, nausea, vomiting, fluctuating hearing loss, and tinnitus in the left ear. At that time she was diagnosed with Ménière's disease and treated with diuretics, antihistamines, and a low-salt diet. Her current spells of vertigo were not associated with fluctuating hearing loss or tinnitus, and were not altered by the use of a diuretic and a low-salt diet. Two years ago she had a visual scintillation that lasted for a few minutes. She had a normal neurological examination, normal caloric test, and normal rotary chair test. She had moderate to severe low-frequency sensorineural hearing defect, and decreased speech discrimination on the left side. Hearing was normal on the right. An MRI of the head with gadolinium was normal.

Comment

This patient started off with Ménière's disease that responded well to treatment. Migraine and Ménière's disease are very common and patients frequently can have both. The peak incidence for migraine is between the ages of 35 and 45.

Management and Outcome

She was diagnosed with migraine aura without headache (IHS classification 1.2.5). She was placed on an antimigraine schedule. Over the next year her spells of vertigo stopped, hearing in the low frequencies became normal, and she developed normal speech discrimination.

CASE STUDY 5

A 33-year-old professor of history is referred for five spells of vertigo beginning several years ago. These spells usually lasted a few minutes and occurred in the morning around the time of her menses. It was unclear whether head movement triggered them. She usually had dysequilibrium for up to 1 hour following the vertigo. She also noted minor right-sided headaches during her menses with queasiness, but denied vomiting, hearing loss, and tinnitus. She recalls having ear infections when she was young. She wondered about anxiety attacks; she lost her husband 2-1/2 years previously to colon cancer. She had normal neurological and neuro-otological examinations. She was reassured that no serious problem was found and was told to come in if she developed another attack. One month later she called and stated the spells returned. She stated that she had just finished her menses and had a minor right-sided headache. On examination she had sustained geotropic nystagmus during the Hallpike-Dix maneuver.

Comment

Migraine is most common during the week prior to menstrual periods. During the migraine aura, head movements usually provoke dizziness. In about 30 percent of patients with migraine-provoked dizziness, true vertigo with the head still occurs. A variety of types of nystagmus can be found, including spontaneous and position induced. Sustained geotropic nystagmus is central. Transient geotropic nystagmus can be due to canalithiasis of the horizontal semicircular canal and sustained ageotropic nystagmus can be due to cupulolithiasis of the horizontal semicircular canal.

Management and Outcome

This patient was also placed on an antimigraine schedule. Her spell and positional nystagmus resolved in a couple of days and she did not have any recurrence of headache or vertigo during the 6 months she was followed.

SUMMARY

It is becoming increasingly recognized that migraine is a common cause of episodic vertigo and dysequilibrium in children and adults. It may present as benign paroxysmal vertigo of childhood, paroxysmal torticollis of infancy, and benign recurrent vertigo in adults. In addition, migraine is associated with motion sickness, Ménière's disease, and BPPV. Migraine is triggered by a number of factors including stress, anxiety, hypoglycemia, fluctuating estrogen, certain foods, and smoking. Episodic vertigo and dysequilibrium from migraine should be treated by reducing these risk factors and, if necessary, by medical therapy.

PATIENT INFORMATION

Glaxo Wellcome (1-800-377-0302) and http://www.healthylives.com/. Obtain free pamphlets including "Chart Your Route to Relief: A Personal Migraine Management Program."

For free newsletters, contact the National Headache Foundation at 1-800-843-2256 and http://www.headaches.org/.

REFERENCES

1. Kayan, A, and Hood, JD: Neuro-otological manifestations of migraine. Brain 107:1123, 1984.
2. Selby, G, and Lance, JW: Observations on 500 cases of migraine and allied vascular headaches. J Neurol Neurosurg Psychiatr 23:23, 1960.
3. Stewart, WF, et al: Migraine headache: Prevalence in the United States by age, income, race and other sociodemographic factors. JAMA 267:64, 1992.
4. Headache Classification Committee of the International Headache Society: Classification and diagnostic criteria for headache disorders, cranial neuralgias and facial pain. Cephalalgia 8 (suppl 7):1, 1988.
5. Fisher, CM: Late-life migraine accompaniments as a cause of unexplained transient ischemic attacks. Can J Neurol Sci 7:9, 1980.
6. Daroff, RB: New headache classification. Neurology 38:1138, 1988.

7. Basser, LS: Benign paroxysmal vertigo of childhood. Brain 87:141, 1964.
8. Fenichel, GM: Migraine as a cause of benign paroxysmal vertigo of childhood. J Pediatr 71:114, 1967.
9. Koenigsberger, MR, et al: Benign paroxysmal vertigo of childhood. Neurology 20: 1108, 1970.
10. Lanzi, G, et al: Benign paroxysmal vertigo of childhood: A long-term follow-up. Cephalgia 14:458, 1994.
11. Parker, W: Migraine and the vestibular system in childhood and adolescence. Am J Otolog 10:364, 1989.
12. Watson, P, and Steele, JC: Paroxysmal dysequilibrium in the migraine syndrome of childhood. Arch Otolaryngol 99:177, 1974.
13. Snyder, CH: Paroxysmal torticollis in infancy. Am J Dis Child 117:458, 1969.
14. Gourley, IM: Paroxysmal torticollis in infancy. Can Med Assoc J 105:504, 1971.
15. Hanukoglu, A, et al: Benign paroxysmal torticollis in infancy. Clin Pediatr 23:272, 1984.
16. Lipson, EH, and Robertson, WC: Paroxysmal torticollis of infancy: Familial occurrence. Am J Dis Child 132:422, 1978.
17. Bickerstaff, ER: Basilar artery migraine. Lancet 1:15, 1961.
18. Eviatar, L: Vestibular testing in basilar artery migraine. Ann Neurol 9:126, 1981.
19. Harker, LA, and Rassekh, CH: Episodic vertigo in basilar artery migraine. Otolaryngol Head Neck Surg 96:239, 1987.
20. Grad, A, and Baloh, RW: Vertigo of vascular origin. Clinical and oculographic features. Arch Neurol 46:281, 1989.
21. Slater, R: Benign recurrent vertigo. J Neurol Neurosurg Psychiatr 42:363, 1979.
22. Harker, LA, and Rassekh, CH: Migraine equivalent as a cause of episodic vertigo. Laryngoscope 98:160, 1988.
23. Moretti, G, et al: "Benign recurrent vertigo" and its connection with migraine. Headache 20:344, 1980.
24a. Ferrari, MD, et al: Treatment of migraine attacks with sumatriptan: The Subcutaneous Sumatriptan International Study Group. New Engl J Med 325:316, 1991.
24b. Schlake, HP, et al: Electronystagmographic investigations in migraine and cluster headache during the pain-free interval. Cephalagia 9:271, 1989.
25. Toglia, JU, et al: Common migraine and vestibular function. Electronystagmographic study and pathogenesis. Ann Otol Rhinol Laryngol 90:267, 1981.
26. Imes, RK, and Hoyt, W: Exercise-induced transient visual events in young healthy adults. J Clin Neuro-ophthalmol 9:178, 1989.
27. Bartleson, JD: Transient and persistent neurological manifestations of migraine. Stroke 15:383, 1984.
28. Bruyn, GW: Complicated migraine. In Vinken, PJ, and Bruyn, GW (eds): vol 6. Handbook of Clinical Neurology, 1968, pp 59–75.
29. Welch, KMA, and Levine, SR: Migraine-related stroke in the context of the International Headache Society Classification of Head Pain. Arch Neurol 47:458, 1990.
30. Coppeto, JR, et al: Vascular retinopathy in migraine. Neurology 36:267, 1986.
31. Weintraub, JM, and Feman, SS: Ischemic optic neuropathy in migraine. Arch Neurol 100:1097, 1982.
32. Viirre, ES, and Baloh, RW: Migraine as a cause of sudden hearing loss. Headache 36:24, 1996.
33. Caplan, LR: Migraine and vertebrobasilar ischemia. Neurology 41:55, 1991.
34. Solomon, GD, and Spaccavento, LJ: Lateral medullary syndrome after basilar migraine. Headache 22:171, 1982.
35. Brandt, Th, and Daroff, RB: The multisensory physiological and pathological vertigo syndromes. Ann Neurol 7:195, 1980.
36. Childs, AJ, and Sweetnam, MT: A study of 104 cases of migraine. Br Industr Med 18:234, 1961.
37. Kuritzky, A, et al: Vertigo, motion sickness and migraine. Headache 21:227, 1981.
38. Baloh, RW: Neuro-otology of migraine. Headache 37:615, 1997.
39. Dornhoffer, JL, and Arenberg, IK: Diagnosis of vestibular Ménière's disease with electrocochleography. Am J Otol 14:161, 1993.
40. Hinchcliffe, R: Headache and Ménière's disease. Acta Otolaryngol (Stockh) 63:384, 1967.
41. Schiller, F, and Hedberg, WC: An appraisal of positional nystagmus. AMA Arch Neurol 2:309, 1960.
42. Baloh, RW, and Honrubia, V: Childhood onset of benign positional vertigo. Neurology 50:1494, 1998.
43. Olesen, J, et al: Focal hyperemia followed by spreading oligemia and impaired activation of rCBF in classic migraine. Ann Neurol 9:344, 1981.
44. Moskowitz, MA, et al: Neocortical spreading depression provokes the expression of c-fos protein-like immunoreactivity within trigeminal nucleus caudalis via trigeminovascular mechanisms. J Neurosci 13:1167, 1993.
45. Peroutka, SJ: Dopamine and migraine. Neurology 49:650, 1997.
46. Goadsby, PJ, and Hoskin, KL: Serotonin inhibits trigeminal nucleus activity evoked by craniovascular stimulation through a 5-HT receptor: A central action in migraine? Ann Neurol 43:711, 1998.
47. Joutel, A, et al: A gene for familial hemiplegic migraine maps to chromosome 19. Nature Genet 5:40, 1993.
48. Ophoff, RA, et al: Familial hemiplegic migraine and episodic ataxia type-2 are caused by mutations in the Ca2+ channel gene CACNL1A4. Cell 87:543, 1996.
49. May, A, et al: Familial hemiplegic migraine locus on 19p13 is involved in the common forms of migraine with and without aura. Hum Genet 96:604, 1995.

50. Elliot, MA, et al: Familial hemiplegic migraine, nystagmus and cerebellar atrophy. Ann Neurol 39:100, 1996.
51. Ducros, A, et al: Mapping of a second locus for familial hemiplegic migraine to 1q21-q23 and evidence of further heterogeneity. Ann Neurol 42:885, 1997.
52a. Diamond, S: Dietary factors in vascular headache. Neurol Forum 2:2, 1991.
52b. Kin, T: Discussion, ideas abound in migraine research: Consensus remains elusive. JAMA 257:9, 1987.
53. Silberstein, SD, and Merriam, GR: Estrogens, progestins, and headache. Neurology 41:786, 1991.
54a. Cooper, KH: The Aerobics Way. Bantam Books, New York, 1997, p 312.
54b. Holroyd, KA, and Penzien, DB: Pharmacological versus non-pharmacological prophylaxis of recurrent migraine headache: A meta-analytic review of clinical trials. Pain 42:1, 1990.
55. Shulman, KI, et al: Dietary restrictions, tyramine, and the use of monoamine oxidase inhibitors. J Clin Psychopharmacol 9:397, 1989.
56. van Den Eeden, SK, et al: Aspartame ingestion and headaches: A randomized crossover trial. Neurology 44:1787, 1994.
57. Capobianco, DJ, et al: An overview of the diagnosis and pharmacologic treatment of migraine. Mayo Clin Proc 71:1055, 1996.
58. Peroutka, SJ: The pharmacology of current anti-migraine drugs. Headache 30(suppl):5, 1990.
59. Bates, D, et al: Subcutaneous sumatriptan during the migraine aura. Neurology 44:1587, 1994.
60. Rice, GPA, and Ebers, GC: Ondansetron for intractable vertigo complicating acute brainstem disorders. Lancet 345:1182, 1995.
61. Bikhazi, P, et al: Efficacy of antimigrainous therapy in the treatment of migraine-associated dizziness. Am J Otol 18:350, 1997.
62. Johnson, GD: Medical management of migraine-related dizziness and vertigo. Laryngoscope 108:1, 1998.
63. Jensen, R, et al: Sodium valproate has a prophylactic effect in migraine without aura. Neurology 44:647, 1994.
64. Athwal, BS, and Lennox, GG: Acetazolamide responsiveness in familial hemiplegic migraine. Ann Neurol 40:820, 1996.
65. Baloh, RW, et al: Familial migraine with vertigo and essential tremor. Neurology 46:458, 1996.

CHAPTER 14

Psychological Problems and the Dizzy Patient

Ronald J. Tusa, MD, PhD

Dizziness can cause extreme stress. This may in turn lead to anxiety (including panic attacks and agoraphobia), depression, and somatoform disorders. These psychological problems can also cause severe dizziness. At times, these psychological causes may become the primary cause of dizziness and replace the initial organic cause. This chapter summarizes the interaction between dizziness and these psychological problems. It also will discuss conversion disorders and malingering. Finally, it presents a practical clinical approach to these topics.

PREVALENCE

Psychological Problems in Patients with Dizziness

GENERAL

There is a high prevalence of unrecognized mood and psychological problems in dizzy patients, especially anxiety disorders.[1,2] Forty percent of all dizzy patients have psychological disorders.[3] Fifteen percent of all dizzy patients meet the DSM-III criteria for panic disorder, agoraphobia or both, and these patients rate themselves as much more disabled by their dizziness than patients with no psychiatric disorder.[4] The prevalence of psychiatric disorders as the primary cause for dizziness declines with increasing patient age.[3,5] In patients over 60 years of age, 38 percent have a psychological diagnosis contributing to dizziness, but of these only 6 percent were felt to have a primary psychological cause. Psychological problems often coexist with a significant balance disorder.

PATIENTS WITH PERIPHERAL VESTIBULAR DEFICITS VERSUS NO VESTIBULAR DEFICITS

Forty percent of patients with vestibular hypofunction presenting to an otolaryngology clinic have an additional panic disorder with and without agoraphobia.[6] Fifty percent of patients with vestibular hypofunction evaluated 3 to 5 years after their original referral still have a significant psychiatric disturbance (panic disorder or major depression).[7] In our own experience, panic attacks occur in a number of patients with vestibular deficits, but not to the same extent as reported in these studies authored by psychiatrists. Chronic anxiety is much more prevalent. The level of anxiety in these patients is usually not high enough to warrant psychotherapy or medication. "Space phobia,"[8] "motorist's disorientation syndrome,"[9] and phobic postural vertigo[10] have also been described as syndromes following vestibular defects. Patients without evidence of peripheral vestibular deficit have a greater mean number of lifetime psychiatric diagnoses, especially major depression and panic disorder, than do those with a vestibular deficit.[2] This group more frequently has a somatization disorder, as well as more current and lifetime unexplained medical symptoms.

Dizziness in Patients with Psychological Disorders

The prevalence of psychological problems in the general population is very high. Table 14–1 lists the prevalence in the United States.

ABNORMALITIES ON VESTIBULAR TESTS

To what extent patients with panic disorder have a vestibular defect is controversial. Several authors have reported abnormalities on a variety of tests used to assess dizziness including caloric, rotary chair, vestibular autorotation, and posturography.[11–15] Few articles have sufficient detail to determine if these deficits are truly due to vestibular dysfunction (low vestibulo-ocular reflex [VOR] gain on rotary chair or decreased response on caloric testing). Of the more detailed articles, one article suggests that as many as 14 percent with panic without agoraphobia and 39 percent of patients with panic with agoraphobia have compensated peripheral vestibular defects.[13] Another article found discrepancies in the VOR but no caloric deficits in patients with panic disorder.[12]

TABLE 14–1 Psychological Disorders in the United States Population (NIMH)

Disorder	Number	Affected (%)
Anxiety disorders	23.2 million	12.6
Phobia		10.9
OCD		2.1
Panic with and without agoraphobia		1.3
Depressive disorders 17.5 million	9.5	
Somatization disorders	400,000	0.2

Abbreviation: OCD, obsessive-compulsive disorder.

TABLE 14–2 Terms Defined by The World Health Organization

Term	Definition
Impairment	Any loss or abnormality of physiologic or anatomical structure or function
Disability	Restriction or lack of ability to perform a task in the manner or within the range considered normal due to an impairment
Handicapped	Social implication of disability

Disability

It is well documented that patients with dizziness suffer a significantly decreased quality of life.[16,17] The definition of disability and related terms by the World Health Organization (WHO) is listed in Table 14–2. Clark et al[16] have evaluated disability in dizzy patients with and without vestibular defects. They found that severe impairment in the ability to function was more strongly associated with the presence of a psychiatric disorder than was the presence of a vestibular disorder. Nausea, vomiting, palpitations, weakness, and difficulty with speech with dizziness were indicators of a psychiatric disorder and not of a peripheral vestibular disorder. This suggests that the clinician should look for comorbid psychiatric disorders in patients with persistent complaints of the symptoms listed above.

PSYCHOLOGICAL DISORDERS

Anxiety

PANIC ATTACKS WITH AND WITHOUT AGORAPHOBIA

Dizziness is the most common symptom in patients with panic disorder, occurring in 50 to 85 percent of all patients.[18,19] **Panic attacks** consist of discrete spells of intense fear or discomfort, in which at least four of the symptoms listed in Box 14–1 develop

---

BOX 14–1   Symptoms of Panic Attack

Dizziness, unsteady feelings or faintness
Nausea or abdominal distress
Shortness of breath (or smothering sensations)
Palpitations or tachycardia
Trembling or shaking
Sweating
Choking
Depersonalization or derealization
Numbness or paresthesias
Flushes (hot flashes) or chills
Chest pain or discomfort
Fear of dying
Fear of going crazy or doing something uncontrolled

abruptly and reach crescendo within 10 minutes. Panic attacks can be unexpected (un-cued) or situation bound (cued). An example of the latter is spells induced when enter-ing a car. Agoraphobia is the aversion of open spaces including leaving the house. Agoraphobia is frequently found in patients with severe panic attacks.

OBSESSIVE-COMPULSIVE DISORDER

An **obsession** is a repetitive intrusive thought, impulse, or image that causes marked anxiety. A **compulsion** is a repetitive ritualistic behavior or mental act that aims to reduce anxiety. Examples of the latter include hand washing and checking to see that doors are locked.

GENERALIZED ANXIETY DISORDER

This is characterized by generalized and persistent anxiety with motor tension, autonomic hyperactivity, apprehensive expectation, and vigilance. An essential feature is unrealistic worry. The duration of these symptoms should be at least 6 months.

Somatoform Disorders

SOMATIZATION

Somatization is defined as the propensity to experience and report somatic symp-toms that have no pathophysiological explanation, to misattribute them to disease, and to seek medical attention for them. Much of general medical practice is devoted to the care of somatizing patients who are symptomatic but not seriously ill.[20]

CONVERSION

Conversion is the development of a symptom or deficit suggestive of a neurologi-cal disorder that affects sensation (including vestibular) or voluntary motor function (including imbalance). There is a temporal relationship between the symptoms or deficits and psychological stressors, conflicts, or needs. There is no conscious intention of producing the symptoms (i.e., factitious disorder or malingering). The symptom or signs cause significant impairment in social or occupational functioning, or marked distress; or they require medical attention or investigation.

Factitious Disorders

A **factitious disorder** is defined as intentional complaint of psychological signs and symptoms or intentional production of physical signs and symptoms motivated by the psychological need to assume a sick role. There must not be external incentives such as economic gain or obtaining better care.

Malingering

Malingering is similar to factitious disorders, but there is an external incentive to be gained from the complaint (usually economic gain).

Phobic Postural Vertigo

Brandt et al[10] have coined the term "phobic postural vertigo" for psychogenic vertigo. In that clinic, it is the most common cause of vertigo second to benign paroxysmal positional vertigo (BPPV). The term is misleading in that these patients do not complain of vertigo but rather complain of vague dizziness with subjective postural and gait instability. This entity mainly occurs in patients with an obsessive-compulsive personality. The patient rarely consults a psychiatrist, but seeks the advice of specialists in the field associated with the relevant physical symptom. In 5 years, 72 percent of the patients had a favorable outcome.

Mal de Debarquement Syndrome

Mal de debarquement literally means "bad feeling after debarking [from a boat]." It consists of the sensation of persistent rocking after returning to a stable environment following motion adaptation.[21,22] It is accompanied by vague unsteadiness and occurs after extended sea voyages, or train or air travel. It usually lasts a few days, but in some cases it persists for years. These same symptoms may occur spontaneously, and are usually relieved when the person is in motion. The physical examination is unrevealing. Patients may show mild functional stance and gait disturbance. Rarely will patients self-rock. Positional nystagmus has been noted in some, but it is very rarely seen in our own clinic or those of others who see a number of these patients. All diagnostic studies are normal, including head MRI, caloric, and rotary chair. When chronic, this disorder may represent as yet an undefined vestibular problem or a type of somatoform disorder. In our own experience, patients who are bothered the most by mal de debarquement syndrome have a pre-existing anxiety or an obsessive-compulsive disorder.

ASSESSMENT

History

There are a number of questionnaires that can be helpful in the diagnosis and assessment of psychological problems. These are listed below.

DIZZINESS HANDICAP INVENTORY-MEASURE

The Dizziness Handicap Inventory-Measure (DHI) is a measure of self-perceived disability attributable to vestibular disease. Twenty-five questions classified into physical, functional, and emotional domains are given (Box 14–2).[23] A "yes" response is

---

BOX 14–2 Items Comprising the Dizziness Handicap Inventory

"P" denotes physical subscale items, "E" denotes emotional subscale items, and "F" denotes functional subscale items.

P1. Does looking up increase your problem?

E2. Because of your problem do you feel frustrated?

F3. Because of your problem do you restrict your travel for business or recreation?

P4. Does walking down the aisle of a supermarket increase your problem?

F5. Because of your problems do you have difficulty getting into or out of bed?

F6. Does your problem significantly restrict your participation in social activities such as going out to dinner, movies, dancing, or parties?

F7. Because of your problems do you have difficulty reading?

P8. Does performing more ambitious activities like sports, dancing, and household chores such as sweeping or putting dishes away increase your problem?

E9. Because of your problems are you afraid to leave your home without having someone accompany you?

E10. Because of your problem have you been embarrassed in front of others?

P11. Do quick movements of your head increase your problem?

F12. Because of your problem do you avoid heights?

P13. Does turning over in bed increase your problem?

F14. Because of your problem is it difficult for you to do strenuous housework or yardwork?

E15. Because of your problem are you afraid people may think you are intoxicated?

F16. Because of your problem is it difficult for you to go for a walk by yourself?

P17. Does walking down a sidewalk increase your problem?

E18. Because of your problem is it difficult for you to concentrate?

F19. Because of your problem is it difficult for you to walk around your house in the dark?

E20. Because of your problem are you afraid to stay home alone?

E21. Because of your problem do you feel handicapped?

E22. Has your problem placed stress on your relationships with members of your family or friends?

E23. Because of your problem are you depressed?

F24. Does your problem interfere with your job or household responsibilities?

P25. Does bending over increase your problem?

---

scored 4 points, "sometimes" is scored 2 points, and "no" is scored 0 points. Thus, the total score ranges from 0 (no perceived disability) to 100 (maximum perceived disability). The test was given to 106 consecutive patients seen for vestibular testing.[23] The mean score and standard deviation was 32.7 ± 21.9. The DHI has a high internal consistency, and could be used to identify specific functional, emotional, or physical problems associated with dizziness. No significant correlation has been found between DHI and the results from caloric or rotary chair testing.[23,24] It is controversial whether there is a correlation between the sensory aspect of posturography and DHI.[24,25] Despite that, this self-assessment inventory is reliable, requires little time to administer, and may be useful to evaluate the efficacy of treatment.

POSITIVE AND NEGATIVE AFFECTIVE SCALE

A good screening scale for anxiety and depression is the Positive and Negative Affective Scale.[28] The patient is given a form similar to the one shown in Box 14–3. The

---

BOX 14–3   Positive and Negative Affective Scale (PANAS)

This scale consists of a number of words that describe different feelings and emotions. Read each item and then mark the appropriate answer in the space next to that word. Indicate to what extent you generally feel this way, that is, how you feel on the average. Use the following scale to record your answers.

1 Very slightly or not at all	2 A little	3 Moderately	4 Quite a bit	5 Extremely

___ interested	(P)	___ irritable	(N)	___ jittery	(N)
___ distressed	(N)	___ alert	(P)	___ active	(P)
___ excited	(P)	___ ashamed	(N)	___ afraid	(N)
___ upset	(N)	___ inspired	(P)	___ hostile	(N)
___ strong	(P)	___ nervous	(N)	___ enthusiastic	(P)
___ guilty	(N)	___ determined	(P)	___ proud	(P)
___ scared	(N)	___ attentive	(P)		

---

only difference is that their form does not contain the (P) and (N) items at the end of each word, which indicates positive and negative terms. The numbers assigned to each (P) term are added up. The mean score for (P) is 35.0 ± 6.4. Depression should be considered if the subject scores below 22 (2 standard deviations below the mean). The numbers assigned to each (N) term are then added up. The mean score for this term is 18.1 ± 5.9. Anxiety should be considered if the subject scores above 29.9 (2 standard deviations above the mean).

OTHER TOOLS

There are other standardized questionnaires listed here; however, they are too long to include in their entirety. We have not used them in our clinic, but they may be useful when assessing the effect of certain forms of therapy on clinical outcome. The *Structured Clinical Interview for DSM IV* is a structured interview in which a series of standard questions are asked in standard order, with options to focus on the most relevant points for that patient.[27] The *Beck Anxiety Inventory*[28] and the *Beck Depression Inventory*[29] are specific screens for anxiety and depression. The *Symptom Checklist-90 (SCL-90-R)* is a standardized questionnaire for medical, functional, and demographic data; there are also anxiety, depression, somatization, and phobic anxiety subscales.

TABLE 14–3 Features on Clinical Examination in Patients with Psychogenic Balance and Gait Disorders

Feature	Percent
Moment to moment fluctuations in the level of impairment	51
Excessive slowness or hesitation	51
Exaggerated sway on Romberg test, often improved by distraction	32
Uneconomical postures with waste of muscular energy	30
Extreme caution with restricted steps ("walking on ice")	30
Sudden buckling of the knees, typically without falling	27

Examinations for Psychogenic Stance and Gait Disorders

CLINICAL EXAMINATION

Lempert et al[29,30] have identified six characteristic features on examination that are useful in the diagnosis of psychogenic balance and gait based on review of video tapes from 37 patients with this disorder (Table 14–3). Table 14–3 also lists the prevalence of each feature in their patients. These authors found psychogenic gait disorders in 9 percent of their neurological inpatients. In 5 years, 47 percent had favorable outcomes.[10]

POSTUROGRAPHY

A number of studies have found characteristic features on dynamic posturography in patients with psychogenic balance disorders.[31–33] Figure 14–1 compares the sensory test in a patient with a vestibular deficit to a patient with a psychogenic balance disorder. Box 14–4 lists the key patterns in patients with psychogenic balance disorders.

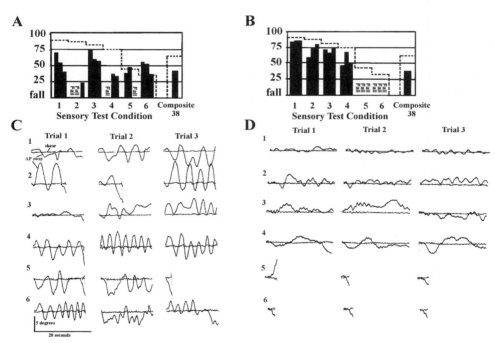

FIGURE 14–1. Sensory tests during dynamic posturography in a patient with psychogenic balance disorder (*A* and *C*) and a patient with an acute unilateral vestibular loss (*B* and *D*). *A* and *B* show the mean sway on the six sensory test conditions repeated three times (100 indicates no sway, 0 indicates sway beyond level of stability or a fall). The patient with psychogenic balance disorder shows better performance for age on the more difficult tests (5 and 6) compared to easier tests (2 and 4). In addition, there is considerable variability from trial to trial within a given test. The patient with the psychogenic balance disorder also shows a regular frequency of sway on all trials suggesting voluntary control (*B*). In contrast, the patient with the unilateral vestibular loss has increased difficulty performing the harder tests (5 and 6), has less variability from trial to trial, and does not have a regular periodicity of sway. The shaded area in *A* and *B* indicates the region where scores are abnormal for age. Note that both subjects were in the same age bracket and that the overall composite scores were equal.

BOX 14–4   Key Patterns on Dynamic Posturography in Patients with Psychogenic Balance Disorders

---

Better performance on harder tests (sensory 5 and 6) compared to easier tests (sensory 1 through 3)

Large intertrial variability

Repetitive large-amplitude anterior-posterior sway without falling (voluntary sway)

Excessive lateral sway compared to anterior-posterior sway

MANAGEMENT

Success in treatment of the psychological problems related to dizziness depends on a positive discussion. Physicians can do this during the first clinic visit. For therapists, this discussion may be delayed until the patient is well into their course of therapy and when a good report has been established. An excellent approach has been outlined by Bursztajn and Barsky.[34] If the opportunity arises, discuss how emotions and stress can cause the same types of symptoms as a vestibular disorder. Try to eliminate any stigma and low self-esteem by stating the prevalence of the psychological disorder. Assure the patient of the therapist's continuing interest and involvement. Include a statement about a possible psychological problem to the referring physician; do not just tell the patient that they need to see a psychiatrist. Patients object to the suggestion of a psychiatric referral for several reasons, including the social stigma of being a psychiatric patient, the creation of low self-esteem, a poor understanding of the role of emotions in causing symptoms, and a feeling of rejection. The term "psychogenic" may be preferred to functional or hysterical because it is diagnostically neutral.

Physicians may want to start the patient on medication (Table 14–4). Those listed under daily medication are nonaddictive, take up to 3 weeks before they are effective, and can be taken for years. They are all antidepressants and FDA approved for anxiety. Parozetine hydrochloride (Paxil) and Sertraline hydrochloride (Zoloft) should be given in the morning as they can impair sleep. Medications listed under intermittent are addictive, can cause sedation, act immediately, and are strictly for anxiety. For patients with severe chronic anxiety or panic attacks, this author usually starts two drugs, one

TABLE 14–4 Medication for Psychological Problems

Medication	Dose	Half-Life (h)
Intermittent medication		
Alprazolam (Xanax)	0.25–1 mg tid	11–15
Lorazepam (Ativan)	0.5–5 mg bid	10–20
Clonazepam (Klonopin)	0.5–10 mg bid	18–50
Diazepam (Valium)	2–10 mg bid	20–50
Daily Medication		
Parozetine hydrochloride (Paxil)	10–20 mg qam	
Sertraline hydrochloride (Zoloft)	50–100 mg qam	
Tofranil (Imipramine)	10–75 mg qd	
Norpramin (Desipramine)	50–300 mg qd	

from the intermittent medication group and one from the daily medication group, using the lowest dose listed in Table 14–4. After three weeks, the intermittent medication is either completely tapered or is limited to 1 to 2 days/week at most.

LONGITUDINAL STUDIES

There are two good longitudinal studies that have assessed the role of psychological problems on dizziness. Kroenke et al[3] examined 94 patients at onset, and then received questionnaires at 4 months and 1 year out. Fifty-one patients improved, symptoms stayed the same for 32, and worsened for 11 patients. Etiology of the dizziness affected outcome. The majority with BPPV, neuritis, migraine, or presyncope improved. Less than half with Ménière's disease, psychiatric, and nonvestibular dysequilibrium improved. There were four multivariate predictors of poor outcome: a primary psychiatric etiology, dysequilibrium, daily dizziness, and the symptom that walking aggravates dizziness.

Yardley et al[35] examined 101 patients evaluated at onset and 7 months. The best longitudinal predictors of poor outcome were autonomic symptoms (heart pounding, excessive sweating, hot or cold spells, feeling faint or short of breath) and somatization (general tendency to complain of a diversity of unrelated health problems ranging from pains in the back to difficulty concentrating). These symptoms had a better prediction of poor outcome than the etiology of true vertigo, severity, duration, test results, and medication. High and persistent handicap arose from psychiatric or psychosocial problems unrelated to the vertigo.

CASE STUDIES

CASE STUDY 1 (O.M.)

A 29-year-old electrician complained of "dizziness for the past 2 years." By dizziness he means trouble walking, poor balance, linear movement, tilt, floating, rocking, and blurred vision as all equal terms for his dizziness. The symptoms started while working on a high lift for 2 hours. He was at a height that caused a sense of rocking on the platform. In addition, he attributes his dizziness to inhalation of fumes of a floor sealant on the job. Since then he has constant dizziness, which is severe when he first awakens in the morning. It is also severe when he is fatigued or walking in a dark room. His head feels heavy. He denied vertigo, hearing loss, and tinnitus. Because of his symptoms, he reduced his exercise program. In the last 6 months he has had loss of strength, energy, and memory, paresthesias, muscle and joint aches, trouble sleeping and speaking, tremor, incoordination, and headaches. His past medical history included surgery to the knee years ago that required IV antibiotic, gonorrhea treated with antibiotics, and anxiety and panic attacks 2 years ago. His mother had been on chronic benzodiazepines for stress. In the last 6 months, the dizziness has interfered with the patient's activities 95 percent of the time and currently it is moderately intense. It has markedly changed his ability to work or do household chores. Dizziness has markedly decreased the amount of satisfaction or enjoyment the patient gets in taking part in family-related or social activities. On the PANAS he scored 34 on positive affect and 19 on negative affect, which is normal.

His physical examination was normal including a visual acuity of 20/26–2 static, 20/30–1 dynamic, normal VOR gain to head thrust, no head-shaking or positional nystagmus, normal pursuit and saccades, normal hearing, normal gait, and balance. He already had a MRI scan with and without gadolinium that included eighth nerve cuts and a caloric. Both were normal.

Comment

This patient has several features consistent with chronic anxiety. His complaints are vague, numerous, and out of proportion to his findings. Complaints of floating and rocking are typical for anxiety or depression. He had a history of panic attacks 2 years ago. There is likely a family history of anxiety as his mother has been on benzodiazepines for "stress." There is frequently a family history of stress, anxiety, or nervousness in patients with anxiety. Exercise is an excellent stress reducer. He stopped all exercise 2 years ago. Even though the PANAS is useful, it was not positive for anxiety in this patient.

Management and Outcome

A tentative diagnosis of chronic anxiety was made. The symptoms from stress and anxiety were discussed with the patient. He was told that these symptoms are very real and can be extreme. The role of his past medical and family history for anxiety was discussed. He was encouraged to restart a regular exercise program to help reduce stress. He was started on parozetine hydrochloride 10 mg qam and clonazepam 0.5 mg qpm; the side effects were explained. He was asked to return in 3 weeks. When he returned to clinic, most of his symptoms had resolved. He was exercising on a regular basis. The clonazepam was tapered over a 3-week period, but the parozetine was continued for 1 year.

CASE STUDY 2 (M.B.)

A 15-year-old girl was referred by her mother for inability to walk for 2 weeks. She could only take a few steps before she had to sit down or her knees would buckle. She started attending a new school 3 weeks prior to her illness. She was doing very well until the dizziness started. She has an older sister who is excelling in the same school. She had a head CT and audiograms, both of which were normal. She had a positive tilt table to isoproterinol suggesting possible orthostatic hypotension and was placed on medication and salt tablets. This may have initially helped, but for only 1 week. Her physical examination was normal except for her stance and gait. There was significant sway at the hips with eyes open and closed, but she did not fall. While walking, she would have sudden buckling of the knees but was able to still walk. There was much side-to-side swaying and waste of muscular energy.

Comment

This patient had a conversion disorder. She had a deficit that suggested a neurological disorder, and yet there was no disorder found. She had a psychogenic stance and gait disorder with several of the features described in Table 14–3. Her symptoms began temporally with the stress of starting a new school—the same school attended by her sister, who was an overachiever. There was no evidence for external economic gain as one would expect for malingering. She did not have a history of assuming a sick role motivated by psychological need as one would expect for a factitious disorder. As in several cases of conversion disorder, this case prompted extensive evaluations and an organic diagnosis (orthostatic hypotension) that proved later to be wrong. The tilt table, especially with isoproterinol, has a number of false-positive outcomes.

Management and Outcome

This diagnosis was not discussed with the child. It was discussed with the mother, but in a way that she could "save face." The social problems with starting a new school attended by an overachieving sister were discussed. School counseling was recommended. Her gait disorder slowly resolved after she was placed in a school that was not attended by her sister. Medications were not used.

CASE STUDY 3 (C.D.)

A 36-year-old lawyer had a chief complaint of light-headedness, nausea, and fatigue. By light-headedness she means "floating or rocking as though I am on a boat." This sensation of rocking goes away when she is in motion (riding in a car) or when she is very busy. It is severe at night when lying down. This all started 2 months ago, after a long train ride in France. She has also been on several cruises. She had seen numerous doctors for this problem including otolaryngologists, neurologists, and ophthalmologists, whose examinations were normal. She had a normal audiogram, caloric, and MRI scan of the head. Her mother had been on benzodiazepines for stress. In her own words she had to have everything correct and was somewhat compulsive. Her physical examination was normal.

Comment

This patient's symptoms fit best with the entity known as mal de debarquement syndrome described in the text. It occurred after prolonged travel; she admitted to compulsive tendencies; there may be a family history of anxiety.

Management and Outcome

This diagnosis was discussed. Parozetine 10 mg qam was added to lorazepam. She was encouraged to begin an exercise program 3 days each week. When she returned in 3 weeks she felt better. The rocking was still there at times, but it was much less noticeable. The lorazepam was tapered over a 2-week period. She called to state she had a recurrence. Lorazepam was restarted and then tapered over the course of 2 months. This resolved her symptoms. The parozetine was continued for 1 year.

SUMMARY

Psychological problems, especially anxiety, are a major contributing factor in all patients with dizziness. This needs to be recognized and dealt with by the therapist for a good outcome. Treatment usually simply requires patient education and reassurance by the referring physician or therapist. Some patients will require medication or stress-reducing programs. If a patient is not progressing during therapy as expected, the therapist should consider a significant psychological problem. A note to or re-evaluation by the physician may be indicated.

REFERENCES

1. Simpson, RB, et al: Psychiatric diagnoses in patients with psychogenic dizziness or severe tinnitus. J Otolaryngol 17:325, 1988.
2. Sullivan, M, et al: Psychiatric and otologic diagnoses in patients complaining of dizziness. Arch Intern Med 153:1479, 1993.
3. Kroenke, K, et al: Causes of persistent dizziness. Ann Intern Med 117:898, 1992.
4. Stein, MB, et al: Panic disorder in patients attending a clinic for vestibular disorders. Am J Psychiatr 151:1697, 1994.
5. Sloane, PD, et al: Psychological factors associated with chronic dizziness in patients aged 60 and older. J Am Geriatric Soc 42:847, 1994.
6. Clark, DB, et al: Panic in otolaryngology patients presenting with dizziness or hearing loss. Am J Psychiatr 151:1223, 1994.
7. Eagger, S, et al: Psychiatric morbidity in patients with peripheral vestibular disorders: A clinical and neuro-otological study. J Neurol Neurosurg Psychiatr 55:383, 1992.
8. Marks, IM: Space "phobia": A pseudo-agoraphobic syndrome. J Neurol Neurosurg Psychiatr 44:387, 1981.
9. Page, NGR, and Gresty, MA: Motorist's vestibular disorientation syndrome. J Neurol Neurosurg Psychiatr 48:729, 1985.
10. Brandt, T, et al: Phobic postural vertigo: A first follow-up. J Neurol 241:191, 1994.
11. Asmundson, GJG, et al: Panic disorder and vestibular disturbance: An overview of empirical findings and clinical implications. J Psychosomatic Res 44:107, 1998.
12. Swinson, RP, et al: Otoneurological functioning in panic disorder patients with prominent dizziness. Compr Psychiatr 34:127, 1993.
13. Jacob, RG, et al: Panic, agoraphobia, and vestibular dysfunction. Am J Psychiatr 153:503, 1996.
14. Hoffman, DL, et al: Autorotation test abnormalities of the horizontal and vertical vestibulo-ocular reflexes in panic disorder. Otolaryngol Head Neck Surg 110:259, 1994.
15. Sklare, DA, et al: Dysequilibrium and audiovestibular function in panic disorder: Symptom profiles and test findings. Am J Otol 11:338, 1990.
16. Clark, MR, et al: Psychiatric and medical factors associated with disability in patients with dizziness. Psychosomatics 34:409, 1993.
17. Fielder, H, et al: Measurement of health status in patients with vertigo. Clin Otolaryngol 21:124, 1996.
18. Aronson, TA, and Logue, CM: Phenomenology of panic attacks: A descriptive study of panic disorder patient's self-reports. J Clin Psychiatr 49:8, 1988.
19. Jacob, RG: Panic disorder and the vestibular system. Psychiatr Clin North Am 11:361, 1988.
20. Barsky, AJ, and Borus, JF: Somatization and medicalization in the era of managed care. JAMA 274:1931, 1995.
21. Brown, JJ, and Baloh, RW: Persistent mal de debarquement syndrome: A motion induced subjective disorder. Am J Otolaryngol 8:219, 1987.
22. Murphy, TP: Mal de debarquement syndrome: A forgotten entity? Otolaryngol Head Neck Surg 109:10, 1993.
23. Jacobson, GP, and Newman, CW: The development of the dizziness handicap inventory. Arch Otolaryngol Head Neck Surg 116:424, 1990.

24. Jacobson, GP, et al: Balance function test correlates of the Dizziness Handicap Inventory. J Am Acad Audiol 2:253, 1991.
25. Robertson, DD, and Ireland, DJ: Dizziness handicap inventory correlates of computerized dynamic posturography. J Otolaryngol 24:118, 1995.
26. Watson, D, et al: Positive and negative affectivity and their relation to anxiety and depressive disorders. J Abnormal Psychol 97:346, 1988.
27. Spitzer, RL, et al: Structured Clinical Interview for DSM-III-R-Non-Patient Version (SCID-NP, Version 1). Washington DC, American Psychiatric Press, 1990.
28. Beck, AT, et al: An inventory for measuring clinical anxiety: psychometric properties. J Consult Clin Psychol 56:893, 1988.
29. Beck, AT, et al: An inventory for measuring depression. Arch Gen Psychiatr 4:561, 1961.
30. Lempert, T, et al: How to identify psychogenic disorders of stance and gait. J Neurol 238:140, 1991.
31. Allum, JHJ, et al: Identifying cases of non-organic vertigo using dynamic posturography. Gait Posture 4:52, 1996.
32. Cevette, MJ, et al: Aphysiologic performance on dynamic posturography. Otolaryngol Head Neck Surg 112:676, 1995.
33. Goebel, JA, et al: Posturographic evidence of nonorganic sway patterns in normal subjects, patients and suspected malingers. Otolaryngol Head Neck Surg 117:293, 1997.
34. Bursztajn, H, and Barsky, AJ: Facilitating patient acceptance of a psychiatric referral. Arch Intern Med 145:73, 1985.
35. Yardley, L, et al: A longitudinal study of symptoms, anxiety and subjective well-being in patients with vertigo. Clin Otolaryngol 19:109, 1994.

Rehabilitation Assessment and Management

CHAPTER 15

Physical Therapy Assessment of Vestibular Hypofunction

Susan L. Whitney, PT, ATC, PhD
Susan J. Herdman, PT, PhD

Patients with peripheral vestibular hypofunction differ with respect to the onset and clinical course of their disability and with respect to the final level of recovery, depending on the type and extent of vestibular deficit. Despite these differences, such patients share many of the same symptoms. These symptoms may include dizziness, light-headedness, vertigo, nystagmus, blurred vision, postural instability, fear of movement, gait disturbances, and occasional falling. In addition, these patients may experience anxiety, depression, and fear related to their disability. In fact, people with vestibular dysfunction report that they are significantly impaired by their disability. As a result of one or more of these symptoms, patients with peripheral vestibular hypofunction often cope with their disability by avoiding certain movements and decreasing their activity level. This habit, if not treated, will lead to the unfortunate results of physical deconditioning and an alteration of the patient's lifestyle.

The purpose of this chapter is to provide the reader with an overview of patient problems and the components of the clinical examination including key elements as well as the comprehensive examination.

FUNCTIONAL DEFICITS

Patients with vestibular hypofunction may express a multitude of symptoms. These symptoms emerge from functional deficits in vestibulo-ocular and vestibulospinal systems (Box 15–1) and from the results of sensory mismatch and physical deconditioning.[1]

BOX 15–1   Questions to Ask a Patient With a Vestibular Disorder

1. Do you experience spells of vertigo (a sense of spinning)? If yes, how long do these spells last?
2. When was the last time the vertigo occurred?
3. Is the vertigo spontaneous, induced by motion, induced by position changes?
4. Do you experience a sense of being off-balance (disequilibrium)? If yes, is the feeling of being off-balance constant, spontaneous, induced by motion, induced by position changes, worse with fatigue, worse in the dark, worse outside, worse on uneven surfaces?
5. Does the feeling of being off-balance occur when you are lying down, sitting, standing, or walking?
6. Do you stumble, stagger, or side-step while walking?
7. Do you drift to one side while you walk? If yes, to which side do you drift?
8. At what time of day do you feel best? _____ worst? _____
9. How many times per day do you experience symptoms?
10. Do you have hearing problems?
11. Do you have visual problems?
12. Have you been in an accident (e.g., motor vehicle)?
13. What medications do you take?
14. Do you live alone?
15. Do you have stairs in your home?
16. Do you smoke? If yes, please indicate how much per day.
17. Do you drink alcohol? If yes, please indicate how much.

Vestibulo-Ocular Dysfunction

The vestibulo-ocular reflex (VOR) is the primary mechanism for gaze stability during head movement. During movements of the head, the VOR stabilizes gaze (eye position in space) by producing an eye movement of equal velocity and opposite direction to the head movement. The ratio of eye velocity to head velocity is referred to as the gain of the VOR. The ideal gain in a normal subject would equal 1. VOR gain has been shown to be reduced to 25 percent in human beings immediately following unilateral labyrinthine lesions for head movements toward the affected side.[2,3] During the acute stage, VOR gain will also be reduced by 50 percent for head movements to the unaffected side.

Normal functioning of the visual-oculomotor systems is also important. Saccadic and pursuit eye movements are not affected by vestibular loss. Pursuit eye movements enable the individual to visually pursue a moving object across the visual field (smooth pursuit) without making compensatory head movements. Saccadic eye movements are rapid voluntary movements that allow refoveation of stationary targets. The vestibulo-ocular and pursuit and saccade systems work cooperatively to stabilize gaze during head movements.[4]

Motion-Induced Disequilibrium

Clinically, patients complain of light-headedness or dizziness associated with particular head or body movements. Norre[5] has referred to this condition as "provoked vertigo," which is attributable to the asymmetry in the dynamic vestibular responses following a unilateral vestibular lesion. According to Norre,[5] when movements are signaled, the disturbed vestibular function produces a sensory input different from the one expected under normal conditions. The abnormal vestibular signal is in conflict with normal signals provided by the visual and somatosensory systems. This "sensory conflict" is thought to produce the symptoms associated with motion misperception.

Postural Instability

Independent and safe ambulation depends on the ability to successfully perceive the relevant features of one's environment. In addition, information about the orientation of the body with respect to the support surface and gravity is essential to postural control. Information necessary for postural control is derived from an integration of sensory inputs from the visual, somatosensory, and vestibular systems.[6]

Impairment in the function of vestibulospinal reflex (VSR) itself is believed to contribute to postural disturbances in patients with peripheral vestibular disorders. Lacour et al[7] have shown that producing a unilateral vestibular neurotomy in baboons induces asymmetrical excitability in ipsilateral and contralateral spinal reflexes. Similarly, Allum and Pfaltz,[8] using support surface rotations, reported that tibialis anterior responses in patients with unilateral peripheral vestibular deficits are enhanced contralateral to and reduced ipsilateral to the side of the lesion. These patients also had reduced neck muscle activity and greater-than-normal head angular accelerations during response to the support surface rotations.

Disturbances in VSR function may account for the locomotor disturbances reported by patients with unilateral peripheral vestibular hypofunction. These patients frequently experience gait instability in situations that require them to walk and move their head, turn, or stop quickly. In addition, clinical observation of their gait frequently reveals deviations such as veering left or right, a widened base of support, decreased gait speed, shortened step lengths, decreased arm swing, a decreased ability to perform multiple tasks while walking, occasional head or trunk tilting, or decreased head and trunk motion. Patients with severe impairments may use an assistive device to serve as a proprioceptive aid in reducing gait stability. Jeka and Lackner's work[9-11] seems to support that an assistive device is a proprioceptive aid to people with severe gait dysfunction.[9-11]

Physical Deconditioning

Changes in a patient's overall general physical condition can be considered the most potentially disabling consequence of vestibular dysfunction. Restriction in cervical range of motion is a common clinical finding in patients with vestibular hypofunction. This finding may be associated with a patient's tendency to restrict movements that potentially provoke symptoms. In addition, patients admit to adopting a more sedentary lifestyle, frequently abandoning premorbid exercise routines or recreational activities. If untreated, such changes could possibly lead to more serious physical and psychosocial consequences.

PHYSICAL THERAPY EVALUATION

History

MEDICAL

Physical therapy usually is initiated following vestibular laboratory testing and the physician's determination of the patient's diagnosis. The diagnosis, vestibular laboratory test, other diagnostic test results, and the patient's current and past medical histories are important pieces of information that should be obtained by the therapist at the initiation of the physical therapy evaluation.

Such information may assist in the identification of problems that could ultimately affect the patient's rehabilitation prognosis and outcome. For example, concurrent disease processes, such as peripheral vascular disease or peripheral neuropathy, could affect and prolong the patient's functional recovery. Diabetes, heart disease, old neck and back injuries, a history of migraines, and lung, kidney, or liver disease are examples of disorders that will affect the ability of the person to compensate for their vestibular loss.

Obtaining a complete medication history from the patient is vitally important because there are many medications that can produce or enhance dizziness (see Chapter 6). Certain medications act to reduce the patient's symptoms by depressing the vestibular system. These medications may also delay or prevent vestibular adaptation, and therefore may prolong the recovery period. Consulting with the physician is advisable to determine the possibility of reducing the dose, or eliminating the medication completely.

SUBJECTIVE HISTORY

The subjective history of the patient's condition is of critical importance in the evaluation of the patient with a peripheral vestibular problem. Questions that go beyond those usually asked by a physical therapist should be considered (see Box 15–1). The use of a questionnaire that the patient can fill out prior to the initial visit is often helpful and saves time (see Appendix 15–A). A complete description of the patient's symptoms should be documented, so that functional progress can be later assessed. Knowing what positions, movements, or situations aggravate the patient's symptoms may be of importance in treatment planning. In addition, the patient should be asked questions regarding the type, frequency, duration, and intensity of symptoms, and whether symptoms are of a fluctuating nature. Knowing the type of onset and frequency of their symptoms is very helpful in determining the physical therapy diagnosis and prognosis. Intensity of symptoms like vertigo and dysequilibrium can be measured using an analog scale similar to that used in the assessment of pain. Some therapists use a 0 to 10 scale and others use a 0 to 100 scale.[12] It is very helpful to have patients rate their symptoms, yet not all patients are able to provide a number. Those who are confused have great difficulty rating their symptoms, and family members often attempt to "help" the patient rate their sensation of dizziness, which is not helpful.

Questions related to the patient's perceived disability and psychosocial status should also be included in the initial assessment. Using the MOS 36-item short-form health survey (SF 36) is one method that could be used to determine if the patient is doing more in their home or community.[13–18] Others may use the Sickness Impact Profile or other health status measures.[19] These tools aid in determining if the patient is feeling better and is more active. Use of health status inventories is an excellent method to determine if the patient has actually improved.[20]

Many patients believe they have a psychological problem, rather than a physical one. The patient's condition is one that cannot be seen by their family and friends. Often, their condition is not well understood and has been misdiagnosed by the medical community.[21] When interacting with these patients, they must be reassured that others share their disorder. This reassurance is essential, because in some cases stress or emotional trauma magnifies symptoms (see Chapter 14). Showing them patient brochures from the Vestibular Disorders Association (VEDA) often validates their condition and they begin to understand that many other people have a similar impairment.

Several attempts have been made to define the patient's subjective symptoms of dizziness in an objective manner.[22] The Dizziness Handicap Inventory (DHI) is a useful clinical tool that can clarify the patient's symptomatic complaints and perceptions of his functional abilities (see Appendix 15–A).[22-26] Items relate to functional, emotional, and physical problems that the patient may have. This inventory can be administered quickly during the initial and discharge visits, in an attempt to quantify whether or not the patient thinks he has improved. The DHI is consistent with high test-retest reliability ($r = .97$).[21]

Shepard et al[27] have suggested the use of a disability scale to objectively document the patient's perceived level of disability (Box 15–2). There has been no published study to examine the reliability or validity of this outcome scale. The six-point scale has descriptors that range from the patient having no disability to having long-term disability. Long-term disability was defined as the inability to work for more than 1 year.[27] This scale can be incorporated into the initial and discharge physical therapy evaluations, in an attempt to document treatment outcome. The Disability Scale is also useful in predicting treatment outcome. Shepard et al[27] found that patients who rated their disability as a 4 or 5 were less likely to show significant improvement with rehabilitation.[27]

BOX 15–2 Disability Scale

Criterion	Score
Negligible symptoms	0
Bothersome symptoms	1
Performs usual work duties but symptoms interfere with outside activities	2
Symptoms disrupt performance of both usual work duties and outside activities	3
Currently on medical leave or had to change jobs because of symptoms	4
Unable to work for over 1 year or established permanent disability with compensation payments	5

Adapted from Shepard, NT, et al: Habituation and balance retraining: A retrospective review. Neurol Clin 8:459, 1990.

FALLS

Some patients with vestibular dysfunction fall. Taking a history of falls is very important because many times individuals misinterpret the question "Have you fallen?" Often when asked, patients will answer "no" but, with probing, it is common to find out that the patient has fallen. A **fall** is defined as involuntarily moving to the ground or floor. Carefully defining what a fall is with your patient will provide the therapist with better data to interpret the patient's condition. People who have fallen two or more times in the last 6 months are at high risk for falling again.[28] Other important issues include determining (1) if the patient has been injured during a fall; (2) the conditions under which the fall(s) occur; and (3) how they have modified their lifestyle after injury.

FUNCTIONAL HISTORY

To obtain a complete picture of the patient's functional status, the patient should be questioned about previous and current activity levels (Box 15–3). A history of the patient's activity level is an important component of the assessment, which often characterizes the extent of the patient's disability. There are patients who have difficulty leaving their home because exposure to highly textured visual stimulation causes disequilibrium. This common experience is referred to as the "shopping aisle syndrome." These patients may have a limited ability to interact with their environment, and over time, tend to adopt a more sedentary lifestyle. Occasionally patients will develop certain phobias associated with their symptoms including fear of elevators and heights.

PATIENT GOALS

At the beginning of the assessment, the patient should be asked about expectations of physical therapy and functional goals. When the therapist concludes the assessment, determining whether these goals are realistic and attainable, or whether they need to be mutually modified by the therapist and patient can be done. The final level of recovery for most patients with unilateral vestibular hypofunction, without other

---

BOX 15–3   Current Functional Status

Are you independent in self-care activities?
Can you drive?
  In the daytime?
  In the nighttime?
Are you working? Occupation: _____
Are you on medical disability?
Can you perform all your normal parenting activities?
Do you have difficulty
  Watching TV?
  Reading?
  Being in stores or malls?
  Being in traffic?
  Using a computer?
Do you have difficulty walking up and down ramps, stairs, walking on grass?

complications, should be a return to full activities. Conditions that may make recovery more difficult that need to be recognized when setting goals include their premorbid physical condition and their personality profile. There are occasionally patients with significant vestibular dysfunction who make remarkable gains based on their premorbid personality.

Clinical Examination

The clinical examination of a patient with vertigo and disequilibrium is usually comprehensive (Box 15–4) and therefore is time consuming. Discretion should be used as to which portions of the examination need to be performed on each patient. We describe the full examination here and have indicated, where possible, when different portions of the examination would be unnecessary. Key elements of the clinical examination are given in Box 15–5.

BOX 15–4   Summary of the Clinical Examination of the "Dizzy" Patient

Oculomotor examination

In room light
- *Nonvestibular*—extraocular movements, pursuit, saccades, VORc, diplopia.
- *Vestibular*—skew, spontaneous and gaze-evoked nystagmus, VOR to slow and rapid head thrusts, visual acuity test with head stationary and during gentle oscillations of the head.
- *With Frenzel lenses*—Spontaneous and gaze-evoked nystagmus, head shaking-induced nystagmus, tragal pressure-induced nystagmus, hyperventilation-induced nystagmus, and positional nystagmus.

Sensation

Somatosensation—proprioception, light touch, vibration; quantified tests: vibration threshold, tuning fork test.
Vision—visual acuity and field.

Coordination

Optic ataxia/past pointing, rebound, diadokokinesia, heel to shin, and postural fixation.

Range of motion: Active and passive

Upper and lower extremity, neck (rotation, extension, flexion, lateral flexion).

Strength (gross)

Grip, upper extremity, lower extremity, trunk.

Postural deviations

Scoliosis, kyphosis, lordosis.

Positional testing

Hallpike-Dix, side-lying test, roll test.

Motion sensitivity

Motion and position induced dizziness.

(Continued)

BOX 15–4   (Continued)

Sitting balance: Active or passive, anterior-posterior, and lateral

Weight shift, head righting, equilibrium reactions, upper and lower extremity, ability to recover trunk to vertical.

Static balance (performed with eyes open and closed)

Romberg, sharpened Romberg, single leg stance, stand on rail, force platform.

Balance with altered sensory cues

Eyes open and closed, foam.

Dynamic balance (self-initiated movements)

Standing reach (Duncan), Functional (Gabell and Simons), Fukuda's stepping test.

Ambulation

Normal gait, tandem walk, walk while turning head, Singleton to right and left, Dynamic Gait Index.

Functional gait assessment

Obstacle course, double-task activities, stairs, ramps, grass, sand.

BOX 15–5   Key Elements of the Clinical Examination

Oculomotor

- *In room light*—skew deviation, spontaneous and gaze-evoked nystagmus, VOR to slow and rapid head thrusts, visual acuity test with head stationary and during gentle oscillations of the head.
- *With Frenzel lenses*—Spontaneous nystagmus, positional nystagmus.

Range of motion

Neck (rotation, extension, flexion, lateral flexion).

Positional testing

Hallpike-Dix, side-lying test, roll test.

Motion sensitivity

Motion- and position-induced dizziness.

Static balance (performed with eyes open and closed)

Romberg, sharpened Romberg, single leg stance.

Balance with altered sensory cues

Eyes open and closed, foam.

Ambulation

Normal gait, tandem walk, walk while turning head, Singleton to right and left, Dynamic Gait Index.

Functional gait assessment

Obstacle course, double-task activities, stairs, ramps, grass, sand.

OCULOMOTOR AND VESTIBULO-OCULAR TESTING

The interaction of the patient's visual and vestibular systems is tested clinically by having the patient perform combinations of head and eye movements. The oculomotor examination is one part of the overall assessment of the "dizzy" patient that may have been performed by a neurologist or otolaryngologist prior to referral for physical therapy and is therefore not always included in the physical therapy assessment.

First, the patient is observed for the presence of *spontaneous nystagmus* in room light. In patients with unilateral peripheral vestibular hypofunction, spontaneous nystagmus will be observable in room light during the acute stage after onset of the lesion. Spontaneous nystagmus occurs because of an imbalance in the tonic or resting firing rate of the vestibular neurons. Within a few days the patient should suppress the nystagmus with visual fixation. Patients in this acute stage often complain of having difficulty reading and watching television.

Smooth pursuit is tested by asking the patient to track a moving object with his or her eyes while the head is stationary. This tracking test should assess the patient's entire visual field. Typically performed in an H-like pattern, this test also assesses the motor function of cranial nerves III, IV, and VI. Inability to perform downgaze is not a sign of vestibular deficits, but can occur with other neurological problems (e.g., progressive supranuclear palsy). Patients with this problem may have difficulty seeing objects on the ground as they walk. During the test of smooth-pursuit eye movements, the presence of *gaze-evoked nystagmus* and the quality of the eye movement should be noted. Saccadic pursuit, especially in younger individuals, or asymmetric pursuit, should be noted. For the patient with nystagmus, however, determining the quality of pursuit eye movements may be difficult. Care must be taken to distinguish gaze-evoked nystagmus from end-point nystagmus. Gaze-evoked nystagmus occurs when the eyes are 30° eccentric. Direction changing, gaze-evoked nystagmus is a sign of a central lesion. End-point nystagmus, which is normal, occurs when the eyes are at the extreme end of their range of motion. It is also important to determine if the patient has any premorbid eye pathology in the initial patient history, including asking about a history of strabismus. Patients with "lazy eye" disorders will have difficulty with smooth pursuit, which can confound the results of the testing.

Patients can also be tested for *ocular alignment*, particularly for skew deviations that can occur during the acute stage of a unilateral vestibular loss. Skew deviations, in which the eye opposite the side of the lesion is elevated, occur because of the loss of the tonic otolith input from one side. Normally, the tonic input holds the eyes level within the orbit; when there is a unilateral loss, the eye on the side of the lesion drops in the orbit and the patient complains of vertical diplopia. By convention, the skew is named by the side of the elevated eye (e.g., right hypertropia means the right eye is elevated, but, in reality, the left eye has dropped).

Saccadic eye movements are tested by simply asking the patient to look back and forth between two horizontal or two vertical targets. In normal individuals, the target can be reached with a single eye movement or with one small corrective saccade.

The patient can then be asked to voluntarily fixate on a moving target while the head is moved in the same direction. This procedure tests *vestibulo-ocular cancellation* (VORc) and is a function of the parietal lobe. Results should agree with the observations made during the smooth-pursuit test.

Next, the VOR itself is tested. The patient is asked to fixate on a stationary target and the head is gently turned several times first horizontally (horizontal canal function) and then vertically (vertical canal function). This procedure should be performed passively, first with slow head movements and then with unpredictable small-amplitude, rapid head thrusts. People without vestibular pathology will be able to maintain fixation during both slow and rapid head movements. People with vestibular deficits often are able to maintain fixation during slow head movements but will make corrective saccades to regain the target with rapid head movements. During the acute stage or with severe deficits, corrective saccades will occur even with slow head rotations.

Another measure of VOR function is to measure the *degradation of visual acuity* that occurs with head movement. In the clinical dynamic visual acuity test, the patient is first asked to read a wall eye chart with the head stationary (we use a modified ETDRS chart with SLOAN letters, Lighthouse Distance Visual Acuity Tests, Long Island City, New York). Then the patient is asked to read the chart while the head is gently oscillated at 2 Hz. Using a metronome helps to standardize the test. In normal individuals, visual acuity changes at most by one line. In patients with uncompensated, unilateral vestibular loss, visual acuity will degrade by three or four lines.

Eye movements can also be observed using *Frenzel lenses*. These magnifying glasses, with light inside them, enable the clinician to observe eye movements but at the same time greatly decrease the patient's ability to stabilize the eyes with visual fixation. Clinical assessment of oculomotor function using Frenzel lenses should include spontaneous and gaze-evoked nystagmus, head-shaking–induced nystagmus, tragal-pressure–induced nystagmus, hyperventilation-induced nystagmus, and positional nystagmus (see Chapter 6).

During this assessment, the patient is asked to report any symptoms of blurred vision or dizziness. Tests that involve repeated head movements (VOR, head-shaking–induced nystagmus) may increase the patient's symptoms. If there is a significant increase in symptoms, the patient may be unable or may refuse to continue with the testing.

SENSORY EVALUATION

Sensation of the extremities and trunk is tested to rule out concurrent pathology and assist in treatment planning. Proprioception, vibration sense, light touch, and pain are tested. Perhaps the most important of these is the assessment of kinesthesia and proprioception, although profound sensory loss affecting touch and pressure sensitivity would obviously affect postural stability.

Proprioception can be assessed by moving the great toes either up or down and asking the patient to identify the position of the toe. Care must be taken to make these relatively small movements or the test becomes too easy. The patient must also be instructed not to guess at the answer. This traditional test of proprioception does not appear to be very sensitive, and patients are quite accurate in perceiving whether the toe is up or down even when other tests indicate sensory deficiencies. *Kinesthesia* can be tested by slowly moving the toe either up or down and asking the patient to state the direction of the movement as soon as they first perceive movement. Again, the patient should be instructed not to guess. Perception of the direction of the movement should occur before the toe is moved more than 10° to 15°, although each clinician will have to develop his or her own internal standard for what is normal. *Vibration* can be tested using a tuning fork applied to a bony prominence. One method is to ask the patient to identify when the vibratory sensation stops, and then to dampen the tuning fork unexpectedly. Another method is to let the vibration diminish naturally and to time the difference between when the patient and the clinician stop feeling the vibration. Again, each clinician will have to develop his or her own sense of normal. Devices are also available that quantify vibration thresholds. These devices enable the clinician to compare the patient with age-matched normal subjects and to follow changes over time.

Visual acuity should be assessed in the clinic using an ETDRS chart. A hand-held Snellen card is not as appropriate because it measures the patient's vision at a distance of only 18 inches, at which distance older patients in particular will have difficulty accommodating. Brandt et al[29] suggest that distance acuity of poorer than 20/50 will have a significant effect on postural stability. Additionally, *visual field* loss can also affect balance[30] and patients with monocular vision may have particular difficulty with depth perception affecting their ability to walk up and down stairs.

The visual, vestibular, and somatosensory systems all show decrements with age, and the clinician should be familiar with these normal changes to differentiate them from pathological changes.[31] Furthermore, certain disorders that can affect perception, such as cataract formation, are more likely to occur in the older person. There is some evidence that a decrease in the gain of the VOR occurs with aging, at least at higher frequencies, and there is a more limited adaptive capability.[3,32]

Multisystem involvement can impede the patient's functional progress. A patient with reduced vestibular function and a deficit in somatosensory cues is likely to compensate by using visual mechanisms. This patient will be limited functionally if placed in a situation void of visual information. For example, many patients with reduced somatosensory cues and a peripheral vestibular deficit have difficulty walking in the dark. A treatment plan that does not consider the patient's sensory loss may be ineffectual and the patient's functional independence could suffer.

COORDINATION

Vestibular deficits per se do not result in poor coordination or in limb ataxia. Assessment of coordination is especially important, however, as part of the preoperative and postoperative examination of patients with cerebellar angle tumors. Finger-to-nose, heel-to-shin, and the ability to perform rapid alternating movements of fingers or feet are gross tests that may be used to subjectively assess the patient's coordination. Other tests of cerebellar function might include truncal stability and tests of tone, such as postural fixation and the rebound phenomenon.

RANGE OF MOTION/STRENGTH

The patient's range of motion and strength must be assessed in the initial evaluation. Although the neck, trunk, and extremities can be included in this assessment, special attention should be paid to neck range of motion. Patients in whom head movement exacerbates symptoms may voluntarily restrict active neck motion and may eventually lose range of motion. Furthermore, many of the other assessments involve passive movement of the neck (VOR during rapid head thrusts, head-shaking–induced nystagmus, positional testing) and any limitations in movement or pain associated with neck movement should be identified before attempting those tests. In some patients, when neck range of motion increases, there appears to be an associated decrease in dizziness symptoms. A detailed examination of extremity strength and range of motion is often unnecessary; however, a quick screen can indicate whether more detailed testing would be appropriate. It is not uncommon in the elderly to see weakness distally that can be recognized in this quick screening and dealt with through use of a home exercise program to "tune up" the system and decrease their risk of falling.

POSTURAL EXAMINATION

In addition to assessment of range of motion, the patient's posture should be evaluated. Predisposing orthopedic conditions or postural deviations may complicate the rehabilitation prognosis. Anterior-posterior and medial-lateral views of both the patient's sitting and standing postures should be assessed. Typically, posture is not affected in people with peripheral vestibular dysfunction. Postural abnormalities are more commonly seen in people with central disorders of the nervous system.

POSITIONAL AND MOVEMENT TESTING

Clinically assessing the positions and movements that provoke the patient's symptoms is important. In this portion of the evaluation, attempts are made to replicate the various positions and movements experienced by the patient throughout the

TABLE 15–1 Typical Positions and Movements*

Baseline Symptoms	Intensity	Duration	Score
1. Sitting to supine			
2. Supine to left side			
3. Supine to right side			
4. Supine to sitting			
5. Left Hallpike-Dix			
6. Return to sit from left Hallpike-Dix			
7. Right Hallpike-Dix			
8. Return to sit from right Hallpike-Dix			
9. Sitting, head tipped to left knee			
10. Head up from left knee			
11. Sitting, head tipped to right knee			
12. Head up from right knee			
13. Sitting, turn head horizontally 5 times			
14. Sitting, move head vertically 5 times (pitch)			
15. Standing, turn 180° to the right			
16. Standing, turn 180° to the left			

*See chapter 23 for further information.

day (Table 15–1). The activities are rated by the patient as to whether they provoke no symptoms or mild, moderate, or severe symptoms. In some situations, the patient may be unable, or unwilling, to perform the task. This reluctance is especially apparent in the patient who develops severe dizziness early in the evaluation. In addition, a patient may refuse to move into or out of a specific posture because of the fear of eliciting symptoms. Every effort should be made to test the patient using those particular positional changes.

One of the most important positional tests is the *Hallpike-Dix maneuver* (Fig. 15–1). This test is most commonly utilized in patients who complain of vertigo only when they move into certain positions, but should be included in almost all assessments. Vertigo and nystagmus occurring when the patient is moved into the Hallpike-Dix position is used to diagnose benign paroxysmal positional vertigo (see Chapter 19). In the Hallpike-Dix maneuver, the patient typically sits with the head turned to one side. The patient then is moved quickly backward so that the head is extended over the end of the table approximately 30° below horizontal. The maneuver is performed to both the right and left sides. The patient should be cautioned in advance that the maneuver can

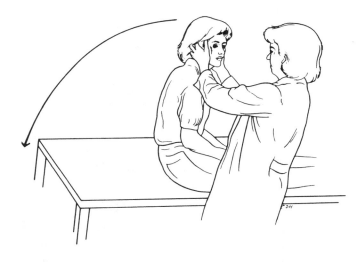

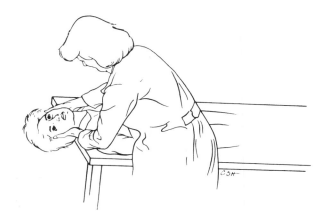

FIGURE 15–1. Hallpike-Dix maneuver used primarily to test for benign paroxysmal positional vertigo. The head is turned to one side and the patient is moved from sitting into a supine position with the head hanging over the end of the table. The patient is then observed for nystagmus, and complaints of vertigo are noted. The patient is then returned to the upright position. (From Physical Therapy 70:381–388, 1990, with permission.)

cause dizziness or vertigo but, nonetheless, should be performed. Two variations of the Hallpike-Dix test, the side lying test and the roll test, should also be performed (see Chapter 19). It is also important to perform the Hallpike-Dix maneuver because some patients will present without a specific diagnosis (i.e., dizziness or vertigo) and after performing the Hallpike maneuver, it is obvious that the patient has benign paroxysmal positional nystagmus.[33] Recognizing benign paroxysmal positional nystagmus and providing the proper intervention can significantly enhance the patient's quality of life.

Benign paroxysmal positional vertigo (BPPV) is a common cause of vertigo. This peripheral vestibular deficit is easily and effectively treated by physical therapy and therefore it should be distinguished from vertebral artery problems (see Chapter 19). Although relatively rare, vertebral artery compression can be distinguished from positional vertigo. One way to distinguish between vertebral artery compression and positional vertigo is to perform the vertebral artery test with the patient sitting and leaning forward slightly. In this position, when the head is extended and turned (the head ends up in an upright position), the posterior canal on that side would not be affected by the pull of gravity. Occlusion of blood flow with compression of the vertebral artery produces other neurological symptoms, such as numbness, weakness, slurred speech, and mental confusion as well as vertigo and nystagmus.

Examples of other movements that can be tested include rolling, supine to sit, reaching in sitting toward the floor, and sit to stand. All of these movements should be tested at various speeds, and with the eyes open and closed. The therapist should exercise care with the standing maneuver with the eyes closed because this is often very difficult for patients and may cause them to lose their balance.

The speed of the activity will often affect the patient's symptoms. For example, a quickly performed movement could increase the patient's symptoms, whereas the same movement done at a slower speed may not. Varying the speed and the conditions under which the patient performs the task may affect the patient's functional ability. Positional and movement testing is limited only by the imagination of the therapist. In one patient seen in the clinic, the only position that increased her symptoms was the all fours position, looking under the bed (Fig. 15–2)!

In addition to testing positions and movements that incorporate multiple body segments, the patient is asked to perform head movements. The head movements are typically tested with the patient sitting. These movements are performed at various speeds and with the eyes open and closed. The patient is asked to report if these movements provoke symptoms, and whether the symptoms are of a mild, moderate, or severe intensity. The same movements are tested in the standing position, if the patient can tolerate further testing.

Balance Assessment

SITTING BALANCE

Although many patients with chronic vestibular disorders do not have difficulty with balance in sitting, for some patients including an assessment of sitting balance may be appropriate. Patients should be tested while they are leaning anteriorly and posteriorly as well as right and left; tests should be performed both actively and passively. The patient can be observed for weight-shifting ability, head righting, equilib-

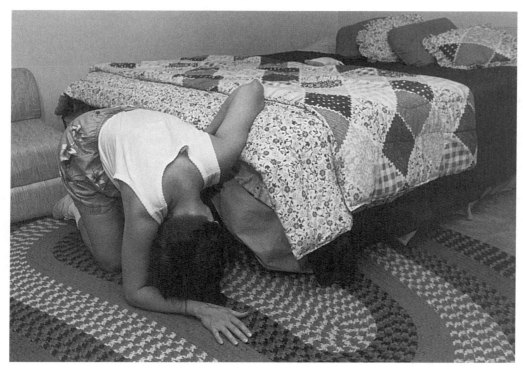

FIGURE 15–2. Patients may experience dizziness or vertigo in positions other than those normally tested. Shown here is the provoking position for one patient who experienced vertigo only when bending over and turning her head.

rium reactions in the upper and lower extremities, and the ability to recover to a trunk vertical position. Having the patient reach in sitting is also valuable information that can be gained in the clinical examination.

STATIC BALANCE

Static balance tasks have been used clinically in an attempt to objectively document balance function.[34–37] Single leg stance (SLS), Romberg, and the sharpened or tandem Romberg are often included in a static balance test battery and can be performed with eyes open or eyes closed.[38–40] Traditionally, the variable of interest in this testing has been the time that the patient maintains the position. Normative data for timed tests have been established for SLS, Romberg, and sharpened Romberg tests.[38] The Romberg test has been shown to have low intrasubject variability when measures are repeated over a 5-day period.[39]

We should remember that patients with vestibular deficits may have normal performance on these tests.[40–42] Tests of static balance, such as the Romberg, are fairly easy. Patients may have difficulty with this test only during the acute stage following onset of their vestibular deficit. Of additional importance is remembering that patients with balance disorders other than from vestibular dysfunction may have difficulty with these tests. Having difficulty maintaining stance with the Romberg test does not necessarily mean the subject has vestibular dysfunction. Table 15–2 gives the expected re-

TABLE 15–2 Expected Test Results in Patients with Unilateral Vestibular Loss

Test	Acute UVL	Compensated UVL
Nystagmus	Spontaneous and gaze-evoked in light and dark; head shaking induced increases nystagmus	Spontaneous in dark; may have head-shaking induced
VOR	Abnormal with both slow and rapid head thrusts	Abnormal with rapid head thrusts toward side of lesion
Romberg	Often, but not always positive	Negative
Sharpened Romberg	Cannot perform	Normal with eyes open; cannot perform with eyes closed
Single leg stance	Cannot perform	Normal
CSTIB—foam, eyes closed	Most cannot perform	Normal
Fukuda's stepping tets	Cannot perform	Normal
Gait	Wide-based, slow cadence, decreased rotation, may need help for a few days	Normal
Turn head while walking	Cannot keep balance	Normal; some may slow cadence

sults for static and dynamic balance tests in patients with acute and compensated unilateral vestibular loss.

MEASURES OF SWAY

During performance of static balance tasks, medial-lateral or anterior-posterior stability can be objectively documented using "high-tech" tools such as force platforms or using simple tools such as a sway grid.[43–44] When assessing and attempting to replicate standing sway measures, the distance the subject stands from a stable visual target, upper extremity positioning, type or lack of footwear, and foot position of the patient should be standardized. Brandt hypothesizes that one explanation for the variability often found on the Romberg test is the inconsistent positioning of the patient with respect to a target used for visual fixation.[29] The distance that the patient stands from the target should be standardized and should be within 1.5 meters. Kirby et al[45] employed five different foot positions to determine the effect of foot position on sway. They determined that subjects, standing in double limb stance, were most stable in the 25°, toe-out position. In addition, they observed that subjects had the greatest medial-lateral sway when their feet closely approximated each other. The standard Romberg position is with heel and toes together.

Postural sway correlates well with measures of the DHI.[23,25,46] Of course, both postural sway and the responses to the DHI questionnaire are under "voluntary control," and what is measured is subject to errors according to what the patient wants to convey. Nevertheless, patients who report the greatest disability on the DHI as a result of their dizziness also demonstrate the highest measures of sway on posturography.[46] Furthermore, the sway patterns of patients with central pathology differed from that of patients with other vestibular diagnoses. Yoneda[47] also reported that sway patterns seem to be different between patients with Ménière's disease, BPPV, vestibular neuronitis and that these patterns differed from those of a normal comparison group.

ALTERING SENSORY CUES

The modified Clinical Test for Sensory Interaction in Balance (CTSIB) should included in the rehabilitation assessment.[48,49] In some ways this test is an extension of the Romberg test, which assessed the effect of removing visual cues on postural stability. Referred to formerly as the "foam and dome" test (Fig. 15–3), the CTSIB assesses the influence of vestibular, somatosensory, and visual inputs on postural control. In the modified version, the "dome" portion of the test is no longer used. In the modified CSTIB, standing on the foam surface and closing the eyes alters somatosensory input and eliminates visual input. In this situation, vestibular input is the most accurate information regarding postural stability. Patients with uncompensated unilateral peripheral vestibular loss may have difficulty maintaining an upright posture when both visual and support-surface information are altered.[6] Subjects with unilateral peripheral vestibular dysfunction often lose their balance when standing on foam with eyes closed using the CTSIB protocol. According to Nashner,[6] symmetry and constancy of vestibular information is critical in providing an absolute reference for reorganization of senses in conflicting conditions. The inability of the vestibular system to provide this information may explain why patients with unilateral vestibular lesions often report postural instability when riding on an escalator or when walking on thick carpet across a dimly lit room. If a patient is unstable when both visual and somatosensory cues are altered, a treatment plan might be designed to improve the function of the remaining vestibular system. Depending on the patient, an alternative treatment strat-

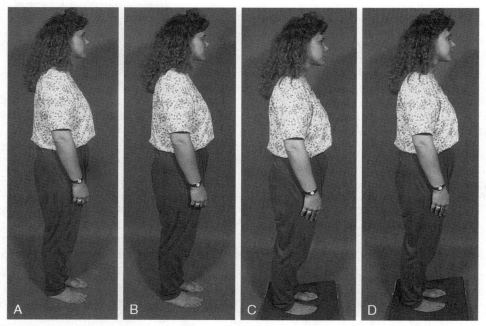

FIGURE 15–3. The modified Clinical Test of Sensory Integration of Balance: The subject is standing on a level support surface with eyes open (*A*), with eyes closed (*B*), a compliant surface with eyes open (*C*), and a compliant surface with eyes closed (*D*). The time the patient performs each task is recorded and the amount of sway and the patient's movement strategy are documented qualitatively. The results of this test help determine if the patient is dependent on certain sensory cues.

egy may focus on altering the patient's environment, so that visual and somatosensory cues are maximized in an effort to overcome the vestibular loss.

SELF-INITIATED MOVEMENTS

In addition to static tests of balance function, self-initiated movements and dynamic tests of balance should be examined. Self-initiated weight shifts performed in different directions can be assessed to determine if the patient moves freely and symmetrically. Self-initiated movements should also be tested in functionally relevant and rich contexts, for example, having the patient reach to pick an object from the floor or placing an object on a high shelf. Altering the environment so that there are many visual distractions may also be a way to make the task more difficult. Reaching for an object on the floor among many objects on the floor might make the task more difficult for the patient.

The standing reach test has been developed as a way to assess balance and willingness to reach outside of the subject's base of support.[50-54] This test functionally and reliably documents performance on a self-initiated task. The subject is asked to reach as far forward as possible. The extent of movement is measured using a simple yard stick (Fig. 15–4). Duncan et al[50] have shown that functional reach, as a measure of a

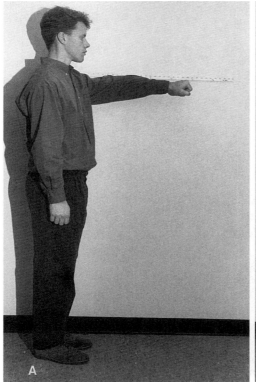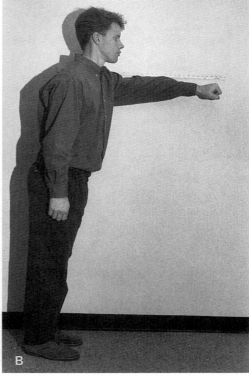

FIGURE 15–4. The distance a patient can reach is one measure of functional balance.[50] The patient's acromion is lined up with the yardstick while the patient's arm is held parallel to the yardstick (*A*). The patient reaches forward as far as possible, while keeping both feet flat on the ground (*B*).

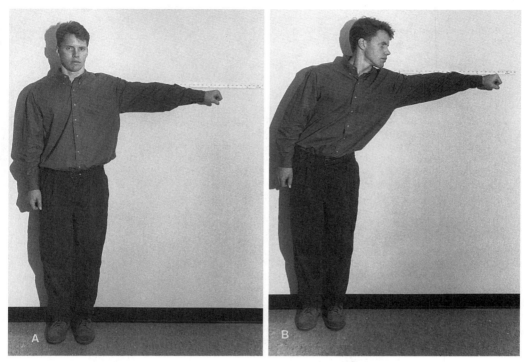

FIGURE 15–5. The distance a patient can reach to the side is another possible functional measure of balance. The patient's acromion is lined up with the edge of the yardstick (*A*). The patient reaches to the side as far as possible, while keeping both feet flat on the floor (*B*).

subject's margin of stability, correlates well with center of pressure measures obtained from a force platform. This test might be modified so that reaches in different directions are documented (Fig. 15–5). Functional reach has also been shown to be related to falls in older male veterans.[51] Generally scores of 6 inches or less indicate that the person is at high risk for falling.[51] It has been shown to have concurrent validity with certain items of the Functional Independence Measure and is useful in determining the risk of falling in older adults. It has also been shown to demonstrate change over the course of rehabilitation.[53]

Gabell and Simons[55] also developed a functional balance test to assess elderly clients at risk for falling. Their assessment examines static positions, and rotational and sagittal movements (Box 15–6) and includes criteria for successful performance of each task. For example, to succeed in one of the rotational stress tasks, the patient must rotate 360° once without staggering or grabbing onto furniture.

Fukuda's stepping test assesses stability during the self-initiated movement of marching which the patient performs first with eyes open and then with eyes closed.[56,57] The test is easily administered in the clinic and can be quantified by using a polar coordinate grid placed on the floor (Fig. 15–6). The test is not specific for vestibular dysfunction, but patients with unilateral vestibular deficits often turn excessively when stepping with the eyes closed.[56] When performing the Fukuda step test, there appear to be many false positives and negatives, so it is important to consider the results as only one aspect of the clinical picture of the patient.

BOX 15–6   Balance Coding
_____

1. Static Stress
    Unsafe while seated   0
    Safe while seated, unsafe standing   1
    Steady while standing for 20 sec with aid   2
    Steady while standing, 20 sec, no aid, wide base   3
    Steady while standing, 20 sec, no aid, narrow base   4
    Steady while standing, 20 sec, no aid, long base   5
    Steady while standing, 20 sec, no aid, long base,
        eyes closed   6
2. Rotational stress
    For those who can stand for 20 sec with or without aid.
    Subject should stand with feet in most stable position.
    Steady while turning head from right to left.   a
    (Tested three times, 5 seconds of rest between each trial)
    Can turn 360° without staggering or grabbing onto
        furniture.   b
3. Sagittal stress
    Subject can arise from chair (with help if necessary),
        is immediately steady and can stand for 20 sec without
        help except for aid if uses one.   x
    (no code given if cannot perform)
4. Directional Preponderance
    Coded if subject tends to fall or overbalance in one
        direction consistently during the above tests.
        Anterior _____ (A) Posterior _____ (P) Right _____ (R) Left _____ (L)

Modified from Gabell, A, and Simons, MA.[55]

The standing reach test,[50] Gabell and Simon's functional assessment[55] and Fukuda's stepping test[56] are administered easily and require very little equipment. Such functional measures of balance can easily be used in the clinic or home care setting to document that the patient has made gains in physical therapy.

MOVEMENT STRATEGY

During the balance assessment, the therapist should observe and document the patient's movement strategy. Three types of movement strategies have been described for controlling anterior-posterior displacements of the center of mass.[58] The *ankle strategy* produces shifts in the center of mass via rotation of the body about the ankle joints. According to Horak and Nashner,[58] the ankle strategy elicits a distal-to-proximal firing pattern of ankle, hip, and trunk musculature. This activation pattern exerts compensatory ankle torques, which are believed to correct for small postural perturbations. The *hip strategy* controls movement of the center of mass by flexing and extending the hips. Unlike the ankle strategy, the muscle activation sequence associated with the hip strategy occurs in a proximal-to-distal fashion. This strategy produces a compensatory horizontal shear force against the support surface. The hip strategy occurs in situations where the ankle is unable to exert the appropriate torque necessary to restore balance. This situation arises when the task of maintaining balance is more difficult, such as when an individual stands on a small, narrow support surface. Finally, a *stepping strat-*

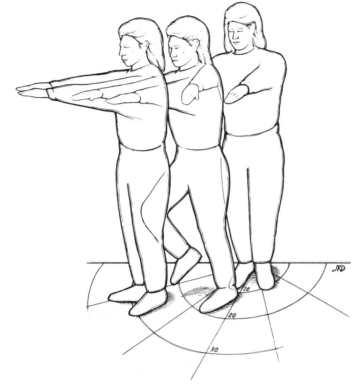

FIGURE 15–6. Fukuda's stepping test assesses balance while the patient marches in place first with eyes open and then with eyes closed. The forward progression of the patient as well as the degree and direction of turning are recorded. Normal subjects will have moved forward less than 50 cm and turned less than 30° at the end of 50 steps. Patients with unilateral vestibular deficits often turn excessively. A polar coordinate grid, placed on the floor, enables easy scoring of the subject's response.

egy is used when the center of mass is displaced outside the base of support. This strategy is employed in response to fast, large postural perturbations.

To function safely and independently throughout the lifespan, humans are required to respond, through their movements, to a variety of task situations and environmental contexts. We should logically assume that postural strategies could be task specific, and therefore categorizing them may prove to be difficult. In addition, individuals vary greatly with respect to body size, proportion, and weight. These considerations, taken together with age-related changes, make the task of categorizing postural strategies difficult. Instead, the physical therapist may be more successful in documenting whether the patient's individual strategy is efficient, safe, and successful with respect to achieving the task goal. With this approach, the clinician's expectations of the patient's responses are not as biased. This notion also has implications for treatment. Current motor learning theory suggests that the learner will be more successful in the task when the learner, not the teacher or therapist, selects the appropriate movement strategy.[59]

Gait Evaluation

Evaluation of the patient's gait provides a dynamic and functional assessment of the patient's postural control mechanism. The gait assessment can be obtained through clinical observation, videotape analysis, or computerized motion analysis. A videotape record of the patient's gait is easily obtained clinically and can be extremely useful for documentation and patient education.

The patient's gait should be assessed in as many situations as are realistically accessible to the therapist. Analysis of the patient walking down a crowded versus a noncrowded hallway may yield very different information about the patient's gait function. Similarly, the patient should be instructed to walk at a normal speed, slowly, and quickly. Common clinical observations indicate that patients with vestibular disorders, like other patients, have greater gait instability when asked to walk at a nonpreferred speed. They also often have difficulty with changing gait speed while they are walking.

During gait assessment, the physical therapist documents the patient's movement strategy, the presence of gait deviations, and whether the patient reports any abnormal sensation of movement. The patient with a peripheral vestibular disorder may select an overall strategy for gait that limits movement of their head and trunk. Clinically, this gait is characterized as being stiff or robotlike, and the patient may use excessive visual fixation while walking. Some of the typical gait deviations demonstrated by these patients include inconsistent step lengths, veering to the right or left, a widened base of support, a listing of the head and/or trunk to one side, decreased rotation through the trunk and neck (and decreased arm swing), and "en bloc" and slow turns. In addition to observable gait deviations, patients with a unilateral peripheral vestibulopathy may associate dizziness with their gait instability.

A complete assessment of the patient's gait function should include having the patient perform a variety of tasks while walking. Many of these tasks will cause the patient to lose balance; therefore, during this portion of the gait assessment, the physical therapist may need to guard the patient but without becoming a part of the patient's postural control system. The goal of this assessment is to learn how the patient, not the therapist, solves the problem of postural control.

One of the gait tasks performed by the patient is to walk while moving the head, either to the left and right or up and down. The therapist documents whether the patient experiences symptoms (dizziness, light-headedness, etc.), loss of balance, or an exaggeration of gait deviations. Such a detailed assessment facilitates documentation of the patient's progress.

Many patients with unilateral peripheral vestibular loss experience difficulty when asked to perform gait tasks that require an anticipatory mode of motor control. One such task requires the patient to walk quickly and then to stop immediately on the therapist's command. To enhance task difficulty, the patient may be asked to perform the same task with eyes closed. Another such task, called the Singleton test, requires the patient to walk quickly and pivot to the right or left immediately on the therapist's command. To maintain a level of uncertainty, the patient should not be informed ahead of time of the required pivot direction. The speed of the pivot is another factor that must be considered. The patient may also slow gait speed as a strategy to avoid disequilibrium during the task. The patient may also slow gait speed to avoid the anticipatory requirements of the task. In such instances, the patient should perform the task at a faster speed, so that the therapist obtains a more complete picture of the patient's gait function.

Observing the ability of the patient to negotiate an obstacle course may also provide the therapist with valuable information about the patient's functional balance (Fig. 15–7). An assessment of the patient's ability to function in an anticipatory mode of control can be obtained. To assess the patient's ability, the patient self selects the path

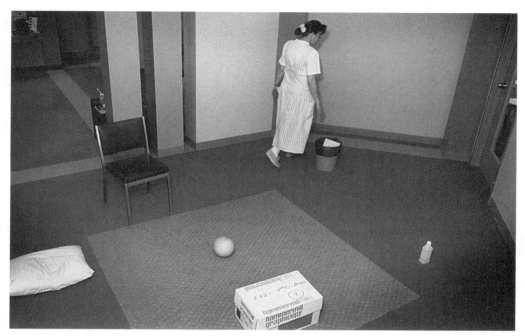

FIGURE 15–7. Patients with vestibular disorders may have difficulty negotiating an obstacle course. The patient selects the path of the course to follow and whether to step over or pick up objects.

to negotiate the obstacle course. In addition, the patient decides whether or not to pick up or step over an object in the course. The patient also decides to negotiate the course quickly or slowly. If, on the other hand, the patient's anticipatory control is of interest, the therapist directs which path the patient should follow. Task variability and uncertainty is manipulated by the therapist. For example, the therapist decides at which point in the course to throw a ball toward the patient (Fig. 15–8). A temporal constraint may also be added to the task. Asking the patient to negotiate the course as quickly as possible enhances task difficulty and provides a means to subjectively document the patient's progress.

The ability of the patient to perform gait tasks while manipulating an object with the hands should also be assessed. Patients with unilateral vestibular loss frequently complain of increased gait instability when carrying a basket of laundry up a flight of stairs or when carrying a bag of groceries. Clinically, the patient's ability to monitor postural control while manipulating an object can be tested in a variety of ways. The patient can be asked to walk, pick up one or more objects off of the floor, and continue walking. Documenting the strategy used by the patient to perform this task is important. Many patients with vestibular loss will bend at the knees and avoid flexing the head or bending at the hips. This strategy may be selected in an attempt to minimize provocation of symptoms or loss of balance. A patient may also be asked to negotiate a flight of stairs while carrying objects of varying weight or size. This task is important to include in the gait assessment, because a patient who demonstrates little difficulty with other gait tasks may express extreme postural instability with this task.

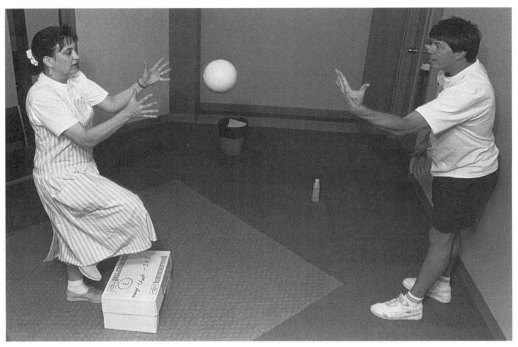

FIGURE 15–8. The obstacle course can also be used to determine how well the patient responds to external perturbations. In this situation, the patient maintains postural control, while simultaneously stepping over a box and catching a ball.

Other gait tasks that can be assessed by the therapist include sidestepping, backward walking, tandem walking, walking in a figure of eight, and marching and/or jogging in place. If feasible, the patient should be asked to perform these tasks at various speeds with the eyes open and eyes closed.

There are additional tests that can be used to assess functional balance in subjects with peripheral vestibular dysfunction. The Dynamic Gait Index, as developed by Shumway-Cook et al,[60,61] is very helpful in quantifying gait dysfunction in people with vestibular disease (Box 15–7). It is an 8-item test that takes less than 10 minutes to perform and requires little equipment (a shoebox, two cones, and stairs). Scoring is based on the concept of no, minimal, moderate, or severe gait dysfunction while performing the eight gait tasks. It has been related to scores on the Berg Balance Scale, which is a tool to assess balance.[60] Scores of 19 or less on the Dynamic Gait Index have been related to falls in older community living elderly adults. In patients with severe vestibular disability, we have seen scores as low as 3 out of 24! The Dynamic Gait Index is very useful for quantifying gait dysfunction in people with vestibular dysfunction and can be easily used as a method of determining if the therapy intervention is effective.

The Berg Balance Scale is also a useful tool to use if the patient has balance dysfunction.[62–66] Not all patients with peripheral vestibular disorders have balance disorders.[67] Scores of 36 and less on this test indicate a 100 percent risk of falling in older adults.[60] The Berg Balance Scale consists of 14 items that include sitting, standing, and reaching activities with a total point value of 56. It has been shown to be a reliable and valid test with many different patient populations and is very useful in assessing change in a patient's balance over time.[62–66,68]

BOX 15–7   Dynamic Gait Index

---

1. Gait Level Surface

   Instructions: Walk at your normal speed from here to next mark (20′).
   Grading: Mark the lowest category that applies.
   - **Normal:** Walks 20′, no assistive devices, good speed, no evidence for imbalance, normal gait pattern.
   - **Mild impairment:** Walks 20′, uses assistive devices, slower speed, mild gait deviations.
   - **Moderate impairment:** Walks 20′, slow speed, abnormal gait pattern, evidence for imbalance.
   - **Severe impairment:** Cannot walk 20′without assistance, severe gait deviations, or imbalance.

2. Change in gait speed

   Instructions: Begin walking at your normal pace (for 5′), when I tell you "go," walk as fast as you can for 5′. When I tell you "slow," walk as slowly as you can (for 5′).
   Grading: Mark the lowest category that applies.
   - **Normal:** Able to smoothly change walking speed without loss of balance or gait deviation. Shows a significant difference in walking speeds between normal, fast, and slow speeds.
   - **Mild impairment:** Is able to change speed but demonstrates mild gait deviations, or no gait deviations but unable to achieve a significant change in velocity, or uses assistive device.
   - **Moderate impairment:** Makes only minor adjustments to walking speed, or accomplishes a change in speed with significant gait deviations, or changes speed but has significant gait deviations, or changes speed but loses balance but is able to recover and continue walking.
   - **Severe impairment:** Cannot change speeds, or loses balance and has to reach for wall or be caught.

3. Gait with horizontal head turns

   Instructions: Begin walking at your normal pace. When I tell you to "look right," keep walking straight, but turn your head to the right. Keep looking to the right until I tell you "look left," then keep walking straight and turn your head to the left. Keep your head to the left until I tell you, "look straight," then keep walking straight but return your head to the center.
   Grading: Mark the lowest category that applies.
   - **Normal:** Performs head turns smoothly with no change in gait.
   - **Mild impairment:** Performs head turns smoothly with slight change in gait velocity (i.e., minor disruption to smooth gait path or uses walking aid).
   - **Moderate impairment:** Performs head turns with moderate change in gait velocity, slows down, staggers but recovers, can continue to walk.
   - **Severe impairment:** Performs task with severe disruptions of gait (i.e., staggers outside 15° path, loses balance, stops, reaches for wall).

4. Gait with vertical head turns

   Instructions: Begin walking at your normal pace. When I tell you to "look up," keep walking straight, but tip your head and look up. Keep looking up until I tell you, "look down." Then keep walking straight and turn your head down. Keep looking down until I tell you, "look straight," then keep walking straight, but return your head to the center.
   Grading: Mark the lowest category that applies.
   - **Normal:** Performs head turns with no change in gait.

(Continued)

BOX 15–7   (Continued)

- **Mild impairment:** Performs task with slight change in gait velocity (i.e., minor disruption to smooth gait path or uses walking aid).
- **Moderate impairment:** Performs tasks with moderate change in gait velocity, slows down, staggers but recovers, can continue to walk.
- **Severe impairment:** Performs task with severe disruption or gait (i.e., staggers outside 15" path, loses balance, stops reaches for wall).

5. Gait and pivot turn

Instructions: Begin walking at your normal pace. When I tell you, "turn and stop," turn as quickly as you can to face the opposite direction and stop.
Grading: Mark the lowest category that applies.

- **Normal:** Pivot turns safely within 3 seconds and stops quickly with no loss of balance.
- **Mild impairment:** Pivot turns safely in >3 seconds and stops with no loss of balance.
- **Moderate impairment:** Turns slowly, requires verbal cuing, requires several small steps to catch balance following turn and stop.
- **Severe impairment:** Cannot turn safely, requires assistance to turn and stop.

6. Step over obstacle

Instructions: Begin walking at your normal speed. When you come to the shoe box, step over it, not around it, and keep walking.
Grading: Mark the lowest category that applies.

- **Normal:** Is able to step over box without changing gait speed; no evidence for imbalance.
- **Mild impairment:** Is able to step over box, but must slow down and adjust steps to clear box safely.
- **Moderate impairment:** Is able to step over box but must stop, then step over. May require verbal cuing.
- **Severe impairment:** Cannot perform without assistance.

7. Step around obstacles

Instructions: Begin walking at your normal speed. When you come to the first cone (about 6' away), walk around the right side of it. When you come to the second cone (6' past first cone), walk around it to the left.
Grading: Mark the lowest category that applies.

- **Normal:** Is able to walk around cones safely without changing gait speed; no evidence of imbalance.
- **Mild impairment:** Is able to step around both cones, but must slow down and adjust steps to clear cones.
- **Moderate impairment:** Is able to clear cones but must significantly slow speed to acomplish task, or requires verbal cuing.
- **Severe impairment:** Unable to clear cones, walks into one or both cones, or requires physical assistance.

8. Steps

Instructions: Walk up these stairs as you would at home (i.e., using the rail if necessary). At the top, turn around and walk down.
Grading: Mark the lowest category that applies.

- **Normal:** Alternating feet, no rail.
- **Mild impairment:** Alternating feet, must use rail.
- **Moderate impairment:** Two feet to stair, must use rail.
- **Severe impairment:** Cannot do safely.

From Shumway-Cook, A: Cook Motor control. Lippincott Williams & Wilkins, Baltimore, 1995, Table 14.2, pp 323–324. (Used with permission.)

BOX 15–8   Red Flags that Indicate a Need to Ask Further Questions

numbness
tingling
weakness
slurred speech
progressive hearing loss
tremors
poor coordination
upper motor neuron signs and symptoms
  positive Babinski
  spasticity
  clonus
loss of consciousness
rigidity
visual field loss
memory loss
cranial nerve dysfunction
spontaneous nystagmus in room light after two weeks
vertical nystagmus (other than BPPV)

Another tool that might be helpful to assess gait over time is the timed "up and go" test.[69] This test includes having the subject rise from a standard height chair with armrests, walk 3 meters, turn, and return to sit in the chair. It is closely related to speed of gait and is a quick method to assess gait performance over time in any physical setting.[70] In people with vestibular dysfunction, it is often helpful to have the subject turn to the right and also to the left to see if any asymmetry exists. The test takes less than one minute to complete and only requires a chair and a stop watch.

RED FLAGS

As the assessment is being performed, certain "red flags" must be recognized. Signs and symptoms of central nervous system pathology must be recognized and reported to the referring physician (Box 15–8). It is possible for individuals to be referred to a balance and vestibular clinic with undiagnosed central nervous system disease. Acoustic neuromas, multiple sclerosis, brainstem TIAs, cerebellar disorders, and migraines are but a few of the pathologies that have presented in our clinic with the diagnosis of dizziness. It is very important that individuals who treat people with vestibular dysfunction become very good at making a physical therapy diagnosis based on the patient's symptoms and physical examination. The patient history gathered early in the assessment will often guide the experienced clinician in deciding which path to follow in further evaluating the patient. Red flags are often identified in the history if the correct questions are asked of the patient.

TRANSITION FROM ASSESSMENT TO TREATMENT

The following points are offered as guidelines in developing a treatment program based on your assessment.

1. *Is there a documented vestibular deficit?* Review the results of the formal vestibular function tests. If the vestibular function tests are normal, you may or may *not* be dealing with a vestibular deficit. The results of the vestibular function tests confirm the presence of horizontal canal deficits. Of course, a patient may have a vertical canal lesion without a horizontal canal problem, but that is most likely to occur in BPPV, which is easily recognized. Otolith and central vestibular lesions are more difficult to identify and we must rely on patient history or on the presence of other deficits that localize the problem to the central nervous system.

2. *What type of vestibular problem does this patient have?* The vestibular function tests indicate whether the patient has a peripheral, unilateral, or bilateral vestibular deficit as well as the degree of the deficit. Some of the exercises for patients with vestibular deficits are designed to improve the remaining vestibular function and therefore are not appropriate for patients with complete vestibular loss. Exercises for benign paroxysmal positional vertigo (see Chapter 19) will not help the patient with a unilateral vestibular loss (see Chapter 17).

3. *Not all dizzy patients have a vestibular lesion.* Although nystagmus and complaints of dizziness and vertigo are common in patients with vestibular deficits, these problems can occur in other, nonvestibular disorders. Nystagmus may be caused by medications, brainstem or cerebral hemisphere lesions, or it may be congenital. Dizziness may occur in patients with peripheral somatosensory deficits (as with patients with peripheral vestibular deficits, these patients feel dizzy when they are standing but not when they are sitting), with central nervous system lesions, with other medical problems such as low blood pressure, or as a side effect of medications. Vertigo, most frequently associated with peripheral vestibular deficits, can occur with central lesions (often patients with central lesions may not complain of vertigo) and with other medical problems such as presyncope. These patients may have balance problems and may need an individualized exercise program but not necessarily exercises designed to improve vestibular function.

4. *Assess and reassess.* The initial assessment is directed at identifying problems associated with the vestibular deficit, such as increased dizziness or decreased visual acuity with head movements, and with the functional limitations of the patient. The exercise plan, therefore, may include vestibular exercises but must also address the specific problems and level of function of the patient. Developing a problem list will enable the therapist to set goals and devise specific exercises for each of those goals. As the patient responds to the exercises, reassessment is necessary to modify the treatment program.

5. *Quantify the assessment.* Although not all components of the assessment yield quantifiable data, many tests do, such as the patient's subjective complaints, dynamic visual acuity, some measures of postural stability, and several of the gait and balance measures. Taking the time to objectively measure the patient's performance is important in order to determine the outcome of the patient's treatment, to modify the treatment, to justify further treatment and to determine when to terminate treatment.

SUMMARY

The physical therapy assessment is multifaceted and aimed toward identifying the patient's specific functional deficits as well as to establish, quantitatively, the effects of the vestibular deficit on the patient's vestibulo-ocular and vestibulospinal systems and subjective complaints of disequilibrium and vertigo. The results of the assessment are used to identify specific patient problems and develop treatment goals for the patient. The results of the assessment also provide the basis for determining whether the treatments used are successful. The use of exercise in the rehabilitation of patients with vestibular disorders is aimed at promoting vestibular compensation and functional recovery.

ACKNOWLEDGMENTS

The authors wish to acknowledge the contribution of Diane F. Borello-France, PhD, PT who co-authored this chapter in the first edition of *Vestibular Rehabilitation*. Supported by NIH grant DC03196 (SJH).

REFERENCES

1. Shumway-Cook, A, and Horak, FB: Rehabilitation strategies for patients with vestibular deficits. Neurol Clin 8:441, 1990.
2. Paige, GD: Nonlinearity and asymmetry in the human vestibulo-ocular reflex. Acta Otolaryngol (Stockh) 108:1, 1989.
3. Allum, JHJ, et al: Long-term modifications of vertical and horizontal vestibulo-ocular reflex dynamics in man. Acta Otolaryngol (Stockh) 105:328, 1988.
4. Baloh, RW: The Essentials of Neurology. F.A. Davis, Philadelphia, 1984.
5. Norre, ME: Treatment of unilateral vestibular hypofunction. In Oosterveld, WJ (ed): Otoneurology. Wiley, New York, 1984, p 23.
6. Nashner, LM: Adaptation of human movement to altered environments. Trends Neurosci 5:358, 1982.
7. Lacour, M, et al: Modifications and development of spinal reflexes in the alert baboon following an unilateral vestibular neurotomy. Brain Res 113:255, 1976.
8. Allum, JHJ, and Pfaltz, CR: Influence of bilateral and acute unilateral peripheral vestibular deficits on early sway stabilizing responses in human tibialis anterior muscles. Acta Otolaryngol (Stockh) 406:115, 1984.
9. Jeka, JJ, and Lackner, JR: Fingertip contact influences human postural control. Exp Brain Res 100:495, 1991.
10. Lackner, JR: Some proprioceptive influences on the perceptual representation of body shape and orientation. Brain 111:281, 1988.
11. Jeka, JJ: Light touch contact as a balance aid. Phys Ther 77:476, 1997.
12. Horak, FB, et al: Effect of vestibular rehabilitation on dizziness and imbalance. Otolaryngol Head Neck Surg 106:175, 1992.
13. Ware, JE, and Sherbourne, CD: The MOS 36-item short-form health survey (SF-36) I. Conceptual framework and item selection. Medical Care 30:473, 1992.
14. McHorney, CA, et al: The MOS 36-item short-form health survey (SF-36) II. Psychometric and clinical tests of validity in measuring physical and mental health constructs. Medical Care 31:247, 1993.
15. McHorney, CA, et al: The MOS 36-item short form survey (SF-36): III. Tests of data quality, scaling assumptions, and reliability across diverse patient groups. Medical Care 32:40, 1994.
16. McHorney, CA, et al: Comparisons of the costs and quality of norms for the SF-36 health survey collected by mail versus telephone interview: Results from a national survey. Medical Care 32:551, 1994.
17. Ware, JE, et al: Comparison of methods for the scoring and statistical analysis of SF-36 health profile and summary measures: Summary of results form the medical outcomes study. Medical Care 33:AS264, 1995.
18. Enloe, LJ, and Shields, RK: Evaluation of health-related quality of life in individuals with vestibular disease using disease-specific and general outcome measures. Phys Ther 77:890, 1997.
19. Bergner, M, et al: The sickness impact profile: Development and final version of a health status measure. Medial Care 19:787, 1981.
20. Patrick, DL and Deyo, RA: Generic and disease-specific measures in assessing health status and quality of life. Med Care 27:5217, 1989.
21. Reishen, S: A career in the balance. Sports Illustrated, 1991, March 18, p 36.
22. Jacobson, GP, and Newman, CW: The development of the dizziness handicap inventory. Arch Otolaryngol Head Neck Surg 116:424, 1990.

23. Mann, GC, et al: Functional reach and single leg stance in patients with peripheral vestibular disorders. J Vestib Research 6:343, 1996.
24. Gill-Body, K, et al: Rehabilitation of balance in two patients with cerebellar dysfunction. Phys Ther 77:534, 1997.
25. Robertson, D, and Ireland, D: Dizziness handicap inventory correlates of computerized dynamic posturography. J Otolaryngol 24:118, 1995.
26. Jacobson, GP, et al: Balance function test correlates of the dizziness handicap inventory. J Am Acad Audiol 2:253, 1991.
27. Shepard, NT, et al: Habituation and balance retraining therapy: A retrospective review. Neurol Clin 8:459, 1990.
28. Studenski, S, et al: Predicting falls: The role of mobility and nonphysical factors. J Am Geriatr Soc 42:297, 1994.
29. Brandt, T, et al: Visual acuity, visual field and visual scene characteristics affect postural balance. In Igarashi, M, and Black, FO (eds): Vestibular and Visual Control on Posture and Locomotor Equilibrium. Karger, Basel, 1985, p 93.
30. Paulus, WM, et al: Visual stabilization of posture. Brain 107:1143, 1984.
31. Kenshalo, DR: Age changes in touch, vibration, temperature, kinesthesis and pain sensitivity. In Birren, JE, and Schaie, KW (eds): Handbook of the Psychology of Aging. New York, Van Nostrand Reinhold, 1977.
32. Paige, GD: Vestibulo-ocular reflex (VOR) and adaptive plasticity with aging. Soc Neurosci Abstr 15:515, 1989.
33. Brandt, T, and Daroff, RB: Physical therapy for benign paroxysmal positional vertigo. Arch Otolaryngol 106:484, 1980.
34. Bohannon, RW, et al: Decrease in timed balance function and the aging process. Phys Ther 64:1067, 1984.
35. Fregly, AR, et al: Walk on floor eyes closed (WOFEC): A new addition to an ataxia battery. Aerospace Med 75:10, 1973.
36. Fregly, AR, et al: Revised normative standards of performance of men on a quantitative ataxia test battery. Acta Otolaryngol 75:10, 1973.
37. Fregly, AR, and Graybiel, A: An ataxia battery not requiring rails. Aerospace Med 39:277, 1968.
38. Ekdahl, C, et al: Standing balance in healthy subjects. Scand J Rehab Med 21:187, 1989.
39. Black, FO, et al: Normal subject postural sway during the Romberg test. Am J Otolaryngol 3:309, 1982.
40. Thyssen, HH, et al: Normal ranges and reproducibility for the quantitative Romberg's test. Acta Neurol Scand 60:100, 1982.
41. Black, FO, et al: Abnormal postural control associated with peripheral vestibular disorders. Progress in Brain Res 76:263, 1988.
42. Horak, FB, et al: Postural strategies associated with somatosensory and visual loss. Exp Brain Res 82:67, 1990.
43. Nashner, LM, et al: Adaptation to altered support and visual conditions during stance: Patients with vestibular deficits. J Neurosci 2:536, 1982.
44. Horak, FB: Clinical measurement of postural control in adults. Phys Ther 67:1881, 1987.
45. Kirby, RL, et al: The influence of foot position on standing balance. Biomechanics 20:423, 1987.
46. Blatchly, CA, et al: Subjective measures of dizziness and objective measures of balance: Is there a relationship? Neurol Rep 14:20, 1990.
47. Yoneda, S, and Tokumasu, K: Frequency analysis of body sway in the upright posture. Acta Otolaryngol (Stockh) 102:87, 1986.
48. Shumway-Cook, A, and Horak, FB: Assessing the influence of sensory interaction on balance: Suggestion from the field. Phys Ther 66:1548, 1986.
49. Weber, PC, and Cass, SP: Clinical assessment of postural stability. Am J Otol 14:566, 1993.
50. Duncan, P, et al: Functional reach: A new clinical measure of balance. J Gerontol 85:529, 1990.
51. Duncan, PW, et al: Functional reach: Predictive validity in a sample of elderly male veterans. J Gerontol 47:M93, 1992.
52. Weiner, DK, et al: Functional reach: A marker of physical frailty. J Am Geriatr Soc 40:203, 1992.
53. Weiner, DK, et al: Does functional reach improve with rehabilitation. Arch Phy Med Rehab 74:796, 1993.
54. Studenski, S, et al: Predicting falls: The role of mobility and nonphysical factors. J Am Geriatr Soc 42:297, 1994.
55. Gabell, A, and Simons, MA: Balance coding. Physiotherapy 68:286, 1982.
56. Fukuda, T: The stepping test: Two phases of the labyrinthine reflex. Acta Otolaryngol 50:95, 1959.
57. Watanabe, T, et al: Automated graphical analysis of Fukuda's stepping test. In Igarashi, M, and Black, FO (eds): Vestibular and Visual Control on Posture and Locomotor Equilibrium. Karger, Basel, 1985, p 80.
58. Horak, FB, and Nashner, L: Central programming of postural movements: Adaptation to altered support-surface configuration. J Neurophysiol 55:1369, 1986.
59. Higgins, S: Motor skill acquisition. Phys Ther 71:123, 1991.
60. Shumway-Cook, A, et al: Predicting the probability for falls in community-dwelling older adults. Phys Ther 77:812, 1997.

61. Shumway-Cook, A, et al: The effect of multidimensional exercise on balance, mobility, and fall risk in community-living older adults. Phys Ther 77:46, 1997.
62. Berg, KO, et al: Clinical and laboratory measures of postural balance in an elderly population. Arch Phys Med Rehab 73:1073, 1992.
63. Berg, KO, et al: Measuring balance in the elderly: Validation of an instrument. Can J Public Health 83:S7, 1992.
64. Berg, K: Balance and its measure in the elderly: A review. Physiother Canada 41:240, 1989.
65. Berg, KO, et al: Measuring balance in the elderly: Preliminary development of an instrument. Physiother Canada 41:304, 1989.
66. Thorbahn, LD, and Newton, RA: Use of the Berg balance test to predict falls in elderly patients. Phys Ther 76:576, 1996.
67. Herdman, SJ: Advances in the treatment of vestibular disorders. Phys Ther 77:602, 1997.
68. Whitney, S, et al: The concurrent validity of the Berg Balance Scale and the Dynamic Gait Index in people with vestibular dysfunction. Neurol Rep 21:167, 1997.
69. Podsiadlo, D, and Richardson, S: The timed "up & go": A test of basic functional mobility for frail elderly persons. J Am Geriatr Soc 39:142, 1991.
70. Watson, D, Clark, LA, and Carey, G: Positive and negative affectivity and their relation to anxiety and depressive disorders. J Abnormal Psychology 97:346, 1988.

APPENDIX A

<u>EVALUATION</u>   Initial: Yes   No   Follow up: Yes   No   Date: _____

Patient: _____ Medical Record #: _____ D.O.B. _____ Age: ____
Referring physicians and physicians to whom we should send report (please give addresses):

Describe the major problem or reason you are seeing us:
When did this problem begin? _____

Specifically, do you experience spells of vertigo (a sense of spinning)?   Yes   No;
   If YES, how long do these spells last? _____
   When was the last time the vertigo occurred _____
   Is the vertigo:
      spontaneous: Yes   No
      induced by motion: Yes   No
      induced by position changes: Yes   No
Do you experience a sense of being off-balance (disequilibrium)?   Yes   No
   If yes, is the feeling of being off-balance:
      constant: Yes   No
      spontaneous: Yes   No
      induced by motion: Yes   No
      induced by position changes: Yes   No
      worse with fatigue: Yes   No   worse in the dark: Yes   No
      worse outside: Yes   No   worse on uneven surfaces: Yes   No
   Does the feeling of being off-balance occur when:
      lying down   Yes   No   sitting   Yes   No
      standing   Yes   No   walking   Yes   No

Do you or have you fallen (to the ground)?   Yes   No
   If yes, please describe _____

How often do you fall? _____
Have you injured yourself?   Yes   No
   If yes, please describe _____

Do you stumble, stagger or side-step while walking?   Yes   No

Do you drift to one side while you walk?   Yes   No
   If yes, to which side do you drift?   Right   Left

PERTINENT Past Medical History:

Do you have:

Diabetes:	Yes	No
Heart Disease:	Yes	No
Hypertension:	Yes	No
Headaches:	Yes	No
Arthritis:	Yes	No
Cervical problems:	Yes	No
Back problems:	Yes	No
Pulmonary problems:	Yes	No
Weakness or paralysis:	Yes	No

Hearing problems: Yes   No   _____

Visual problems: Yes   No   _____

Have you been in an accident?   Yes   No

If yes, please describe _____

_____

When did it occur? _____

What medications do you take?: _____

_____

Social History:

Do you live alone?   Yes   No   If NO, who lives with you? _____

Do you have stairs in your home?   Yes   No   If YES, how many? _____

Do you smoke?:   Yes   No;   If yes, please indicate how much per day _____

Do you drink alcohol?   Yes   No;   If yes, please indicate how much _____

Do you have trouble sleeping?   Yes   No

The scale below consists of a number of words that describe different feelings and emotions. Read each item and then mark the appropriate answer in the space next to that word. Indicate to what extent you generally feel this way. That is, how do you feel on the average. Use the following scale to record your answers:

1	2	3	4	5
very slightly or not at all	a little	moderately	quite a bit	extremely

_____ interested	_____ irritable	_____ jittery	_____ strong	_____ nervous
_____ enthusiastic	_____ distressed	_____ alert	_____ active	_____ excited
_____ ashamed	_____ afraid	_____ upset	_____ inspired	_____ hostile
_____ guilty	_____ determined	_____ proud	_____ scared	_____ attentive

How would you describe your functional level of activities before this problem developed?

_____

Current functional status:

Are you independent in self-care activities: Yes   No

Can you drive?   In the daytime?   Yes   No   In the nighttime?   Yes   No

Are you working?   Yes   No   Not applicable;   occupation: _____

Are you on Medical Disability?   Yes   No

Can you perform all your normal parenting activities?   Yes   No   Not applicable

Are you able to:

Watch TV comfortably?	Yes	No
Read?	Yes	No
Go shopping?	Yes	No
Be in traffic?	Yes	No
Use a computer?	Yes	No

Initial visit:

For the following, please pick the one statement that best describes how you feel (from Shepard et al[27]):

_____ Negligible symptoms

_____ Bothersome symptoms

_____ Performs usual work duties but symptoms interfere with outside activities

_____ Symptoms disrupt performance of both usual work duties and outside activities

_____ Currently on medical leave or had to change jobs because of symptoms

_____ Unable to work for over one year or established permanent disability with compensation payments

Final visit:

For the following, please pick the one statement that best describes how you feel (from Shepard et al[27]):

_____ No symptoms remaining at the end of therapy

_____ Marked improvement remaining at the end of therapy

_____ Mild improvement, definite persistent symptoms

_____ No change in symptoms relative to therapy

_____ Symptoms worsened with therapy activities on a persistent basis relative to pre-therapy period

(Modified) Jacobson's DHI Scale[22]: Below are a series of questions that pertain to your problem.

You should respond "yes, sometimes, no."   Yes   Sometimes   No

1. Does looking up increase your problem?   ____   ____   ____
2. Because of your problem, do you feel frustrated?   ____   ____   ____
3. Because of your problem do you restrict your travel?   ____   ____   ____
4. Does walking down the aisle of a supermarket increase
    your problem?   ____   ____   ____
5. Because of your problem, do you have difficulty getting
    into or out of bed?   ____   ____   ____
6. Does your problem significantly restrict your   ____   ____   ____
    participation in social activities?
7. Because of your problem do you have difficulty
    reading?   ____   ____   ____
8. Does performing more ambitious activities increase
    your problem?   ____   ____   ____
9. Because of your problem, are you afraid to leave home
    without having someone with you?   ____   ____   ____
10. Because of your problem, are you embarrassed in front
    of others?   ____   ____   ____
11. Do quick head movements increase your problem?   ____   ____   ____
12. Because of your problem, do you avoid heights?   ____   ____   ____
13. Does turning over in bed increase your problem?   ____   ____   ____
14. Because of your problem is it difficult for you to do
    strenuous work?   ____   ____   ____
15. Because of your problem, do you avoid driving your
    car in the daytime?   ____   ____   ____
16. Because of your problem, are you afraid people think
    you are intoxicated?   ____   ____   ____
17. Because of your problem, is it difficult for you to go for
    a walk by yourself?   ____   ____   ____
18. Does walking down a sidewalk increase your problem?   ____   ____   ____
19. Because of your problem, is it difficult for you to
    concentrate?   ____   ____   ____
20. Because of your problem, is it difficult for you to walk
    around your house in the dark?   ____   ____   ____
21. Because of your problem, are you afraid to stay home
    alone?   ____   ____   ____
22. Because of your problem, do you feel handicapped?   ____   ____   ____
23. Because of your problem, do you avoid driving your
    car in the dark?   ____   ____   ____
24. Has your problem placed stress on your relationships
    with members of your family or friends?   ____   ____   ____
25. Because of your problem, are you
    depressed?   ____   ____   ____

ASSESSMENT
SUBJECTIVE COMPLAINTS
    PANAS scale[69]: score/significance: _____

1) Vertigo: (0–10) _____ Disequilibrium: (0–10) _____ Oscillopsia (0–10) _____
2) Time of day patient feels best _____ worse _____
3) How many times per day does patient experience symptoms? _____
4) DHI score: _____
    Major problems: _____
5) Disability score: _____ (pre-therapy) _____ (post-therapy)

MOTION SENSITIVITY QUOTIENT (from Shepard et al[27]) _____
Duration: 5–10 secs = 1 point; 1–30 secs = 2 points; >30 secs = 3 points
MSQ = {(Total score) $\times$ (# of positions with symptoms)} / 20.48. Don't forget to adjust for baseline intensity so MSQ is based on change in Intensity. MSQ: 0–10 is mild; 11–30 is moderate; 31–100 is severe

	Intensity (0–5)	Duration	Score (Intensity + Duration in points)
Baseline Symptoms			
1. Sitting to supine			
2. Supine to left side			
3. Supine to right side			
4. Supine to sitting			
5. Left Hallpike-Dix			
6. Return to sit from left Hallpike-Dix			
7. Right Hallpike-Dix			
8. Return to sit from right Hallpike-Dix			
9. Sitting, head tipped to left knee			
10. Head up from left knee			
11. Sitting, head tipped to right knee			
12. Head up from right knee			
13. Sitting, turn head horizontally 5 times			
14. Sitting, move head vertically 5 times			
15. Standing, turn 180° to the right			
16. Standing, turn 180° to the left			

OCULOMOTOR EXAMINATION
Room light: A. spontaneous nystagmus   Y   N
               B. gaze holding nystagmus   Y   N
               C. Smooth pursuit _____
               D. Saccadic eye movements _____
               E. VORc _____
               F. VOR slow _____
               G. VOR rapid head thrusts _____
               H. Visual acuity stationary: _____   Dynamic _____

Frenzel / IR (recorded   Y   N)
               A. spontaneous nystagmus?   Y   N
               B. gaze holding nystagmus?   Y   N
               C. Horizontal head-shaking–induced nystagmus? _____
               D. Vertical head-shaking–induced nystagmus? _____
               E. R Hallpike-Dix maneuver: nystagmus _____ vertigo _____
               F. L Hallpike-Dix maneuver: nystagmus _____ vertigo _____
               G. Supine roll head right: nystagmus _____ vertigo _____
               H. Supine roll head left: nystagmus _____ vertigo _____
               I. Pressure test _____

QUANTITATIVE DVA: static _____   right _____   left _____

CALORIC/ VAT/ HEAD THRUSTS: _____

STANCE POSTURAL CONTROL
     A. Alignment eyes open: _____ (erect, head still, B of S?)
     B. Self-initiated weight-shifting: _____ (strategy)
     C. Reactive responses (sternal shove): _____ (strategy)

BALANCE TESTS   (video-taped?   Y   N)
     A. Romberg: eo _____   ec _____ Normal / abnormal for age? _____
     B. Sharpened Romberg: eo _____   ec _____
         Normal / abnormal for age? _____
     C. Single leg stance: eo _____   ec _____
         Normal / abnormal for age? _____
     D. Functional reach: _____ (normal = >12 inches)
     E. Fukuda's stepping test: eo _____ (FP, turn)   ec _____
         (FP, turn) Normal? _____

GAIT   Assistive devices: _____ Orthoses? _____
     A. At self-initiated pace:
         Cadence: _____   Base of support: _____
         Step length: _____ (equal, each foot passes the other)
         Arm swing: _____
         Head and trunk rotation: _____
         Path: Straight?   Y   N,   Swerves: R   L,   Staggers: Y   N
             Side-steps: Y   N
     B. At increased pace: Can perform   Cannot perform

Cadence: _____   Base of support: _____
Step length: _____ (equal, each foot passes the other)
Arm swing: _____
Head and trunk rotation: _____
Path: Straight?   Y   N,   Drifts: R   L,   Staggers: Y   N
      Side-steps: Y   N

C. Gait deviations: (20 foot path, 12 inches wide) _____

D. Walk turn head: Can perform   cannot perform
      Cadence: _____   Base of support: _____
      Path: Straight?   Y   N,   Drifts: R   L,   Staggers: Y   N
            Side-steps: Y   N

E. Walk move head vertically
      Cadence: _____   Base of support: _____
      Path: Straight?   Y   N,   Drifts: R   L,   Staggers: Y   N
            Side-steps: Y   N

F. Walk, turn head and count backwards out loud by _____:
      Cadence: _____   Base of support: _____
      Path: Straight?   Y   N,   Drifts: R   L,   Staggers: Y   N
            Side-steps: Y   N

G. Walk, turn around rapidly:
      Normal: _____
      Has difficulty / loses balance turning right _____
      turning left _____

H. Singleton test: To Right _____   To Left _____

FUNCTIONAL GAIT: Independent   min / mod / max assist
dependent   slow, cautious
      Stairs _____   Inclines _____   Uneven surfaces _____ Carpet _____

SUBSYSTEMS
A. ROM:
      Cervical_____
      R- UE _____   L- UE _____   R- LE _____   L- LE _____
B. Strength: R- UE _____   L- UE _____   R- LE _____   L-LE _____
C. Soft tissue problems: Y   N   location: _____   nature: (spasm?) _____
D. Sensation: (vibration, proprioception, kinesthesia)   LEs _____
E. Muscle tone: UEs _____   LEs _____
F. Cerebellar: Finger to nose   R _____   L _____
              Rapid alternating movement: R _____   L _____
              Optic ataxia   R _____   L _____
              Tremor   R _____   L _____
              Heel to shin—looking   R _____   L _____
              Heel to shin—not looking   R _____   L _____
              Rapid alternating movement   R _____   L _____
G. Pain: Y   N   location _____

Created by Susan J. Herdman, PhD, PT, Dizziness and Balance Center, Bascom Palmer Eye Institute and Division of Physical Therapy, University of Miami.

APPENDIX B: DIZZINESS INVENTORY

Name: _____ **Date:** _____

The purpose of this scale is to identify difficulties that you may be experiencing because of your dizziness or unsteadiness. Please answer "Yes," "No," or "Sometimes" to each question. *Answer each question as it pertains to your dizziness or unsteadiness only.*

		Yes	No	Sometimes
P1.	Does looking up increase your problem?	____	____	____
E2.	Because of your problem, do you feel frustrated?	____	____	____
F3.	Because of your problem, do you restrict your travel for business or recreation?	____	____	____
P4.	Does walking down the aisle of a supermarket increase your problem?	____	____	____
F5.	Because of your problem, do you have difficulty getting into or out of bed?	____	____	____
F6.	Does your problem significantly restrict your participation in social activities such as going out to dinner, the movies, dancing, or to parties?	____	____	____
F7.	Because of your problem, do you have difficulty reading?	____	____	____
P8.	Does performing more ambitious activities like sports or dancing or household chores such as sweeping or putting dishes away increase your problem?	____	____	____
E9.	Because of your problem, are you afraid to leave your home without having someone accompany you?	____	____	____
E10.	Because of your problem, are you embarrassed in front of others?	____	____	____
P11.	Do quick movements of your head increase your problem?	____	____	____
F12.	Because of your problem, do you avoid heights?	____	____	____
P13.	Does turning over in bed increase your problem?	____	____	____
F14.	Because of your problem, is it difficult for you to do strenuous housework or yardwork?	____	____	____
E15.	Because of your problem, are you afraid people may think you are intoxicated?	____	____	____
F16.	Because of your problem, is it difficult for you to walk by yourself?	____	____	____
P17.	Does walking down a sidewalk increase your problem?	____	____	____
E18.	Because of your problem, is it difficult for you to concentrate?	____	____	____
F19.	Because of your problem, is it difficult for you to walk around your house in the dark?	____	____	____

E20. Because of your problem, are you afraid to stay
home alone?   _____   _____   _____

E21. Because of your problem, do you feel
handicapped?   _____   _____   _____

E22. Has your problem placed stress on your
relationships with members of your family or
friends?   _____   _____   _____

E23. Because of your problem, are you depressed?   _____   _____   _____

F24. Does your problem interfere with your job or
household responsibilities?   _____   _____   _____

P25. Does bending over increase your problem?   _____   _____   _____

                                            Total   _____   _____   _____
                                                     (×4)   (×0)   (×2)

Total: _____ F _____ E _____ P _____
                  (38)   (36)   (28)

From Jacobson, GP, and Newman, CW: The development of the dizziness handicap inventory. Arch Otolaryngol Head Neck Surg 116:424, 1990. Copyright © 1990 The American Medical Association.

CHAPTER 16

Disability in Vestibular Disorders

Helen S. Cohen, EdD, OTR, FAOTA

Disorders of the vestibular system cause a variety of symptoms, including vertigo, oscillopsia, disequilibrium, disorientation, and autonomic signs such as nausea, sweating, and increased heart rate and respiration. These symptoms cause discomfort. They also cause secondary problems such as fatigue and headache, fear of falling or having a driving accident, social embarrassment, and decreased activity level. People with vestibular disorders have decreased independence in activities of daily living including self-care skills and instrumental activities, decreased job performance, decreased participation in family responsibilities, and reluctance to participate in social activities outside of the home. Thus, even though most vestibular disorders are relatively benign and not life-threatening, they can have serious consequences, which are not predicted by performance on diagnostic tests[1] (Fig. 16–1).

The functional consequences of vestibular disorders are poorly understood, even by health care providers who are familiar with vestibular disorders. A recent study provided an interesting insight into some physicians' understanding of disability in the vestibularly impaired population. Patients with a variety of vestibular disorders and their physicians were surveyed about the effect of vestibular disorders on quality of life. Patients' perceptions of the effect of vestibular impairments on the quality of life correlated poorly with their physicians' perceptions, particularly if the patients had high levels of anxiety.[2] Not surprisingly, patients considered themselves more incapacitated than did their physicians.

People are complex systems; to understand the ramifications of disease, we must understand the different levels of the system. The symptoms and secondary problems mentioned above represent many different levels of the person as a system. Together, these problems are all encompassed under the umbrella term, *disablement*.[3] We can use existing taxonomies to understand the manifestations of disablement at different levels of the system. First, we need a common language and frame of reference. The following section provides operational definitions of terms used in current taxonomies and

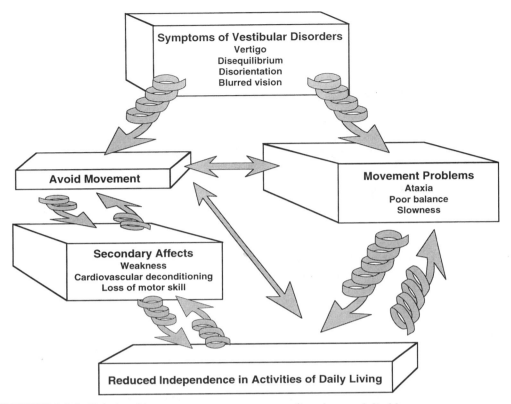

FIGURE 16–1. Relationships among symptoms, motor disorders, and disablement.

explains how different problems fit at different levels of the system. Each version of the taxonomy of disablement addresses the same issue: that a problem at one level of the system has consequences at succeeding higher levels of the system. The taxonomies vary with each attempt to refine the expression of that idea.

TAXONOMIES OF DISABLEMENT

World Health Organization System

Nagi[4] published the first taxonomy of disablement in 1969. He described several levels of disablement comparable to different levels of the person/society system.[4] Later, in response to the need for a classification system of disablement, the World Health Organization (WHO) published the International Classification of Impairments, Disabilities, and Handicaps (ICIDH).[5] A revised version is now being tested. The current version uses the following definitions:

• **Impairment** is any loss or abnormality of psychological, physiological, or anatomic structure or function

- **Disability** is a decrement or a restriction in the ability to perform an activity within normal limits
- **Handicap** is a disadvantage in role performance caused by an impairment or disability.

In this taxonomy, **impairment** refers to function of body parts. **Disability** refers to function of the whole person. **Handicap** refers to function of the whole person in society. All of the taxonomies carry through these distinctions, including the concept of handicap as imposed by society. An example of the distinction between disability and handicap is the integration of early twentieth-century deaf residents in the communities on Martha's Vineyard, an island off the coast of Cape Cod.[6] Because most islanders spoke the local dialect of sign language, the preferred mode of verbal communication was often sign. Therefore, hearing loss was an impairment and occasionally a task-specific disability, but not a handicap.

The ICIDH uses a classification system similar to the International Classification of Diseases, Injuries and Causes of Death (ICD).[7] The ICD assigns numerical and descriptive codes to different diseases. In the United States, physicians often write diagnoses with the ICD codes, which are internationally accepted. This system has been so useful that a similar system was adopted for the ICIDH, although with somewhat less success in North America. The ICIDH, which was adopted by the American Medical Association,[8] lists separate codes for impairment, disability, and handicap. Using the ICIDH manual, a patient with chronic vertigo caused by viral labyrinthitis (ICD code 386.10, peripheral vertigo), who is a secretary in a busy office, lives in New York, and rides the subway to go to work, could be described with the Impairment codes I48.0 (vertigo), I48.1 (impairment of labyrinthine function), I48.2 (impairment of locomotion related to vestibular or cerebellar function), and I48.4 (other impairment of vestibular function).

Because people with vestibular disorders have many levels of disability,[9] discussed later in this chapter, many disability codes could apply. Owing to reduced gain of the vestibulo-ocular reflex (VOR), this patient could have difficulty with tasks requiring fine visual discrimination when the head is not stabilized against a headrest (i.e., D26.0, disability in detailed visual tasks). This person might also have difficulty with bathtub transfers (i.e., D33.0, bathing disability associated with transfer difficulty). The detailed disability codes also include other personal care tasks such as upper- and lower-extremity dressing, codes for locomotion disabilities including walking on a flat surface (D40) and climbing stairs (D42), and codes for situational disabilities such as D76, disability relating to tolerance of work stresses, including the inability to cope with the speed of work. The disability codes include a 10-point ordinal scale for rating the severity of the problem and a 10-point ordinal scale for rating the potential for improved functional performance. This **Assessment of Outlook** scale is a rating of the prognosis for rehabilitation that does not address the prognosis for improvement from the original disease process. This distinction is useful because the physical damage causing a vestibular impairment is usually permanent, but the individual may compensate behaviorally and become less disabled.

The handicap codes are less detailed. They include codes that might be relevant to our hypothetical patient, such as H3 (mobility handicap), including H3.2 (impaired mobility), such that the ability to get around takes longer because the individual has difficulty coping with public transportation, but nevertheless *is* able to cope with public transportation. Our patient might arrange an alternate work schedule and take the subway—an efficient and relatively inexpensive way to travel about such a large and dense city—only during off-peak times: When taking the subway at rush hour, entering and leaving the subway car require split-second predictive timing. Riders must also move out of the way of other subway patrons crowding into the car at the same time. Standing during the rush hour ride requires good dynamic balance, and reading the station signs in time to get off at the correct stop requires good dynamic visual acuity, complicated by the need to look around other people. During off-peak times, predictive timing is still needed but can be more leisurely, seats are more likely to be available, and the view through the window is less likely to be obscured by other riders. That New Yorkers perform this feat at rush hour so easily every day suggests they are remarkable people!

National Institutes of Health Taxonomy

The Nagi taxonomy and the ICIDH needed further refinement. Also, the term "handicap" had itself taken on a negative connotation in some circles. Therefore, the Institute of Medicine refined the existing taxonomies[10] but retained the concept of nested levels of disablement such that physiological impairment has consequences for functional behavior and social role. Then the National Institutes of Health (NIH) added some levels to the system and removed the offending term "handicap."

In the document describing their research program the National Center for Medical Rehabilitation Research/ National Institute for Child Health and Human Development/ NIH published the revised taxonomy.[11] In this taxonomy

- **Pathophysiology** means the interruption or interference of function in normal processes or structures
- **Impairment** means loss or abnormality of function at the level of the organ or organ system
- **Functional limitation** means the decrease or inability to perform an action normally
- **Disability** means a limitation in performing tasks at normal or socially expected levels
- **Societal limitation** means a restriction in role fulfillment owing to social policy or other externally imposed barriers.

Note that in the NIH taxonomy the word "handicap" has been eliminated, although the level of analysis that includes the attitudes and expectations of society has been retained and augmented (Table 16–1).

Consider our hypothetical patient. The pathophysiological mechanism is a viral infection affecting the labyrinth. The impairment is evident as decreased gain and increased phases on low frequency, sinusoidal tests of the VOR in darkness, an asymmetry between the two ears on caloric testing, and decreased performance on dynamic posturography tests. Functional limitations include requiring assistance for bathtub transfers, requiring more time for performing all self-care skills, having difficulty climbing the steps to ride the bus or descending to the subway, having difficulty maintaining balance while riding the subway, and using safety guarding when performing many other activities of daily living (ADLs). The disability is the difficulty in performing socially defined roles, such as performing the requirements for her job.[12] The soci-

TABLE 16–1 NIH Taxonomy of Disablement

Term	Definition	Example
Pathophysiology	Interruption or loss of function of the anatomical structure	Gentamicin causes loss of vestibular hair cells.
Impairment	Abnormal function of the organ system	Reduced postural stability. Decreased VOR gain. Oscillopsia.
Functional limitation	Decreased behavioral performance	Ambulation with a cane. Inability to read while moving.
Disability	Deficit in performing social role due to constraints of the individual's condition	Inability to hold a particular job, e.g., emergency room nurse.
Societal limitation	Deficit in maintaining social role owing to constraints placed by external society	Inability to work as a nurse because the hospital fears liability.

etal limitations include constraints on holding a job when vertigo occurs suddenly and unexpectedly. Our patient's supervisor, a busy executive, may believe that the patient is malingering and she may be required to explain the nature of her disorder to the director of personnel, confirmed by a letter from her physician.

FUNCTIONAL LIMITATIONS AND DISABILITY IN ACTIVITIES OF DAILY LIVING

Many papers in the clinical literature discuss changes in motor behaviors controlled by the vestibular system, such as the parameters of the VOR (e.g., VOR gain). VOR gain, however, is an indicator of impairment; it is not an indicator of functional limitations or disability. The goal of rehabilitation is to make the patient feel better (reduce vertigo), and to reduce or eliminate functional limitations and disability, or to make the patient more independent in ADLs. **ADLs** are the routine tasks performed in the course of our daily lives. These tasks include self-care tasks, instrumental ADLs, and mobility skills.

Assessments

The standard diagnostic tests of vestibular impairment (e.g., caloric tests, rotatory tests, and posturography) are not appropriate to evaluate functional limitations and disability. These issues should be assessed directly. The literature includes, at last count, approximately 100 assessments of activities of daily living (Kathlyn L. Reed, PhD, OTR, MLIS, FAOTA, personal communication, October 1995). Few of them, however, are appropriate for assessment of patients with vestibular disorders. The scales developed for other patient populations, including such well-known assessments as the Barthel Index,[13] Functional Independence Measure,[14] and Klein-Bell Scale,[15] are not appropriate for patients with vestibular disorders; vestibularly impaired patients usually move their limbs well and often have no other sensory impairments. Many have no central nervous system disorders of the type that would impair fine motor performance and manipulative skills, and they are often able to move about the environment, albeit slowly. Therefore the problems of this population may be too subtle to be detected by scales normed for other patient populations who have more overt physical limitations. Other instruments, such as the admirably client-centered Canadian Occupational Performance Measure (COPM),[16,17] are not diagnosis-specific or omit some tasks that are problematic for this population, and therefore may not detect some of the subtle problems associated with vestibular disorders.

The client-centered aspect of the COPM is a unique strength of that assessment. The concept of asking the patient which tasks or skills are actually important to that individual's life is unusual among the many ADL scales. This concept can be incorporated easily in routine clinical use of any scale and may add to the clinician's understanding of the patient's level of disablement. Most people are unconcerned about eliminating tasks that are unimportant to them, but find adaptive ways to perform tasks that are essential to their lives. Such tasks may not be obvious from a standard listing of ADLs, but may only be discovered by discussing the patient's individual lifestyle needs. For example, our hypothetical patient rides the subway and has no need to drive a car on a regular basis although she has a driver's license. Therefore, although she may have difficulty driving, this functional limitation may not be disabling to her and may not present a societal limitation; using mass transit is a more efficient way to travel about many parts of New York, anyway. If, however, she travels to care for her elderly grandmother in the suburbs every weekend, she may need to drive a car on those occasions. Likewise, another patient with the same deficit may live in a suburb of a midwestern city in a community with little public transportation. This patient may have to drive to work downtown in the city; at home she may have to drive several miles to go to the grocery store or run errands. For that individual, a functional limitation in driving is severely disabling and presents a societal limitation.

Few performance assessments have been described in the literature for patients with vestibular disorders, including only two that address ADLs,[9,18] both self-administered questionnaires with ordinal scales. The Dizziness Handicap Inventory, a three-point, 25-item questionnaire covers self-care, higher level skills, psychological issues, and mobility skills. This scale was the first designed for the vestibularly impaired population. In contrast, Cohen's questionnaire has five levels and more tasks, and does not include assessment of psychological issues. It is currently being updated.[19] The new version, currently being normed, is more sensitive and eliminates questions that do not differentiate normals from patients with vestibular impairments. The psychosocial problems and related deficits of this population can be assessed with Yardley's well-normed Vertigo Handicap Questionnaire and Vertigo Symptom Scale.[20]

Self-Care Tasks

Self care tasks are the tasks needed to prepare ourselves for the day, meet personal needs and assure the ability to continue to function throughout the day. These tasks include eating, bathing, dressing, toileting, and grooming. They may include motor skills such as transferring on and off of a seat or in and out of the bathtub, standing up from a bed or chair, bending down, reaching for objects, and manipulation of small closures such as buttons. Vestibular impairments that cause blurred vision, oscillopsia, postural instability, and spatial disorientation can interfere with performance of these tasks. Patients with a wide range of vestibular impairments have difficulty with tasks such as lower extremity dressing, bathtub transfers, hair washing, and shaving.[9,19,21–23]

Instrumental Tasks

More complex, less personal ADLs known as instrumental ADLs[24] are common, but not necessarily universal. These tasks include: home-management skills, such as meal preparation, washing floors, and gardening; communication skills, such as using a telephone or word processor; transportation tasks, such as driving or riding the bus; and community activities, such as participation in social functions outside the home, shopping, voting, and participating in sports or other recreational activities. Instrumental ADLs also include occupational role (paid or unpaid work), although occupational role is a special case.

Occupational role includes employment in a profession or job, unpaid family-related work such as child care, and unpaid volunteer work. This task category has particular significance for social status and sense of psychological well-being as well as for providing for the needs of oneself and family members. The requirements of many occupational roles vary widely. Many roles, such as caretaker for a child or elderly parent, involve many kinds of task. Some paid jobs have specific or unique tasks associated with them, such as use of a welding torch or a microscope. For many other roles, however, tasks that are generic to many kinds of work are involved. For example, many people (e.g., scientists, secretaries, teachers, and therapists) all use word processors. When assessing the impact of vestibular impairment on occupational role performance the unique nature of vocational tasks should be considered.

Many patients have difficulty performing a variety of home-management tasks, such as cleaning floors, making beds, gardening, caring for the family car, and putting away groceries or dishes in cupboards. Patients also report having difficulty doing the grocery shopping, participating in some social and recreational activities, going to a car wash, and performing some job-specific tasks.[9,19,21–23,25–27] Depending on the nature of the individual's job, these kinds of problems may be moderately to severely disabling.[12,25]

Mobility Skills

PERSONAL MOBILITY

Independence in walking, use of stairs, and generally moving about the environment is achieved in most people by age 3. Functional limitations in personal mobility can be psychologically devastating. Vestibular disorders, because they cause vertigo, disequilibrium, and deficits in spatial orientation, cause deficits in personal mobility. Many people have difficulty walking and tend to move more slowly and carefully than usual. When use of a cane is necessary, the patient may perceive use of the cane as having a social stigma. As a visible reminder of the problem, the cane may also represent impending infirmity. Thus, many patients prefer to avoid using their canes, moving more slowly or with greater difficulty. People also have difficulty ascending or descending stairs, particularly in the absence of a handrail, and they may avoid use of escalators. Reduced personal mobility may be the reason for reduced participation in community activities, such as going to church, doing volunteer work, attending sports events, and attending social gatherings. Because walking in a busy airport is difficult for some people, they may avoid business trips, which can have implications for their job performance. Interpersonal relationships can be affected, too. Many patients complain of veering into walls or off sidewalks. One patient told of trying to avoid bumping into her husband when they went out for their daily walk together, which caused him to think she was avoiding him. Other patients have reported avoiding social gatherings or being embarrassed by the comments of people who are unaware of their vestibular impairments, and mistake the ataxia for drunkenness.

COMMUNITY MOBILITY

The ability to travel around the community independently is essential for most adults. In some cities community mobility may involve use of public transportation, such as buses or trains. In many communities, however, public transportation is either unavailable or difficult to use and most people rely on automobiles. Therefore in many places in North America, the ability to drive is essential. Recent surveys of Canadian and American otolaryngologists suggest that the standards for safe driving are confusing and vary widely.[28,29] These physicians considered the most problematic disorder for driving safety to be Ménière's disease with Tumarkin's drop attacks, which is rare. They considered benign paroxysmal positional vertigo (BPPV) to be least problematic. These ideas, however, have not yet been correlated with opinions of patients, or with actual data on the incidence of driving problems.

Other reports suggest that patients with vestibular disorders often consider driving problematic. Patients with Ménière's disease are most likely to be dependent for driving while having an exacerbation and many of these patients decrease their driving for fear of having an episode of vertigo unexpectedly.[12] Many other patients with peripheral vestibular disorders use safety guarding; they drive more slowly than usual and avoid highway driving if possible.[9] In the acute period following a labyrinthectomy or resection of an acoustic neuroma, many patients are not allowed to drive. But, even after they resume driving, many of these patients drive only on local roads, only drive after rush hour, stay in the right-hand lane, or drive slowly.[30]

Limitations in community mobility limit participation in the same community events affected by limitations in personal mobility. Aside from a paucity of handicapped-only parking spaces in some places, people tend to avoid traveling to events that are nonessential because they fear having vertigo while driving, the subsequent consequences for their safety and that of others, and because they fear the social consequences of being seen in public while having an episode of vertigo or while walking with an ataxic gait. Thus, otherwise simple, local trips, such as a clinic visit, can require considerably more advanced planning than usual, such as timing the visit to avoid driving in rush hour, and arranging the trip so that a relative or friend can take off work to drive.

Psychosocial Consequences

Most patients prefer not to go out without a companion for fear of becoming incapacitated or falling.[27,31] They also fear being embarrassed. For example, as mentioned, they may be ridiculed by people who mistake an ataxic gait for evidence of alcohol consumption. Panic disorder may be associated with vestibular impairment because going out in public may provoke panic attacks.[32,33] People may become so uncomfortable leaving the home that they may be diagnosed with agoraphobia.[26,34] Although these patients may have mild impairments in self-care skills, the difficulty in leaving the home can cause severe deficits in instrumental ADLs. Therefore, they are often depressed, sometimes clinically, and feel a sense of isolation.[26,35,36] Compounding the problem, many patients report that employers, physicians not familiar with vestibular disorders, friends, and family members may not understand the signs and symptoms of a vestibular impairment and may accuse them of malingering or having psychosomatic problems.

Diagnosis-Specific Problems

Although many functional deficits are common across vestibular impairments, some conditions are associated with special problems. For example, because Ménière's disease is characterized by hearing loss and often tinnitus as well as vertigo,[37,38] during episodes of symptom exacerbation Ménière's patients have difficulty using a telephone and performing other tasks that require good hearing; they also have particular difficulty with tasks that require good balance[12] (Fig. 16–2). Many Ménière's patients

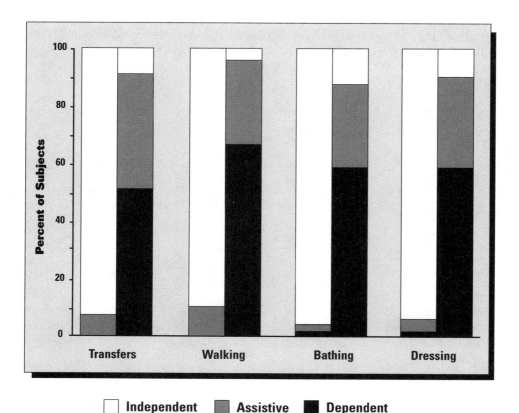

FIGURE 16–2. Percentage of Ménière's patients who are independent, assistive, and dependent for transfers, walking on level surfaces, bathing, and dressing in between Ménière's attacks (left half of each pair) and during Ménière's attacks (right half of each pair). Independent, lightest bar; assistive, medium shaded bar; dependent, darkest bar. From Cohen et al.[12] Used by permission.

report that tasks requiring good balance or good dynamic visual acuity, which would be affected by an impaired VOR, are either difficult or dangerous to perform. Therefore, they try to avoid or adapt those tasks. Also, for many patients the hearing loss is as disabling as the vertigo.

The disabling effect of Ménière's disease has significant social and economic consequences. The vertigo, hearing loss, or the combination of both problems can be severe enough to cause patients to change or modify their jobs. When surveyed, 86 percent of people with Ménière's disease reported that the symptoms hindered their job performance; 70 percent had to modify the way they performed their jobs; and 40 percent had to change jobs. Of 17 people who changed jobs, 2 had to stop working altogether.

Bilateral vestibular loss also causes significant disablement. These patients have oscillopsia,[39,40] which interferes with the ability to see clearly while moving and even while standing still.[41] Oscillopsia causes difficulty reading signs or identifying faces while moving[42]; such a problem can interfere with the ability to read the instrument panel on the dashboard of a car or road signs that must be viewed while driving; several patients with bilateral vestibular impairment have commented on these problems in particular. The oscillopsia and balance impairments can have significant effect on occupational role. Of seven patients seen in this investigator's clinical practice recently, each of whom had minimal or no caloric or rotatory responses bilaterally, four had to stop working and one worked only part time.

BPPV causes vertigo that is usually specific to pitch rotations of the head. Patients with this disorder often have difficulty performing tasks requiring pitch rotations of the head, such as reaching up to take an object off a shelf, or reaching down to tie shoes or pick up an object from the floor.[43,44]

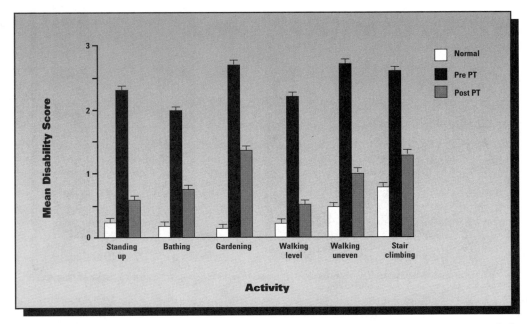

FIGURE 16–3. Performance of six activities of daily living, before and after developing a vestibular disorder, and after vestibular rehabilitation. The disability scale is from 0 (no disability) to 4 (dependent). Tasks: standing up from a chair; bathing; gardening; walking on level surfaces; walking on uneven surfaces; climbing stairs. Adapted from Cohen.[9] Used by permission.

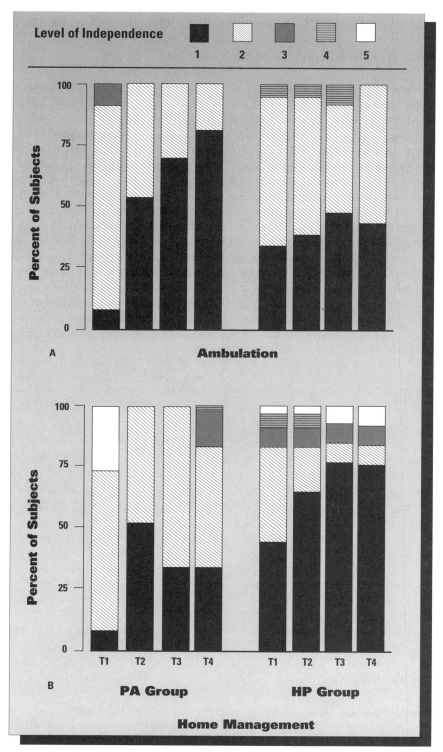

FIGURE 16–4. Improvements in independence in ambulation and home management skills with 6 weeks of either biweekly occupational therapy plus 5 days of home habituation exercises or daily home habituation exercises. Level of independence: 1, independent; 5, dependent. Test dates were pretest (T1), 6-week post-test (T2), 1-month follow-up (T3), 3-month follow-up (T4). PA indicates purposeful activities; HP indicates habituation. (From Cohen et al.[45] Used with permission.)

EFFECTS OF VESTIBULAR REHABILITATION

The evidence from two studies indicates that patients perceive they have greater independence in self-care and instrumental ADLs after participation in vestibular rehabilitation programs. A 1992 study surveyed patients with a variety of vestibular disorders after they had participated in a physical therapy program incorporating both habituation exercises and balance training. They reported having had significantly reduced independence in activities of daily living compared to their premorbid levels before starting physical therapy. After vestibular rehabilitation, however, they had significantly greater ADL independence, approaching their premorbid levels[9] (Fig. 16–3).

A later prospective study of patients with chronic, peripheral vestibular impairments assigned subjects to one of two 6-week programs: (1) habituation exercises and (2) occupational therapy using purposeful activities. The treatments in both groups incorporated rapid, repetitive head rotations and visual/vestibular interaction. In both treatment groups, ADL independence improved significantly as compared to their premorbid levels[45] (Fig. 16–4). Thus, after developing a vestibular disorder most patients perceive themselves to be disabled. They feel they are less independent than before. After participating in either physical therapy or occupational therapy programs that are based on the principles of vestibular rehabilitation patients perceive themselves as more independent and less disabled.

SUMMARY

Patients with vestibular pathologies present with measurable impairments in the motor behaviors controlled by the vestibular system (postural control, oculomotor control, and spatial orientation) and by perceptual illusions, such as vertigo. Discomfort, decreased motor skills, and the related psychological distress lead to functional limitations in self-care skills and instrumental ADLs, especially during performance of tasks that require good balance, rapid head rotations, and good dynamic visual acuity. These problems are disabling and affect their ability to function normally in society. Fortunately, however, the disabling effects of vestibular impairment can be remediated with vestibular rehabilitation.

ACKNOWLEDGMENTS

Supported by the Clayton Foundation for Research and NIH grant DC02412.

REFERENCES

1. Cohen, H: Defining disablement in otolaryngology. Ear Nose Throat J 74:233, 1995.
2. Honrubia, V, et al: Quantitative evaluation of dizziness characteristics and impact on quality of life. Am J Otol 17:595, 1996.
3. Jette, AM: Physical disablement concepts for physical therapy research and practice. Phys Ther 74:380, 1994.
4. Nagi, SZ: Disability and Rehabilitation. Ohio State Univ. Pr., Columbus, 1969.
5. International Classification of Impairments, Disabilities, and Handicaps. World Health Organization, Geneva, 1980.

6. Groce, NE: Everyone Here Spoke Sign Language: Hereditary Deafness on Martha's Vineyard. Harvard Univ. Pr., Cambridge, 1985.
7. International Classification of Diseases, Injuries and Causes of Death, 10 ed. World Health Organization, Geneva, 1992.
8. Guides to the Evaluation of Permanent Impairment. American Medical Association, Chicago, 1990.
9. Cohen, H: Vestibular rehabilitation reduces functional disability. Otolaryngol Head Neck Surg 107:638, 1992.
10. Pope, AM, and Tarlov, AR (eds): Disability in America: Toward a National Agenda for Prevention. National Academy Press, Washington, D.C., 1991.
11. Research Plan for the National Center for Medical Rehabilitation Research. U.S. Department of Health and Human Services/Public Health Service/National Institutes of Health/National Institute of Child Health and Human Development. NIH Publication No. 93-3509., Bethesda, 1993.
12. Cohen, H, et al: Disability in Ménière's disease. Arch Otolaryngol 121:29, 1995.
13. Mahoney, FI, and Barthel, DW: Functional evaluation: The Barthel Index. Maryland State Med J 14:61, 1965.
14. Hamilton, BB, et al: A uniform national data system for medical rehabilitation. In Fuhrer, MJ (ed): Rehabilitation Outcomes: Analysis and Measurement. Brookes, Baltimore, 1987.
15. Klein, RM, and Bell, B: Self-care skills: Behavioral measurements with the Klein-Bell ADL Scale. Arch Phys Med Rehab 63:335, 1982.
16. Law, M, et al: The Canadian Occupational Performance Measure: An outcome measure for occupational therapy. Can J Occupational Ther 57:82, 1990.
17. Law, M, et al: Canadian Occupational Performance Measure. Canadian Association of Occupational Therapists, Toronto, 1991.
18. Jacobson, GP, and Newman, CW: The development of the Dizziness Handicap Inventory. Arch Otolaryngol 116:424, 1990.
19. Cohen, H, and Downs, A: A new assessment of independence in activities of daily living for patients with vestibular impairments. ARO Abstr 19:54, 1996.
20. Yardley, L, and Hallam, RS: Psychosocial aspects of balance and gait disorders. In Bronstein, AM, et al (eds): Clinical Disorders of Balance, Posture and Gait. Arnold, London, 1996.
21. Morris, PA: A habituation approach to treating vertigo in occupational therapy. Am J Occupational Ther 45:556, 1991.
22. Farber, SD: Living with Meniere disease: An occupational therapist's perspective. Am J Occupational Ther 43:341, 1989.
23. Cohen, H: Vestibular rehabilitation improves daily life function. Am J Occupational Ther 48:919, 1994.
24. Lawton, MP, and Brody, EM: Assessment of older people: Self-maintaining and instrumental activities of daily living. Gerontologist 9:179, 1969.
25. Shepard, NT, et al: Habituation and balance retraining therapy: A retrospective review. Neurol Clin 8:459, 1990.
26. Eagger, S, et al: Psychiatric morbidity in patients with peripheral vestibular disorder: A clinical and neuro-otological study. J Neurol Neurosurg Psychiat 55:383, 1992.
27. Yardley, L, et al: A longitudinal study of symptoms, anxiety and subjective well-being in patients with vertigo. Clin Otolaryngol 19:109, 1994.
28. Parnes, LS, and Sindwani, R: Impact of vestibular disorders on fitness to drive: A consensus of the American Neurotology Society. Am J Otol 18:79, 1997.
29. Sindwani, R, and Parnes, LS: Reporting of vestibular patients who are unfit to drive: Survey of Canadian otolaryngologists. J Otolaryngol 26:104, 1997.
30. Cohen, H: Functional improvements and vestibular rehabilitation following acoustic neuroma resection. Abstracts of the XIXth Barany Society Satellite Meeting on Vestibular Compensation, Hamilton Island, Australia, 1996, p 19.
31. Cawthorne, T: The physiological basis for head exercises. J Chart Soc Physiother 29:106, 1994.
32. Stein, MB, et al: Panic disorder in patients attending a clinic for vestibular disorders. Am J Psychiatr 151:1697, 1994.
33. Sklare, DA, et al: Dysequilibrium and audiovestibular function in panic disorder: Symptom profiles and test findings. Am J Otol 11:338, 1990.
34. Yardley, L, et al: Relationship between balance system function and agoraphobic avoidance. Behav Res Ther 33:435, 1995.
35. Coker, NJ, et al: Psychological profile of patients with Meneire's disease. Arch Otolaryngol Head Neck Surg 115:1355, 1989.
36. Yardley, L, and Putman, J: Quantitative analysis of factors contributing to handicap and distress in vertiginous patients: A questionnaire study. Clin Otolaryngol 17:231, 1992.
37. Alford, BR: Meniere's disease: Criteria for diagnosis and evaluation of therapy for reporting. Trans Am Acad Ophthalmol Otol 76:1462, 1972.
38. Pearson, BW, and Brackmann, DE: Committee on hearing and equilibrium guidelines for reporting treatment results in Meniere's disease. Otolaryngol Head Neck Surg 93:579, 1985.
39. Dandy, WE: The surgical treatment of Meniere's disease. Surg Gynecol Obstet 72:421, 1941.

40. Bender, MB: Oscillopsia. Arch Neurol 13:204, 1965.
41. Hillman, EJ, et al: Dynamic visual acuity while walking: A measure of oscillopsia. J Vestib Res 9:49, 1999.
42. J. C.: Living without a balancing mechanism. New Engl J Med 246:458, 1952.
43. Cohen, H, and Jerabek, J: Effectiveness of liberatory maneuvers for treatment of benign paroxysmal positional vertigo. Barany Society Meeting Abstracts, 1996, p 19.
44. Cohen, HS, and Jerabek, J: Efficacy of treatments for posterior canal benign paroxysmal positional vertigo. Laryngoscope 109:584, 1999.
45. Cohen, H, et al: Occupation and visual/vestibular interaction in vestibular rehabilitation. Otolaryngol Head Neck Surg 112:526, 1995.

CHAPTER 17

Treatment of Vestibular Hypofunction

Susan J. Herdman, PT, PhD
Susan L. Whitney, PT, ATC, PhD

Vestibular rehabilitation is now accepted as an appropriate and valuable treatment approach for patients with vestibular hypofunction. The use of exercises to treat patients with vestibular dysfunction is not new, but recent studies have documented the effectiveness of these exercises.[1-4] New information about how the nervous system works and about the mechanisms of recovery following vestibular loss has led to the development of more specific exercises than those proposed by Cawthorne and Cooksey in the 1940s.[5,6] This chapter provides the reader with the background necessary to treat patients with vestibular hypofunction. The similarities and differences among the various treatment approaches are examined. Several case studies are provided to illustrate the decision making process in developing exercise programs.

MECHANISMS OF RECOVERY

Several different mechanisms are involved in the recovery of function following unilateral vestibular loss. These mechanisms include cellular recovery, spontaneous reestablishment of the tonic-firing rate centrally, vestibular adaptation, the substitution of other strategies, and habituation.

Cellular Recovery

Cellular recovery suggests that the receptors or neurons that were damaged and initially stopped functioning may recover. This has been demonstrated for vestibular hair cells in nonprimate mammals following aminoglycoside-induced loss.[7,8] There appears to be some functional recovery related to the anatomic recovery although there is a persistent deficit.[9] It is unclear at this time whether recovery of hair cells is a significant factor in recovery of vestibular function in human beings.

Spontaneous Recovery

Unilateral disturbances of static vestibular function (nystagmus, skew deviation, and postural asymmetries in stance) recover spontaneously.[10,11] These symptoms and signs are caused by the disruption of tonic vestibulo-ocular and vestibulospinal responses. In the normal individual, when the head is stationary, the tonic firing of the neurons in the vestibular nuclei on each side of the brainstem is balanced. Unilateral loss of the input from the semicircular canals results in an asymmetry in that activity. That asymmetry is interpreted as head movement. For example, loss of the signal from the semicircular canals on one side results in a slow-phase eye movement away from the intact side as if the intact side were excited by movement. The slow-phase eye movement is interrupted by a quick-phase eye movement in the opposite direction. This quick-phase eye movement resets the eye position, creating a spontaneous nystagmus. Unilateral loss of utricular inputs results in a skew deviation in which the eye on the side of the lesion drops in the orbit. Patients with skew deviations complain of a vertical diplopia.[12] Disruption of the tonic vestibulospinal responses produces an asymmetry in the muscle activity in the lower extremities, as measured electromyographically, while the patient is standing,[13] and in a postural asymmetry, which can be detected clinically.[14] These signs and symptoms resolve within 3 to 14 days following onset of the unilateral vestibular deficit. The timing of the disappearance of these symptoms parallels the recovery of the resting firing rate of the vestibular nucleus neurons.[15] Although visual cues can also be used to suppress spontaneous nystagmus and the postural asymmetry, several studies have demonstrated that recovery of spontaneous nystagmus is not dependent on visual inputs per se.[16] Nystagmus decreases at the same rate in animals kept in the dark immediately after unilateral labyrinthectomy as in animals kept in a lighted environment. Spontaneous recovery is probably due to the development of denervation supersensitivity and to axonal sprouting.

Vestibular Adaptation

Unilateral vestibular loss also results in disequilibrium and visual blurring, especially during head movements. These symptoms are due to the disruption of the vestibular response to head movement. This results in a dramatic decrease in vestibulo-ocular reflex (VOR) gain during head movements. During the acute stage, the gain of the VOR is decreased by as much as 75 percent for head movements toward the side of the lesion and by 50 percent for head movements away from the side of the lesion in patients with unilateral vestibular deficits.[17] Disturbances of the *dynamic vestibulospinal response* are distinguished by a gait ataxia. Typically, patients ambulate with a widened base of support, frequently side-step, and may drift from one side to another while walking. They decrease trunk and head rotation while walking because these rotations would make them less stable. Head movement would result in an asymmetric vestibular signal that increases their sense of disequilibrium and the ataxia. Recovery of the dynamic vestibulo-ocular responses probably is due to the adaptive capability of

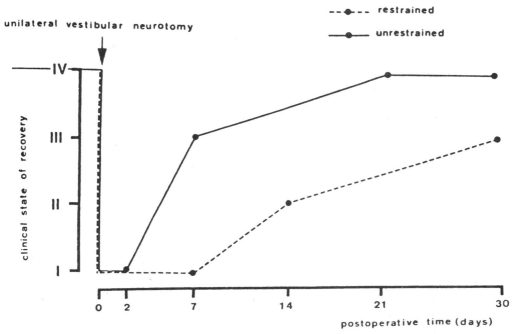

FIGURE 17–1. Effect of restricting mobility on rate of recovery following unilateral transection of vestibular nerve. Baboons that were restrained after unilateral vestibular nerve section had a delayed onset of recovery and a more prolonged recovery than those animals that were allowed free movement. Reprinted with permission from Lacour, M, Roll, JP, and Appaix, M: Modifications and development of spinal reflexes in the alert baboon (papio papio) following an unilateral vestibular neurectomy. (From Brain Res 113:255, 1976, with permission.)

the vestibular system; that is, the ability of the vestibular system to make long-term changes in the neuronal response to input.

The signal for inducing vestibular adaptation is **retinal slip**, or the movement of a visual image across the retina.[18] This slip results in an error signal that the brain attempts to minimize by increasing the gain of the vestibular responses. There is a wealth of evidence that recovery from the dynamic disturbances of vestibular function requires both visual inputs and movement of the body and head.[11,19–22] The gain of the vestibulo-ocular response does not recover when cats or monkeys are kept in the dark following unilateral labyrinthectomy.[16,21] Recovery of vestibulo-ocular gain begins when the animals are returned to a lighted environment. Similarly, if animals are prevented from moving after unilateral vestibular nerve section, there is a delay in the onset of the recovery of postural stability and the recovery period is prolonged[22] (Fig. 17–1).

Substitution

The fourth mechanism involved in recovery following vestibular lesions is the substitution of other strategies to replace for the lost function. Sensory inputs from muscles and joint facets in the neck produce a slow-phase eye movement, the cervico-ocular reflex (COR), that complements the VOR during very low frequency, brief head movements.[23,24] Maoli and Precht[25] suggest that neck proprioceptive inputs have increased influence on gaze stability after unilateral vestibular loss. Smooth pursuit and saccadic eye movements may also contribute to gaze stability.[23,26,27]

Recovery of postural stability may be due to the use of visual and somatosensory cues instead of remaining vestibular cues. Although the substitution of visual or somatosensory cues as a strategy may provide sufficient information for postural stability in many situations, the patient will be at a disadvantage if trying to walk when those cues are inaccurate or even not available, such as in the dark. At an extreme, some patients may modify their behavior to avoid situations where visual or somatosensory cues are diminished, such as going out at night.

These mechanisms do not adequately substitute for the lost vestibular function (Fig. 17–2). The VOR needs to function across frequencies of up to 20 Hz[28,29] for activities such as walking and running. In contrast, the COR works only up to 0.5 Hz and

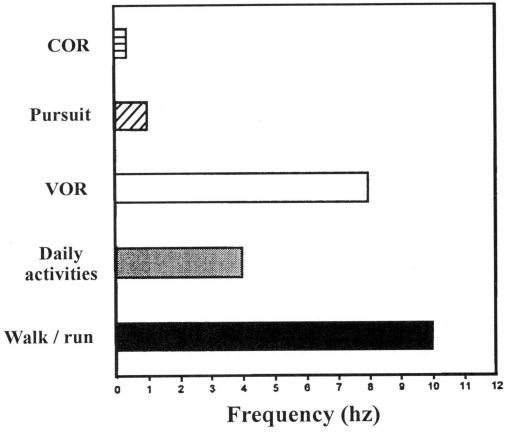

FIGURE 17–2. Frequency range over which the COR, smooth-pursuit eye movements, and the VOR can contribute to gaze stability compared with the frequency and velocity ranges for daily activities, walking, and running. Only the normal VOR operates over the frequency and velocity ranges of normal activities. Modified from Herdman, SJ: The role of adaptation in vestibular rehabilitation. (From Otolaryngol Head Neck Surg 119:49–54, 1998, with permission.)

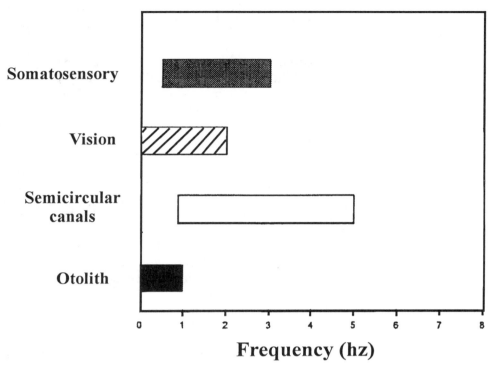

FIGURE 17–3. Frequency ranges over which somatosensory, visual, semicircular canal, and otolith inputs contribute to postural stability. This information has been determined only for stability during quiet stance and following sudden perturbations. Modified from Herdman, SJ: The role of adaptation in vestibular rehabilitation. (From Otolaryngol Head Neck Surg 119:49–54, 1998, with permission.)

with a maximum gain of 0.3.[23,24,30] Pursuit eye movements are limited to less than 1 Hz and a maximum eye velocity of 60° per second.[27] Saccadic eye movements would not be a particularly useful alternative for a poor VOR because patients would not be able to see the target clearly during the actual eye movements.[26] Similar limitations exist for the substitution of somatosensory and visual cues for lost vestibular function (Fig. 17–3). Again, the vestibular system operates through a wider frequency and velocity range than does vision and somatosensation.[31–33]

Patients may also restrict head movements as a means of seeing clearly or maintaining their balance. This strategy is not particularly desirable because it would result in limited activity but would not provide a mechanism for seeing clearly or for maintaining balance during head movements.

Habituation

Habituation refers to a reduction in symptoms produced by specific movements. It occurs through repetitive exposure to the movement and presumably is a central process. The mechanism and neural circuitry are not well known.

EVIDENCE THAT EXERCISE FACILITATES RECOVERY

The use of exercises, especially if supervised, adds to the health care costs of the patient. It is necessary, therefore, to be able to demonstrate the effectiveness of these exercise approaches in the rehabilitation of patients with vestibular hypofunction. Animal studies support the concept that visuomotor experience facilitates the rate of recovery and improves the final level of recovery following vestibular dysfunction.[16,20–22] Several animal studies have suggested that exercise may facilitate the process of vestibular compensation. Igarashi et al[34] found that, following unilateral labyrinthectomy, squirrel monkeys exercising in a rotating cage had less spontaneous nystagmus than a nonexercise control group. In another similar study, Igarashi et al[20] found locomotor equilibrium compensation occurred faster (7.3 days as compared to 13.7 days) in a group of squirrel monkeys exercising in a rotating cage compared to a nonexercise group. Similar findings have been observed in cats following unilateral labyrinthectomy.[19]

Several studies of patients with unilateral vestibular deficits also support the benefits of exercise for improving recovery. Horak et al[1] compared the effectiveness of vestibular rehabilitation (customized programs consisting of gaze stability, habituation, and balance exercises), general conditioning exercises, and vestibular suppressant medications on dizziness and imbalance in patients with chronic vestibular dysfunction. In this prospective, blinded study, patients were randomly assigned to one of the groups and were followed for 6 weeks. Dizziness was assessed using a calculation of movement sensitivity based on intensity and duration of symptoms provoked by specific movements and positions, and by indicating whether the symptoms had improved, worsened, or were unchanged. Postural stability was assessed by measuring peak to peak anterior-posterior (AP) sway under different sensory conditions. A functional balance measure, single leg stance (SLS), was also used. They found a significant decrease in dizziness only in the group of patients receiving vestibular rehabilitation. Similarly, only the vestibular exercise group had a significant improvement in postural stability as indicated by decreased AP sway and increased SLS time. It is understandable that the group receiving medications did not show improvement; both meclizine and diazepam are vestibular suppressants. A more recent study has shown that chronic use of these medications actually prolongs the recovery period.[35] One criticism of this study is that it did not use an untreated group of patients for comparison with the group performing vestibular exercises. An untreated group, however, would not be an appropriate control because the subjects would clearly know they were not being treated and they would not have parallel contact with the physical therapists.

In another study of patients with chronic vestibular deficits, Shepard and Telian[2] examined the efficacy of customized vestibular exercise programs to a more generic exercise program. They did not use a control group but instead used a delayed treatment paradigm. All subjects were assessed at baseline and again at 1 month before initiating any exercises to serve as a control for spontaneous recovery. Subjects who did not show spontaneous recovery were then stratified by age and pretreatment disability levels to assure that the two groups were similar. After 3 months of therapy, both groups reported a decrease in self-reported levels of dizziness with 85 percent of those in the vestibular rehabilitation group and 64 percent in the generic exercise group reporting complete or dramatic improvement. Only the vestibular rehabilitation group, however, showed a significant reduction in dizziness during routine daily activities. The vestibular rehabilitation group also showed a significant improvement on both static and dynamic posturography, a reduction in motion sensitivity, and a decrease in asymmetry of vestibular function. The generic exercise group improved only in their performance of static balance tests.

Herdman et al[3] examined whether patients with acute unilateral vestibular loss following resection of acoustic neuroma would benefit from vestibular rehabilitation. This prospective, double-blinded study compared the effect vestibular adaptation exercises with exercises designed to be "vestibular neutral" (smooth pursuit eye movements performed with the head still). Both groups were instructed in safe ambulation every day. Exercises were initiated on postoperative day 3 in both groups. They found no difference in subjective complaints of vertigo between the groups over the course of the study. This was expected, because vertigo occurs as a result of the asymmetry in the tonic firing rate of the vestibular system and recovers spontaneously. There was, however, a significant difference in the complaints of disequilibrium by postoperative days 5 and 6. As a group, patients performing the vestibular adaptation exercises had significantly less disequilibrium than did patients in the control group. Differences between the groups were also noted for gait pattern, especially with horizontal head movement. All of the control subjects had increased ataxia or developed some ataxia when asked to turn their head while walking. In contrast, only 50 percent of the vestibular exercise group showed this gait disturbance. One criticism of this study is that the extent of vestibular dysfunction and vestibular compensation prior to surgery was not known. There was no difference, however, between the two groups based on clinical examination preoperatively.

The original Cawthorne-Cooksey exercises, developed to treat patients with vestibular deficits, were not customized for the individual patient.[5,6] These exercises are often given as a handout to patients who are simply instructed to "go home and do them." Szturm et al[4] compared the effectiveness of an unsupervised program of Cawthorne-Cooksey exercises to a customized, supervised program of vestibular adaptation exercises. They found that a greater percentage of patients improved in the vestibular adaptation exercise group than in the Cawthorne-Cooksey exercise group.

PREDICTORS OF OUTCOME

An important part of treatment is the education of the patient about the possible final level of recovery. This enables the patient (and the therapist) to set realistic goals. As one might expect, patients with less initial disability and those seen earlier after onset will have a better recovery.[2,36] Patients with stable unilateral vestibular deficits, or those partially compensated patients with symptoms provoked only by movement also have a better prognosis.[37] Studies also indicate that patients with head injury associated with a vestibular deficit show less improvement with treatment.[36,37] This finding does not necessarily extend to all central injuries, however. Keim et al[38] found that patients with central vestibular deficits showed the same improvement as those with peripheral vestibular lesions. These findings were based on standing and walking balance as well as self-report of resumed activities. Shepard et al[35] found that patients with mixed central and peripheral lesions had a more prolonged recovery period than did patients with peripheral lesions only.

The relationship of patient age to the potential for recovery is also not clear. Shepard et al[35] reported that age was not a factor based on the length of the recovery period and on the final level of recovery. In contrast, Norre and Beckers[39] found that patients age 60 years and older recovered more slowly than younger subjects. Vestibular suppressant medications appear to prolong the recovery period but do not actually prevent recovery.[35]

GOALS OF TREATMENT

The goals of physical therapy intervention are to (1) improve the patient's functional balance especially during ambulation; (2) improve the patient's ability to see clearly during head movement; (3) improve the patient's overall general physical condition and activity level; (4) reduce the patient's social isolation; and (5) decrease the patient's disequilibrium (sense of being off-balance) and oscillopsia (visual blurring during head movement). Patients are usually seen by the physical therapist on an outpatient basis, although, in some cases, the initial treatments will occur while the patient is in the hospital. An important part of the rehabilitation process is the establishment of a home exercise program. The physical therapist must motivate the patient and obtain compliance. To do so, the physical therapist must identify the patient's own goals and clarify to the patient the treatment goals as well as the potential effects of exercise.

IS RECOVERY MAINTAINED AFTER THE EXERCISES ARE STOPPED?

Both anecdotal evidence and systematic studies suggest that recovery following vestibular loss may be "fragile." Symptomatic relapse may occur with extreme fatigue or stress, prolonged periods of inactivity, illness, or even a change in medication.[2] Patients need to be aware of this possibility and should understand that it does not indicate a worsening of the underlying pathology.

TREATMENT APPROACHES

Several different approaches have been advocated in the management of patients with vestibular hypofunction. Four different approaches are presented, although there are elements common to all. Table 17–1 provides a summary and comparison of these different approaches. Two case studies are used to demonstrate the basis for specific exercises used in treatment and the progression of the patient's exercise program.

Adaptation

Vestibular adaptation refers to the long-term changes that occur in the response of the vestibular system to input. Adaptation is important during development and maturation, and in response to disease and injury. Exercises that facilitate adaptation can be used in patients with vestibular hypofunction as a mechanism to induce recovery. There is evidence that the vestibular system can be modified during the acute stage after unilateral vestibular loss. VOR adaptation can be induced after unilateral labyrinthectomy in cats as early as the third day after surgery.[25] The vestibular system in human beings also can be adapted during the acute stage after unilateral vestibular

TABLE 17–1 Comparison of Different Exercise Approaches
for the Patient with a Peripheral Vestibular Disorder

Movement	Adaptation	Substitution	Cawthorne-Cooksey	Habituation
Incorporates head and neck exercises into the treatment approach	X	X	X	X
Uses a functional evaluation to assess the symptoms of the patient	X	X	X	X
Incorporates principles of motor control and learning into designing a treatment program	X			X
Practices mental exercises to increase concentration	X		X	X
Has the patient work in a variety of environments and task contexts	X	X	X	X

loss. Pfaltz[40] found an increase in the VOR gain in patients with unilateral vestibular loss stimulated optokinetically compared to untreated patients. More recently, Szturm et al[4] reported increased VOR gain in patients following a course of vestibular adaptation exercises but not in a control group.

GUIDELINES FOR DEVELOPING EXERCISES

The following points should be considered when developing exercises based on adaptation for the patient with a unilateral peripheral lesion.

1. As mentioned before, *the best stimulus to induce adaptation is one producing an error signal* that the central nervous system attempts to reduce by modifying the gain of the vestibular system. The best stimuli appear to be those that incorporate movement of the head and a visual input. Optokinetic stimulation (movement of visual world only) by itself also can increase the gain of the vestibular system although, perhaps not be as effectively as head movement combined with a visual stimulus.[18,41–43] Figure 17–4 shows two simple exercises that can be used as the basis for an exercise program for patients with unilateral vestibular lesions. In each, the patient is required to maintain visual fixation on an object while the head is moving.

2. *Adaptation takes time.* The early studies on vestibular adaptation used paradigms in which the stimulus was present for several hours or more.[44,45] This situation would not be appropriate for patients, especially during the acute stage. We now know that vestibular adaptation can be induced with periods of stimulation as brief as 1 to 2 minutes.[40,46] During the time in which the brain is trying to reduce the error signal, the patient may experience an increase in symptoms and must be encouraged to continue to perform the exercise without stopping. Each exercise shown in Figure 17–4, for instance, should be performed for 1 minute without stopping. The time for each exercise can then be gradually increased to 2 minutes.

3. *Adaptation of the vestibulo-ocular system is context specific.* Therefore, for optimal recovery, exercises must stress the system in different ways.[46] For example, adaptation

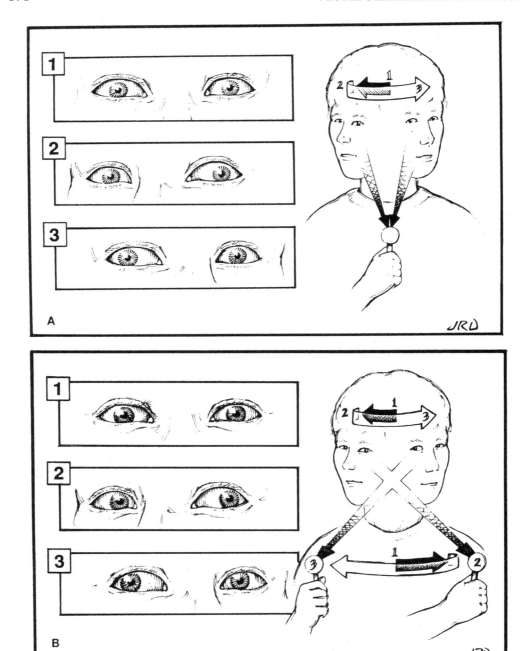

FIGURE 17–4. Exercises to increase the gain of the vestibular system can include an ×1 viewing paradigm (A) and an ×2 viewing paradigm (B). In the ×1 viewing paradigm, the visual target is stationary and the subject moves his head back and forth while trying to maintain visual fixation on the target. In the ×2 viewing paradigm, the target and the head move in opposite directions while the subject again keeps the target in focus. These exercises are performed using a small visual target (foveal stimulus) and a large visual target (full-field stimulus) with the head moving either horizontally or vertically. (Modified from Tusa, RJ, and Herdman, SJ: Vertigo and disequilibrium. In Johnson, R, and Griffin, J (eds): Current Therapy in Neurological Disease, ed 4. Mosby Year-Book, St. Louis, 1993, p 12, with permission.)

of the vestibular system is frequency dependent.[47,48] If the system is adapted at a specific frequency, gain will improve most at that frequency. Because normal movement occurs over a wide range of frequencies of head movement, the patient should perform the head movement exercises at many different frequencies for optimal effects. Different head positions can also be used to vary the exercise.

4. *Adaptation is affected by voluntary motor control.*[49,50] VOR gain can be increased even in the dark if the subject simply imagines that he is looking at a stationary target on the wall while the head is moving. Although not increasing the gain as much as head movement plus vision combined, these results suggest that mental effort will help improve the gain of the system. Patients should be encouraged to concentrate on the task and should not be distracted by conversation and other activities.

5. *Patients should always work at the limit of their ability.* Although the patient's morale can be lifted through activities that they can perform relatively easily, most exercises should stress the patient's ability. For example, with the eye-head exercises, the speed of the head movement should be increased *as long as the patient can keep the visual target in focus.*

Substitution

Mechanisms other than adaptation are involved in recovery, and should be included in a well-rounded exercise program. Exercises should synthesize the use of visual and somatosensory cues with the use of vestibular cues as well as the possibility of central preprogramming to improve gaze and postural stability. For example, balance exercises should "stress" the system by having the patient work with and without visual cues or while altering somatosensory cues by having the patient stand on foam. Removing or altering cues forces the patient to use the remaining cues. Thus, if the patient is asked to stand on foam with eyes closed, the use of vestibular cues will be fostered.

Cawthorne-Cooksey Exercises

The Cawthorne-Cooksey[5,6] exercises were developed in the 1940s. At the time, Cawthorne was treating patients with unilateral vestibular deficits and postconcussive disorders. In conjunction with Dr. Cooksey, a physiotherapist, Cawthorne developed a series of exercises that addressed their patients' complaints of vertigo and impaired balance. The Cawthorne-Cooksey exercises include movements of the head, tasks requiring coordination of eyes with the head, total body movements, and balance tasks (Box 17–1).

GUIDELINES FOR DEVELOPING EXERCISES

The following points should be considered when using the Cawthorne-Cooksey exercises in the treatment of the patient with a unilateral peripheral lesion.

1. Cawthorne and Cooksey recommended that the exercises be performed in various positions and at various speeds of movement.
2. In addition, patients were required to perform the exercises with their eyes open and closed. According to Cawthorne and Cooksey,[5,6] performing the exercises with

---

BOX 17–1   Cawthorne-Cooksey Exercises for Patients with Vestibular Hypofunction

A. In bed
  1. Eye movements—at first slow, then quick
     a. up and down
     b. from side to side
     c. focusing on finger moving from 3 ft to 1 ft away from face
  2. Head movements at first slow, then quick; later with eyes closed
     a. bending forward and backward
     b. turning from side to side

B. Sitting (in class)
  1. and 2 as above
  3. Shoulder shrugging and circling
  4. Bending forward and picking up objects from the ground

C. Standing (in class)
  1. as A1 and A2 and B3
  2. Changing from sitting to standing position with eyes open and shut.
  3. Throwing a small ball from hand to hand (above eye level).
  4. Throwing ball from hand to hand under knee.
  5. Changing from sitting to standing and turning round in between.

D. Moving about (in class)
  1. Circle round center person who will throw a large ball and to whom it will be returned.
  2. Walk across room with eyes open and then closed.
  3. Walk up and down slope with eyes open and then closed.
  4. Walk up and down steps with eyes open and then closed.
  5. Any game involving stooping and stretching and aiming such as skittles, bowls, or basket-ball.

  Diligence and perseverance are required but the earlier and more regularly the exercise regimen is carried out, the faster and more complete will be the return to normal activity.

Cawthorne-Cooksey exercises for patients with vestibular hypofunction. Reprinted with permission from Dix, MR: The rationale and technique of head exercises in the treatment of vertigo. Acta Oto-rhino-laryng (Belg) 33:370, 1979.

---

the eyes closed decreased the patient's reliance on visual information and possibly forced more effective compensation by vestibular and somatosensory mechanisms.
3. Cawthorne and Cooksey also recommended that patients be trained to function in noisy and crowded environments. These situations may be very difficult for patients with vestibular disorders to manage.
4. To encourage active participation, Cawthorne and Cooksey had patients exercise together in daily group sessions. Cawthorne and Cooksey believed a group exercise format would be more economical and more fun for the patient, and would make it easier to identify a malingerer.

Hecker et al[51] utilized the Cawthorne-Cooksey exercises to treat a group of patients with vestibular disorders and reported that 84 percent of the patients responded favorably. They also emphasized the importance of performing the exercises regularly.[51] In addition, they noted that emotional stress seemed to affect the patient's progress.

Cooksey[6] stressed that patients should be encouraged to move into positions that provoke symptoms. She believed that with repeated exposure to a stimulus, the patient would eventually tolerate the position without experiencing symptoms. This treatment philosophy is remarkably similar to the philosophy supported by many physical therapists today who use habituation exercises. Most physical therapy clinics that treat patients with vestibular deficits use some component of the Cawthorne-Cooksey exercises.

Habituation Exercises

This exercise approach is based on the concept that repeated exposure to a provocative stimulus will result in a reduction in the pathological response to that treatment. In 1979, Norre[30] proposed the use of vestibular habituation training for the treatment of patients with unilateral peripheral vestibular loss. According to Norre and De Weert,[52] an asymmetry in labyrinth function results in a "sensory mismatch." The disturbed vestibular signal produces an input to the brain that conflicts with information received from intact visual and somatosensory systems. This conflict, they believed, produced the symptoms experienced by patients with unilateral peripheral vestibular loss.

The Motion Sensitivity Test, developed by Shepard and Telian, uses a series of movements and positions as the basis for establishing an individualized exercise program for patients with chronic unilateral vestibular hypofunction (Table 17–2).[2,35,37] Again, the patient rates the intensity of their symptoms and indicates the duration of symptoms.

GUIDELINES FOR DEVELOPING EXERCISES

The following points should be considered when developing exercises based on habituation for the patient with a unilateral peripheral lesion.

1. Up to four movements are chosen from the test results to form the basis for these exercises. The patient performs these movements 2 or 3 times, twice a day.
2. It is important that the patient perform the movements quickly enough and through sufficient range to produce mild to moderate symptoms.
3. As habituation occurs, the movements can be performed more rigorously.
4. The patient should rest between each movement for the symptoms to stop. The symptoms should decrease within a minute after each exercise or within 15 to 30 minutes after all exercises have been performed.
5. It may take 4 weeks for the symptoms to begin to decrease. The exercises are usually performed for at least 2 months and then can be gradually decreased to once per day.
6. This treatment approach is not advocated for all patients. The elderly especially should not perform movements in which they rise quickly. Precautions include orthostatic hypotension and orthostatic intolerance. If treatment fails, counseling is advisable regarding changing activities or reorganizing the work area.

TABLE 17–2 Motion Sensitivity Quotient Test for Assessing
Patients With Dizziness

Baseline Symptoms	Intensity	Duration	Score
1. Sitting to supine			
2. Supine to left side			
3. Supine to right side			
4. Supine to sitting			
5. Left Hallpike-Dix			
6. Return to sit from left Hallpike-Dix			
7. Right Hallpike-Dix			
8. Return to sit from right Hallpike-Dix			
9. Sitting, head tipped to left knee			
10. Head up from left knee			
11. Sitting, head tipped to right knee			
12. Head up from right knee			
13. Sitting, turn head horizontally 5 times			
14. Sitting, move head vertically 5 times (pitch)			
15. Standing, turn 180° to the right			
16. Standing, turn 180° to the left			

From Shepard, NT, and Telian, SA: Programmatic vestibular rehabilitation. Otolaryngol Head Neck Surg 112:173, 1995.

EXPECTATIONS FOR RECOVERY

Recovery from unilateral vestibular lesions is usually quite good and patients should expect to return to normal activities. Several factors can affect the final level of recovery and should be kept in mind when talking to patients about their progress and anticipated recovery.

1. Recovery may be delayed or limited if the patient restricts head movement or if visual inputs are minimized.[16,21,22] Patients with vestibular lesions often prefer to keep their eyes closed and their heads still to minimize symptoms. Another factor that may delay recovery or limit the final level of recovery may be the use of medications that suppress vestibular function.[53]
2. Recovery following unilateral vestibular deficits can also be affected by the presence of other disorders affecting the peripheral or central nervous systems. Central nervous system deficits that affect the vestibular nuclei or the cerebellum may affect vestibular adaptation[54,55] whereas other lesions can affect structures involved in the

substitution of alternative strategies, such as using visual or somatosensory cues for balance. The same is also true for lesions in the peripheral nervous system. To have adequate postural stability, an individual needs two sensory cues. Patients with vestibular deficits plus visual or lower-extremity somatosensory changes generally do not do as well as patients with vestibular deficits alone. Predicting the final level of recovery is even more difficult in patients with combined central nervous system and vestibular deficits.

3. The rate and final level of recovery can be affected by age-related changes in the vestibular, visual, and somatosensory systems.[56–64] There is evidence that the adaptive capability of the vestibular system itself is reduced in the older person.[60] There is also an increased likelihood that there will be a loss or decrement of more than one sensory cue, which would have a significant impact on postural stability. An individual has good stability with eyes closed (loss of one sensory cue) but is less stable if he stands with eyes closed and has a vestibular lesion. Diminished visual and somatosensory cues may affect the useful substitution of alternative strategies to improve postural stability.

TREATMENT

General Considerations

1. Treatment should begin early. As mentioned, when visuomotor experience is prevented during the early stages after unilateral vestibular loss, there is a delay in recovery.[16,21] Furthermore, the initiation of the recovery of postural responses is delayed, and the course of recovery is prolonged when motor activity is restricted.[22]

2. Exercise can be for brief periods of time initially. Pfaltz's study[40] is also important for showing that even brief periods of stimulation can produce VOR gain changes that would be particularly useful in the treatment of patients during the acute stage of recovery.

3. Although patients with chronic vestibular deficits often do not have vertigo or vomiting (the exception being those patients with episodic vestibular disorders, such as Ménière's disease), they frequently have limited their movements, or at least their head movements, in an attempt to avoid precipitating the symptoms of disequilibrium and nausea. Head movements must be encouraged in these patients both to induce vestibular adaptation (and thereby improve the function of the remaining vestibular system) and to habituate the symptoms provoked by movement.

4. Many of the exercises provided to the patient may, at first, increase the patient's symptoms. This is because the exercises involve head movement, which the patient has been avoiding, because moving the head provokes the patient's dizziness. This situation may be threatening to patients who are extremely fearful of experiencing their symptoms. Nevertheless, patients should be told that during physical therapy, there might be a period when they may feel worse before they feel better. To assist the patient through this period, the physical therapist should be accessible. For example, the patient should be instructed to telephone the therapist if the symptoms become severe or long lasting. In such instances, the physical therapist determines if the exercises can be modified or if the exercises should be discontinued until the patient is formally re-evaluated.

Excessive exacerbation of the patient's symptoms can also be avoided by careful exercise prescription. Initially, the patient may be provided with only a few key exercises. The patient is instructed to attempt the exercises 3 to 5 times per day; the number of repetitions is based on the therapist's assessment of the patient's exercise tolerance. It is a good idea to have the patient perform all exercises completely during the clinic visit in order to assess the response to the exercises. Patients who become excessively "dizzy" while performing the exercises may think the exercises are making them worse and may refuse to continue with rehabilitation. On subsequent visits, the patient is re-evaluated and the exercise program expanded, so that all of the initial physical therapy goals are addressed.

5. It is reasonable to expect improved function within 6 weeks in patients who are compliant about doing their exercises but, anecdotally at least, the longer the problem has existed, the longer the time needed to see improved function. Once the patient is able to perform the initial vestibular exercises, it may be necessary to take the chronic patient through more complex movements in order to habituate the response to movement or at least to make them less fearful that movement will precipitate vertigo. Cawthorne's exercises, such as moving from sitting to standing and turning around in between, and the habituation exercises are very useful at this stage (see Box 17–1 and Table 17–2).

PROBLEM-ORIENTED APPROACH

In a problem-oriented treatment approach, the physical therapy program is based on (1) the problem areas identified during the evaluation, (2) the patient's diagnosis and (3) the patient's medical history. For example, the physical therapy program for a patient with Ménière's disease would differ from that provided to a patient with vestibular neuronitis. Specifically, the treatment program for a patient with Ménière's disease would not address the symptom of vertigo. Compensation of vertigo in Ménière's disease is difficult to achieve because of the fluctuating nature of the disease process itself. Instead, the physical therapy program would focus on improving the patient's balance function in a variety of task and environmental situations, preventing physical de-conditioning, and if indicated, education in environmental modification and safety awareness.

A problem-oriented treatment approach can incorporate adaptation, substitution, habituation, and the Cawthorne-Cooksey exercises according to what is needed. In addition, it should incorporate functional activities and contemporary principles of motor learning and motor control. As with many of the other approaches, the general treatment progression includes the following:

1. Increasing and alternating the speed of the exercises.
2. Performing exercises in various positions and activities (i.e., head movements performed while sitting, then standing, during walking, and during walking with upper extremity manipulation).
3. Performing exercises in situations of decreasing visual and/or somatosensory input (i.e., balance exercises with eyes open and eyes closed).
4. Exposing the patient to a variety of task and environmental situations and contexts (i.e., walking in the home to walking at a shopping mall).

Problem: Visual Blurring and Dizziness When Performing Tasks that Require Visual Tracking or Head Stabilization

Visual blurring and dizziness when performing tasks that require visual tracking or gaze stabilization during head movements is most likely due to decreased VOR gain resulting in visual blurring during head movement and also visual-vestibular sensory mismatch. Adaptation exercises can be used to improve the gain of the VOR and therefore improve gaze stabilization. Some caution should be taken when adaptation exercises are used during the acute stage following unilateral vestibular loss. In this stage, the patient may complain of severe vertigo and may be nauseated and vomiting. Head movement will make these symptoms worse and the patient usually prefers to lie quietly, often in a darkened room or with eyes closed. At this stage, the patient may also be taking medications to suppress these vegetative responses and may be receiving intravenous fluid replacement. Slow, easy head movements, such as turning the head to look at someone, should be encouraged. Good visual inputs (bright room lights, curtains open) also should be encouraged during the first days after the acute onset of a vestibular deficit.

After 1 to 3 days, the symptoms of nausea and vertigo should resolve and the spontaneous nystagmus should be decreasing as the resting state of the vestibular neurons recovers. Patients can begin exercises to facilitate adaptation of the vestibular system as early as 1 or 3 days after the onset of the vestibular loss using gentle, active head movement. Horizontal head movement while fixating a small (foveal), stationary target is performed for only 1 minute followed by a period of rest ($\times 1$ viewing; see Fig. 17–4 and Box 17–2). The exercise is then repeated using vertical head movements. As the patient improves, he or she should try to perform the exercises for up to 2 minutes each. Although the patient may complain of increased vertigo or disequilibrium with head movements, neither is a reason to stop the exercises. Vomiting or significant nausea, however, are reasons for terminating or modifying the exercises.

VOR gain in the acute stage after unilateral vestibular loss is poor (.25 to .5) and relatively slow head velocities and low frequencies should be used so that the patient can keep the visual target in focus at all times. As the patient improves (within a few days to a week or more), the exercises can be expanded to include use of a full-field stimulus (checkerboard) in addition to the small target they had been using. Within 1 or 2 weeks after onset, patients can begin the vestibular adaptation exercises that requires them to maintain fixation on a visual target that is moving in the opposite direction as their head movement ($\times 2$ viewing; see Fig. 17–4 and Box 17–2). This exercise should be performed with somewhat smaller head movements (and comparably small target movements) because the target cannot be kept in focus while viewing out of the corner of an eye. The head movements may have to be slower as well for the patient to maintain fixation. Both the $\times 1$ and the $\times 2$ viewing paradigms should be performed at increasing head velocities as the patient improves. Within two or three days after onset, patients can begin to perform the VOR adaptation exercises while standing as a preparation for walking and turning the head as well.

Ultimately, the adaptation paradigms should be incorporated into gait and other functional activities. Patients with vestibular deficits should also be instructed to perform functional tasks or games that require visual tracking or gaze fixation. For example, laser tag requires the patient to move the head while focusing eyes on a moving target. Bouncing and catching a ball may be another appropriate task for some pa-

BOX 17–2   Exercises to Improve Postural Stability

There are many different balance exercises that can be used. These exercises are devised to incorporate head movement (vestibular stimulation) or to foster the use of different sensory cues for balance.

1. The patient stands with his feet as close together as possible with both or one hand helping maintain balance by touching a wall if needed. He then turns his head to the right and to the left horizontally while looking straight ahead at the wall for one minute without stopping. The patient takes his hand or hands off the wall for longer and longer periods of time while maintaining balance. The patient then tries moving his feet even closer together.
2. The patient walks, with someone to assist him if needed, as often as possible (acute disorders).
3. The patient begins to practice turning his head while walking. This will make the patient less stable, so the patient should stay near a wall as he walks.
4. The patient stands with his feet shoulder width apart with eyes *open*, looking straight ahead at a target on the wall. He progressively narrows his base of support from feet apart to feet together to a semi–heel-to-toe position. The exercise is performed first with arms outstretched, then with arms close to the body and then with arms folded across the chest. Each position is held for 15 seconds before the patient does the next most difficult exercise. The patient practices for a total of 5 to 15 minutes.
5. The patient stands with his feet shoulder-width apart with eyes open, looking straight ahead at a target on the wall. He progressively narrows his base of support from feet apart to feet together to a semi–heel-to-toe position. The exercise is performed with eyes *closed*, at first intermittently and then for longer and longer periods of time. The exercise is performed first with arms outstretched, then with arms close to the body and then with arms folded across the chest. Each position is held for 15 seconds and then the patient tries the next position. The patient practices for a total of 5 to 15 minutes.
6. A headlamp can be attached to the patient's waist, shoulders, or head and the patient can practice shifting his weight to place the light into targets marked on the wall. This home "biofeedback" exercise can be used with the feet in different positions and with the patient standing on surfaces of different densities.
7. The patient practices standing on a cushioned surface. Progressively more difficult tasks might be hard floor (linoleum, wood), thin carpet, shag carpet, thin pillow, sofa cushion. Graded density foam can also be purchased. Backward walking can be attempted cautiously.
8. Make walking more difficult by asking the patient to count backwards as they walk. This can be made progressively more difficult by having the patient perform the exercise while walking on different surfaces.
9. The patient practices walking with a more narrow base of support. The patient can do this first touching the wall for support or for tactile cues, and then gradually touching only intermittently, and then not at all.
10. The patient practices turning around while he walks, at first making a large circle but gradually making smaller and smaller turns. The patient must be sure to turn in both directions.
11. The patient can practice standing and then walking on ramps, either with a firm surface or with more cushioned surface.
12. The patient can practice maintaining balance while sitting and bouncing on a swedish ball or while bouncing on a trampoline. This exercise can be incorporated with attempting to maintain visual fixation of a stationary target thus facilitating adaptation of the otolith-ocular reflexes.
13. Out in the community, the patient can practice walking in a mall before it is open and therefore quiet. They can practice walking in the mall while walking in the same direction as the flow of traffic, or walk against the flow of traffic.

tients. The patient could be advised to bounce the ball off the floor, wall, and/or ceiling in an attempt to vary the task by changing direction of object motion and/or neck position. Using multicolored or highly patterned balls may also increase task difficulty, because the moving pattern or high color contrast may greatly increase the patient's symptoms. Electronic "Simon Says" requires the patient to watch and remember a sequence of lights that flash in rapid succession in front of the patient. This task incorporates Cawthorne's suggestion to include mental exercises into the exercise regimen.

Exposing the patient to highly textured visual environments may also assist in the remediation of visuo-vestibular interaction deficits. For example, the patient may be instructed to gradually perform tasks, such as grocery shopping or walking through a shopping mall.

Problem: Exacerbation of Symptoms

If a patient experiences exacerbation of symptoms during the head movement assessment, habituation exercises are incorporated into the exercise program. During the physical therapy assessment, positions or movements that provoke the patient's symptoms are identified based on the results of the Motion Sensitivity Test (see Chapter 15). These positions and movements are then incorporated into the patient's exercise program. Movements, such as rolling, supine to sit, and sit to stand frequently exacerbate the patient's symptoms (see Table 17–2). If the patient has significant symptoms, these exercises may be performed initially in the supine or sitting position. Later, the patient can perform these exercises in standing or during walking. If straight plane movements of the head produce few symptoms, neck diagonals, with or without a combination of trunk movement, are prescribed. During the head movement/position exercises, the patient is instructed to hold the position for at least 10 seconds, or until the symptoms dissipate. In addition, the patient is instructed to perform each exercise 3 to 5 times. It is particularly important that the initial prescription of these exercises should avoid those movements/positions that produce severe symptoms. Many therapists have experienced that too aggressive an approach initially may lead to patient noncompliance. Instead, therapists should select movements and positions that produce a minimal to moderate level of symptoms.

Attempts are also made to include habituation exercises into the patient's daily routine. For example, the patient is instructed to incorporate neck diagonals into the task of loading and unloading the dishwasher. This task requires the patient to focus on the object and move the body, head and arm synchronously to either pick up or place the object on a high shelf (Fig. 17–5).

Problem: Static and Dynamic Postural Instability

The balance and gait exercises prescribed for a patient are based on the problems identified during assessment and will vary considerably depending on patient history and medical diagnosis. Recovery from unilateral vestibular neuronitis, labyrinthitis, or from a surgical procedure, such as vestibular nerve section, typically takes 6 weeks, although recovery may take up to 6 months in some patients. Patients with vestibular nerve section, for example, often return to work within 3 weeks. Recovery from resection of acoustic neuroma typically takes longer, although most of the recovery occurs

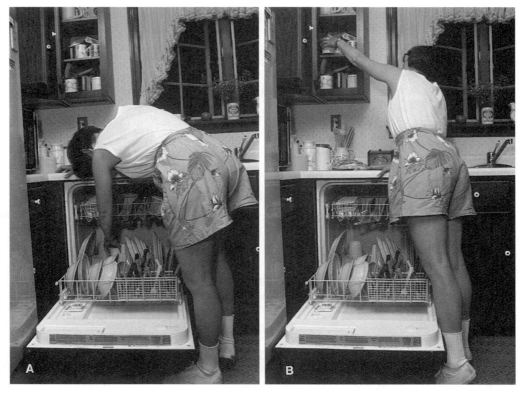

FIGURE 17–5. Neck movements are incorporated into the patient's normal daily routine. In this example, the patient is instructed to incorporate a neck diagonal when loading and unloading the dishwasher.

within the first few weeks. After the first 2 or 3 weeks, the main complaints are fatigue, instability when turning quickly, and some increased difficulty walking in the dark. Patients may also complain of greater instability when walking on uneven surfaces or when there is a change in light intensity (opening a door to the outside, walking through intermittent shadows, such as trees).

Although many patients with peripheral vestibular hypofunction perform below the norm on static tests of balance during the acute stage, the most common complaint is imbalance during dynamic activities such as walking. Rarely do these patients report an inability to stand on one leg. Instead, they may complain of difficulty walking on an uphill grade, through a cluttered room, or into a movie theater. Because of the nature of the patient's deficits, balance training should address the dynamic aspects of gait and be task directed. Balance and gait training are inseparable and therefore considered together in this discussion.

Based on the evaluation, the therapist identifies the patient's functional balance deficits. Therapeutic exercise prescription should address the patient's specific deficits. For example, a patient may experience disequilibrium when the opportunity to use visual and/or somatosensory input for balance is minimized. In this situation, emphasizing exercises and tasks that require the patient to focus on vestibular, instead of vi-

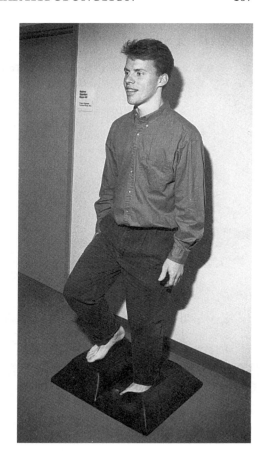

FIGURE 17–6. Activities that promote use of vestibular information for balance are frequently included in the patient's home exercise program. In this example, the patient marches in place on a foam cushion, with the eyes open or closed. Closing the eyes maximizes the importance of vestibular information.

sual or somatosensory, input is important. Such exercises include walking backward, sidestepping, and braiding performed with the eyes closed, marching in place on foam performed with the eyes open and later with the eyes closed (Fig. 17–6 and Box 17–3), and walking across an exercise mat or mattress in the dark.

Another functional deficit is the instability experienced by patients when faced with situations that require movements of the head during gait. For instance, many patients indicate having difficulty shopping for groceries. To scan the grocery shelves for the desired item, the patient must walk while moving the head left, right, or diagonally. At the same time, the patient must continue to monitor the environment to prevent a collision with another shopper. As a result, this rather ordinary task creates an overwhelming challenge to the patient's postural control system. To overcome this challenge, the patient is first instructed to walk down a corridor while moving the head left and right, or up and down. Later, the patient performs the same task, while avoiding objects placed in the walking path. The most difficult condition would be to perform this exercise in an area with a complex visual environment (similar to a shopping aisle with people and carts).

The last deficit to be discussed is the difficulty patients with vestibular deficits experience when their gait is unexpectedly disrupted. One seldom walks through a busy

---

BOX 17–3   Exercises to Improve Gaze Stability

Acute stage (also used with chronic, uncompensated patients):

1. A business card, or other target with words on it (foveal target), is taped on the wall in front of the patient so he can read it. The patient moves his head gently back and forth horizontally for one minute while keeping the words in focus.
2. This is repeated moving the head vertically for one minute.
3. Depending on whether this induces any nausea, the exercise is then repeated using a large pattern such as a checkerboard (full-field stimulus), moving the head horizontally.
4. The exercise with the checkerboard is then repeated moving the head vertically.

The patient should repeat each exercise at least three times a day.
The duration of each of the exercises is extended gradually from one to two minutes. Patients should be cautioned that the exercises may make them feel dizzy or even nauseated but that they should try to persist for the full one to two minutes of the exercise, resting between exercises.

Sub-acute stage:

1. The patient holds a business card in front of him so that he can read it. He moves the card and his head back and forth horizontally in *opposite* directions keeping the words in focus for one minute without stopping.
2. This is repeated with vertical head movements and with a large, full-field stimulus.

The duration is gradually extended from one to two minutes. The patient should repeat each exercise at least three times each day.

Chronic stage:

1. The patient fixates on a visual target placed on the wall in front of them while gently bouncing up and down on a trampoline (otolith stimulation).

---

shopping mall without experiencing a sudden head-on encounter with another person. Such tasks require the postural control system to respond quickly. In some cases, the patient may need to improve the ability to anticipate forthcoming events. As indicated in the gait evaluation, an obstacle course can be devised to assess the patient's ability to anticipate or respond quickly to changes in task context. The obstacle course can also be used in treatment. The patient should be instructed to vary the course in as many ways as possible. Having a family member verbally direct the patient on the path to follow is helpful. Commands are given at the moment the patient must encounter or avoid an obstacle, thereby maintaining a level of task uncertainty. Another task that requires the patient to respond quickly to externally imposed constraints is walking and pivoting to the left or right. Again, a family member directs the patient on when and in what direction to pivot. Family members can also quickly give the command to "stop."

Patients with vestibular disorders can experience difficulty with many different balance and gait tasks. This discussion considered only a few. With a thorough evaluation, the therapist may identify the patient's specific motor control problem. In such cases, the therapy program should not be limited to specific balance or gait exercises. Instead the therapist should provide the patient with balance and gait activities that challenge the patient's postural control system in a variety of ways.

Progression of Balance and Gait Exercises

Recovery of postural stability occurs more gradually than recovery of gaze stability. Following acute onset of vestibular loss, patients need assistance to get out of bed for 1 to 2 days after the onset, sometimes longer. They usually, although not always, need assistance with ambulation for the first few days. Patients with unilateral vestibular loss usually can stand with feet together and their eyes closed within 4 to 5 days after the onset, although they still will have increased sway. Gait will be grossly ataxic for the first week, but patients should be walking independently, albeit with a widened base of support, within 1 week. During this initial stage of recovery, several different balance and gait exercises are appropriate. Goals include increasing the patient's endurance while walking, improving stability while standing with a more narrow base of support (Romberg position) with eyes open and closed, and beginning to turn the head while walking. Exercises to improve balance in sitting or other positions are usually not necessary and for postoperative patients, bending over must be avoided.

Gait exercises can be more challenging for patients with chronic vestibular disorders, although, again, the starting point depends upon the problems identified during the assessment (see Box 17–3). Patients can be taken through a series of exercises that stress their balance by gradually decreasing their base of support or by altering visual and somatosensory cues. Even if they are unable to maintain the position successfully for the required period of time, practicing will improve their balance. Patients with complete unilateral vestibular loss, however, rarely perform the sharpened Romberg with eyes closed at any age. More difficult dynamic balance exercises may include walking and turning suddenly or walking in a circle while gradually decreasing the circumference of the circle, first in one direction and then in another. The patient needs the practice of walking in different environments, such as on grass, in malls (walking in an empty mall is easier than in a crowded mall, walking with the crowd is easier than against the crowd), and walking at night. Precautions to prevent falls should always be taken until the patient no longer needs them but it is important to avoid letting the patient become dependent on assistive devices for walking.

Problem: Physical Deconditioning

Physical deconditioning because of inactivity may be a significant problem for many patients with unilateral vestibular loss. Many patients are advised to begin a regular walking program. The purpose of the walking program is two-fold: First, to prevent deconditioning of the patient; second, to provide realistic balance challenges to the patient's central nervous system. Tasks such as walking on uneven terrain, walking through a shopping mall, or crossing the street challenge the patient in ways that cannot be simulated by a therapeutic exercise program (Fig. 17–7). When crossing the street, the patient must conform to the temporal constraints imposed by moving vehicles. Specifically, the patient must determine at what moment to step off of the curb to avoid confronting a vehicle. When crossing the street at a busy intersection, this requirement becomes more difficult to fulfill. In addition, the patient's postural control system must make quick adjustments to offset perturbations caused by changes in terrain or motion of other people.

The initial program requires the patient to walk for 15 to 20 minutes four times per week. Over the subsequent weeks, the patient is instructed to increase to a 30-minute

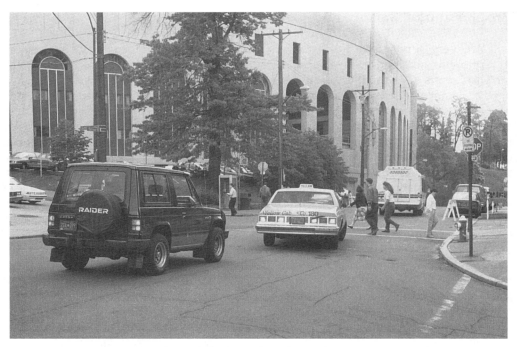

FIGURE 17–7. Patients may have difficulty with walking when they must conform to temporal constraints such as when crossing a street before the light changes.

walk. Initially, the patient may be advised to walk in a familiar environment with few challenges. Later, the therapist encourages the patient to expand the walking program to other situations and contexts. Walking in a park and at a shopping mall are frequently recommended. When walking in these situations, patients are advised to experience as many challenges as possible. For example, riding an escalator in a shopping mall may provide an interesting challenge to the patient. The patient must remain balanced while standing on a moving support surface. In addition, the motion of other people toward or to the side of the patient may create a sense of dizziness or imbalance, enhancing the difficulty of the task. Such challenges are necessary to overcome if the patient is to manage safely in a variety of contexts without experiencing an exacerbation of symptoms.

Patients can also be encouraged to return to other activities, such as tennis or golf, which will help improve their overall fitness. These activities need to be added gradually. Activities such as using a stationary bike, although it should help improve fitness, will not help improve postural stability except indirectly by increasing strength or range of motion. Swimming can be safely performed by patients with unilateral vestibular loss and is a good fitness exercise. If the patients want to return to ocean swimming, they should be advised that they might have some difficulty initially walking on the sand or standing on the sand in the water. (Patients with bilateral vestibular loss must be more cautious because without visual cues, they will have difficulty knowing 'which way is up' when under water. Ocean swimming in particular may not be advisable. Swimming with goggles will help, but not in murky water.) For all patients, the precautions we all should follow need to be observed: never swim alone.

Problem: Return to Driving

One of the more commonly asked questions is when the patient may begin to drive again. The legal ramifications may vary from state to state, but essentially patients should not drive if they cannot see clearly during head movements or if head movements result in significant dizziness (or disorientation). One guideline, that patients should be able to see clearly when making rapid and abrupt head movements, can be tested using the dynamic visual acuity test. If a patient decides to return to driving, he or she should be encouraged to begin on quiet, local streets or in a parking lot when it is empty. Driving at night and driving on high-speed roads should be delayed until the patient is comfortable with the quieter roads. Drivers' training is often beneficial and may be covered through insurance.

SUMMARY

Patients with unilateral vestibular deficits can be expected to recover from the vertigo and/or disequilibrium they first experience. The final level of recovery should be to return to all or most activities. Other nervous system disorders can delay or limit the level of recovery. Animal studies and anecdotal evidence in human beings suggest that exercises facilitate recovery of vestibular system function. Early intervention also seems to be important in optimizing recovery. Restricting movement, preventing visual inputs and the use of vestibular suppressant medications may delay the onset of recovery and may limit the final level of recovery.

This chapter has presented treatment strategies for the physical therapy management of patients with unilateral peripheral vestibular hypofunction. Patients with unilateral peripheral vestibular hypofunction may present with a variety of functional deficits. The physical therapy treatment program should address all of the patient's functional deficits. The use of exercise in the rehabilitation of patients with vestibular disorders is aimed at promoting vestibular compensation. Several case studies were presented to illustrate the rehabilitation management of patients with unilateral peripheral vestibular hypofunction.

CASE STUDIES

CASE STUDY 1

A 74-year-old woman developed severe vertigo with nausea and vomiting 6 months ago. At that time, the vertigo appeared to be positional. She reports she had to crawl to the bathroom and that she "passes out" for an unknown period of time. She was hospitalized for 8 days. A caloric test performed at that time showed right canal paresis. She had a course of vestibular rehabilitation at a different site, which she states was not beneficial. Presently she complains of light-headedness and dizziness with head movement. She is using a cane for ambulation which she did not need prior to the onset of the vertigo. Review of records from 6 months ago show that at that time the patient was ambulating with a walker, could not perform the Fukuda's Stepping Test, and that her clinical visual acuity was 20/20 with her head stationary and increased to 20/200 during 2-Hz horizontal head oscillations.

Past Medical and Social History

Significant weight gain in last 6 months. No history of trauma, exposure to ototoxic medications, no heart disease, diabetes, thyroid disorder, hypertension, arthritis or treatment by psychiatrist.

Comment

This patient had a unilateral vestibular loss 6 months ago (based on the caloric); the description of the vertigo as being "positional" is misleading, but may indicate a superior vestibular artery lesion resulting in horizontal canal hypofunction and utricular degeneration with sparing of the posterior canal. This would result in canal paresis and posterior semicircular canal BPPV. It is not clear why the patient believes the previous course of vestibular rehabilitation was not beneficial. If the exercise program were too aggressive, it may have provoked excessive dizziness and therefore the patient may have not been compliant with the exercises. It is clear that she had made some improvement since the onset of the problem—she is walking now with a cane instead of a walker.

Subjective Complaints

The patient rates her disequilibrium as a 6.0 on an analogue scale from 0 (normal) to 10 (worst it could be). She rates her oscillopsia during ambulation as an 8.4 on a similar scale.

Neurological Examination

Normal except as follows:

1. Visual acuity was 20/25–4 OU (both eyes viewing) with head stationary and decreases to 20/63 - 3 during 2-Hz horizontal oscillations of the head.
2. VOR is normal during slow head rotation but patient makes large corrective saccades with head thrusts to the right.
3. Patient has decreased response to vibration (125 Hz) and abnormal kinesthesia in her toes. Ankle jerk responses are absent bilaterally.
4. She walks with a slow cadence, widened base of support, and decreased rotation through trunk and neck. She is unable to turn her head while walking and keep her balance.
5. Fukuda's Stepping Test results in excessive translation to the left.

Comment

The decrease in visual acuity during head movement is consistent with an uncompensated vestibular deficit. The presence of corrective saccades with head thrusts to the right is consistent with a right deficit. The normal-appearing VOR with slow head movements may be due to the function of the intact left side or to substitution of gaze stability by the pursuit system. The peripheral neuropathy, although mild, may affect her postural stability, especially in the dark, as well as the final level of functional recovery. Her gait pattern is typical of a person with an uncompensated vestibular deficit.

Oculomotor Examination

Oculomotor examination using an infrared recording system to prevent fixation suppression of nystagmus reveals:

1. No spontaneous or gaze-holding nystagmus.
2. Horizontal head-shaking resulted in a left-beating nystagmus; there was no vertical head-shaking–induced nystagmus.
3. Movement into the Hallpike-Dix position to the left was negative but to the right the patient developed a mild left beating nystagmus without vertigo.

Comment

Head-shaking–induced nystagmus is not always present in patients with unilateral vestibular deficits. The presence of a left-beating nystagmus following horizontal head shaking is consistent with her right-sided lesion. The left-beating nystagmus, without vertigo, when the patient was moved into the right Hallpike-Dix position, is from the asymmetry in the utricular signal produced by movement into that position and is not uncommon in patients with unilateral vestibular loss. It may explain why an earlier diagnosis of positional vertigo was made.

Plan for Vestibular Rehabilitation

Problems

1. Disequilibrium and postural instability induced by head movement.
2. Decrement in visual acuity with head movement.
3. Ambulation with a cane.
4. Decreased activity level.
5. Social isolation.

Plan

The patient was placed on vestibular adaptation exercises, static and dynamic balance exercises, and some exercises based on functional activities. The exercises consisted of the $\times 1$ viewing paradigm, which the patient performed for 1 minute each using a foveal target held in her hand. Initially, the patient performed these exercises sitting down. She used both horizontal and vertical head movements. This exercise was to be performed five times daily. The goals of these exercises was to increase the gain of the remaining vestibular system, decrease her symptomatic response to head movement and encourage the patient to make head movements. Functionally, the exercises should improve her visual acuity during head movement and habituate the dizziness induced by head movement. She was also instructed in static balance exercises performed with eyes open and then with eyes closed. She was instructed to practice walking without her cane. This latter exercise she was to perform in her house in the hallway for 5 minutes, twice daily. The goal of these exercises was to decrease her reliance on visual cues for balance and decrease her reliance on her cane while walking. The patient was also asked to begin a walking exercises program, increasing her walks to 20 minutes daily. The patient performed all exercises at least once during this initial clinic visit to ensure that she was able to perform the exercises correctly and that the exercises did not make her so dizzy that she would stop performing them. Follow-up was scheduled for 1 week later and the patient was told to call if she had questions or difficulty performing the exercises. After the initial follow-up visit, the patient was seen in clinic every 2 weeks.

One-Month Re-evaluation

Subjective Complaints
The patient rated her disequilibrium as a 3.0 on an analogue scale from 0 (normal) to 10 (worst it could be). She rated her oscillopsia during ambulation as a 2.9 on a similar scale. This was a marked improvement over her initial visit.

Balance and Gait
Fukuda's Stepping Test resulted in a 4-inch forward progression and an 85° turn to the left. She still could not perform the sharpened Romberg with eyes open. She no longer was using her cane. During ambulation, her cadence, base of support, step length, and rotation through trunk and neck were normal. When asked to turn her head from side to side while walking, there was a slight decrease in cadence but the patient could perform the task with only a slight deviation from a straight path. She was able to walk safely on ramps, stairs and on grass with and without head rotation.

Comment

This patient showed excellent recovery following her unilateral vestibular loss. The persistence of an abnormal Fukuda's Stepping Test (performed with eyes closed) is not unusual. Her inability to perform the sharpened Romberg with eyes open is normal for age (although some people in her age range can perform this test).

CASE STUDY 2

A 44-year-old woman is referred for treatment of her acoustic neuroma. For the past year she has had complaints of disequilibrium and difficulty seeing clearly when walking or riding in a car, but was otherwise in good health. She also complained of a gradual loss of hearing in her left ear. Her audiogram showed a Speech Reception Threshold of 65 and no identifiable speech discrimination. She had normal hearing on the right with 100 percent discrimination. MRI with gadolinium showed a 4-cm tumor in the left cerebellar-pontine angle, which was compressing the lower midbrain, pons, upper medulla, and cerebellum. Facial nerve function appeared to be symmetrical and normal. She had decreased light touch sensation on the midportion of the left face to cotton. Corneal reflex was decreased on the left. She had direction changing, gaze-evoked nystagmus. Pursuit, saccades, and VOR cancellation were normal. VOR to slow head movement was normal in both directions. VOR to rapid head thrusts to the right was normal but resulted in corrective saccades with head movements to the left. With Frenzel lenses, gaze-evoked nystagmus was more pronounced to the right than to the left. After head shaking there was only a single drift of the eyes to the left and a single corrective saccade. No nystagmus was elicited with vertical head shaking. Visual acuity with the head stationary was 20/20 corrected. Quantified visual acuity during active head oscillations at 150° per second degraded to 20/34.

Her Romberg was normal and the patient could maintain the sharpened Romberg with eyes open for 30 seconds. She could not perform the sharpened Romberg with eyes closed. Fukuda's Stepping Test with eyes open resulted in a 22-inch forward progression with no turn. With eyes closed she had a 40-inch forward progression with no turn. The patient ambulated with a normal cadence, stride length, base of support, trunk and neck rotation, and arm swing. She did not appear to use excessive visual fixation to maintain her balance while ambulating. Posturography tests showed that the patient had difficulty maintaining her balance when both visual and somatosensory cues were absent (eyes closed) or altered. She showed mildly increased reliance on visual cues for balance. The latency to force development, gain, and symmetry of her automatic postural responses were within normal limits bilaterally. Short-, middle-, and long-latency responses as measured by EMG were within normal limits bilaterally. Vibration threshold in her left foot was normal but elevated in her right foot ($\bar{x}$ + 3SD). At the time of her initial physical therapy evaluation, the patient was also oriented to the postoperative rehabilitation care.

Comments

This patient is typical of many patients with acoustic neuromas (AN) in that her main complaint was decreased hearing. She additionally had developed some balance problems but many patients with AN do not notice any changes in balance preoperatively. The absence of vertigo or even disequilibrium in these patients is because of the gradual vestibular loss occurring as the tumor grows rather than an abrupt onset as would occur with vestibular neuronitis. This tumor was quite large and was compressing brainstem structures and the cerebellum without producing many symptoms or signs other than decreased sensation in the face and a decreased corneal reflex. The direction changing gaze-evoked nystagmus may have been due to compression of the brainstem or cerebellum. The patient made corrective saccades with head movements toward the involved side which indicates an inadequate vestibular response. In addition, her dynamic visual acuity was abnormal (normal is little or no change in acuity with head movement). The fact that she had no head-shaking–induced nystagmus, in spite of having a unilateral vestibular deficit, may be due to poor velocity storage related to the brainstem compression. Several abnormal findings were found with assessment of her balance including inability to perform the sharpened Romberg with eyes closed, abnormal Fukuda's Stepping Test with eyes closed, and difficulty maintaining her balance on the posturography tests when both visual and somatosensory cues are altered. We have found that the sharpened Romberg test with eyes closed is sensitive to unilateral vestibular loss but not specific for vestibular deficits. Her ability to perform Fukuda's Stepping Test without turning is a little unusual in a patient with a unilateral deficit but may reflect compensation.

Intervention

Surgical resection of the acoustic neuroma was performed using a suboccipital approach (see Chapter 10). A large tumor, approximately 5 cm in diameter that filled the posterior fossa and eroded the posterior lip of the internal auditory canal, was found. The seventh cranial nerve was monitored throughout the procedure and was intact. The patient did well postoperatively. She had no complaints of vertigo or of diplopia. She had a right-beating nystagmus when she looked to the right or upward. She did have a prominent VIIth palsy and evidence of involvement of cranial nerves IX and X.

On postoperative day 3, she still had a right-beating nystagmus. Her active neck range of movement was limited by 50 percent because of pain at the surgical site, which she described as a pulling sensation. She was beginning to ambulate with contact guarding only. She walked with a widened base of support and minimized rotation through her trunk. Her gait was slow and she occasionally side-stepped. Her balance when turning appeared to be less secure. She appeared to use excessive visual fixation while she walked for balance. She could not turn her head while walking without an increase in her ataxia. She had a negative Romberg. Sharpened Romberg was not tested. Posturography showed that she was unable to maintain her balance when both visual and somatosensory cues were altered, and she had increased difficulty when somatosensory inputs alone were altered. Her balance was within normal limits on the other tests. There was no asymmetry in stance. Vestibular adaptation exercises were initiated on postoperative day 3. The initial exercise used was the $\times 1$ viewing paradigm, which the patient was to perform both while sitting and while standing. While standing she was to gradually decrease her base of support and bring her feet closer together. The exercise was to be performed using a foveal stimulus with horizontal and vertical head movements. The patient was instructed to perform the exercises three to five times a day for one minute each. In addition, she was to practice walking, gradually increasing the distance walked.

Comment

This patient's postural instability and her performance on the various balance tests are typical of patients following resection of AN. Many patients experience vertigo immediately after the surgery, but this patient probably had lost most of her vestibular function unilaterally because of the size of the tumor. The loss of vestibular function prior to surgery may also account for the minimal nystagmus and the absence of a skew deviation in this patient.

Early Postoperative Course

By postoperative day 6, she still had a direction-changing gaze-evoked nystagmus, but it had decreased. Her quantitative dynamic visual acuity was 20/60. She had a normal sharpened Romberg with eyes open but could not perform it with eyes closed. She was ambulating independently but still had an increased base of support. Her gait was less ataxic and she no longer used excessive visual fixation to maintain balance. She was independent on stairs with a railing. Her exercise program consisted of the ×1 and the ×2 viewing paradigms, using both a foveal and a full-field stimulus, that she was to perform in sitting and in standing three times a day. She was to perform each exercise for 2 minutes. She also was instructed to begin practicing turning her head while walking, being careful because it would make her less stable. Each exercise period would take approximately 45 minutes. At this stage, patients are still not allowed to bend over or lift anything more than 5 pounds (risk of cerebrospinal fluid leak). The patient was discharged from the hospital on postoperative day 7.

Comment

Rapid recovery for patients with unilateral vestibular loss is typical. The effect of the vestibular loss is still obvious (dynamic visual acuity is degraded to 20/60, her gait is still abnormal especially when she turns her head). Most patients with unilateral vestibular loss are never able to perform the sharpened Romberg with eyes closed. We typically do not give these patients any kind of assistive device to use when walking. There are 2 or 3 days while they are in the hospital when walking with a cane might be helpful for some patients. Purchasing a cane for these patients is difficult to justify, because the cane will not be needed at discharge. There are exceptions to this rule, of course, but in over 200 patients only three or four have needed an assistive device for walking.

Outpatient Follow-up

The patient was next seen in the outpatient clinic 3 weeks after surgery. Romberg was normal and sharpened Romberg with eyes open was normal, but patient could not perform the sharpened Romberg with eyes closed. Posturography showed that the patient could maintain her balance within normal limits when both visual and somatosensory cues were altered. Motor tests showed normal latency, gain, and symmetry of response. The patient ambulated with a normal cadence and a normal base of support. She could turn without loss of balance, but did slow down slightly. When asked to turn her head repeatedly while walking, her base of support widened and her gait became slightly ataxic. Her exercise program now included ×1 and ×2 viewing exercises in stance only, using both a foveal and a full-field stimulus, with both horizontal and vertical head movements. She was to perform the exercises with her feet positioned so that her balance was challenged as well (for example in a semi-tandem position). She was also to practice standing with and without visual cues while gradually decreasing her base of support (see Box 17–3). She continued to practice walking and turning her head because that was still a problem. She began a walking program to improve her exercise tolerance and was encouraged to walk in different environments such as outdoors, on uneven surfaces, or in a mall.

Comment

The goals for this patient are that she return to full activities, probably within 6 weeks of surgery. Other patients require a longer recovery period, and may not return to work for 3 months. The full recovery period following this surgery is 1 year with fatigue being the main problem. Within 6 months (and usually earlier), patients should be able to participate in sports such as tennis, racquetball, and golf, all of which are also good vestibular and balance exercises. They may have to change how they play and may have to shift to doubles tennis games. Patients will be aware of a sense of imbalance when they turn rapidly toward the side of the deficit, but usually do not have any loss of balance. Some patients complain that they have difficulty when balance is stressed, such as when walking in the dark on uneven surfaces or if they have to step backwards suddenly.

Patients who do not do well should be carefully screened for other problems that would complicate their recovery, such as the coexistence of visual changes, sensory changes in the feet, or central nervous system lesions that would prevent vestibular adaptation. Some patients are fearful of moving their head. These patients may still benefit from vestibular exercises even several months after surgery, but will need to be on a more closely supervised program to ensure compliance.

This patient also had a facial palsy after surgery. The potential for recovery is good because the nerve was intact after surgery. We do not initiate facial exercises until the patient has more than faint voluntary movements and then patients are cautioned to practice gentle facial movements rather than forceful movements. Another approach would be to send the patient for EMG biofeedback instruction. In patients with significant synkinesis, we use biofeedback training to improve the quality of the facial movements. Of main concern for patients with facial paresis or palsy is protection of the eye. If lid closure is absent or poor, patients may use either a cellophane moisture chamber or an eye patch to prevent drying of the eye and corneal damage. Patients using either type of patch should be advised to be careful when walking because they have only monocular depth perception cues.

CASE STUDY 3

A 46-year-old woman is referred to physical therapy with a diagnosis of a right peripheral vestibulopathy. The physician's report indicated that her symptoms appeared suddenly, for no apparent reason. Symptomatic complaints included disequilibrium with rapid head movements, blurred vision, and veering to the right during ambulation. Although somewhat improved, these symptoms had persisted for 2 months. The patient was unable to drive and was on a medical leave from her job. Her past medical history was significant for hypertension and thyroid disease.

Comment

This patient's history is interesting because most patients with unilateral vestibular deficits present with a history of a specific episode of vertigo rather than of disequilibrium. Her complaints of disequilibrium with head movement, blurred vision and a gait disturbance reflect the disturbance of the dynamic vestibular responses.

Examinations

The neurological examination was normal. Her MRI scan and audiogram were unremarkable. Vestibular laboratory testing included an oculomotor screening battery, static positional testing, caloric testing, rotational testing, and posturography. Test results showed a left gaze-evoked nystagmus, a left-beating nystagmus on positional testing, a right vestibular paresis on caloric testing, a left directional preponderance on rotational testing, and abnormal posturography (abnormal response for all six sensory organization conditions and abnormal adaptation to toes up rotation on movement coordination).

Comments

The left-beating, gaze-evoked nystagmus, the left-beating nystagmus on positional testing, and the directional preponderance most likely reflect right vestibular paresis. The increased difficulty experienced by the patient on all six of the sensory organization tests is unusual, but not unheard of, during the chronic stage following unilateral vestibular deficits. In some patients, this finding may reflect a functional component to the patient's complaints. Difficulty maintaining balance to sudden toes-up rotations of the support surface may signify a tendency toward retropulsion in some patients, but is a nonspecific finding in many patients with balance problems. It may indicate that the patient will have difficulty walking on uneven surfaces.

Intervention

The patient was assessed in physical therapy 3 days after her neurotological evaluation. She reported that looking up, reading, and quick head movements worsened her symptoms. She reported a decreased activity level and an inability to do grocery shopping or heavy housework. The patient indicated that her symptoms, which occurred several times per day, lasted 2 to 3 minutes.

On clinical evaluation, she reported disequilibrium when moving from the supine to sitting position. Head movements (flexion, extension, left and right rotation, and left and right lateral flexion), tested in the sitting position with eyes open and closed, provoked disequilibrium. Disequilibrium and blurred vision occurred when she was asked to track a moving target, while keeping her head stationary. In addition, she experienced disequilibrium and blurred vision when asked to move her head, while focusing her eyes on an object that was either stationary or moving.

During tests of static balance performance, she maintained SLS with her eyes open for 14 seconds on the left foot and 18 seconds on the right foot. With her eyes closed, she could only perform SLS for 3 seconds on either foot. On the CT-SIB[65,66] (see Chapter 15), she maintained all conditions for 30 seconds. However, she experienced disequilibrium during the test, especially for the condition requiring her to stand on foam with her eyes closed.

The patient could ambulate independently, but considerable veering to the right and left, decreased trunk rotation, and decreased arm swing were noted during gait. Disequilibrium was produced when the following advanced gait tasks were performed: walking with right and left head movements, walking and stopping quickly, and walking with pivot turns to the right or left. She was able to tandem walk five steps with her eyes open and one step with her eyes closed, before losing her balance.

Comments

The patient complaints of disequilibrium were almost always associated with movement of the head that reflects the persistent defect in the dynamic VSRs and VORs. Her complaint of disequilibrium during pursuit eye movements with her head stationary may be related to her nystagmus, although many patients are unaware of nystagmus. The age of the patient must be considered when interpreting whether or not a timed balance test, such as SLS, is normal. In this case, the patient should have been able to maintain SLS with eyes open and closed for at least 28 and 16 seconds, respectively.

Management

The patient was given a home exercise program that consisted of head movements in sitting with eyes open, eye/head exercises, and a walking program. She was told to perform the head and eye/head exercises twice a day for 2 weeks. She was advised to walk 4 times a week. She was seen on two subsequent visits, each 2 weeks apart, upon which she was re-evaluated and given a progression in her home exercise program. The following exercises were added to her home program: head movements in sitting with eyes closed, walking with head movements, walking with pivots, and circle walking. She was also given additional eye/head exercises.

After 2 months, the patient was retested in preparation for discharge. She had no symptoms when moving from the supine to sitting position. Head extension and left rotation, performed with the eyes closed, were the only head movements that continued to produce mild disequilibrium. The patient continued to have mild disequilibrium when asked to track a moving object while maintaining a stable head position. Other tasks, which required movement of her head with fixation of her eyes on a stationary or moving object, no longer produced symptoms of disequilibrium and blurred vision.

Timed static balance measures, performed with eyes open, improved to 22 seconds and 29 seconds, for left and right SLS, respectively. The same tasks performed with eyes closed were unchanged from the initial physical therapy evaluation. The patient no longer complained of symptoms when performing the CT-

SIB. Her gait no longer revealed any abnormalities. She was able to tandem walk 15 steps with her eyes open and 3 steps with her eyes closed. In addition, walking and moving the head left and right was the only advanced gait task that continued to produce mild disequilibrium.

At discharge, her activity level had improved. She was walking for 25 minutes four times a week. She was able to drive and perform heavy housework without difficulty. She felt that her symptoms had significantly improved. Her symptoms typically occurred once a week, lasting only 1 minute. At discharge, the patient was instructed in a maintenance home program that consisted of head movements, eye/head movements, and a walking program.

The patient underwent vestibular testing approximately 1 month after her discharge from physical therapy. At the time of retesting, she indicated that she had returned to work part-time. Vestibular testing was much improved as compared to her initial test results. She no longer had a gaze-evoked nystagmus or a left-beating nystagmus on positional testing. Repeated posturography revealed normal adaptation to toes up rotation on movement coordination testing. On sensory organization testing, only condition 5 continued to reveal an abnormal response. Rotational testing indicated a reduction in the left directional preponderance seen on initial testing.

Comment

Although it is considered preferable to begin treatment of patients with vestibular deficits as soon as possible after onset of the vestibular deficit, in many cases exercises are not needed and patients will recover on their own. This patient, however, continued to have disequilibrium and was unable to function at work or around the home. The exercise program, and perhaps time, resulted in improvement in her sense of disequilibrium and in her postural stability that was documented both subjectively and objectively.

ACKNOWLEDGMENTS

This work was supported by NIH grant DC 03196. The authors also wish to acknowledge the contribution of Diane Borello-France, PhD, PT.

REFERENCES

1. Horak, FB, et al: Effects of vestibular rehabilitation on dizziness and imbalance. Otolaryngol Head Neck Surg 106:175, 1992.
2. Shepard, NT, and Telian, SA: Programmatic vestibular rehabilitation. Otolaryngol Head Neck Surg 112:173, 1995.
3. Herdman, SJ, et al: Vestibular adaptation exercises and recovery: Acute stage after acoustic neuroma resection. Otolaryngol Head Neck Surg 113:77, 1995.
4. Szturm, T, et al: Comparison of different exercise programs in the rehabilitation of patients with chronic peripheral vestibular dysfunction. J Vestib Res 4:461, 1994.
5. Cawthorne, T: The physiological basis for head exercises. Journal of the Chartered Society of Physiotherapy 30:106, 1944.

6. Cooksey, FS: Rehabilitation in vestibular injuries. Proc Royal Soc Med 39:273, 1946.
7. Meza, G, et al: Recovery of vestibular function in young guinea pigs after streptomycin treatment. Glutamate decarboxylase activity and nystagmus response assessment. Int J Devel Neurosci 10:407, 1992.
8. Forge, A, et al: Ultrastructure evidence for hair cell regeneration in the mammalian inner ear. Science 259:1616, 1993.
9. Jones, TA, and Nelson, RC: Recovery of vestibular function following hair cell destruction by streptomycin. Hear Res 62:181, 1992.
10. Precht, W: Recovery of some vestibuloocular and vestibulospinal functions following unilateral labyrinthectomy. Prog Brain Res 64:381, 1986.
11. Fetter, M, et al: Effect of lack of vision and of occipital lobectomy upon recovery from unilateral labyrinthectomy in Rhesus monkey. J Neurophysiol 59:394, 1988.
12. Halmagyi, GM, et al: Diagnosis of unilateral otolith hypofunction. Diagnostic Neurotology 8:313, 1990.
13. Allum, JHJ, and Pfaltz, CR: Postural control in man following acute unilateral peripheral vestibular deficit. In Igarashi, M, and Black, FO (eds): Vestibular and Visual Control on Posture and Locomotor Equilibrium. Karger, Basel, 1985, p 315.
14. Halmagyi, GM, et al: Vestibular neurectomy and the management of vertigo. Curr Opinion Neurol Neurosurg 1:879, 1988.
15. Yagi, T, and Markham, CH: Neural correlates of compensation after hemilabyrinthectomy. Exp Neurol 84:98, 1984.
16. Fetter, M, and Zee, DS: Recovery from unilateral labyrinthectomy in Rhesus monkeys. J Neurophysiol 59:370, 1988.
17. Allum, JHJ, et al: Long-term modifications of vertical and horizontal vestibulo-ocular reflex dynamics in man. Acta Otolaryngol (Stockh) 105:328, 1988.
18. Miles, FA, and Eighmy, BB: Long-term adaptive changes in primate vestibuloocular reflex. I. Behavioral observations. J Neurophysiol 43:1406, 1980.
19. Mathog, RH, and Peppard, SB: Exercise and recovery from vestibular injury. Am J Otolaryngol 3:397, 1982.
20. Igarashi, M, et al: Further study of physical exercise and locomotor balance compensation after unilateral labyrinthectomy in squirrel monkeys. Acta Otolaryngol 92:101, 1981.
21. Courjon, JH, et al: The role of vision on compensation of vestibulo ocular reflex after hemilabyrinthectomy in the cat. Exp Brain Res 28:235, 1977.
22. Lacour, M, et al: Modifications and development of spinal reflexes in the alert baboon (Papio papio) following an unilateral vestibular neurectomy. Brain Res 113:255, 1976.
23. Kasai, T, and Zee, DS: Eye-head coordination in labyrinthine-defective human beings. Brain Res 144:123, 1978.
24. Bronstein, AM, and Hood, JD: The cervico-ocular reflex in normal subjects and patients with absent vestibular function. Brain Res 373:399, 1986.
25. Maoli, C, and Precht, W: On the role of vestibulo-ocular reflex plasticity in recovery after unilateral peripheral vestibular lesions. Exp Brain Res 59:267, 1985.
26. Segal, BN, and Katsarkas, A: Long-term deficits of goal-directed vestibulo-ocular function following total unilateral loss of peripheral vestibular function. Acta Otolaryngol (Stockh) 106:102, 1988.
27. Leigh, RJ, et al: Supplementation of the vestibulo-ocular reflex by visual fixation and smooth pursuit. J Vestib Res 4:347, 1994.
28. Grossman, GE, et al: Frequency and velocity of rotational head perturbation during locomotion. Exp Brain Res 70:470, 1988.
29. Grossman, GE, et al: Performance of the human vestibuloocular reflex during locomotion. J Neurophysiol 62:264, 1989.
30. Sawyer, RN, et al: The cervico-ocular reflex of normal human subjects in response to transient and sinusoidal trunk rotations. J Vestib Res 4:245, 1994.
31. Diener, HC, et al: The significance of proprioception on postural stabilization as assessed by ischemia. Brain Res 296:103, 1984.
32. Diener, HC, et al: Stabilization of human posture during induced oscillations of the body. Exp Brain Res 45:126, 1982.
33. Dichgans, J, and Brandt, T: Visuo-vestibular interaction. Effects on self-motion perception and postural control. In Held, R, et al (eds): Handbook of Sensory Physiology. Springer, Berlin, 1978, p 755.
34. Igarashi, M, et al: Effect of physical exercise upon nystagmus and locomotor dysequilibrium after labyrinthectomy in experimental primates. Acta Otolaryngol 79:214, 1975.
35. Shepard, NT, et al: Vestibular and balance rehabilitation therapy. Ann Otol Rhinol Laryngol 102:198, 1993.
36. Telian, SA, et al: Habituation therapy for chronic vestibular dysfunction: Preliminary results. Otolaryngol Head Neck Surg 103:89, 1990.
37. Shepard, NT, et al: Habituation and balance retraining therapy. Neurol Clin 5:459, 1990.
38. Keim, RJ, et al: Balance rehabilitation therapy. Laryngoscope 102:1302, 1992.
39. Norre, ME, and Beckers, A: Vestibular habituation training for positional vertigo in elderly patients. J Am Geriatr Soc 36:425, 1988.

40. Pfaltz, CR: Vestibular compensation. Acta Otolaryngol 95:402, 1983.
41. Istl-Lenz, Y, et al: Response of the human vestibulo-ocular reflex following long-term 2X magnified visual input. Exp Brain Res 57:448, 1985.
42. Davies, P, and Jones, GM: An adaptive neural model compatible with plastic changes induced in the human vestibulo-ocular reflex by prolonged optical reversal of vision. Brain Res 103:546, 1976.
43. Collewijn, H, et al: Compensatory eye movements during active and passive head movements: Fast adaptation to changes in visual magnification. J Physiol 340:259, 1983.
44. Jones, GM, et al: Changing patterns of eye-head coordination during 6 h of optically reversed vision. Exp Brain Res 69:531, 1988.
45. Demer, JL, et al: Adaptation totelescopic spectacles: Vestibulo-ocular reflex plasticity. Investigative Ophthalmology and Visual Science 30:159, 1989.
46. Collewijn, H, et al: Compensatory eye movements during active and passive head movements: Fast adaptation to changes in visual magnification. J Physiol 340:259, 1983.
47. Lisberger, SG, et al: Frequency- selective adaptation: Evidence for channels in the vestibulo-ocular reflex. J Neurosci 3:1234, 1983.
48. Goodaux, E, et al: Adaptive change of the vestibulo-ocular reflex in the cat: The effects of a long-term frequency-selective procedure. Exp Brain Res 49:28, 1983.
49. Baloh, RW, et al: Voluntary control of the human vestibulo-ocular reflex. Acta Otolaryngol (Stockh) 97:1, 1984.
50. Furst, EJ, et al: Voluntary modification of the rotatory-induced vestibulo-ocular reflex by fixating imaginary targets. Acta Otolaryngol (Stockh) 103:231, 1987.
51. Hecker, HC, et al: Treatment of the vertiginous patient using Cawthorne's vestibular exercises. Laryngoscope 84:2065, 1974.
52. Norre, ME, and De Weerdt, W: Treatment of vertigo based on habituation. I. Physio-pathological basis. J Laryngol Otol 94:689, 1980.
53. Zee, DS: The management of patients with vestibular disorders. In Barber, HO, and Sharpe, JA (eds): Vestibular Disorders. Year Book, Chicago, 1987, p 254.
54. Lisberger, SG: Role of the cerebellum during motor learning in the vestibulo-ocular reflex. Trends Neurosci 5:437, 1982.
55. Galiana, HL, et al: A reevaluation of intervestibular nuclear coupling: Its role in vestibular compensation. J Neurophysiol 51:242, 1984.
56. Bergstrom, B: Morphology of the vestibular nerve. II. The number of myelinated vestibular nerve fibers in man at various ages. Acta Otolaryngol 76:173, 1973.
57. Richter, E: Quantitative study of human scarpa's ganglion and vestibular sensory epithelium. Acta Otolaryngol (Stockh) 90:199, 1980.
58. Rosenhall, U: Degenerative patterns in the degenerating human vestibular neuro-epithelia. Acta Otolaryngol (Stockh) 76:208, 1973.
59. Wall, C, et al: Effects of age, sex and stimulus parameters upon vestibulo-ocular responses to sinusoidal rotation. Acta Otolaryngol (Stockh) 98:270, 1984.
60. Paige, GD: Vestibulo-ocular reflex (VOR) and adaptive plasticity with aging. Soc Neurosci Abstr 15:515, 1989.
61. Kosnik, W, et al: Visual changes in daily life throughout adulthood. J Gerontol Psychol Sci 43:63, 1988.
62. MacLennan, S, et al: Vibration sense, proprioception, and ankle reflexes in old age. J Clin Exp Gerontol 2:159, 1980.
63. Perret, E, and Regli, F: Age and the perceptual threshold for vibratory stimuli. Euro Neurol 4:65, 1970.
64. Kenshalo, DR: Age changes in touch, vibration, temperature, kinesthesis and pain sensitivity. In Birren, JE, and Schaie, KW (eds): Handbook of the Psychology of Aging. New York, Van Nostrand Reinhold, 1977, p 562.
65. Shumway-Cook, A, and Horak, FB: Assessing the influence of sensory interaction on balance: Suggestion from the field. Phys Ther 66:1548, 1986.
66. Horak, FB: Clinical measurement of postural control in adults. Phys Ther 67:1881, 1987.

CHAPTER 18

Assessment and Treatment of Complete Vestibular Loss

Susan J. Herdman, PT, PhD
Richard A. Clendaniel, PT, PhD

The loss of vestibular function bilaterally results in difficulty maintaining balance, especially when walking in the dark or on uneven surfaces, and in a decrease in the patient's ability to see clearly during head movements. Patients with bilateral vestibular loss (BVL) also complain of severe disequilibrium and dizziness, especially when standing or walking. Because of these problems, patients with BVL often restrict their activities and can become socially isolated.

Vestibular rehabilitation can improve postural stability and decrease the sense of disequilibrium in many patients, enabling them to resume a more normal life.[1] Preliminary evidence exists that visual acuity during head movement also improves (personal observation). The exercises used must be aimed at fostering the substitution of alternative strategies to compensate for the lost vestibular function as well as at improving any remaining vestibular function. This chapter presents the assessment and physical therapy treatment of these patients. Case studies are used to illustrate different points.

PRIMARY COMPLAINTS

Balance

Patients with bilateral vestibular loss are primarily concerned with their balance and gait problems. During the acute stage they may feel off balance even when lying or sitting down. More typically, however, their balance problems are obvious only when they are standing or walking. Patients who develop the problem following use of an ototoxic medication, the most common cause of bilateral vestibular loss, often do not know they have a balance problem until they get out of bed. Typically, these patients have been treated with the ototoxic medication because of a serious infection. They are often debilitated and their balance problems are attributed to weakness.

Even with full compensation, balance problems will persist. Although the other sensory and motor systems do help compensate for the vestibular loss, these systems cannot substitute completely for the loss of vestibular function (see Chapter 17, Figs. 17–2 and 17–3). Normal postural stability while walking requires the combined use of at least two of three sensory cues (visual, vestibular, somatosensory). Patients who have no vestibular function, therefore, will have difficulty when either visual or somatosensory cues are also significantly decreased (e.g., walking in the dark). Although balance may be poor, it is not known what the actual frequency of falling is for patients with BVL. Most patients are able to prevent falls even though they may side-step or stagger occasionally.

Oscillopsia

Another problem for patients with bilateral vestibular loss is the visual blurring that occurs during head movements. Initially, loss of vestibular function results in a decrement in visual acuity even when the patient is stationary, if the head is not supported.[2] Even following the best compensation, patients say that objects that are far away appear to be jumping or bouncing. This visual blurring or oscillopsia increases with irregular or unpredictable head movements such as would occur while walking. As a result, patients may not be able to read street signs or identify people's faces as they walk, or they may have difficulty seeing clearly while in a moving car. Severe oscillopsia will also impact postural stability because decreased visual acuity will affect the person's ability to use visual cues for stability.[3]

Sense of Disequilibrium or Dizziness

Patients often complain of "dizziness," "heaviness," or a sense of being "off-balance" that is separate from their actual postural instability. This feeling lessens or disappears when the person is lying or sitting down with the head supported. It increases dramatically when the person is moving. Although this dizziness or disequilibrium may decrease as a result of compensation, for many patients it remains a serious and debilitating problem. It can lead to decreased physical activity, social isolation, and depression.

Physical Deconditioning

Poor physical condition can be a significant problem for patients with BVL. This can be caused directly by a decreased activity level because of the patient's fear of loss of balance or because of the increased dizziness that occurs with movement. It is especially a problem for patients whose vestibular loss is secondary to ototoxic medications. These patients are already debilitated because of severe infection. Many patients on peritoneal dialysis, for example, develop infections that are treated with gentamicin, a vestibulotoxic aminoglycoside.

ASSESSMENT

The assessment of patients with BVL is similar to that for patients with unilateral vestibular deficits; therefore only certain aspects of the assessment will be described here. Physical therapy assessment of patients with BVL must address the postural instability and oscillopsia, the patient's overall physical condition, and their ability to perform activities of daily living (ADLs). This assessment must also identify other factors that might affect recovery, especially visual and somatosensory deficits. A summary of the assessment and the usual findings for patients with bilateral vestibular loss is presented in Box 18–1.

BOX 18–1   Test Results on Patients with BVL

Oculomotor examination
- *Abnormal findings in room light including:* poor VOR to slow and rapid head thrusts; visual acuity with head stationary is usually normal but during gentle oscillation of the head, acuity would change to 20/100 or worse.
- *With Frenzel lenses:* No spontaneous, gaze-evoked, head-shaking–induced, tragal-pressure–induced, hyperventilation-induced, or positional nystagmus.

Sensation
 Somatosensory and visual information is critical to functional recovery and must be carefully evaluated.

Coordination
 Should be normal.

Range of motion
 Should be normal, but patients will voluntarily restrict head movements because head movement makes them less stable and also results in poor vision.

Strength (gross)
 Should be normal.

Postural deviations
 Should be normal.

Positional and movements testing
 Should not result in vertigo.

Sitting balance
 Patients may have difficulty maintaining their balance during weight-shifting in sitting during the acute stage, but should not have difficulty during the compensated stage.

Static balance
- *Romberg:* Abnormal during acute stage in many patients.
- *Sharpened Romberg:* Patients with complete or severe bilateral loss will not be able to perform this with eyes closed.

(Continued)

(BOX 18–1   Continued)

Static balance (continued)

- *Single leg stance:* Difficult to perform even during compensated stage, with eyes open.
- *Stand on rail:* Usually not tested.
- *Standing on foam surface:* Difficult to perform with decreasing base of support. Should not be attempted in many patients.
- *Force platform:* Normal or close to normal anterior-posterior sway with eyes open or closed during compensated stage on stable surface.

Balance with altered sensory cues

Increased sway when visual *or* somatosensory cues are altered, loss of balance when *both* visual and somatosensory cues are altered.

Dynamic balance (self-initiated movements)

- *Fukuda's Stepping Test:* Normal with eyes open during compensated stage; cannot perform with eyes closed (rapid loss of balance).
- *Functional reach:* May be decreased with eyes closed.

Ambulation

The patient's gait is usually at least slightly wide-based during compensated stage. There is a tendency to use visual fixation while walking and to turn "en bloc." Tandem walk cannot be performed with eyes closed.

- *Walk while turning head:* Gait slows and becomes ataxic.
- *Singleton:* Expect loss of balance. Uneven surfaces or poor light will result in increased ataxia and possibly loss of balance.

History

Bilateral loss of vestibular function can occur for several reasons (see Chapter 5). Most common is the effect of an ototoxic medication such as gentamicin. Considered to be an idiosyncratic response, less than 3 percent of people who receive gentamicin develop a vestibular deficit.[4] The prevalence is as great as 10 to 20 percent, however, in those patients with renal impairment, over the age of 65 years, taking loop diuretics, or with previous vestibular loss, although that percentage increases to 20 percent among persons on renal dialysis who receive gentamicin. The significance of knowing the underlying etiology of the BVL is in the accompanying problems the patient may have. The patient who has a spontaneous or sequential BVL is less likely to have other health problems that will affect their recovery than a patient who had a severe infection and was treated with an ototoxic medication. Furthermore, the patient who has a loss of vestibular function, with its resultant balance and visual problems, because they received an ototoxic medication, may have to deal with significant anger and depression.

While taking the patients' histories, the clinician should identify the presence of progressive disorders such as macular degeneration and cataracts. These disorders result in a gradual decrease in available visual cues and will have an adverse effect on balance in the future. Similarly, disorders that frequently result in peripheral neuropathies should be noted, such as diabetes or chronic alcohol abuse.

Subjective Complaints

The patient's complaints of disequilibrium and oscillopsia can be assessed using a visual analogue scale. The Dizziness Handicap Inventory[5] and the Activities of Daily Living Assessment for Vestibular Patients[6] are useful tools to assess the patient's perception of disability or handicap and the patient's functional abilities and problems.

Vestibular Function

One important consideration in designing a treatment program is whether there is any remaining vestibular function. Vestibular function can be documented using tests such as the rotational chair and caloric tests. This information is then used to determine which exercises to give the patient. If there is no remaining vestibular function, the exercises must be directed at the substitution of visual and somatosensory cues to improve gaze and postural stability.

The presence of remaining vestibular function can be used as a guide in predicting the final level of recovery for patients. Patients with incomplete bilateral vestibular loss are often able to return to activities such as driving at night and to some sports. Patients with severe bilateral loss may not be able to drive at night and some patients will not be able to drive at all because of the gaze instability. Activities such as sports and dancing may be limited because of the visual and the balance problems.

Vestibular function tests can also be used to follow the course of the vestibular loss and of any recovery of vestibular function that might occur.[7,8] Certain aminoglycoside antibiotics are selectively taken up by vestibular hair cells and result in a gradual loss of vestibular function. Typically, there is continued loss of vestibular function even after the medication is stopped. Some improvement in vestibular function may occur if there are hair cells that were affected by the ototoxic drug but not killed. Potentially, an increase in gain may also occur with the use of vestibular adaptation exercises. This has been demonstrated in patients with unilateral vestibular loss but not in patients with BVL.[9]

Visual System

Assessment of visual function should include at least a gross test of visual field and a measure of visual acuity, because both of these can affect postural stability.[3] Measuring visual acuity during head movement is particularly important. The vestibulo-ocular system normally stabilizes the eyes during head movements; when there is no vestibulo-ocular reflex (VOR) to stabilize the eyes during head movement, small amounts of retinal slip (movement of image across the retina) will degrade vision. For instance, $3°$ per second of retinal slip would cause visual acuity to change from 20/20 to 20/200.[10] The movement of the head that occurs when in a moving car can cause a degradation of visual acuity that would make driving a car unsafe.

Assessment of visual acuity during head movement (dynamic visual acuity [DVA]) can be performed either clinically or using a computerized system. The advantage of the computerized system is that the test is standardized and more reliable.[11] Clear difference in DVA scores occur among normal subjects, those with dizziness from nonvestibular causes, and patients with known vestibular loss (Table 18–1). The

**TABLE 18–1 Distribution of Normal and Abnormal DVA Scores
Based on Computerized System**

Subject	DVA (LogMAR)	Normal DVA (%)	Abnormal DVA (%)
Normal (*n* = 51)	0.040 + .045	96.1	3.9
Dizzy, nonvestibular (*n* = 16)	0.097 + .099	87.5	12.5
Unilateral vestibular loss (*n* = 53)	0.282 + .140	11.3	88.7
Bilateral vestibular loss (*n* = 34)	0.405 + .134	0	100

results of the DVA test are both sensitive (90 percent for those over 65 years old and 97 percent for those under 65 years old) and specific (94 percent) for vestibular loss. The clinical DVA, however, is easy to perform and is sufficiently reliable to be useful as a guide to treatment and to treatment efficacy[12] (Fig. 18–1).

Somatosensory System

Particular attention should be made to assess vibration, proprioception, and kinesthesia in the feet. Although mild deficits in sensation in the feet may have no effect on postural stability in otherwise normal individuals, in patients with vestibular loss, somatosensory deficits may have profound effects on balance and on the potential for functional recovery. As with visual system disorders, being aware of potentially progressive disorders affecting somatosensory information is important.

Balance and Gait

Patients with BVL must be given a detailed assessment of balance and gait. Obviously, static balance should be assessed first. In the acute stage, patients with bilateral vestibular deficits may have positive Romberg tests. In the compensated stage, the Romberg is usually normal. Patients will not be able to perform the Sharpened Romberg with eyes closed, although some patients will be able to perform the Sharpened Romberg with eyes open. Patients with bilateral vestibular deficits will also have difficulty performing tests in which both visual and somatosensory cues are altered. An example of this would be Fukuda's Stepping Test in which the eyes are closed and the patient is marching in place. Patients may have normal tests with eyes open but will fall with eyes closed.

Determining how well patients use different sensory cues to maintain balance and whether they are dependent on particular sensory cues is critical. It is important to recognize that this may vary considerably from patient to patient and that it can change over the course of recovery. Bles et al[13] have shown that patients with BVL initially are more dependent on visual cues than on somatosensory cues for balance. With time, there is an improvement in the ability of patients to use somatosensory cues. This improvement varies from patient to patient, however, and needs to be carefully assessed (Fig. 18–2).

The gait of patients with bilateral vestibular deficits is wide-based and ataxic. Patients decrease their trunk and neck rotation in an effort to improve stability by avoid-

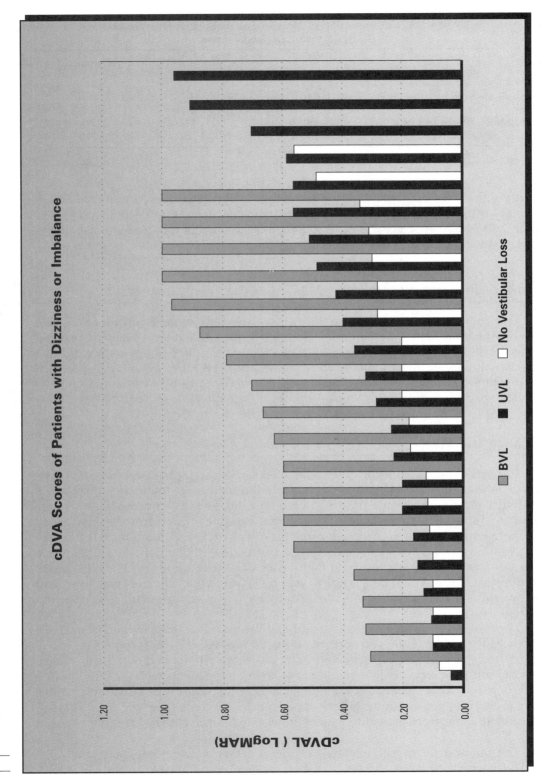

FIGURE 18–1. Distribution of dynamic visual acuity scores (LogMAR) using the clinical test in patients with unilateral and bilateral vestibular loss and in normal subjects. (From Venuto, P, with permission.)

A

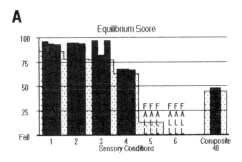

B

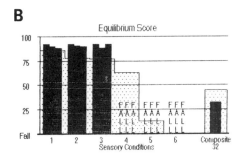

C

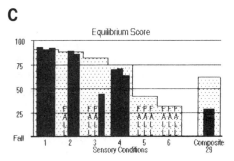

D

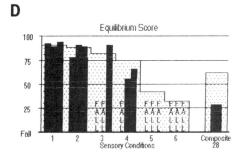

FIGURE 18–2. Posturography test results from patients with bilateral vestibular loss demonstrating the differences in ability to maintain postural stability when different sensory cues are altered or removed. Patients are tested using six different conditions:

	Available cues	Unavailable or altered cues
Test 1	Vision, vestibular somatosensory	—
Test 2	Vestibular, somatosensory	No vision
Test 3	Vestibular, somatosensory	Vision altered
Test 4	Vision, vestibular	Somatosensory altered
Test 5	Vestibular	No vision, somatosensory altered
Test 6	Vestibular	Vision and somatosensory altered

Results show patients who have difficulty when both visual and somatosensory cues are altered (*A*), when somatosensory cues only are altered (*B*), when visual cues only are altered (*C*), and when either visual *or* somatosensory cues are altered (*D*).

ing head movements. Arm swing is similarly decreased. Usually patients use excessive visual fixation and therefore have increased difficulty if asked to look up while walking. Patients typically turn "en bloc" and may even stop before they turn. Asking patients to turn their heads while walking results in increased ataxia and, often, loss of balance.

MECHANISMS OF RECOVERY

The mechanisms used to stabilize gaze in the absence of vestibular inputs have been well studied (Box 18–2).[6–8] The mechanisms involved in maintaining postural stability are still somewhat less well understood, although research is being done in that area.

BOX 18–2   Mechanisms Used to Stabilize Gaze

Change amplitude of saccades
Use corrective saccades
Modify pursuit eye movements
Central preprogramming of eye movements

Gaze Stability

Subjects without vestibular function must develop different mechanisms to keep the image of the target on the fovea during head movements (see Box 18–2). Central preprogramming is probably the primary mechanism by which gaze stability is improved in patients with BVL. It is assessed by comparing the gain of compensatory eye movements during active and passive head movements.[14,15] The difficulty with central preprogramming as a substitute for the loss of vestibular function is that it would not be effective in situations in which head movements are unpredictable, such as while walking.

Other mechanisms used to improve gaze stability include modifications in saccadic and pursuit eye movements.[14] Patients with complete BVL may make hypometric saccades toward a visual target. Then, as the head moves toward the target, the eyes would be moved passively into alignment with the target. They may also make accurate saccadic eye movements during combined eye and head movements toward a target, and then make corrective saccades back to the target as the head movement pulls the eyes off the target. These strategies enable the patient to recapture a visual target following a head movement. Pursuit eye movements can be used during low-frequency (and low-velocity) head movements to stabilize the eyes. Pursuit eye movements work at frequencies of up to 1 Hz and at velocities of up to 30° per second.[14]

Potentiation of the cervico-ocular reflex (COR) was initially thought to contribute significantly to the recovery of gaze stability in patients with BVL.[14,16,17] In the COR, sensory inputs from neck muscles and facet joints act to produce a slow phase eye movement that is opposite to the direction of the head movement during low-frequency, brief head movements. The COR, therefore, complements the VOR, although in normal subjects it is often absent and when present contributes, at most, 15 percent of the compensatory eye movement. In patients with complete BVL, the COR operates at frequencies of head movements of up to 0.3 Hz, well below the frequency range of head movements during normal activities. Therefore, although the COR is increased in patients with BVL, in reality it does not operate at frequencies that would contribute significantly to gaze stability during the head movements that would occur during most activities.

Kasai and Zee[14] found that different patients with complete BVL use different sets of strategies to compensate for the loss of VOR. Therefore, exercises to improve gaze stability should not be designed to emphasize any particular strategy, but instead should provide situations in which patients can develop their own strategies to maintain gaze stability (see Box 18–2). No mechanism to improve gaze stability fully compensates for the loss of the VOR, however, and patients will continue to have difficulty seeing during rapid head movements.

Postural Stability

A study on the course of recovery of patients with complete bilateral vestibular deficits over a 2-year period has shown that patients switch the sensory cues upon which they rely.[13] Initially, they rely on visual cues as a substitute for the loss of vestibular cues, but over time they become more reliant on somatosensory cues to maintain balance. In this study, patients were required to maintain balance when facing a moving visual surround. Over the 2-year study, they recovered the ability to maintain their balance to within normal limits in the testing paradigm except at high frequencies. The vestibular system functions at higher frequencies than do the visual or somatosensory systems, which would account for why neither visual nor somatosensory cues can substitute completely for loss of vestibular cues.

The contribution of somatosensory inputs from the cervical region to postural stability in patients with complete BVL is not clearly understood. Bles et al[19] found that changes in neck position did not affect postural stability in patients with complete BVL. They concluded that somatosensory signals from the neck do not contribute to postural stability. We do not know, however, if kinesthetic signals from the neck, which would occur during head *movement*, would affect postural stability. Certainly patients with bilateral vestibular dysfunction become less stable when asked to turn their heads while walking. This observation may indicate that kinesthetic cues do not contribute significantly to *dynamic* postural stability and/or that these patients are more reliant on visual cues to maintain postural stability and thus, when the head moves and visual cues are degraded, their balance becomes worse. The contribution of somatosensory cues from the lower extremities to postural stability in patients with BVL is also not well understood. Certainly some patients are dependent on somatosensory cues rather than on visual cues. Perhaps more importantly, we do not yet know how the degree of somatosensory loss affects postural stability in these patients.

The loss of either visual or somatosensory cues in addition to vestibular cues has a devastating effect on postural control. Paulus et al[20] reported a case in which the patient had a complete bilateral vestibular loss plus a loss of lower extremity proprioception. This patient relied on visual cues to maintain his balance. When the effectiveness of the visual cues was degraded (i.e., by fixating on a visual target more than 1 meter away), his postural stability deteriorated significantly. Visual and somatosensory cues will not substitute fully for the lost vestibular contribution to postural stability (see Chapter 17).[21-23]

Compensatory Strategies

Patients can be taught, and often develop on their own, strategies to use when in situations in which their balance will be stressed. For example, they learn to turn on lights at night if they have to get out of bed. They may also wait, sitting at the edge of the bed, before getting up in the dark to allow themselves to awaken more fully and for their eyes to adjust to the darkened room. They should be advised to use lights that come on automatically and to have emergency lighting inside and outside the house in case of a power failure. Patients may need to learn how to plan to move around places with busy visual environments such as shopping malls and grocery stores. For some patients, moving in busy environments may require the use of some type of assistive device, such as a shopping cart or a cane, but for many patients with BVL, no assistive devices are needed after the patient becomes comfortable walking in that environment.

EVIDENCE THAT EXERCISE FACILITATES RECOVERY

There is some evidence that experience facilitates recovery following bilateral ablation of the labyrinth. Igarashi et al[24] trained monkeys to run along a straight platform. Performance was scored by counting the number of times the monkeys moved off the straight line. A two-stage ablation of the labyrinth was then performed. After the unilateral ablation, animals given specific exercises recovered faster than nonexercised animals, but all animals eventually achieved preoperative functional levels. After ablation of the second labyrinth, all monkeys had difficulty with the platform run task. The control group reached preoperative balance performance levels in 81 days whereas the exercise group reached preoperative levels in 62 days. This result actually was not significantly different because of the large variation in individual animals. Igarashi et al[24] also looked at how long the animals took to have eight consecutive trial days in a row in which they could keep their balance at preoperative levels. The exercise group achieved this criterion in 118 days. The control group took longer. One animal took 126 days, another took 168 days, and one animal had not achieved that criterion at 300 days. The conclusions from this study are (1) recovery from bilateral deficits occurs more slowly than does recovery from unilateral lesions; (2) exercise impacts that rate of recovery in bilateral and unilateral lesions; and (3) the final level of function may be improved if exercises are given after bilateral lesions.

Krebs et al[1] studied the effectiveness of vestibular exercises on postural stability during functional activities for patients with chronic bilateral vestibular deficits. In a double-blinded, placebo-controlled trial, they found those patients performing customized vestibular and balance exercises had better stability while walking and during stair climbing than did patients performing isometric and conditioning exercises, such as using an exercise bicycle. Furthermore, the patients who had vestibular rehabilitation were able to walk faster. They used vestibular adaptation and eye-head exercises as well as balance and gait training. Not all exercise approaches are appropriate for patients with BVL, however. Telian et al[25] studied the effectiveness of a combination of balance exercises, vestibular habituation exercises, and general conditioning exercises for patients with bilateral vestibular deficits. They were unable to demonstrate a significant change in functional activity in these patients following treatment. Thus, vestibular habituation exercises do not appear to be appropriate for these patients. This makes sense, because habituation exercises are designed to decrease unwanted responses to vestibular signals rather than improve gaze or postural stability.

TREATMENT

The treatment approach for patients with complete loss of vestibular function involves the use of exercises that foster the substitution of visual and somatosensory information to improve gaze and postural stability and the development of compensatory strategies that can be used in situations where balance is stressed maximally (Boxes 18–3 and 18–4). Patients with some remaining vestibular function may benefit

---

BOX 18–3   Exercises to Improve Gaze Stability

---

1. To improve remaining vestibular function and central preprogramming

Tape a business card on the wall in front of you so that you can read it.

Move your head back and forth sideways, keep the words in focus.

Move your head faster but keep the words in focus. Continue to do this for 1 to 2 minutes without stopping.

Repeat the exercise moving your head up and down.

Repeat the exercises using a large pattern such as a checkerboard (full-field stimulus).

- *Note:* When training the patient to perform this exercise, watch the eyes closely. If the patient is making corrective saccades, the patient should slow the head movement down.

2. To foster the use of saccadic or pursuit strategies and central preprogramming

Active eye-head movements between two targets

- *Horizontal targets:* Look directly at one target being sure that your head is also lined up with the target. Look at the other target with your eyes and then turn your head to the target (saccades should precede head movement). Be sure to keep the target in focus during the head movement. Repeat in the opposite direction. Vary the speed of the head movement but always keep the targets in focus.
- *Note:* Place the two targets close enough together that when you are looking directly at one, you can see the other with your peripheral vision. Practice for 5 minutes, resting if necessary. This exercise can also be performed with two vertically placed targets.

3. To foster central preprogramming

- *Imaginary targets*
  Look at a target directly in front of you.
  Close your eyes and turn your head slightly, imagining that you are still looking directly at the target.
  Open your eyes and check to see if you have been able to keep your eyes on the target.

Repeat in the opposite direction. Be as accurate as possible.

Vary the speed on the head movement.

Practice for up to 5 minutes, resting if necessary.

---

from vestibular adaptation exercises to enhance the remaining vestibular function (Fig. 18–3). For both groups, postural stability can be improved by fostering the use of visual and somatosensory cues. This approach is also used in the treatment of patients with vestibular hypofunction (see Box 18–4).

Once the patient's specific problems have been identified, the exercise program can be established. During the initial sessions, particular attention should be paid to the degree to which the exercises increase the patient's complaints of dizziness. The patient's perception of dizziness can be the major deterrent (limiting factor) to the patient's eventual return to normal activities. Head movement, a component of all exercises, increases that dizziness. Also, the home exercise program typically requires that the patient perform exercises many times daily. Patients may find that they become increasingly dizzy with each performance of the exercises. It is important to explain to

---

BOX 18–4   Exercises to Improve Postural Stability

The purpose of these exercises is to force you to develop strategies of performing daily activities even when deprived of vision, proprioception, or normal vestibular inputs. The activities are supposed to help you develop confidence and establish your functional limits. **On all of these exercises you should take extra precautions so you do not fall.**

1. _____ Stand with your feet as close together as possible with both hands helping you maintain your balance by touching a wall. Take your hand or hands off the wall for longer and longer periods of time while maintaining your balance. Try moving your feet even closer together. Repeat this for _____ minutes twice each day.

   _____ Repeat exercise #1 with eyes closed, at first intermittently and then continuously, all the while making a special effort to mentally visualize your surroundings.

2. _____ Stand with your feet shoulder width apart with eyes open, looking straight ahead at a target on the wall. Progressively narrow your base of support from:
   feet apart to
   feet together to
   a semi–heel-to-toe position to
   heel almost directly in front of the toes
   - change your foot position one inch at a time.

   Do the exercise first _____ with arms outstretched and then
   _____ with arms close to your body and then
   _____ with arms folded across your chest.

   Hold each position for 15 seconds and then move on to the next most difficult exercise.

   _____ Repeat exercise #2 with eyes closed, at first intermittently and then continuously, all the while making a special effort to mentally visualize your surroundings.

3. _____ Repeat #_____ above but while standing on a foam pillow (*Note:* unusual for patients with BVL).

4. _____ Walk close to a wall with your hand braced available for balancing. Walk with a narrower base of support. Finally, walk heel to toe. Do this with eyes _____ (open/closed). Practice for _____ minutes.

5. _____ Walk close to a wall and turn your head to the right and to the left as you walk. Try to focus on different objects as you walk. Gradually turn your head more often and faster. Practice for _____ minutes.

6. _____ Walk and turn your head to the right and to the left as you walk while you count backwards out loud from 100. Try to focus on different objects as you walk. Gradually turn your head faster. Practice for _____ minutes.

7. _____ Practice turning around while you walk. At first, turn in a large circle but gradually make smaller and smaller turns. Be sure to turn in both directions.

---

the patient that some increase in dizziness is expected when they begin the exercises and with any increase in the intensity of the exercises. Limit the exercises that involve head movement to only one exercise initially. Other exercises can be added and the frequency and duration of the exercises can be increased as the patient improves. Have the patient perform at least one set of all the exercises at the time of the clinic visit.

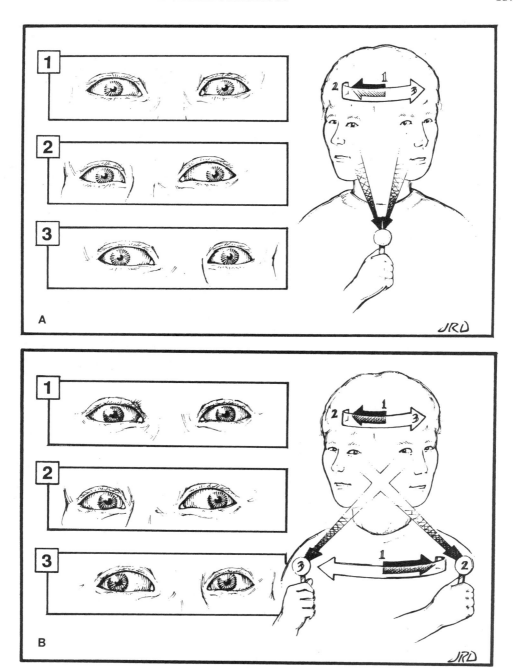

FIGURE 18–3. Exercises that enhance the adaptation of the vestibular system should be used with any patient who has remaining vestibular function. These exercises should be performed many times a day and can be performed in sitting or eventually while standing. (Modified from Tusa, RJ, and Herdman, SJ: Vertigo and disequilibrium. In Johnson, R, and Griffith, J (eds): Current Therapy in Neurological Disease, ed 4. Mosby Year-Book, St. Louis, 1993, p 12, with permission.)

BOX 18–5   Adjustments to Exercises Because of Severe Dizziness

Decrease the number of times they perform the exercises each day.
Move the head more slowly.
Perform each exercise for a shorter period of time.
Rest longer between each exercise.

Patients should also be taught how to modify the exercises if the dizziness becomes overwhelming (Box 18–5). They should be strongly encouraged to contact the therapist if they are having difficulty. In those patients in whom dizziness continues to be a problem, we suggest meditation and relaxation techniques to try to reduce the effect of the dizziness on the patient's life.

Progression of Exercises

Changing the duration of any given exercise, the frequency of performance, and how many different exercises are given (Table 18–2) can modify the intensity of the exercise program to improve gaze stability. Patients will find the exercises more challenging if they have to perform them while standing as opposed to sitting. Exactly which exercises are given initially and the progression itself will depend on the individual patient. Concurrent with the exercises to improve gaze stability, of course, the patient should be instructed in exercises to improve postural stability. Again, the initial exercise program and the rate of progression should be customized for each patient.

Guidelines to Treatment and Prognosis

There are several factors to remember when working with patients with bilateral vestibular deficits.

1. The patient's perception of dizziness can be the major deterrent to the patient's return to normal activities.
2. Recovery following bilateral deficits is slower than for unilateral lesions and can continue to occur over a 2-year period.
3. Recovery is easily upset by other medical problems such as having a cold or receiving chemotherapy.
4. To maintain recovered function, patients may always need to be doing some exercises, at least intermittently.
5. Postural stability will never be completely normal. The patient may have a negative Romberg and may be able to maintain the Sharpened Romberg position with eyes open, but not with eyes closed.
6. Initially, the patient may need to use a cane or a walker while ambulating. Some patients, especially older patients, need to use a cane at least some of the time. Most patients, however, are eventually able to walk without any assistive devices. Ambulation during the acute stage will be wide-based and ataxic with shortened stride length and side-stepping to the right and left. The patient will turn en bloc and turn-

TABLE 18-2 Suggested Progression for Gaze Stability Exercises

Exercise	Duration	Frequency	Position
X1 viewing paradigm against plain stationary background; horizontal or horizontal and vertical head movement	Maybe for <1 minute each time	Two or three times daily	Sitting until can perform the head movements easily and then standing
X1 viewing paradigm against plain stationary background; horizontal or horizontal and vertical head movement	Increase to 1 minute each exercise	Increase to five times daily	Standing[a]
X1 with target held in hand against a plain background; horizontal and then vertical head movements;	1 minute each exercise	Up to five times daily	Standing[a]
Add eye-head exercises, horizontally and vertically	No specific duration	Two to three times daily	Sitting at first and then standing
X1 with target held in hand and also with target at distance	1 minute each exercise	Two or three times daily	Standing[a]
Eye-head exercises, horizontally and vertically	No specific duration	Two or three times daily	Standing[a] if possible
X1 with target held in hand and also with target at distance	1 minute each exercise	Four times daily	Standing[a]
Eye-head exercises, horizontally and vertically	No specific duration	Four times daily	Standing[a]
Add imaginary target exercise	No specific duration	Four times daily	Sitting at first and then standing
X1 with target held in hand and also with target at distance	1 minute each exercise	Four times daily	Standing[a]
Eye-head exercises, horizontally and vertically	No specific duration	Four times daily	Standing[a]
Imaginary target exercise	No specific duration	Four times daily	Standing[a]
Some patients may be able to progress to X2 with target held in hand and also with target at distance	1 minute each exercise	Four times daily	Standing[a]
Eye-head exercises, horizontally and vertically	No specific duration	Four times daily	Standing[a]
Imaginary target exercise	No specific duration	Four times daily	Standing[a]
X1 with target held in hand and also with target at distance	1 minute each exercise	Four times daily	Standing[a]
Eye-head exercises, horizontally and vertically	No specific duration	Four times daily	Standing[a]
Imaginary target exercise	No specific duration	Four times daily	Standing[a]
Add finding numbers written randomly on large (6 ft by 5 ft) checkerboard pattern placed on wall	No specific duration	Twice daily	Stand and step to touch number

[a]The exercise can be made more difficult by changing the base of support (e.g., from feet apart to feet together).

ing the head will cause increased instability. Ambulation will improve but, again, it will not be normal.

7. Patients will be at increased risk for falls when walking in low-vision situations, over uneven surfaces, or when they are fatigued.

SUMMARY

Patients with bilateral vestibular problems can be expected to return to many activities but will continue to have difficulties with balance in situations in which visual cues are absent or diminished. The degree of disability is in part dependent on the degree of the vestibular loss but also reflects involvement of the visual and somatosensory systems. Treatment approaches include increasing the function of the remaining vestibular system, inducing the substitution of alternative mechanisms to maintain gaze stability and postural stability during head movements, and modifications of the home and working environment for safety. Patients should be able to return to work and most of them will be able to ambulate without the use of a cane or walker, at least when they are in well-lighted environments.

CASE STUDIES

CASE STUDY #1

A 64-year-old woman with a history of acute unsteadiness is referred for treatment. Six weeks prior to this clinic visit, she had a chronic bladder infection that had not responded to other antibiotics and was placed on IV gentamicin at home q8h for 10 days. There was no history of renal failure, nor was she on other antibiotics or a loop diuretic at that time. She began to complain of imbalance 2 days after the last dose of gentamicin. She had no complaints of hearing loss, tinnitus, or vertigo. Her imbalance was severe and she was using a walker. She was unable to walk independently. Standing, walking or moving her head exacerbated her balance problem.

Comment

Her history suggests an ototoxic reaction to gentamicin. Fewer than 3 percent of all individuals treated with gentamicin develop a BVL, and she had no known risk factors that would increase the likelihood of an ototoxic reaction such as renal failure or being on a loop diuretic.[4]

Pertinent History

Patient had been treated for depression and anxiety. Current medications include Zoloft, Valium, Premarin.

Neurological Examination

Normal except for visual acuity of 20/20-3 OU with head stationary that increases to 20/80-4 during to Hz head oscillations (clinical DVA test). Patient makes corrective saccades with slow and rapid head thrusts, worse to the right. She has a positive Romberg. Gait is extremely slow and cautious without the walker. She stops frequently and cannot turn around without stopping. Patient also has a significant scoliosis.

Comment

The large decrease in visual acuity during head movement (greater than 4 lines) is consistent with a severe vestibular deficit. The presence of corrective saccades with slow head rotations as well as with rapid head thrusts also suggests a profound deficit. Although gentamicin was given systemically, her vestibular loss appears to be asymmetric. She does not appear to have compensated at this time based on the positive Romberg test as well as the poor VOR during slow head rotations. Her gait pattern may reflect fear as well as the vestibular deficit. Her history of depression may be a factor in the final level of recovery.

Caloric Test

No response to either cool or warm irrigation of either ear. Ice water irrigation of both the right and left ears resulted in nystagmus with peak slow phase eye velocities of 8° per second. The direction of the nystagmus reversed when the patient was moved from supine to prone.

Comment

Ice water is a stronger stimulus than either cool or warm water. The nystagmus generated by ice water irrigation may represent either a response of the peripheral vestibular system or an alerting response to the extreme cold. If the nystagmus were due to excitation of the hair cells in the inner ear, the direction of the nystagmus would reverse when the patient is moved from supine to prone because the direction of endolymph flow would reverse. If the nystagmus were due to an alerting response, it would not reverse when the patient was moved from supine to prone. The test results for this patient suggest there is some residual function in each ear.

Vestibular Rehabilitation

The patient was seen 1 week later to institute a vestibular rehabilitation program. At that time she was still using a walker. She reported that her imbalance was induced by movement, occurred only while walking, and was worse in the dark. She denied any falls but reported that she did stagger and side-step while walking, and tended to drift to both the right and the left if she tried to walk without her walker.

Social History

She lived with her husband. Her home had no stairs. She did not smoke or use alcohol.

Current Functional Level

She was independent in self-care activities. She was no longer driving. She had been inactive since the onset of this problem.

Subjective Complaints

She stated her symptoms disrupted her performance of both her usual work and outside activities (rated a 3 on the Disability Scale). She scored a 56 on Jacobson's Dizziness Handicap Index, indicating that she would not go for a walk by herself, could not walk in the dark, and was limited in her ability to travel or participate in social activities. She also reported feeling frustrated, embarrassed in front of others, and handicapped. She rated her disequilibrium as a 9.3 on an analogue scale of 0 to 10 (10 worse). She rated her oscillopsia as a 5.7 on a similar scale.

Quantitative Dynamic Visual Acuity

Her visual acuity during 120° per second horizontal head movements was LogMAR = .450 (approximately 20/50-3; normal LogMAR = 0.000).

Gait

When asked to walk without the walker, her cadence was slow and she had a widened base of support. Her step length was decreased but symmetrical. Arm swing and head and trunk rotation were markedly decreased, especially when she turned. She could not walk a straight path but had no side-stepping or foot crossover. Her gait pattern was affected by her scoliosis (arm swing asymmetry). She was able to walk more rapidly without a significant change in her base of support or gait pattern. When asked to try to turn her head horizontally while walking, her cadence slowed significantly and she side stepped occasionally.

Comment

The patient's Disability Scale score and her Dizziness Handicap Index score both indicate a moderate perception of disability/handicap. Shepard et al[26] have shown that patients who score a 5 on the Disability Scale are less likely to show improvement with vestibular rehabilitation than those who rate themselves as a 3 or lower, as she did (see Chapter 15). Although she has been using a walker, she was able to ambulate safely without the walker. Head movements (turning her head or turning around) both increased her instability. Her dynamic visual acuity was consistent with other patients with bilateral vestibular loss.

Goals

The short-term goals for this patient were (1) to perform the vestibular adaptation exercises without a significant increase in her symptoms; (2) to walk daily; and (3) to no longer use her walker in her home. The long term goals were (1) to return to all normal activities except possibly driving; (2) to improve her visual acuity during head movements by two lines on the quantitative DVA test and to 20/50 on the clinical DVA test; and (3) to decrease her symptoms by 50 percent during head movements.

Plan

The patient was placed on a home exercise program, which included the ×1 viewing paradigm to be performed with both horizontal and vertical head movements for 1 minute each four times a day. The target was to be placed against a plain wall. Initially, she was to perform this exercise seated and then was to perform the exercise standing with her feet apart. She was also instructed to practice walking in a hallway twice daily for 5 minutes each time, with rests without touching the walls. Finally, she was told to walk for 20 minutes daily outside with her husband. She was given a calendar to fill in to help assure compliance. The total duration of her exercises at this point was 36 minutes. The program was limited until the patient's response could be determined. The patient was seen at 1-week intervals.

On the first follow-up, the patient was doing well with the exercises and was no longer using her walker at all. Her exercise program was changed to include the eye-head exercises both vertically and horizontally and the ×1 paradigm using a near target held in the hand was added to her program. She was to practice walking and turning her head horizontally for 5 minutes, twice daily. She was also instructed in a static balance exercise in which she would stand while gradually decreasing her base of support. This was to be performed with eyes open and then eyes closed. She was to continue walking for 20 minutes daily. Total exercise time was increased to 45 minutes.

On next follow-up visit, the patient reported that she initially had difficulty with the exercises involving head movements, all of which increased her dizziness. However, she reported that after 2 days of performing the exercises, she was able to perform them without a significant increase in dizziness. Review of the exercises showed that she was performing them all correctly and was maintaining fixation on the ×1 viewing paradigms, although her head movements were slow. Her exercise program was modified to include performing the ×1 paradigm using a target on a checkerboard and the "imaginary target" exercise was added. For these exercises, she was instructed to attempt to move her head more rapidly while maintaining focus on the target. She was also instructed to add walking and moving her head vertically. The ×1 viewing paradigm using a target placed against the wall was discontinued. Eventually in her program, she was instructed in the ×2 viewing paradigm.

One month after the initiation of her exercise program, the patient was walking with an increased cadence and a narrower base of support. She still had difficulty walking a straight line, but she was able to turn her head while walking and turn around without stopping. She no longer used a walker at any time. Her rating of her subjective complaints of disequilibrium was a 0.6 (down from 9.3) and of oscillopsia was a 1.5 (down from 5.7). Her quantitative DVA score was Log-MAR 0.143 (initial DVA was LogMAR 0.450), a three-line improvement. The plan was for the patient to continue with the rehabilitation process to further improve her gait and to enable her to return to more of her normal activities. On her next visit, 1 week later, she came in complaining of increased difficulty with her balance and increased dizziness. She reported that the exercises were okay but she was dizzy while walking and even when she rolled over in bed.

Comment

The patient was making good progress and both her balance and dynamic visual acuity had improved considerably when she suddenly had increased difficulty walking and increased complaints of dizziness. Her complaint that she has increased dizziness when she rolls over in bed sounds like benign paroxysmal positional vertigo (BPPV). Eye movements were recorded while the patient was moved into the right and left Hallpike-Dix positions. She developed an upbeating nystagmus, concurrent with complaints of vertigo, when moved into the left Hallpike-Dix position. The latency and duration of the nystagmus and vertigo were consistent with posterior canal canalithiasis. This indicated that although the patient had a bilateral vestibular deficit, there was remaining function in the left posterior canal. The caloric test had previously shown that there was remaining function in the left horizontal canal. The patient was treated for left posterior canal BPPV using the canalith repositioning maneuver. After successful remission of her positional vertigo, she resumed her exercises for the effect of her bilateral vestibular deficit.

CASE STUDY #2

A 34-year-old woman with a history of diabetes and renal failure has been on peritoneal dialysis for 1-1/2 years. She had been treated with gentamicin 9 and 6 months ago for peritonitis. She had no complaints of disequilibrium after either of those drug courses. Two months later she again developed peritonitis and again received IV gentamicin. After a few days, she complained of vertigo and tinnitus, developed disequilibrium and could not walk unassisted. She also complained that she was not able to see clearly when her head was moving. She was admitted to the hospital for a work-up of her vertigo and disequilibrium.

Clinical Examination

Significant findings on clinical examination included a spontaneous nystagmus with fast phases to the left, poor VOR to slow head movements, and large corrective saccades with rapid head movements bilaterally, worse with head movements to the right than to the left. The test for head-shaking nystagmus was not performed because the patient complained of severe nausea following even gentle head movements and vomited. She also had a positive Romberg. Sharpened Romberg and Fukuda's Stepping Test were not performed. The patient could not ambulate without the assistance of two people.

Comment

This patient's signs and symptoms (vertigo, disequilibrium, oscillopsia, spontaneous nystagmus, and poor VOR) certainly were suggestive of a vestibular disorder. Furthermore, her history included multiple treatments with gentamicin, an ototoxic medication. With bilateral dysfunction owing to treatment with an ototoxic drug, the symptoms of oscillopsia and disequilibrium develop over time and may not appear until after the drug treatment is finished. Once the symptoms appear, they may continue to become worse for several weeks. With some patients there is a partial reversal of symptoms with time. Often the vestibular symptoms are accompanied by hearing loss. Typically, however, the vestibular loss is symmetric and patients do not develop vertigo or spontaneous nystagmus, both of which are associated with unilateral vestibular loss or with asymmetric bilateral vestibular deficits. Although gentamicin usually results in BVL, symptoms of asymmetric effects on the vestibular and auditory systems have been reported.[3] Her poor VOR to slow head movements and the presence of corrective saccades during rapid head thrusts bilaterally suggested a bilateral vestibular deficit, which was confirmed by the rotational test results. This patient's gait disturbance appeared to be unusually severe and further testing showed a moderate loss of proprioceptive and kinesthetic perception in her feet, which would contribute significantly to her problem. This sensory loss was probably due to her diabetes. This finding was particularly important in developing her exercise program and in predicting her final level of recovery.

A CT and MRI were ordered, both of which were normal. Audiogram showed an asymmetric sensorineural hearing loss, right worse than left (Fig. 18–4). Caloric tests showed a poor response bilaterally to warm or cool water although ice water in the left ear did result in a weak but appropriate response. There was a directional preponderance to the right. Rotational chair test showed a severe bilateral vestibular deficit (Fig. 18–5). There was little optokinetic after-nystagmus and the VOR Tc was 2.4 seconds to 60° per second step rotations. At

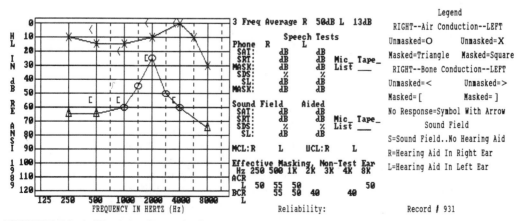

FIGURE 18–4. Hearing test results from patient with gentamicin ototoxicity. Circles and triangles indicate right ear and X and squares indicate left ear respectively. Note asymmetry in hearing loss for this patient.

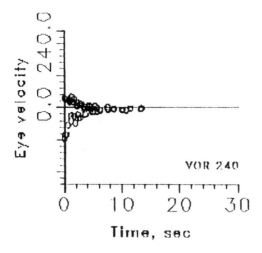

FIGURE 18–5. Plot of the decay in slow-phase eye velocity with time during VOR after nystagmus. Patient is first rotated in a chair in complete darkness for 2 minutes and then the chair is stopped. The slow-phase eye movements that occur are due to the discharge of the velocity storage system and represent the function of the vestibular system. These results show the poor peak slow phase eye velocity (35° per second) and the short time constant (<2 sec) in a patient with bilateral vestibular loss. A step rotation at 240° per second was used. Eye movements were recorded using electro-oculography.

240° per second step rotation, some vestibular response was evident—the gain of the response was 0.15 and the Tc was 2.4 seconds.

Treatment

At this point, the patient was started on a vestibular rehabilitation program. She performed the ×1 viewing paradigm exercise (see Fig. 18–3) first with horizontal head movements for 1 minute and then vertical head movements for 1 minute. Because head movement exacerbated her nausea, she rested for 10 minutes or more between each of these exercises. Initially she performed these exercises while sitting, up to five times a day. She also practiced standing unsupported, first with her feet apart and her eyes open and then gradually moving her feet together and briefly closing her eyes. She was instructed on how to use a walker and an emphasis was placed on increasing her endurance. Initially, she needed contact guarding while using the walker and would occasionally lose her balance, especially when trying to turn or if she moved her head too quickly. After 4 days, she was able to walk independently with the walker and was discharged from the hospital. At that time, she no longer had nausea with gentle head movements.

Comments

Although this patient had a bilateral vestibular deficit, the caloric and rotary chair tests showed that she had remaining vestibular function (response to ice water caloric on the left and a Tc of 2.4 seconds at 60° per second rotations). Her initial exercise program, therefore, consisted of vestibular adaptation exercises, because she had remaining vestibular function, and ambulation training. Her balance exercises were designed to gradually increase the difficulty of maintaining balance by slowly decreasing her base of support, changing her arm positions (arms out, arms at side, arms across the chest) and then altering her use of visual cues. Although she had decreased sensation in her feet, subtracting visual cues was used as a treatment approach in order to facilitate her ability to use the remaining somatosensory and vestibular cues.

Follow-Up

The patient continued to be followed as an outpatient. Exercises designed to facilitate the substitution of alterative strategies to maintain gaze stability as well to improve her static and dynamic balance were added to her program. The patient no longer needed to use a walker but she had a wide-based gait and had to stop walking before turning around. She had a negative Romberg but could not perform a sharpened Romberg. Although her vision improved and she could read if she was sitting quietly, she could not see clearly while in a car and had not resumed driving. Approximately 2 months later, the patient had a retinal hemorrhage in her left eye. She already had retinal damage in the right eye from her diabetes which essentially meant that she had only partial visual, vestibular, and somatosensory cues for balance and, as a result, she could no longer keep her balance even in well-lighted conditions. For 1 week she either used a wheelchair or, at home, a walker. Fortunately, her vision recovered and she was again able to walk independently. On her last visit she reported that she had returned to most activities except driving. Her base of support while walking was more narrow and her stability while turning had improved. Her Romberg was clinically normal but she could not perform a sharpened Romberg with eyes open. She was seeking part-time employment and was waiting for a kidney transplant.

CASE STUDY #2

A 61-year-old man is referred by a neurologist for treatment of disequilibrium secondary to BVL. The patient had been hospitalized for a subarachnoid hemorrhage 18 months previously. During his hospitalization, he developed several systemic complications including renal failure, pulmonary infiltrates, and ventriculitis, and was treated with two courses of vancomycin, gentamicin, and ceftazidime. The neurologist saw him 7 months after this hospitalization because of the patient's persistent disequilibrium. At that time, the patient complained that he stumbled occasionally and that he had increased difficulty walking on uneven surfaces, in the dark, or when he moved his head quickly. He denied nausea, vertigo, or a rocking sensation, although he did state that he had a feeling of being tilted when he walked. He stated that his disequilibrium began following his hospitalization. He also had bilateral hearing loss but had no complaints of tinnitus, pressure, or fullness in the ears. The remainder of his history was noncontributory.

The neurological examination was normal except for (1) visual acuity, as assessed using a wall chart, increased from 20/20 with the head stationary to 20/100 during gentle (2 Hz) oscillations of the head; (2) right Horner's syndrome; (3) staircase saccades downward from the midposition; (4) decreased vestibuloocular gain based on visualization of the optic nerve head and on the presence of compensatory saccades during rapid head thrusts; (5) mild decrease in vibration sensation in his feet, right more than left; (6) inability to perform tandem walking, sharpened Romberg or Fukuda's Stepping Test; and (7) bilateral hearing loss.

Quantitative testing of the oculomotor system showed low VOR gain (0.2 and 0.13 to the right and left, respectively) and short time constant (2.2 seconds bilaterally) to a 60° per second step rotation and low gain (0.19 and 0.34) and time constants (1.9 and 1.2 secs) to 240° per second rotations. It was concluded that the patient had BVL, probably from the gentamicin and he was referred for vestibular rehabilitation.

Treatment

Prior to establishing an exercise program, additional testing was performed. Dynamic posturography showed that the patient had an inability to maintain his balance when both visual and somatosensory cues were altered and a decreased ability to maintain his balance when visual cues were inappropriate (Fig. 18–6). Quantitative visual acuity testing showed that his acuity changed from 20/20 when his head was stationary to 20/40 during 150° per second head movements using a forced-guess paradigm. (The apparent discrepancy between the clinical dynamic visual acuity test, 20/100, and the quantitative dynamic visual acuity test, 20/40, are due to the use of a forced guess paradigm in the latter test.) Quantitative vibration threshold confirmed the moderate loss of vibration perception in his feet. The patient's gait was wide-based and he frequently side-stepped while walking. He appeared to use excessive visual fixation to maintain his balance during ambulation. The patient was started on a program of exercises designed to (1) enhance his remaining vestibular function; (2) develop alternative mechanisms to improve gaze stability; (3) improve his static balance in the absence of visual cues; and (4) improve his balance while ambulating.

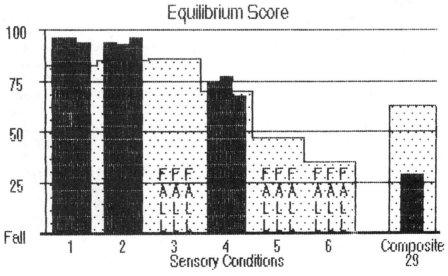

FIGURE 18–6. Results from posturography test in patient with bilateral vestibular loss. Test conditions were those used in Figure 18–2.

Follow-Up

Six weeks later, his Romberg was normal but he still could not perform a sharpened Romberg with his eyes open, nor could he perform Fukuda's Stepping Test with eyes closed. He continued to walk with a widened base of support. Quantitative testing of the oculomotor system was unchanged from the previous test. Quantitative visual acuity testing showed an acuity of 20/30 during 150° per second head movements, which was a marked improvement over his previous test. The patient wished to return to driving and we suggested that should he decide to drive, he should start first in local traffic and even in an empty parking lot on a weekend. He was advised that driving at night and high-speed driving would still be hazardous. One month later the patient reported that he had returned to driving during the day and that he was working part-time. He still could not walk in the dark or with his eyes closed without assistance. Several suggestions were made to the patient concerning modifications in his home to assure safety including emergency lighting that would come on automatically if there were a power failure, railings for all stairways and safety bars in the bathroom.

ACKNOWLEDGMENTS

This work was supported by NIH grant DC 03196 (SJH).

REFERENCES

1. Krebs, DE, et al: Double-blind, placebo-controlled trial of rehabilitation for bilateral vestibular hypofunction: Preliminary report. Otolaryngol Head Neck Surg 109:735, 1993.
2. JC: Living without a balance mechanism. New Engl J Med 246:458, 1952.
3. Brandt, T, et al: Visual acuity, visual field and visual scene characteristics affect postural balance. In Igarashi, M, and Black, FO (eds): Vestibular and Visual Control on Posture and Locomotor Equilibrium. Karger, Basel, 1985, p 93.
4. Hewitt, WL: Gentamicin toxicity in perspective. Postgrad Med J 50(suppl 7):55, 1974.
5. Jacobson, GP, and Newman, CW: The development of the dizziness handicap inventory. Arch Otolaryngol Head Neck Surg 116:424, 1990.
6. Cohen, H: Vestibular rehabilitation reduces functional disability. Otolaryngol Head Neck Surg 107:638, 1992.
7. Black, FO, et al: Vestibular reflex changes following aminoglycoside induced ototoxicity. Laryngoscope 97:582, 1987.
8. Esterhai, JL, et al: Gentamicin-induced ototoxicity complicating treatment of chronic osteomyelitis. Clin Orth Related Res 209:185, 1986.
9. Szturm, T, et al: Comparison of different exercise programs in the rehabilitation of patients with chronic peripheral vestibular dysfunction. J Vestib Res 4:461, 1994.
10. Westheimer, G, and McKee, SP: Visual acuity in the presence of retinal-image motion. J Optical Soc Am 65:847, 1975.
11. Herdman, SJ, et al: Computerized dynamic visual acuity test in the assessment of vestibular deficits. Am J Otol 19:790, 1998.
12. Venuto, PJ, et al: Interrater reliability of the clinical dynamic visual acuity test. Scientific Meeting and Exposition of the American Physical Therapy Association. Orlando, FL, June 6, 1998.
13. Bles, W, et al: Compensation for labyrinthine defects examined by use of a tilting room. Acta Otolaryngol 95:576, 1983.
14. Kasai, T, and Zee, DS: Eye-head coordination in labyrinthine-defective human beings. Brain Res 144:123, 1978.

15. Barnes, GR: Visual-vestibular interaction in the control of head and eye movement: The role of visual feedback and predictive mechanisms. Prog Neurobiol 41:435, 1993.
16. Bronstein, AM, and Hood, JD: The cervico-ocular reflex in normal subjects and patients with absent vestibular function. Brain Res 373:399, 1986.
17. Chambers, BR, et al: Bilateral vestibular loss, oscillopsia, and the cervico-ocular reflex. Otolaryngol Head Neck Surg 93:403, 1985.
19. Bles, W, et al: Postural and oculomotor signs in labyrinthine-defective subjects. Acta Otolaryngol (Stockh) 406:101, 1984.
20. Paulus, WM, et al: Visual stabilization of posture. Brain 107:1143, 1984.
21. Diener, HC, et al: The significance of proprioception on postural stabilization as assessed by ischemia. Brain Res 296:103, 1984.
22. Diener, HC, et al: Stabilization of human posture during induced oscillations of the body. Exp Brain Res 45:126, 1982.
23. Dichgans, J, and Brandt, T: Visuo-vestibular interactions. Effects on self-motion perception and postural control. In Held, R, et al (eds): Handbook of Sensory Physiology. Springer, Berlin, 1978, pp 755–804.
24. Igarashi, M, et al: Physical exercise and balance compensation after total ablation of vestibular organs. In Pompeiano, O, and Allum, JHJ (eds): Progress in Brain Research. Elsevier, Amsterdam, 1988, p 395.
25. Telian, SA, et al: Bilateral vestibular paresis: Diagnosis and treatment. Otolaryngol Head Neck Surg 104:67, 1991.
26. Shepard, NT et al: Vestibular and balance rehabilitation therapy. Ann Otol Rhinol Laryngol 102:198, 1993.

CHAPTER 19

Assessment and Treatment of Patients with Benign Paroxysmal Positional Vertigo

Susan J. Herdman, PT, PhD
Ronald J. Tusa, MD, PhD

Twenty-five years ago, only one treatment was used for patients with benign paroxysmal positional vertigo (BPPV).[1] More recently, new understanding of the pathophysiology underlying the signs and symptoms of BPPV has led to different treatments, each designed specifically for the particular canal involved and for the mechanism underlying the signs and symptoms (canalithiasis versus cupulolithiasis). These recent developments have significantly improved our ability to treat this disorder. This chapter will review the underlying mechanisms of BPPV, as well as the assessment tools and treatments now available for its management.

CHARACTERISTICS AND HISTORY

BPPV is the most common cause of vertigo due to a peripheral vestibular disorder.[2,3] It is characterized by brief episodes of vertigo when the head is moved into certain positions. Although BPPV has been reported in adults of all ages (Table 19–1), it is uncommon in children.[3,4] BPPV occurs spontaneously in many patients but may follow head trauma, labyrinthitis, or ischemia in the distribution of the anterior vestibular artery.[4] Spontaneous remission is common. For those patients in whom the episodic vertigo persists, this disorder can be annoying, disruptive, and often results in significant changes in normal activities.

Patients with BPPV commonly report vertigo triggered by lying down, rolling over in bed, bending over, and looking up. Common situations in which vertigo is provoked include getting out of bed, gardening, washing hair in the shower, and going to

TABLE 19–1 Age Distribution of BPPV

Age (y)	With Complaints of Dizziness (n)	BPPV (%)	BPPV (n)
0–9	9	0.0%	0
10–19	32	3.1%	1
20–29	64	3.1%	2
30–39	191	17.8%	34
40–49	261	16.5%	43
50–59	207	22.2%	46
60–69	298	26.2%	78
70–79	376	23.7%	89
80–89	176	33.1%	58
90–99	14	50.0%	7

Cases seen at the Dizziness and Balance Center, University of Miami Dept of Physical Therapy and Bascom Palmer Eye Institute 1994–98.

the dentist or beauty parlor. Other complaints associated with BPPV include balance problems that may last for hours or days after the episodic vertigo has stopped as well as more vague sensations such as lightheadedness or a feeling of floating (Table 19–2).

Mechanism

Schuknecht,[5] in 1969, proposed that degenerative debris from the utricle (possibly fragments of otoconia) adhered to the cupula of the posterior canal making the ampulla gravity sensitive. This theory, *cupulolithiasis*, was supported by the presence of basophilic deposits on the cupula of the posterior canal in patients with a history of BPPV. Presumably, the presence of the debris adhering to the cupula significantly increases the density of the cupula and therefore produces an inappropriate deflection of the cupula of the posterior canal when the head is positioned with the affected ear below the horizon (Fig. 19–1). The result is vertigo, nystagmus, and nausea. Because the cupula remains deflected as long as the patient is in the provoking position, the nys-

TABLE 19–2 Frequency of Complaints in 100 Consecutive Patients With BPPV

Poor balance	57%
Sense of rotation (vertigo)	53%
Trouble walking	48%
Lightheaded	42%
Nausea	35%
Queasy	29%
Spinning inside head	29%
Sense of tilt	24%
Sweating	22%
Sense of floating	22%
Blurred vision	15%
Jumping vision	13%

Tusa RJ, Herdman SJ. Adapted from Canalith Repositioning for Benign Paroxysmal Positional Vertigo. American Academy of Neurology 3B5.002.

A Head upright-sitting   to Hallpike-Dix position

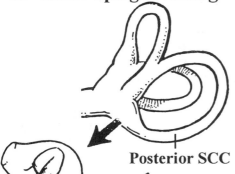
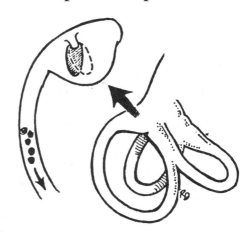

Posterior SCC

B Head upright-sitting   to Hallpike-Dix position

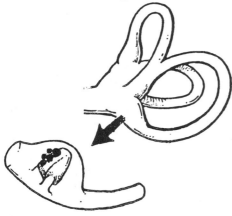
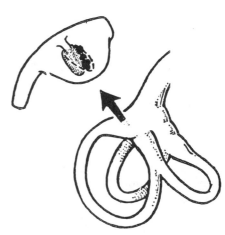

FIGURE 19–1. In canalithiasis (*A*), the calcium carbonate crystals are floating freely in the long arm of the canal (shown here for posterior canal). When the head is moved into the head-hanging position (Hallpike-Dix), the debris moves to the most dependent portion of the canal. The movement of the debris causes the endolymph to move which in turn overcomes the inertia of the cupula and an abnormal signal is sent to the central nervous system. In cupulolithiasis (*B*), the debris is adhering to the cupula of the semicircular canal (shown here for posterior canal). Movement into the head-hanging position, gravity displaces the weighted cupula again resulting in an abnormal signal from that canal. (Modified from Herdman, SJ, et al, 1993, with permission.)

tagmus and vertigo will persist although the intensity may decrease slightly because of central adaptation.[6] Thus cupulolithiasis is characterized by (1) immediate onset of vertigo when the patient is moved into the provoking position, (2) the presence of a nystagmus, which appears with the same latency as the complaints of vertigo, and (3) persistence of the vertigo and nystagmus as long as the person's head is maintained in the provoking position. This form of BPPV is relatively uncommon.

A second theory, *canalithiasis*, was proposed by Hall et al[7] who suggested that the degenerative debris is not adherent to the cupula of the posterior canal but instead is floating freely in the endolymph of the canal. Freely moving debris has been visualized through a microscope in patients in whom the membranous labyrinth has been exposed during surgery.[8] When the head is moved into the provoking position, the otoconia move to the most dependent position in the canal (see Fig. 19–1). The movement of the otoconia results in movement of the endolymph, which in turn pulls on the cupula and increases the firing rate of the neurons of that canal. The latency of the response is related to the time needed for the cupula to be deflected by the pull of the endolymph. The vertigo and nystagmus are related to the relative deflection of the cupula. The decrease in vertigo and nystagmus as the position is maintained is due to cessation of endolymph movement. Thus, BPPV from canalithiasis is characterized by: (1) delay in the onset of the vertigo of 1 to 40 seconds after the patient has been placed in the provoking position; (2) the presence of a nystagmus, which appears with the same latency as the complaints of vertigo; and (3) a fluctuation in the intensity of the vertigo and nystagmus which increases and then decreases, disappearing within 60 seconds. BPPV from canalithiasis is the most common form of this disorder.

Canal Involvement

Initially BPPV was believed to involve only the posterior semicircular canal. This was because the most commonly observed nystagmus, upbeating and torsional, would be produced by excitation of the posterior canal. More recently it has been recognized that the anterior and horizontal canal involvement also occurs.[9–13] The frequency of BPPV in each of the canals is shown in Table 19–3.

The identification of canal involvement usually is based on the direction of the nystagmus observed when the patient is moved into the provoking position (Table 19–4). Careful observation of the direction of the reversal phase of the nystagmus and the direction of the nystagmus when the patient returns to a sitting position can also be used to identify which canal is involved (see Table 19–4). Proper identification of the involved canal and determination of whether cupulolithiasis or canalithiasis is the underlying problem dictates which treatment will be appropriate.

Diagnosis

Three different maneuvers can be used to provoke the vertigo and nystagmus. Because observation of the direction and duration of the nystagmus is critical to develop-

TABLE 19–3 Canal Involvement in BPPV

Canal	Patients (*n*)	Patients (%)
Posterior SCC	49	63.6
Anterior SCC	9	11.7
Horizontal SCC	1	1.3
Posterior or anterior SCC?	18	23.4

In 77 consecutive patients (Herdman et al[9]).

TABLE 19–4 Identification of Canal Involvement Based on Direction
of Nystagmus During Right Hallpike-Dix Test

Canal	Right Hallpike-Dix	Reversal Phase	Return to Sitting
Right posterior	Upbeat, right torsion[a]	Down and left torsion	Down and left torsion
Right Anterior	Downbeat, right torsion	Up and left torsion	Up and left torsion
Left Anterior	Downbeat, left torsion	Up and right torsion	Up and right torsion

[a]Torsion is defined as the direction movement of the superior pole of the eyes (in right torsion, the superior poles of both eyes move to the patient's right [quick phase]).

ing a treatment plan, it is important that the patient understand what to expect. The patient should keep their eyes open and should try to stay in the provoking position. Explaining to the patient that the vertigo will stop or decrease if they stay in the position usually is reassuring and enables the patient to complete the test. If the patient's history suggests which side is affected, it is best to test the presumed unaffected side first to minimize nausea. For patients with severe nausea and a history of emesis associated with vertigo, the testing maneuvers should be performed more slowly, although this decreases the likelihood of provoking the nystagmus.

All of these tests can be performed in room light but the use of Frenzel lenses or of infrared camera system to prevent fixation suppression of horizontal and vertical nystagmus will increase the likelihood of observing nystagmus. Torsional nystagmus is not suppressed by fixation.

HALLPIKE-DIX TEST

Also called the Barany maneuver and the Nylen-Barany maneuver, this is the most commonly used test to confirm the diagnosis of BPPV.[14] In this test, the patient's head is turned 45° horizontally while the patient is in the sitting position (Fig. 19–2, position 1). The patient then quickly lies down with the head hanging over the edge of the treatment table approximately 30° below the horizontal (Fig. 19–2, position 2). This places the posterior canal on the downside ear in the plane of the pull of gravity. Debris adhering to the cupula or free-floating in the long arm of the canal will shift and result in vertigo and nystagmus. The patient should be kept in this position for at least 30 seconds because of the possible latency to onset of the vertigo. If the patient has BPPV, vertigo and nystagmus will be provoked when the affected ear is inferior. Then the patient can be slowly returned to a sitting position. If vertigo was provoked when the patient was moved into the head-hanging position, the patient may experience vertigo again when returned to a sitting position. The test can then be repeated with the patient's head turned to the other side. Note that the anterior canal of the downside ear is also in a more dependent position and this maneuver may also trigger vertigo due to anterior canal involvement of the downside ear (see Fig. 19–2, position 2). The nystagmus in anterior canal BPPV will be downbeating and torsional.

SIDELYING TEST

In this test, the patient sits on the side of the treatment table (Fig. 19–3, position 1). The head is turned 45° to one side and the patient then quickly lies down on the opposite side (Fig. 19–3, position 2). This again puts the posterior canal on the downside ear

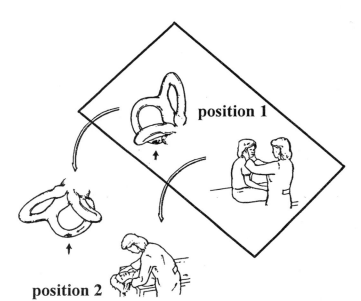

FIGURE 19–2. Position testing for anterior or posterior canals BPPV: Hallpike-Dix Test. The patient sits on the examination table and the head is turned 45° horizontally toward the labyrinth to be tested (position 1). The head and trunk are quickly brought straight back "en bloc" so that the head is hanging over the edge of the examination table by 20° to 30° (position 2). The patient is asked if they have vertigo and is observed for nystagmus. The patient is then brought up slowly to a sitting position with the head still turned 45° and nystagmus is looked for again (not shown). This test then is repeated with the head turned 45° in the other direction. This figure also shows the right labyrinth with free-floating otoconia in the right posterior SCC (*large black arrows*). During the Hallpike-Dix test, the debris would move resulting in nystagmus and vertigo when the test is performed to the right side, but not when the test is performed to the left side. (Modified from Tusa, RJ, and Herdman, SJ: Canalith repositioning for benign positional vertigo. Education Program Syllabus 3BS.002, Am Acad Neurol, Minnesota, 1998, p 6, with permission.)

in the plane of the pull of gravity and may provoke a response in either canalithiasis or cupulolithiasis. Similarly, debris in the anterior canal of the downside or inferior ear will also move, provoking vertigo and downbeating and torsional nystagmus. The patient then returns to sitting and after waiting to be sure that the patient does not experience any vertigo in sitting, the test is repeated to the opposite side.

ROLL TEST

In horizontal canal BPPV, the Hallpike-Dix test may not provoke vertigo and nystagmus.[11] The best maneuver would be one that moves the patient's head in the plane of the horizontal canal. The patient lies supine with the head flexed 20° (Fig. 19–4A). Then the head is quickly rolled to one side and kept in that position for up to one minute to see if the patient experiences any vertigo (Fig. 19–4B). The head is then slowly rolled back to midline (still in slight flexion) (Fig. 19–4C) and then quickly rolled to the other side (Fig. 19–4D). In horizontal canal BPPV, vertigo and nystagmus

FIGURE 19–3. Position testing for anterior or posterior canals BPPV: Sidelying Test. The patient sits on the bed with the legs over the side and the head is rotated 45° horizontally *away from* the labyrinth to be tested (position 1). The patient is then quickly brought down on their side opposite to the direction the head is turned (position 2). The patient is asked to report any vertigo and is observed for nystagmus. The patient is then brought to a sitting position with the head still turned 45° and nystagmus and vertigo is rechecked (not shown). The head is then rotated 45° horizontally to the opposite side and the patient is quickly brought down on their side opposite to the direction the head is turned. Nystagmus and vertigo are checked. The patient then sits up and nystagmus and vertigo are checked again. This figure also shows the right labyrinth with free-floating otoconia in the right posterior SCC (*large black arrows*). During the Hallpike-Dix test, the debris would move resulting in nystagmus and vertigo when the test is performed to the right side, but not when the test is performed to the left side. This test is also useful for anterior canal BPPV, because debris in this canal would move when the test is done on the right side. (Modified from Tusa, RJ, and Herdman, SJ: Canalith repositioning for benign positional vertigo. Education Program Syllabus 3BS.002, Am Acad Neurol, Minnesota, 1998, p 6, with permission.)

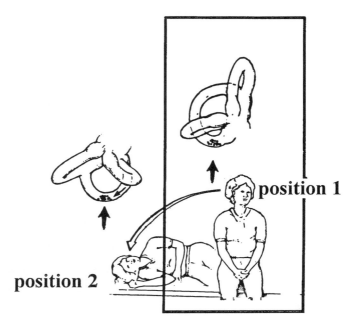

position 1

position 2

will occur when the head is turned to both the right and the left because the debris moves back and forth within the canal. The slow-phase eye velocity, duration of the nystagmus, and the patient's subjective complaints are believed to be worse toward the affected ear.[11] The direction of nystagmus in horizontal canal BPPV depends on whether the debris is free-floating (canalithiasis) or adhering to the cupula (cupulolithiasis)[11] (Fig. 19–5). In canalithiasis of the horizontal canal, the nystagmus is geotropic and will fatigue while in cupulolithiasis, the nystagmus is ageotropic and persistent.

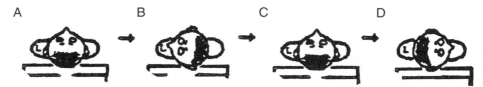

FIGURE 19–4. Roll Test for horizontal canal BPPV. (*A*) The patient is laid supine with the head flexed 20°. (*B*) The head is quickly rolled to one side, and nystagmus is looked for and the patient is asked to report any vertigo. (*C*) The head is then slowly rolled back to a supine position. (*D*) The head is then quickly rolled to the other side, and nystagmus is looked for and the patient is asked to report any vertigo. (Modified from Tusa, RJ, and Herdman, SJ: Canalith repositioning for benign positional vertigo. Education Program Syllabus 3BS.002, Am Acad Neurol, Minnesota, 1998, p 8, with permission.)

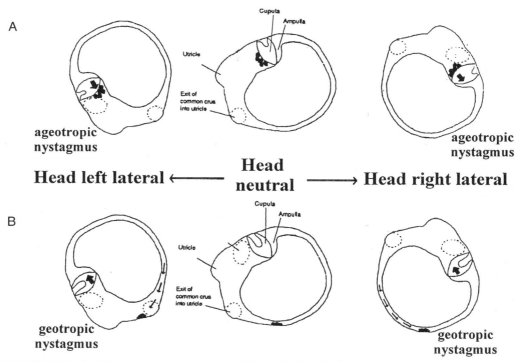

FIGURE 19–5. Direction of nystagmus in HC BPPV. For both HC cupulolithiasis (*A*) and HC canalithiasis (*B*), the patient would have nystagmus and vertigo when they are rolled to either side, but the duration and direction of the nystagmus would differ in these two types of BPPV. For cupulolithiasis, the nystagmus is persistent and the direction of the quick phases is away from earth (ageotropic). For canalithiasis, the nystagmus is transient and the direction of the quick phases is towards the earth (geotropic). (Modified from Baloh, et al, 1993.)

TREATMENT

Successful treatment depends on identifying which canal is involved and whether the debris is free-floating or adhering to the cupula. There are three basic bedside treatments for BPPV, each with its own indications for use: canalith repositioning, and liberatory and Brandt-Daroff habituation exercises. Variations of these treatments have been developed depending upon which canal is involved. Studies on the efficacy of these treatments indicate that all three treatments facilitate recovery.[1,15–23] The results of these studies must be interpreted cautiously, however, because of the high incidence of spontaneous remission that occurs in patients with BPPV. Several authors have reported spontaneous recovery within 3 to 4 weeks[21,24] although Brandt et al[1] suggest that the vertigo may disappear spontaneously after several months even if left untreated.

The choice of which exercise is most appropriate for the patient depends on which canal is involved as well as whether the patient has the canalithiasis or cupulolithiasis form of BPPV (Table 19–5). We typically use the canalith repositioning treatment (for canalithiasis) or the liberatory maneuver (for cupulolithiasis) first. The Brandt-Daroff habituation exercises are used for more mild residual complaints.

Canalith Repositioning Treatment: Posterior and Anterior Canal Canalithiasis

This treatment is based on the theory of canalithiasis.[7,25] It is a single maneuver in which the patient is taken through a series of head positions to move the head around the debris. Note that the same maneuver would be effective for both posterior and anterior canal BPPV. During canalith repositioning treatment (CRT), the patient is first moved into the Hallpike-Dix position toward the side of the affected ear (shown here for left) and kept down for 1 to 2 minutes (Fig. 19–6A,B). Then, the head is slowly rotated through moderate extension toward the unaffected side and kept in the new position briefly (Fig. 19–6C) before the patient is rolled on a sidelying position with the head turned 45° down (toward the floor) (Fig. 19–6D). In this last position the patient may develop a short spell of vertigo and nystagmus with the same characteristics, which indicates the debris is moving inside the posterior canal. Keeping the head devi-

TABLE 19–5 Treatment Options and Indications

	Canalithiasis (Severe)	Canalithiasis (Mild)	Cupulolithiasis
Posterior Canal BPPV	CRT[a] Liberatory Brandt-Daroff	Brandt-Daroff[a] CRT Liberatory	Liberatory[a] Brandt-Daroff
Anterior Canal BPPV	CRT[a] Liberatory_A Brandt-Daroff	Brandt-Daroff[a] CRT Liberatory_A	Liberatory_A[a] Brandt-Daroff
Horizontal Canal BPPV	CRT_Hcanal	CRT_Hcanal	Brandt-Daroff_Hcupulo

[a]Indicates treatment of first choice.

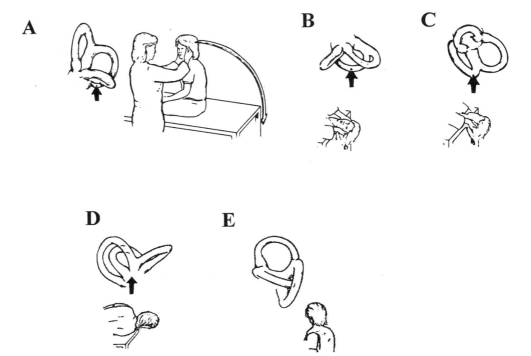

FIGURE 19–6. Canalith repositioning treatment for treatment of posterior or anterior SCC BPPV. During CRT the patient is first moved into the Hallpike-Dix position towards the side of the affected ear (shown here for left) and kept down for 1 to 2 minutes (*A* to *B*). Then, the head is slowly rotated through moderate extension toward the unaffected side and kept in the new position briefly (*C*) before the patient is rolled on a sidelying position with the head turned 45° down (toward the floor) (*D*). In each of these positions, the patient may develop a short spell of vertigo and nystagmus with the same characteristics as the original nystagmus indicating the debris is moving through the posterior canal. Keeping the head deviated toward the unaffected side and the head pitched down, the patient then slowly sits up (*E*). To make certain the debris stays in the utricle after the treatment, the patient is fitted with a soft collar and told not to bend over, lie back, move their head up or down, or tilt their head to either side for the rest of the day. The traditional follow-up treatment is to have the patient to keep their head upright even during sleep for 48 hours and then not to sleep on the affected ear until follow-up assessment 5 days later. *Filled arrows* indicate location of free-floating debris in the posterior semicircular canal. Note that the movement of the patient's head will gradually shift the debris away from the cupula and into the common crus. (Modified from Tusa, RJ, and Herdman, SJ: Canalith repositioning for benign positional vertigo. Education Program Syllabus 3BS.002, Am Acad Neurol, Minnesota, 1998, p 13, with permission.)

ated toward the unaffected side and the head pitched down, the patient then slowly sits up (Fig. 19–6*E*). The nystagmus should be in the same direction throughout the treatment if the debris is moving through the canal and into the common crus. Observation of a reversal of the nystagmus would suggest that the debris moved back toward the cupula. To make certain the debris stays in the utricle after the treatment, the patient is fitted with a soft collar and told not to bend over, lie back, move their head up or down, or tilt their head to either side for the rest of the day. The traditional follow-up treatment is to have the patient keep their head upright, even while sleeping, for 48 hours and then not to sleep on the affected ear until follow-up assessment

5 days later. More recent studies have suggested that it is not necessary to have the patient sleep upright and we now recommend that patients sleep on extra pillows to keep the head elevated.[22] Epley[15] suggests using vibration over the mastoid during the treatment to facilitate the movement of the debris. A comparison of studies in which vibration was applied over the mastoid bone during treatment with studies in which vibration was not used shows no difference in outcome.[16–20,22]

TREATMENT EFFICACY

In patients in whom the BPPV is due to canalithiasis, the most commonly used treatment appears to be CRT. There is some controversy as to the efficacy of this treatment, however. Early studies reported 85 to 95 percent remission of symptoms in patients with posterior canal BPPV, but did not use control groups.[15,16] Because there is a significant spontaneous remission of the symptoms of BPPV, at least some of the effects attributed to the treatment could have been due to spontaneous recovery. More recently, studies have compared the treatment effects using untreated control groups[17,20,26] but reached different conclusions. The first study concluded that there was no difference between the remission rates in patients treated using the canalith repositioning maneuver ($n = 16$) and the control group ($n = 22$) 1 month after treatment.[26] This study, however, did not replicate the maneuver as it is typically performed. Additionally, it assessed the treatment effect at 1 month posttreatment by which time recurrence of symptoms, which can occur in up to 30 percent of all subjects, may have been a factor. Advocates of CRT emphasize that one of the benefits of this treatment is the *rapid* relief of vertigo. The second study, using the canalith repositioning maneuver as originally proposed, reported that 70 percent of the treated group ($n = 27$) had no nystagmus when evaluated 1 week after treatment compared to none of the untreated control group ($n = 23$).[17] The difference in the findings of these two studies may be due to the precise maneuver used. Herdman et al[16] found that if patients with posterior canal BPPV ($n = 30$) were moved from the original provoking position (see Fig. 19–6B) to the contralateral Hallpike-Dix position (see Fig. 19–6C) and then returned to sitting without rolling over onto their side so the head was turned 45° down, the remission rate was only 50 percent. In comparison, the remission rate was 83 percent in a similar group of patients ($n = 30$) who were rolled onto the contralateral side with the head turned 45° toward the floor (see Fig. 19–6B–D) before sitting up. The last part of the treatment maneuver results in the movement of the debris into the common crus. The third study was a double-blind, controlled study.[20] They compared CRT without vibration to a placebo maneuver. They found a significant difference in outcome between the two groups, with 88.9 percent of the CRT-treated patients having full remission of symptoms compared to only 26.7 percent of the control group. The remission of symptoms following CRT appears to be due to the maneuver itself, not to the period during which the subjects stay upright.[27] One variable in these studies may be which canal was involved, as many of the studies do not identify the direction of the nystagmus as part of the inclusion criteria. That is, we do not know if the correct maneuver was performed based on which canal was involved. Only preliminary work has examined the efficacy of CRT in patients with anterior canal canalithiasis. Tusa et al[28] reported an 88.2 percent remission rate in patients with anterior canal BPPV ($n = 17$) following one treatment.

COMPLICATIONS

In a study of 85 consecutive patients with posterior canal canalithiasis treated with CRT, two had developed anterior canal and three developed horizontal canal BPPV when tested 7 days later.[29] The authors speculated that some of the debris moved into the canals either during the treatment or after the treatment when the patients lay down. This secondary BPPV was treated successfully in these patients (personal communication). Baloh[11] has also described this as a cause of horizontal canal BPPV. Careful observation of nystagmus during the treatment and during reevaluation of the patient will ensure identification of this complication of CRT and proper treatment.

Another complication is neck stiffness and muscle spasm from keeping the head upright. Patients should be advised to take off the soft collar and move the head horizontally periodically. Finally, some patients experience severe vertigo and nausea during the testing and treatment. They should be asked to sit quietly for a period of time before leaving the clinic.

Canalith Repositioning Treatment: Horizontal Canal Canalithiasis

The canalith repositioning treatment has been modified to move the head in the plane of the horizontal canal so that free-floating debris will move through the long arm of the horizontal canal into the vestibule (CRT_Hcanal).[30,31] The patient is moved into supine with the head turned toward the affected side. The patient's head is then slowly rolled away from the affected side in 90° increments until the head has been moved 360°, waiting in each position until the dizziness stops (Fig. 19–7). As with the

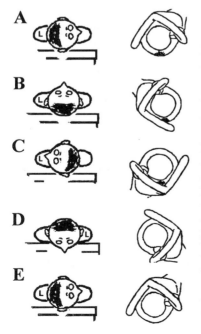

FIGURE 19–7. Canalith Repositioning Treatment (CRT) for horizontal SCC BPPV. The patient lies supine on the exam bed with the affected ear down (shown here for right HC BPPV) (*A*). The patient's head is then slowly rolled away from the affected ear until the face is pointed up, this position is maintained for about 15 seconds or until any vertigo stops (*B*). The patient then continues to roll the head in the same direction until the affected ear is up. This position is also maintained for 15 seconds or until the dizziness stops (*C*). The patient then rolls the head and body in the same direction until the face is down and stays in that position for 15 seconds (*D*). Finally, the head and body are rolled in the same direction to the original position with the affected ear down (*E*). After 15 seconds, the patient slowly sits up, keeping the head level or pitched down 30°. As with the regular CRT, the patient is fitted with a soft collar and told not to bend over, lie back, move the head up or down, or tilt the head to either side for the rest of the day. The follow-up treatment is the same as regular CRT. (Modified from Tusa, RJ, and Herdman, SJ: Canalith repositioning for benign positional vertigo. Education Program Syllabus 3BS.002, Am Acad Neurol, Minnesota, 1998, p 15, with permission.)

regular CRT, the patient is fitted with a soft collar and told not to bend over, lie back, or move their head up or down. Additionally, the patient is advised not to tilt their head to either side for the rest of the day. The follow-up treatment is the same as for regular CRT. A variation of this treatment can be used for horizontal canal cupulolithiasis by moving the patient's head more abruptly from one position to another (see Table 19–5).

Liberatory Maneuver: Posterior Canal

This is a single treatment approach developed by Semont et al.[21] Once the side of involvement has been identified, the patient is quickly moved into the provoking side-lying position with the head turned into the plane of the posterior canal and is kept in that position for 2 to 3 minutes (Fig. 19–8). The patient is then rapidly moved up through the sitting position and down into the opposite side lying position with the therapist maintaining the alignment of the neck and head on the body. (The face is then angled down toward the bed). Typically, nystagmus and vertigo reappear in this second position. If the patient does not experience vertigo in this second position, the head is abruptly shaken once or twice, through a small amplitude, presumably to free the debris. The patient stays in this position for 5 minutes. The patient is then slowly taken into a seated position. He must remain in a vertical position for 48 hours (including while sleeping) and must avoid the provoking position for 1 week following the treatment. Like CRT, the liberatory maneuver usually requires only a single treatment. Reportedly, this approach works by floating the debris through the canal system to the common crus but may also dislodge debris adhering to the cupula.

The liberatory maneuver must be modified if it is to be used to treat patients with anterior canal BPPV (liberatory_ A). In this modification, the head is turned toward the involved side and the patient rapidly lies down on the involved side so the nose is pointed 45° down toward the floor. After a few minutes the patient is rapidly moved through the sitting position onto the other side (note the nose will now be pointing 45° up). The remainder of the treatment is the same as for posterior canal BPPV.

TREATMENT EFFICACY

Semont et al[21] reported a series of 711 patients with BPPV treated over an 8-year period. Their paper did not identify if patients had other neurotological problems. They state only that some of the patients had slightly increased or decreased responses on caloric testing but their criteria for normal were not given. Statistically significant abnormal responses to caloric testing have been reported to occur in up to 47 percent of patients with BPPV.[4] Semont et al[21] reported a "cure" rate of 84 percent after a single treatment and 93 percent after two treatments. Again, recurrence of the symptoms was infrequent (4 percent). Other studies have reported somewhat lower remission rates.[22,32] We have used the Semont maneuver on much smaller population. Of 30 subjects treated, the Semont maneuver resulted in remission of symptoms or in significant improvement in 90 percent of the cases after a single treatment.[16] More recently, one study examined the effectiveness of the liberatory maneuver on a series of patients using the patients as their own control.[22] The patients were first treated with the liberatory maneuver but on the *unaffected* side. None of the patients had any relief from their

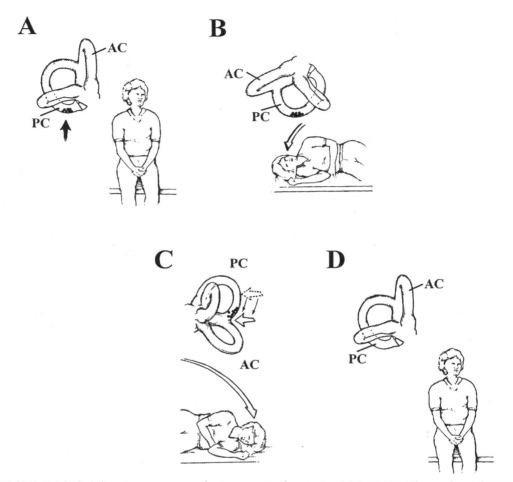

FIGURE 19–8. Liberatory maneuver for treatment of posterior SCC BPPV. (Shown for right PC BPPV) The patient sits on the examination table sideways and the head is rotated 45° towards the *unaffected* side (*A*). The patient is then moved quickly onto their affected side (parallel to the plane of the affected posterior canal) until the head is hanging 20° (*B*). After 1 minute, the patient is rapidly moved through the initial sitting position to the opposite side while the head is still positioned 45° toward the unaffected side (*C*) (nose will now be 45° down toward the floor). The patient holds this position for 1 minute and then moves slowly to a sitting position (*D*). The patient is then placed in a soft collar and given the same instructions as that described for the CRT. (Modified from Tusa, RJ, and Herdman, SJ: Canalith repositioning for benign positional vertigo. Education Program Syllabus 3BS.002, Am Acad Neurol, Minnesota, 1998, p 17, with permission.)

vertigo. The patients were then treated using only the routine post-maneuver instructions to keep the head upright for 48 hours, including sleeping in a sitting position. Again, at the end of 1 week, all patients were symptomatic. Then the patients were treated using the liberatory maneuver on the affected side. At the end of 1 week, all patients were symptom-free. Although the number of subjects in this study is small (*n* = 10), the results do support the earlier claims that this maneuver is an effective treatment for BPPV.

Brandt-Daroff Habituation Exercises: Posterior Canal Cupulolithiasis

Proposed by Brandt et al,[1] this treatment requires the patient to move into the provoking position repeatedly, several times a day. The patient first sits and then is moved rapidly into the position that causes the vertigo (Fig. 19–9). A torsional and/or upbeating nystagmus occurs with the onset of the vertigo. The severity of the vertigo will be directly related to how rapidly the patient moves into the provoking position. The patient stays in that position until the vertigo stops and then sits up again. Usually moving to the sitting position will also result in vertigo, although this will be less severe and of a shorter duration. Nystagmus, if reoccurring, will be in the opposite direction. The patient remains in the upright position for 30 seconds and then moves rapidly into the mirror-image position on the other side, stays there for 30 seconds, and then sits up. The patient then repeats the entire maneuver until the vertigo diminishes. The entire sequence is repeated every 3 hours until the patient has 2 consecutive days without vertigo. It is not clear why these exercises result in a decrease in the vertigo and nystagmus. One explanation is that the debris becomes dislodged from the cupula of the posterior canal and moves to a location no longer affecting the cupula during head movement. A second possibility is that central adaptation occurs, reducing the nervous system response to the signal from the posterior canal. Brandt argues against central adaptation as a mechanism for recovery because many patients recover abruptly.[7]

The Brandt-Daroff exercises for PC BPPV can be modified for horizontal canal cupulolithiasis by applying the same concept and having the patient perform rapid, repetitive movements in the plane of the horizontal canal (Brandt-Daroff_ Hcupulo). Although this appears to be an effective treatment, only anecdotal evidence exists at this time because of the relatively low occurrence of this form of BPPV. Presumably this treatment works by dislodging the debris from the cupula.

TREATMENT EFFICACY

Brandt et al[1] studied a series of 67 patients with histories of BPPV of 2 days' to 8 months' duration. None of these patients had evidence of other neurological or neurotological disease. They reported that 98 percent of the subjects had no symptoms after 3 to 14 days of exercises. The only subject who did not respond to treatment had a perilymph fistula requiring surgical repair. Recurrence was low, affecting only 3 percent of the patients. In our experience with a series of 20 BPPV patients treated with exercises similar to those advocated by Brandt et al,[1] the time until the patients were symptom-free ($n = 12$) or had at least a moderate reduction in symptoms ($n = 7$) was more protracted, extending from 1 week to 6 months (this latter case being a patient who was afraid to lie down, which extended the treatment course several extra months while he worked at home just to achieve the supine position). Patients in whom there was only partial recovery complained most frequently of an intermittent "swimming" sensation rather than of true vertigo. One patient experienced no change in his vertigo. These patients had histories of BPPV extending from a few days to 35 years. The more protracted the course, the more resistant the BPPV may be to treatment. We also noted that many patients having a more prolonged recovery course had additional nervous system disorders that may have compounded the course of recovery.

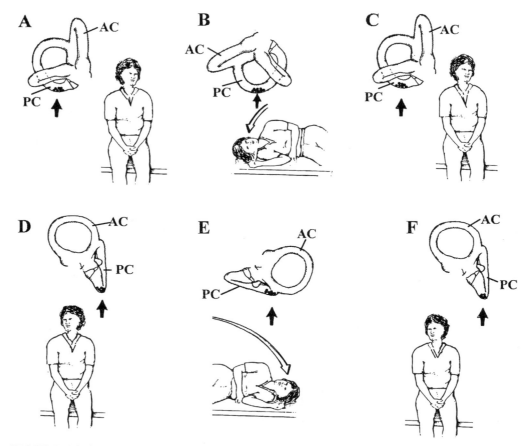

FIGURE 19–9. Brandt-Daroff treatment for treatment of posterior SCC BPPV. The patient is moved quickly into the sidelying position on the affected side (shown here as right side) and stays in that position until the vertigo stops plus an additional 30 seconds. The patient then sits up and again waits for the vertigo to stop. The patient then repeats the movement to the opposite side, stays there for 30 seconds, and sits up. The entire treatment is repeated 10 to 20 times, three times a day until the patient has two days in a row with no vertigo. (Modified from Tusa, RJ, and Herdman, SJ: Canalith repositioning for benign positional vertigo. Education Program Syllabus 3BS.002, Am Acad Neurol, Minnesota, 1998, p 18, with permission.)

Treatment Guidelines

Figure 19–10 illustrates a paradigm for arriving at the appropriate treatment for BPPV. Identification of the side, which canal is involved (based on direction of nystagmus) and whether the problem is due to canalithiasis or cupulolithiasis lead to specific treatments.

OTHER EXERCISES

Several different treatments have been advocated for patients who complain of disequilibrium associated with head movements. Although these patients may have had BPPV, they often have more generalized motion sensitivity rather than a vestibular

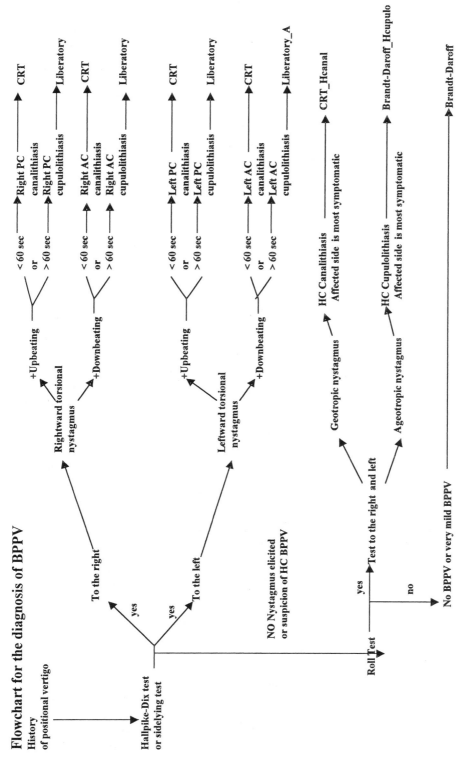

FIGURE 19–10. Schematic for assessment leading to treatment. Identification of the direction and duration of the nystagmus leads to the identification of which canal is involved and whether the BPPV is from canalithiasis or cupulolithiasis. This information directs the appropriate choice of treatment.

disorder (see Chapter 15). Tests to determine the provoking positions are important in developing the appropriate treatment protocol and monitoring the progress of the patient. Measurement of the latency and the duration of the vertigo as well as the intensity (scaled 1–5 or 1–10) should be kept for each of the position changes (see Chapter 15). The provoking positions used are specific for each patient and are not limited to the Hallpike-Dix maneuver.[33,34]

NONEXERCISE TREATMENT

Medications are not indicated in the treatment of BPPV other than to relieve the nausea that can accompany the episodic vertigo. As such, phenergan or compazine can be given prior to treatment in those patients with severe nausea or emesis. Surgical management includes vestibular nerve section, section of the singular nerve (which innervates the posterior canal), and occlusion of the affected canal.[35–37] Today, surgery is rarely used because of the successful management using exercises.

Postural Disturbances

Several studies have documented the postural instability of patients with BPPV.[38–40] Black and Nashner[38] found decreased postural stability in BPPV patients and suggested that they rely excessively on visual cues to maintain balance. Unfortunately, Black and Nashner do not report how many of the 11 patients showed this pattern of increased reliance on visual cues. Thirty-seven percent of a group of 19 patients with BPPV studied by Voorhees[39] had abnormal posturography tests. He found that these BPPV patients could not use vestibular cues effectively to maintain balance but did not find the increased reliance on visual cues suggested by Black and Nashner. Blatt et al[40] found that approximately 66 percent of subjects with posterior canal BPPV had increased sway or loss of balance on posturography testing when somatosensory cues were altered (SOT 4, 5, and 6). In addition, they reported that, for most patients, improved postural stability did occur with remission of vertigo following CRT.

The postural instability of patients with BPPV may not be related to debris in the semicircular canal itself. Many patients with BPPV have a history of head injury or have horizontal canal hypofunction as well as positional vertigo. Either of these factors could result in postural instability. Assessment of postural stability, therefore, would be an important part of the assessment of these patients in order to develop an appropriate treatment plan.

Because patients with BPPV complain of postural instability and have documented instability that does not resolve fully with resolution of their vertigo and nystagmus, balance should also be assessed in these patients. Many different clinical tests can be used for assessing postural stability (see Chapter 15). These tests are not specific for the vestibulospinal system but are simply ways of assessing postural stability. Assessment of balance should include tests of static (quiet stance) and dynamic (moving) stability under conditions which stress balance, such as decreasing the base of support or requiring head movement, and under conditions that assess the patient's ability to maintain balance using only certain sensory cues. Normal values by age are available for many of these tests. Among the tests are the Romberg and sharpened or tandem Romberg tests, and measurement of one-legged standing balance, all with eyes open and eyes closed. Patients can be required to maintain balance with eyes open and eyes closed while standing on foam to distort somatosensory feedback. Postural stability can be assessed under more dynamic conditions by observing the patient's ability to perform tandem walking (walk-on-floor-eyes-closed test), the Singleton test, and Fukuda's Stepping Test. The patient might also be asked to walk while turning the head from side to side as such movements frequently result in ataxia.

Balance can also be assessed using a force platform. With a force platform, quantifying anterior-posterior and lateral sway while the patient is standing on a stationary surface (static posturography) is possible. A system is also available that quantifies the patient's ability to maintain balance when visual and/or somatosensory cues are either absent or inappropriate (Neurocom International, Inc).

Management

1. Patients, especially those with long histories of BPPV, may have anxiety about moving into the provoking position. Careful explanation to the patient of the test or the treatment and what the patient can expect will bring better cooperation from the patient, especially if they can be reassured that the vertigo will stop. Some patients prefer the single-treatment approaches but for others, Brandt's exercises may be modified so that the patient has more control over the position change and gradually becomes less fearful of provoking the vertigo and nausea. Also, patients may be more comfortable performing the exercises on the floor rather than on the bed because they know they will not fall. The anxious patient, however, may tend to move out of the provoking position too quickly when attempting to do the exercises on his own. The extent of anxiety patients can experience should not be underestimated; one patient with a long history of BPPV became so fearful of provoking the vertigo that he tied one arm down at night to keep from rolling over onto the "bad side."

   Patients who are especially fearful of the sensation of the vertigo may be unwilling to perform exercises in which they must repeatedly provoke the vertigo. These patients may be successfully treated using the single treatment approaches (CRT and liberatory) knowing that they will only experience the vertigo one or two times.

2. Patients may not be able to keep their head relatively upright as required by CRT and by the liberatory maneuver. We still encourage patients to sleep with extra pillows for 2 nights, but explain that they may shorten that time period if they would like. Patients with posterior or anterior canal BPPV are advised to avoid bending over or moving the head vertically for 5 subsequent days. Some patients may have difficulty avoiding bending over (e.g., parents with small children, certain work-related activities). For these patients, Brandt-Daroff habituation exercises would be more appropriate.

3. The success of the Brandt-Daroff habituation exercises depends on the compliance of the patient. Some improvement may occur within a few days after initiating the treatment, but treatment may have to be continued for extended periods of time. Weekly clinic visits may help to improve patient compliance, but in patients with poor compliance, CRT or the liberatory maneuver may be a more appropriate choice.

4. With the Brandt-Daroff habituation exercises, the patient must perform the exercise even though it may provoke vertigo and nausea. Usually the vertigo and nausea disappear quickly when the patient is moved out of the provoking position. Re-

peated positional changes, however, may cause a prolonged and generalized disequilibrium with persistent nausea. The disequilibrium and nausea may be disturbing enough that the patient stops the exercises. Patients should be warned that this may occur, but that it is only a temporary effect. Usually all that is needed is to modify the exercises (e.g., decrease the repetitions for a while) or regulate the time during the day when the exercises are performed but medication, such as phenergan, may be taken 30 minutes before the exercises are performed. Brandt-Daroff habituation exercises are usually performed with the eyes closed to minimize the visual-vestibular conflict contributing to the nausea. Opening the eyes may result in an increase in the nausea but may also facilitate adaptation and therefore recovery.

5. Cervical and back pain may preclude the use of CRT or the liberatory maneuver, or may be aggravated by the repeated positional changes of Brandt-Daroff habituation exercises. Older patients may be less tolerant of CRT or the liberatory maneuver, especially if they move cautiously because of other conditions such as arthritis. The use of a tilt table can reduce the amount of neck extension needed during CRT. The positional changes used in the Brandt-Daroff habituation exercises may be modified to enable the patient to perform them but the other maneuvers can not be modified.

6. There is a slight risk of soft tissue neck injury when performing CRT or the liberatory maneuver. This risk is small, however, because the head is supported at all times. We have had no neck injuries associated with these procedures. Care should be taken, however, in using any of these procedures in patients with osteoporosis or with previous neck injury or surgery.

7. Bilateral BPPV, like BPPV affecting the labyrinth unilaterally, has been reported in idiopathic cases and after head injury.[41] If either CRT or the liberatory maneuver is used, the most symptomatic side is treated first. Many times this will result in resolution of symptoms on both sides indicating that the patient had a unilateral BPPV mimicking bilateral BPPV.[41] The Brandt-Daroff habituation exercises may also be an appropriate choice for bilateral BPPV if it involves the posterior canal bilaterally.

8. Patients with BPPV and horizontal canal hypofunction are given exercises for both disorders. If CRT or the liberatory maneuver are used, delaying initiation of the vestibular adaptation exercises until after the BPPV is treated is necessary. In this way there is less risk that the patient may move the head inappropriately during the BPPV treatment. If the Brandt-Daroff habituation exercises are used, vestibular adaptation exercises may be used concurrently. Exercises to improve postural stability in these patients must be considered.

9. Central positional nystagmus can be mistaken for the nystagmus of BPPV. This is especially true for persistent down-beating nystagmus, which may be due to either cerebellar degeneration, Chiari malformation, and selective lesions involving the cerebellar flocculus or the medial longitudinal fasciculus in the floor of the fourth ventricle, or can be due to anterior canal cupulolithiasis. Up-beating nystagmus can also occur with central lesions although it is less common.[42]

CONCLUSION

BPPV is a common disorder that results in what can be disabling episodes of vertigo. There are now several different treatments that can be used to relieve the patient's symptoms and enable the patient to return to normal activities. Which treatment is used depends on many factors, including which canal is involved and whether the patient has canalithiasis or cupulolithiasis as well as the presence of other vestibular deficits and the willingness of the patient to make himself "dizzy." Given the different treatments available, however, patients should no longer be told that they must "learn to live with vertigo."

CASE STUDIES

CASE #1
History

The patient with a history had an episode of vertigo 1 week ago when she was at the beauty parlor and lay back to have her hair washed. She continued to have vertigo with nausea and vomiting for several hours afterwards. Presently she notes vertigo when she bends forward and then straightens up. She also has complaints of feeling off-balance but has not fallen. Examination showed nystagmus with the fast phases upbeating and rightward torsional when she was moved into the right Hallpike-Dix position. The latency and duration of the nystagmus, and the concurrent vertigo, was consistent with canalithiasis.

Comment

The direction of the nystagmus indicates involvement of the posterior canal on the right. The most appropriate treatment would be CRT. The patient was treated with the CRT and during the treatment, she had upbeating nystagmus and vertigo with all position changes but when she returned to a sitting position, the nystagmus became down-beating. The treatment was immediately repeated and again she had down-beating nystagmus when she returned to sitting. On the second repetition of the treatment, she had no nystagmus or vertigo when she returned to sitting.

Comment

Down-beating nystagmus indicates that the debris did not move out of the common crus into the vestibule when the patient moved into a sitting position but instead moved back into the posterior canal. This can occur because of the variation in the orientation of the canals or because of inappropriate head positions during the treatment. For that reason, the treatment was immediately repeated until there was no nystagmus (or until the direction of the nystagmus is appropriate throughout the entire treatment, in this case upbeating and rightward torsional). On follow-up visit, the patient was without nystagmus or vertigo.

CASE #2
History

Patient had a history of brief episodes of vertigo when looking up or rolling over in bed at night. The patient was in a car accident 2 months prior to the reported onset of the vertigo. He had orbital and nasal fractures and was semicomatose and heavily sedated for 4 days following the accident. Furthermore, he had a thoracic spine injury and was braced until recently. This restricted his movement. Examination showed vertigo and nystagmus with the fast phase eye movement rightward torsional when the patient was moved into the right Hallpike-Dix position. The vertical component of the nystagmus could not be discerned. There was a latency of a few seconds to onset of the vertigo and nystagmus and the duration was less than 20 seconds.

Comment

Head injury or even a sudden acceleration/deceleration of the head is known to result in BPPV.[4] In this case, the onset of BPPV may have been masked by the limitation in the patient's movements because of the immobilization for the spinal injury. The latency and duration of the vertigo and nystagmus are consistent with canalithiasis. The direction of the nystagmus elicited in the right Hallpike-Dix position suggests either posterior or anterior canal involvement on the right. Therefore the most appropriate treatment would be the canalith repositioning treatment for the right side.

Treatment

The patient was successfully treated with CRT but had a recurrence 3 months later. Examination showed right posterior canal canalithiasis. As the patient returned to the sitting position in the last phase of the treatment (CRT), the direction of the nystagmus changed from upbeating and rightward torsional to geotropic.

Comment

The change in the direction of the nystagmus suggests that the free-floating debris moved from the posterior canal into the horizontal canal. The direction of the horizontal nystagmus, geotropic, indicates horizontal canal canalithiasis. The patient was immediately treated with the canalith-repositioning maneuver modified for horizontal canal canalithiasis. Follow-up visit 1 week later showed that this treatment was successful.

CASE #3

History

A 73-year-old female complains of balance problems intermittently over the past few years and was referred for treatment of positional vertigo. Five months prior to this visit, she began having severe episodes of vertigo when she was in bed. She states that the vertigo lasts approximately 1 minute. She also reports that her balance has become worse. Three months ago, she had an episode of vertigo while working outside in her garden and fell, injuring her ankle and calf. The injury is still healing. She notes that she can no longer bend over to pick something up without experiencing some vertigo. Her most recent episode of vertigo was this morning. Examination today revealed no nystagmus when moved into either the right or left Hallpike-Dix position nor when moved into the right or left side-lying positions. Remainder of oculomotor examination was also normal.

Comment

The brief episodes of vertigo when in bed or when bending over are consistent with BPPV. This disorder has a high incidence in older individuals. Being unable to elicit the vertigo and nystagmus during the examination is not unusual. Balance problems are also commonly associated with BPPV. Because the canal and side of involvement could not be determined, the patient was instructed in the Brandt-Daroff habituation exercises. She was to perform the exercises twice a day.

Follow-up

The patient returned 2 weeks later and reported no further episodes of vertigo but she had complaints of a worsening sense of imbalance, especially immediately after moving from sitting to standing. She denied falling but stated that she had to hold on occasionally. Examination showed no nystagmus or vertigo. The patient did complain of imbalance when she returned to a sitting position during the Hallpike-Dix tests.

Comment

The patient appears to be in remission with respect to her BPPV. Her continued imbalance may be due to a residual BPPV but it is unusual for BPPV to cause extreme dizziness when the patient moves from supine to sitting or standing and no other signs or symptoms. This patient's blood pressure was tested supine and then, after 10 minutes of lying down, upon standing up. Her blood pressure while supine was 112/58 and decreased to 90/64 when standing. She was also symptomatic while standing. This drop in blood pressure could account for her imbalance and dizziness when standing. It also raised the issue whether the patient had BPPV at all, even though her history was consistent with BPPV, because nystagmus was never observed. The patient's primary care physician was contacted and the patient was scheduled to see her.

ACKNOWLEDGMENTS

Supported by NIDCD Grant DC03196.

REFERENCES

1. Brandt, T, and Daroff, RB: Physical therapy for benign paroxysmal positional vertigo. Arch Otolaryngol. 106:484, 1980.
2. Mizukoshi, K, et al: Epidemiological studies on benign paroxysmal positional vertigo. Acta Otolaryngol (Stockh) (suppl) 447:67, 1988.

3. Froehling, DA, et al: Benign positional vertigo: Incidence and prognosis in a population-based study in Olmsted county, Minnesota. Mayo Clin Proc 66:596, 1991.
4. Baloh, RW, et al: Benign positional vertigo: Clinical and oculographic features in 240 cases. Neurology 37:371, 1987.
5. Schuknecht, HF: Cupulolithiasis. Arch Otolaryngol 90:765, 1969.
6. Boumans, LJJM, et al: Gain of the adaptation mechanism in the human vestibulo-ocular reflex system. Otorhinolaryngology 50:319, 1988.
7. Hall, SF, et al: The mechanisms of benign paroxysmal vertigo. J Otolaryngol 8:151, 1979.
8. Parnes, LS, and McClure, JA: Free-floating Endolymph Particles: A new operative finding during posterior semicircular canal occlusion. Laryngoscope 102:988, 1992.
9. Herdman, SJ, et al: Eye movement signs in vertical canal benign paroxysmal positional vertigo. In Fuchs, AF, et al (eds): Contemporary Ocular Motor and Vestibular Research: A Tribute to David A. Robinson. Stuttgart, Thieme, 1994, pp 385–387.
10. McClure, J: Horizontal canal BPV. J Otolaryngol 14:30, 1985.
11. Baloh, RW, et al: Horizontal semicircular canal variant of benign positional vertigo. Neurology 43:2542, 1993.
12. De la Meilleure, G, et al: Benign paroxysmal positional vertigo of the horizontal canal. J Neurol Neurosurg Psychiatr 60:68, 1996.
13. Nuti, D, et al: Benign Paroxysmal Positional Vertigo of the Horizontal Canal: A form of canalithiasis with variable clinical features. J Vestib Res 6:173, 1996.
14. Dix, MR, and Hallpike, CS: Pathology, symptomatology and diagnosis of certain disorders of the vestibular system. Proc Roy Soc Med 45:341, 1952.
15. Epley, JM: The canalith repositioning procedure: For treatment of benign paroxysmal positional vertigo. Otolaryngol Head Neck Surg 107:399, 1992.
16. Herdman, SJ, et al: Single treatment approaches to benign paroxysmal positional vertigo. Arch Otolaryngol Head Neck Surg 119:450, 1993.
17. Li, JC: Mastoid oscillation: A critical factor for success in the canalith repositioning procedure. Otolaryngol Head Neck Surg 112:670, 1995.
18. Harvey, SA, et al: Modified liberatory maneuver: Effective treatment for benign paroxysmal positional vertigo. Laryngoscope 104:1206, 1994.
19. Welling, DB, and Barnes, DE: Particle repositioning maneuver for benign paroxysmal positional vertigo. Laryngoscope 104:946, 1994.
20. Lynn, S, et al: Randomized trial of the canalith repositioning procedure. Otolaryngol Head Neck Surg 113:712, 1995.
21. Semont, A, et al: Curing the BPPV with a Liberatory maneuver. Adv Otorhinolaryngol 42:290, 1988.
22. Ireland, D: The Semont maneuver. Proceedings of the XVIth Barany Society Meeting, Prague Czechoslovakia, 1994, pp 367–370.
23. Parnes, LS, and Price-Jones, RG: Particle repositioning maneuver for benign paroxysmal positional vertigo. Ann Otol Rhinol Laryngol 102:325, 1993.
24. Gyko, K: Benign paroxysmal positional vertigo as a complication of bedrest. Laryngoscope 98:332, 1988.
25. Epley, JM: New dimensions of benign paroxysmal positional vertigo. Otolaryngol Head Neck Surg 88:599, 1980.
26. Blakley, BW: A randomized, controlled assessment of the canalith repositioning maneuver. Otolaryngol Head Neck Surg 110:391, 1994.
27. Massoud, EAS, and Ireland, DJ: Post-treatment instructions in nonsurgical management of benign paroxysmal positional vertigo. L Otolaryngol 25:121, 1996.
28. Tusa, RJ, and Herdman, SJ: Assessment and treatment of anterior canal benign paroxysmal positional vertigo using the canalith repositioning maneuver (CRM). Neurology 48:A384, 1997.
29. Herdman, SJ, and Tusa, RJ: Complications of the canalith repositioning procedure. Arch Otolaryngol Head Neck Surg 122:281, 1996.
30. Lempert, T, and Tiel-Wilck, K: A positional maneuver for treatment of horizontal-canal benign positional vertigo. Laryngoscope 106:476, 1996.
31. Herdman, SJ: Physical therapy in the treatment of patients with benign paroxysmal positional vertigo. Neurol Report 20:46, 1996.
32. Pagnini, P, et al: La rieducazione vestibolare: Aspetti clinici e reseltati. Giornate Italiane de Otoneurologia 8:81, 1989.
33. Norre, ME, and Beckers, A: Vestibular habituation training: Exercise treatment for vertigo based upon the habituation effect. Otolaryngol Head Neck Surg 101:14, 1989.
34. Tangeman, PT, and Wheeler, J: Inner ear concussion syndrome: Vestibular implications and physical therapy treatment. Top Acute Care Trauma Rehab 1:72, 1986.
35. Gacek, RR: Singular neurectomy update. Ann Otol Rhinol Laryngol 91:469, 1982.
36. Gacek, RR: Techniques and results of singular neurectomy for the management of benign paroxysmal positional vertigo. Acat Otolaryngol (Stockh) 115:154, 1995.

37. Parnes, LS, and McClure, JA: Posterior semicircular canal occlusion for intractable benign paroxysmal positional vertigo. Ann Otol Rhinol Laryngol 99:330, 1990.
38. Black, FO, and Nashner, LM: Postural disturbances in patients with benign paroxysmal positional nystagmus. Ann Otol Rhinol Laryngol 93:595, 1984.
39. Voorhees, RL: The role of dynamic posturography in neurotologic diagnosis. Laryngoscope 99:995, 1989.
40. Blatt, PJ, et al: Postural instability in benign paroxysmal positional vertigo—Does it resolve with canalith repositioning? Am J Otology, 1999. Submitted.
41. Steddin, S, and Brandt, T: Unilateral mimicking bilateral benign paroxysmal positioning vertigo. Arch Otolaryngol Head Neck Surg 120:1339, 1994.
42. Fisher, A, et al: Primary position upbeating nystagmus: A variety of central positional nystagmus. Brain 106:949, 1983.

CHAPTER 20

Vestibular Rehabilitation of the Patient with Traumatic Brain Injury

Anne Shumway-Cook, PT, PhD

This chapter will discuss the confounding influence of traumatic brain injury (TBI) on the assessment, treatment, and recovery of function in patients with peripheral vestibular system pathology. The array of vestibular pathologies associated with TBI are similar to those commonly found in most neurotological practices. What distinguishes the patient with TBI from other patients with peripheral vestibular disease is the mechanism of vestibular injury and the high incidence of other neurological deficits complicating the recovery process.

Recognizing and treating symptoms of vestibular dysfunction including dizziness and imbalance is an essential part of TBI rehabilitation. Many therapists involved in rehabilitating the patient with TBI are familiar with approaches to treating imbalance but lack strategies to treat complaints of dizziness. As a result, therapists often try to avoid provoking dizziness when treating patients with TBI. However, avoiding the movements that provoke dizziness can actually delay recovery from vestibular system dysfunction, resulting in persisting symptoms.[1,2] Persisting symptoms complicate recovery and contribute to long term loss of functional independence.[3–5]

The objectives of this chapter are to discuss mechanisms of traumatic injury producing peripheral vestibular system pathology in TBI. Strategies for assessing and treating symptoms of peripheral vestibular system dysfunction will be reviewed. In addition, the chapter will discuss the effect of other traumatically induced sensory, motor, and cognitive deficits on strategies for treating the patient with TBI and associated vestibular system pathology.

VESTIBULAR PATHOLOGY

As many as 30 to 65 percent of patients with TBI suffer symptoms of traumatic vestibular pathology at some point during their recovery.[4-9] Symptoms of peripheral vestibular system dysfunction can include vertigo, eye-head dyscoordination affecting the ability to stabilize gaze during head movements, and imbalance affecting the ability to maintain stability when standing and walking.[10] The specific constellation of symptoms found in individual patients will vary depending on the type and extent of injuries to both vestibular and central neural structures. Understanding peripheral vestibular pathology and its effect on gaze, postural, and perceptual functions is essential because treatment varies according to the patient's symptoms and diagnosis.[11]

Mechanism of injury and resulting vestibular pathologies reported to occur frequently following TBI are summarized below.

Concussion

Inner ear concussion injury is the most common vestibular sequelae of TBI.[8,12,13] Symptoms of concussive-type vestibular injury can include high frequency sensorineural hearing loss, benign paroxysmal positional nystagmus and vertigo (BPPN/V), postural dyscontrol, and gait ataxia. BPPV in TBI is believed to occur because of the intense acceleration of the utricular otolithic membrane resulting in displacement of otoconia to the posterior semicircular canal. Displaced otoconia, adhering to the cupula or free-floating in the long arm of the posterior canal, may result in displacement of the cupula in response to gravity in specific positions.[14] BPPV produces a transient positional nystagmus and vertigo in a characteristic head-dependent position. In addition, patients with BPPV complain of transient vertigo when lying down and rolling over to the affected side, or when looking up or down (see Chapter 19).

Fractures

Traumatic fractures of the temporal bone can produce unilateral or bilateral vestibular hypofunction. Transverse fractures account for approximately 20 percent of all temporal bone fractures, and are reported to result most frequently from blows to the occiput.[12,15] Transverse fractures of the temporal bone produce a unilateral loss of vestibular function, which can be either partial or complete. Functional effects of a unilateral loss of vestibular function include spontaneous nystagmus (acute stage only) and provoked vertigo, problems with gaze stabilization, and dysequilibrium affecting the ability to maintain stability in sitting, standing and walking.[16] Functional effects of a bilateral loss of vestibular function include oscillopsia (inability to stabilize gaze during head movements) and severe imbalance affecting stance and gait.

Longitudinal fractures account for approximately 80 percent of all temporal bone fractures and are associated primarily with blows to the parietal and temporal regions of the skull.[12,15] Anatomic damage associated with longitudinal fractures is primarily to middle ear structures leading to conductive hearing loss. Associated vestibular symptoms are considered secondary to a concussive injury to the membranous labyrinth.

Intracranial Pressure and Hemorrhagic Lesions

Changes in intracranial pressure can produce ruptures in the round or oval window and a perilymph fistula (PLF) between the middle and inner ear.[8,11,17–19] PLF can result in fluctuating hearing loss, episodic vertigo, and gait and balance disturbances. In addition, patients with PLF may have a number of cognitive symptoms, including memory, concentration, and attention deficits.[20] The incidence of PLF in head-injured patients is uncertain.[18,20–22]

Vascular injuries, including hemorrhage into the membranous labyrinth, can injure the endolymphatic system producing a posttraumatic hydrops or Ménière-type syndrome, with corresponding symptoms of tinnitus, hearing loss, vertigo and imbalance.[8,11]

Central Vestibular Lesions

Traumatic head injury can also produce damage to central vestibular structures.[3,13,23] Multiple petechial hemorrhages in the brainstem, which damage central vestibular structures have been reported in both the mildly (no loss of consciousness) and moderately head-injured patient. Symptoms include spontaneous nystagmus and oculomotor problems including ocular dysmetria, cogwheeling during smooth-pursuit eye movements, and marked optokinetic asymmetries. Spontaneous and/or provoked vertigo may or may not occur in the patient with central vestibular lesions.

VESTIBULAR REHABILITATION

Vestibular rehabilitation is a comprehensive approach to assessing and treating symptoms of vestibular system pathology.[21,22,24] The overall goal of assessment is to document the patient's functional problems, and the many sensory, motor, and cognitive limitations contributing to loss of functional independence. Specific evaluation of vestibular system pathology, summarized in Box 20–1, focuses on assessment of vertigo, control of eye-head coordination for stabilizing gaze, and musculoskeletal and neural components of postural control underlying the ability to maintain stability and orientation when sitting, standing and walking. Sorting out the relative contribution of vestibular system pathology to overall loss of function can be difficult because functional deficits following TBI are usually due to a combination of many interacting factors.

Vestibular rehabilitation uses exercise to decrease dizziness, improve gaze stabilization, and retrain sensory and motor aspects of postural control. In most instances exercises are designed to facilitate central nervous system (CNS) compensation rather than alter underlying vestibular pathology. The exception to this is treatment of BPPV, which is aimed at altering the underlying mechanism producing symptoms, rather than facilitating CNS adaptation. Strategies for treating vestibular system dysfunction are individualized to each patient's problems, and focus on both remediating underlying impairments and improving functional skills.[21,22] Vestibular rehabilitation programs are often modified in the patient with TRI owing to the frequency of both physical and cognitive problems following trauma. Modifications include:

BOX 20–1   Vestibular Rehabilitation Assessment

Vertigo

> Spontaneous
> Provoked
> > Positional
> > Movement

Eye-head coordination

> Oculomotor control—saccade and smooth pursuit
> Gaze stabilization during head movements
> Gaze fixation suppression

Postural control in sitting, standing, and walking

> Functional Status
> Underlying Impairments
> > Biomechanical constraints
> > Neuromuscular constraints
> > Sensory/perceptual constraints

Other Limitations

> Pain
> Cognitive and behavioral constraints

---

1. Providing physical assistance to accommodate movement problems.
2. Providing increased supervision to accommodate cognitive and behavioral problems.
3. Progressing the patient more slowly owing to multiplicity of problems.

The following sections discuss clinical strategies for assessing and treating symptoms of vestibular system pathology including vertigo, eye-head coordination, and postural dyscontrol in the patient with TBI.

Vertigo

ASSESSMENT

When assessing vertigo the therapist notes whether dizziness symptoms are spontaneous or provoked, and determines the situations and conditions that precipitate complaints of dizziness.[21,22,25] Characteristics of vertigo are noted, such as onset latency, duration, intensity, and the effect of repeating the movement. Associated autonomic symptoms, such as nausea, sweating, and pallor are noted. The presence and type of nystagmus are recorded. Head movements are repeated in sitting, standing, and walking. In addition to subjective complaints of dizziness, episodes of staggering and dysequilibrium associated with complaints of dizziness are recorded, particularly in standing and walking.

The patient with unilateral vestibular hypofunction (partial or complete) will experience both spontaneous and provoked vertigo in the acute stage. Often by the time a patient with TBI and concomitant unilateral loss of vestibular function enters a rehabilitation program, spontaneous complaints have resolved. Patients will, however, continue to complain of vertigo, lasting from seconds to minutes, which is provoked by head movements in all planes. Vertigo in the patient with BPPV lasts 30 to 45 seconds and is provoked by placing the patient in the Hallpike position. Patients with BPPV may also report vertigo when lying down and rolling to the affected side, when looking up or when leaning over.[26,27]

TREATMENT

Habituation exercises are used to decrease dizziness in patients who have movement-provoked symptoms of vertigo. Habituation exercises involve repeating the movements that provoke vertigo between 5 and 10 times, two to three times a day. When a patient is residing in an inpatient rehabilitation facility, habituation exercises are incorporated into twice-daily physical therapy treatments, usually at the end of each exercise session. As mentioned previously, habituation exercises are routinely modified to accommodate both movement and cognitive limitations in the patient with TBI. Written exercise sheets are used, and patients are provided logs to record exercise sessions. Because of the high frequency of behavioral and cognitive problems, including attention and memory deficits, closer supervision and physical assistance are more often required when treating vestibular dysfunction in the patient with TBI, than in other types of patients.

In our clinic the canalith repositioning maneuver (CRM) developed by John Epley is used almost exclusively to treat patients with BPPV[26] (see Chapter 19). Because of the success of the CRM, we rarely use the liberatory maneuver described by Semont et al for management of BPPV.[27] When the CRM is used on an inpatient on rehabilitation, it is essential to provide the nursing staff with information regarding the necessary follow-up precautions in order to insure that the patient is consistent in adhering to these precautions (see Chapter 19). Inability to adhere to follow-up precautions can make the procedure ineffective.[28]

Eye-Head Coordination

ASSESSMENT

Eye movements from both the visual and vestibular systems used to keep gaze stable during voluntary and involuntary movements of the head are also examined.[22,24] Testing gaze stabilization is done with the patient seated, standing unsupported, and walking. Visually generated eye movements including smooth-pursuit and saccadic eye movements are assessed. The patient's ability to maintain a stable gaze during horizontal and vertical head motions of varying speed is examined. Finally the patient's ability to keep gaze fixed on an object moving in phase with the head is used to test visual suppression of vestibular-driven eye movements. Subjective complaints of dizziness, blurred vision, or oscillopsia are noted.

Following TBI, eye-head dyscoordination can result from (1) damage to the vestibular system disrupting vestibulo-ocular reflex (VOR) function; (2) deficits within the visual system including loss of ocular motility, visual acuity/field deficits, or visual perceptual deficits; (3) orthopedic injuries limiting cervical motion; and (4) damage to cerebellar structures resulting in loss of visual suppression of the VOR.[29,30]

TREATMENT

Exercises are used to improve gaze stabilization when the head is still and in motion. Saccadic and smooth-pursuit tracking exercises are performed initially if the patient has dizziness during these eye movements. Next the patient is asked to keep the gaze fixed on a central target while moving the head either horizontally or vertically for a progressively longer period of time. Finally, patients are given exercises to improve visual modulation of vestibulo-ocular responses (see Chapter 17).[16,24,31] The patient repeats these exercises first in a supported sitting position, and progresses to standing and walking.

Because so many of the exercises used to treat symptoms of vestibular system pathology involve movement of the head and neck, treatment of cervical complaints is essential to recovery of function. Vestibular rehabilitation exercises combined with physical modalities and orthopedic manual skills have produced excellent results.[32]

Postural Control Underlying Stability

The ability to maintain a stable position is critical to independence in most functional skills. **Stability** is defined as the ability to maintain the center of body mass within limits determined principally by the extent of the support base.[33] Stability requires a continuous interaction between the individual and the environment, and involves many bodily subsystems collectively referred to as the postural control system (see Chapter 2).

ASSESSMENT

Because postural control is complex, involving the interaction of many systems, assessment of postural control must be multidimensional. Assessment focuses on documenting the ability to perform functional skills requiring posture control, and investigating the underlying impairments that constrain the maintenance of postural stability. Impairments are limitations within the individual that restrict sensory and motor strategies for postural control.[34] As shown in Figure 20–1, impairments affecting postural stability following TBI can be musculoskeletal, neuromuscular, sensory/perceptual, or cognitive.

The information gained through assessment is used to develop a comprehensive list of problems, establish short- and long-term goals, and formulate a plan of care for retraining posture control. A thorough assessment must include a review of the patient's medical and social history, as well as a review of current symptoms and concerns.[34] Procedures for assessing the multiple levels of postural control have been described in detail elsewhere, and so will only be briefly reviewed here.[34–36]

FUNCTIONAL STATUS

There are a number of tests available to measure functional skills related to postural control. Our outpatient program uses three tests to document functional balance and mobility skills. The Berg Balance Scale shown in Box 20–2 rates performance from 0 (cannot perform) to 4 (normal performance) on 4 different tasks including ability to sit, stand, reach, lean over, turn and look over each shoulder, turn in a complete circle,

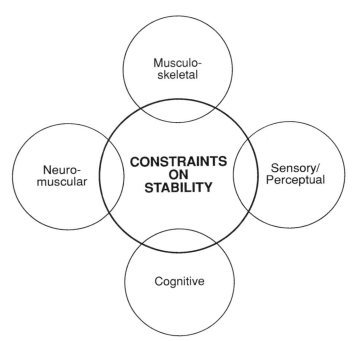

FIGURE 20–1. Categories of constraints on stability following traumatic brain injury.

and step.[37] The total possible score on the Berg Balance Scale is 56, indicating excellent balance. The Berg Balance Scale has been shown to have excellent interrater reliability and relatively good concurrent validity. It has shown to be an effective predictor of fall risk in community-dwelling older adults.[38] Its ability to predict fall risk in patients with TBI is unknown.

Self-selected walking speed has been used as a measure of a patient's ability and confidence in walking.[39] There is a paucity of information on what constitutes independent functional mobility. One study reported that in order to perform instrumental activities of daily living (ADL) skills the average person must be able to walk a minimum of 1000 feet, be able to achieve 80 meters per minute velocity for 13 to 27 meters in order to cross a street safely, be able to negotiate a 7- to 8-inch curb independently, and be able to walk and turn the head without loss of balance.[40] In our clinic, two methods are used to assess functional mobility. The first is the Three-Minute Walk Test, which requires subjects to walk at their preferred pace for 3 minutes over a 524-foot indoor course.[34] The course is carpeted, and involves four different turns. Distance walked in the 3 minutes is recorded, as is the number of times the patient moves outside a 15-inch walking path. The second test of functional mobility is the Dynamic Gait Index, which is used to evaluate the ability to adapt gait to changes in task demands including changing speeds, head turns in the vertical or horizontal direction, stepping over or around obstacles, and stair ascent and descent. The test includes eight tasks which are scored from 0 to 3, for a total of 24 points.[34]

New research suggests that dual-task methods for assessing balance and mobility may be more sensitive indicators of functional mobility problems than tests which focus on single-task performance.[41,42] The use of dual-task measures may be particularly

BOX 20–2 Berg Balance Scale

1. **Sitting to standing.**

   Instruction: Please stand up. Try not to use your hands for support.
   Grading: Please mark the lowest category that applies.

   (4) Able to stand, no hands and stabilize independently.
   (3) Able to stand independently using hands.
   (2) Able to stand using hands after several tries.
   (1) Needs minimal assistance to stand or to stabilize.
   (0) Needs moderate or maximal assistance to stand.

2. **Standing unsupported.**

   Instruction: Stand for 2 minutes without holding on.
   Grading: Please mark the lowest category that applies.

   (4) Able to stand safely 2 minutes.
   (3) Able to stand 2 minutes with supervision.
   (2) Able to stand 30 seconds unsupported.
   (1) Needs several tries to stand 30 seconds unsupported.
   (0) Unable to stand 30 seconds unassisted.

If subject is able to stand 2 minutes safely, score full marks for sitting unsupported.
Proceed to position change standing to sitting.

3. **Sitting unsupported, feet on floor.**

   Instruction: Sit with arms folded for 2 minutes.
   Grading: Please mark the lowest category that applies.

   (4) Able to sit safely and securely 2 minutes.
   (3) Able to sit 2 minutes under supervision.
   (2) Able to sit 30 seconds.
   (1) Able to sit 10 seconds.
   (0) Unable to sit without support, 10 seconds.

4. **Standing to sitting.**

   Instruction: Please sit down.
   Grading: Please mark the lowest category that applies.

   (4) Sits safely with minimal use of hands.
   (3) Controls descent by using hands.
   (2) Uses back of legs against chair to control descent.
   (1) Sits independently but has uncontrolled descent.
   (0) Needs assistance to sit.

5. **Transfers.**

   Instruction: Please move from chair to bed and back again. One way toward a
   seat with armrests and one way toward a seat without armrests.
   Grading: Please mark the lowest category that applies.

   (4) Able to transfer safely with only minor use of hands.
   (3) Able to transfer safely with definite need of hands.
   (2) Able to transfer with verbal cueing and/or supervision.
   (1) Needs one person to assist.
   (0) Needs two people to assist or supervise to be safe.

(Continued)

(BOX 20–2   Continued)

6. Standing unsupported with eyes closed.

Instruction: Close your eyes and stand still for 10 seconds.
Grading: Please mark the lowest category that applies.

(4) Able to stand 10 seconds safely.
(3) Able to stand 10 seconds with supervision.
(2) Able to stand 3 seconds.
(1) Unable to keep eyes closed 3 seconds but stays steady.
(0) Needs help to keep from falling.

7. Standing unsupported with feet together.

Instruction: Place your feet together and stand without holding on.
Grading: Please mark the lowest category that applies.

(4) Able to place feet together indep and stand 1 minute safely.
(3) Able to place feet together indep and for 1 minute with supervision.
(2) Able to place feet together indep but unable to hold for 30 seconds.
(1) Needs help to attain position but able to stand 15 seconds feet together.
(0) Needs help to attain position and unable to hold for 15 seconds.

The following items are to be performed while standing unsupported.

8. Reaching forward with outstretched arm.

Instruction: Lift arm to 90°. Stretch out your fingers and reach forward as far as you can. (Examiner places a ruler at end of fingertips when arm is at 90°. Fingers should not touch the ruler while reaching forward. The recorded measure is the distance forward that the fingers reach while the subject is in the most forward lean position.)
Grading: Please mark the lowest category that applies.

(4) Can reach forward confidently >10 inches.
(3) Can reach forward >5 inches safely.
(2) Can reach forward >2 inches safely.
(1) Reaches forward but needs supervision.
(0) Needs help to keep from falling.

9. Pick up objects from the floor.

Instruction: Pick up the shoe/slipper placed in front of your feet.
Grading: Please mark the lowest category that applies.

(4) Able to pick up slipper safely and easily.
(3) Able to pick up slipper but need supervision.
(2) Unable to pick up but reaches 1–2 inches from slipper and keeps balance independently.
(1) Unable to pick up and needs supervision while trying.
(0) Unable to try/needs assistance to keep from falling.

10. Turning to look behind/over left and right shoulders.

Instruction: Turn to look behind you over/toward left shoulder. Repeat to the right.
Grading: Please mark the lowest category that applies.

(4) Looks behind from both sides and weight shifts well.
(3) Looks behind one side only; other side shows less weight shift.
(2) Turns sideways only but maintains balance.
(1) Needs supervision when turning.
(0) Needs assist to keep from falling.

(Continued)

(BOX 20–2 Continued)

---

11. **Turn 360°.**

    Instruction: Turn completely around in a full circle. Pause. Then turn a full circle in the other direction.
    Grading: Please mark the lowest category that applies.

    - (4) Able to turn 360° safely in <4 seconds each side.
    - (3) Able to turn 360° safely one side only in <4 seconds.
    - (2) Able to turn 360° safely but slowly.
    - (1) Needs close supervision or verbal cueing.
    - (0) Needs assistance while turning.

Dynamic weight shifting while standing unsupported

12. **Count number of times step touch measured stool.**

    Instruction: Place each foot alternately on the stool. Continue until each foot has touched the stool four times.
    Grading: Please mark the lowest category that applies.

    - (4) Able to stand indep and safely and complete 8 steps in 20 seconds.
    - (3) Able to stand indep and complete 8 steps in >20 seconds.
    - (2) Able to complete 4 steps without aid, with supervision.
    - (1) Able to complete >2 steps needs minimal assistance.
    - (0) Needs assistance to keep from falling/unable to try.

13. **Standing unsupported, one foot in front.**

    Instruction: (Demonstrate to subject.) Place one foot directly in front of the other. If you feel that you cannot place your foot directly in front, try to step far enough ahead that the heel of your forward foot is ahead of the toes of the other foot.
    Grading: Please mark the lowest category that applies.

    - (4) Able to place foot tandem independently and hold 30 seconds.
    - (3) Able to place foot ahead of other independently and hold 30 seconds.
    - (2) Able to take small step independently and hold 30 seconds.
    - (1) Needs help to step but can hold 15 seconds.
    - (0) Loses balance while stepping or standing.

14. **Standing on one leg.**

    Instruction: Stand on one leg as long as you can without holding on.
    Grading: Please mark the lowest category that applies.

    - (4) Able to lift leg indep and hold >10 seconds.
    - (3) Able to lift leg indep and hold 5–10 seconds.
    - (2) Able to lift leg indep and hold >3 seconds.
    - (1) Tries to lift leg; unable to hold 3 seconds but remains standing independently.
    - (0) Unable to try or needs assistance to prevent fall.

(Reprinted with permission: Berg, K, Measuring balance in the elderly: Validation of an instrument. Dissertation, McGill University, Montreal, 1993)

---

important in patients with TBI owing to the frequency of cognitive impairments such as disorders in attention, memory, and judgment. Kerns and Mateer[43] report an example of a traumatically brain injured patient who when given the task of grating cheese, was noted to progressively slump down and forward until his forehead touched the counter. This patient was unable to successfully divide attention between two tasks, that of maintaining a vertical posture and grating cheese.[44] We have found that in patients with mild to moderate head injury, postural control is particularly compromised during the simultaneous performance of cognitive tasks requiring visual processing.[43] The development of dual task methods for assessing functional balance and mobility skills is just beginning.[41] However, their usefulness in documenting functional limitations in patients with TBI is very promising.

IMPAIRMENTS LIMITING POSTURAL STABILITY

Evaluation of motor impairments include an assessment of muscle tone, strength, range of motion, cerebellar coordination, static postural alignment in sitting and standing, and examining coordinated multijoint movements used to recovery stability following perturbations of different size, amplitudes, and directions.[34] Although not performed routinely in the clinic, electromyography and kinematic analysis of associated body movements can be used to quantify dyscoordination in stance and gait, and improvements during the course of recovery.

Weakness, particularly, hemiparesis, is frequently a primary neuromuscular impairment affecting balance in the patient with TBI. Traumatic injury to the cerebellum or deep hemorrhagic lesions in the basal ganglia can affect the timing and scaling of muscles working synergistically for postural control. Clinical indicators of muscular dyscoordination during postural tasks include asymmetrical use of limbs for movement control and excessive movements at the joints, including excessive flexion of the hip and loss of knee control.

Assessment of sensory impairments includes evaluating sensation (vibratory sense, stereognosis, and peripheral visual acuity), determining the patient's ability to remain oriented under different sensory conditions, and assesses whether perceptions relevant to stability are accurate.[22,23] Moving platform posturography is one approach to examining the organization and selection of senses for postural control.[45] Posturography uses a moving force plate in conjunction with a moving visual surround to determine the patient's ability to correctly select from among visual, somatosensory and vestibular inputs, the most appropriate sense for orientation (see Chapter 2).

Alternatively, the Clinical Test for Sensory Interaction in Balance (CTSIB) tests the patient's use of alternative sensory cues for orientation, using procedures similar to those of posturography.[46] This test, originally described in 1986, used six sensory conditions to examine a person's ability to maintain stability under altered sensory contexts. These six sensory conditions are shown in Figure 20–2. In our clinic, we have modified this test and now use only four sensory conditions, eliminating the dome conditions (3 and 6), but maintaining the two foam conditions of 4 and 5. The dome was originally created to identify patients with visual motion sensitivity. **Visual motion sensitivity** is a heightened sensitivity to motion in the environment, such as is found in crowded shopping centers. The dome has not proven to be sensitive or specific enough in identifying visual motion sensitivity.[47] Compliant foam (medium-density Sunmate Foam) is used to reduce the effectiveness of support surface somatosensory inputs for orientation. Procedures for administering the CTSIB are detailed elsewhere.[48]

Sensory impairments affecting orientation following TBI can result from pathology within the peripheral vestibular system or within central structures which organize sensory information for postural orientation. Although both posturography and the CTSIB test can identify and quantify functional problems in selecting sensory in-

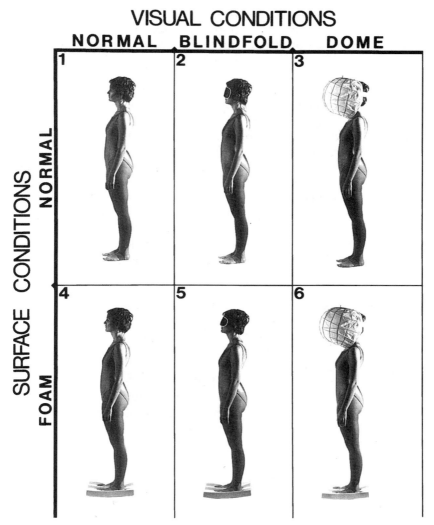

FIGURE 20–2. The six positions used to test sensory interaction in balance. (From Shumway-Cook, A, and Horak, F: Assessing the influence of sensory interaction on balance. Phys Ther 66:1548, 1986, with permission.)

puts for postural control, they cannot determine the anatomic location of the injury producing these functional problems.

TREATMENT

Treatment of instability involves remediating impairments and improving sensory and motor strategies essential to ensuring stability in functional tasks performed in sitting, standing and walking.[21,22,24] Biomechanical limitations and movement disorders are a particular concern in patients with vestibular pathology because they limit a patient's ability to move in ways that are necessary for compensation.

Treatment of biomechanical limitations includes physical modalities, such as heat and ultrasound, as well as exercises to improve range of motion, joint flexibility and body alignment.[34,49] Treatment of neuromuscular problems varies depending on the nature of the problem. Strengthening exercises are used to improve impaired force generation. Therapy for muscular dyscoordination includes functional electrical stimulation, electromyographic biofeedback, and neuromuscular facilitation exercises.[34]

Exercises to improve sensory function for orientation require the patient to maintain balance during progressively difficult movement tasks while the therapist varies the availability and accuracy of one or more senses for orientation.[21,22] For example, during exercises to decrease sensitivity to visual motion cues the patient performs balance and movement tasks when visual cues are reduced or absent (eyes closed or while wearing blinders or a blindfold), or inaccurate for orientation (prism glasses, optokinetic stimuli, and within a large moving visual surround).[50] During these exercises accurate orientation cues from the surface are essential.

In contrast, exercises to improve use of vestibular inputs for postural control in the patient with partial loss of vestibular function involve decreasing the availability of *both* visual and somatosensory input for orientation. An example would be asking the patient to reach for an object while wearing blinders and standing unsupported on a piece of foam or a thick piece of carpet.

Patients who have had a complete bilateral loss of vestibular function are taught to rely on visual and or somatosensory cues for postural control. Because these patients have no residual vestibular function available to them, the goal of therapy is sensory substitution, rather than enhancement, of remaining vestibular function.

In summary, treatment of postural dyscontrol in the patient with TBI and associated vestibular system pathology is directed at helping the patient to reestablish effective sensorimotor strategies for balance control. Therapy focuses on practicing functional tasks such as standing unsupported while reaching, leaning or turning, or moving from sit to stand. In addition, treatment seeks to remediate specific deficits in musculoskeletal and sensorimotor systems underlying postural dyscontrol.

Time Course for Recovery

The time course for recovery from traumatic vestibular lesions is different from that of vestibular lesions of other etiologies.[51] In the patient with TBI and vestibular system pathology, concomitant CNS lesions impair the compensatory process itself. As a result recovery from traumatic vestibular lesions is often protracted. Pfaltz and Kamath[51] compared recovery in patients with a unilateral loss of vestibular function due to various pathologies including trauma, Ménière's disease, labyrinthectomy, and other diseases. At 6 months only one-third of the patients with unilateral loss owing to trauma were symptom free; the majority of other patients had achieved compensation and were symptom free. At 18 months many of the trauma patients continued to show persisting symptoms of vestibular system pathology.

Berman and Fredrickson[3] studied 321 mildly and moderately head-injured patients with vestibular system pathology. Vertigo was reported in 34 percent of mildly head-injured patients, and in 50 percent of moderately head-injured patients. Sixty to 70 percent of those patients with central vestibular dysfunction had persisting symptoms 5 years postinjury. Almost half of these patients never returned to work.

These and other studies suggest that the typical time course for recovery from vestibular system pathology in patients with TBI is protracted, requiring 1 to 3 times longer than in patients with vestibular system pathology owing to other causes. Usually many patients with traumatic vestibular dysfunction show persisting symptoms of dizziness and dysequilibrium several years following trauma. The degree to which specific exercise interventions can influence the time course of recovery from vestibular system dysfunction in the patient with TBI is an important theoretical and clinical question currently under study.

CASE STUDY

S.D. is a 31-year-old male admitted for rehabilitation 1 month following a closed head injury. He fell 40 feet, striking the left side of his head, and experienced a brief (less than 5 minutes) loss of consciousness. He was admitted to the hospital with a Glasgow Coma Score of 13. Computed tomography showed multiple left parietal-occipital cerebral contusions. Associated trauma included three fractured ribs and a contusion of the left hip. There was no previous history of medical or neurological problems.

Otological evaluation included both a clinical examination, and electronystagmography, including tests for gaze and positional nystagmus, oculomotor function (saccade, smooth-pursuit, and optokinetics), and VOR function using rotational chair testing. Results from this examination indicated the presence of posttraumatic BPPV. Other test results were within normal limits, suggesting no evidence for vestibular hypofunction, or a central vestibular lesion.

ASSESSMENT

On assessment the patient was found to have moderate to severe imbalance (score of 46 of 56 on the Berg Balance Scale). The patient had difficulty maintaining stability when moving from sit to stand, when standing with eyes closed or with a reduced base of support, and when reaching, leaning or turning while standing. The patient used a cane and required stand-by assistance for safety when walking. On the Three-Minute Walk test he walked 135 feet, and had four significant path deviations. Gait pattern abnormalities included an equinovarus foot position at foot strike, circumduction of the right leg during swing phase of gait, and hyperextension of the right knee during the stance phase of gait. He had significant problems with adapting gait to changing task demands scoring 13 of 24 on the Dynamic Gait test. He required minimal assist to maintain his balance when walking with head turns (horizontal or vertical) and when stepping over obstacles.

Sensorimotor constraints included:

1. Positional vertigo in the left Hallpike position, as well as vertigo during gait with vertical head motions
2. Postural dyscontrol including
   Right hemiparesis and dyscoordination
   Limitation of range in right ankle

Asymmetries in weight bearing primarily in stance and during gait
Difficulty organizing sensory inputs for balance and effectively using vestibular inputs for orientation in the absence of visual and somatosensory cues.
3. Other Problems
Pain owing to fractured ribs and contusions on the left hip
Moderate cognitive impairments including memory and attention deficits
Decreased awareness of his limitations raising a number of safety issues.

TREATMENT

Treatment focused on eliminating positional vertigo, balance retraining to improve ability to perform functional skills in sitting and standing, and gait retraining to improve gait pattern, endurance and adaptive capability when walking.

The canal repositioning maneuver was used to eliminate BPPV. Balance retraining included exercises to improve strength, range of motion, and coordination in the right extremities; and postural sway biofeedback to reduce weight-bearing asymmetries in standing and to improve range of center of mass movements over the hemiparetic leg. Manual cues and feedback were used to improve joint coordination at the knee and hip while the patient practiced voluntary sway in standing, while moving from sit to stand, and during gait. The patient also practiced maintaining balance during such functional tasks as reaching, leaning, and turning in the standing position. In order to improve the ability to use vestibular inputs for postural control, the patient practiced a variety of stance balance tasks while standing on foam or various grades of carpets, with blinders or with eyes closed.

Outcomes following four months of rehabilitation (1 month as an inpatient, 3 months as an outpatient) were as follows: the BPPV was successfully eliminated using the Epley. Postural control underlying stability in sitting, standing and walking had improved, the patient was transferring and walking independently, and no longer needed a cane to walk. Results of posturography testing examining sensory aspects of postural control in SD prior to and following rehabilitation are shown in Figure 20–3.

Figure 20–3 compares performance on balance tasks under altered sensory conditions at 1 month and 6 months post-TBI. Peak-to-peak center-of-gravity angle, in degrees, is plotted for individual trials in the six conditions, conditions 3 through 6 have three trials each (see Chapter 2). Encompassing individual trials is a larger histogram that shows the upper limits of normality, established using the 95th percentile from 250 normal controls ages 8 to 70.[52] At one month S.D. lost balance (indicated in Fig. 20–3 by "test stopped") when either visual or surface cues for orientation were reduced or inaccurate (conditions 3, 4, 5, and 6). At 6 months post injury he fell on the first trial only when deprived of both visual and surface cues simultaneously (conditions 5 and 6).

SUMMARY

Assessment and treatment of vestibular system pathology are essential parts of rehabilitating the patient with TBI. However, following TBI, injuries to other parts of the CNS can complicate recovery from vestibular system pathology in several ways: (1) as-

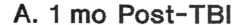

A. 1 mo Post-TBI

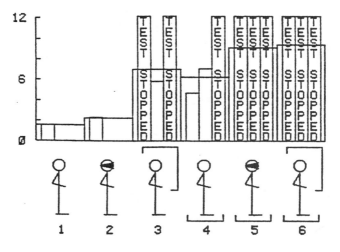

B. 6 mos Post-TBI

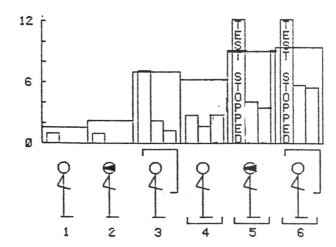

FIGURE 20–3. Recovery of sensory organization aspects of postural control is shown by comparing body sway during altered sensory conditions at 1 month and 6 months post-TBI. See text for details.

sociated trauma can produce pain and restrict movements; (2) musculoskeletal and neuromuscular problems can affect the patient's ability to move in ways that are necessary to achieve CNS compensation; (3) damage to visual and somatosensory systems may limit the availability of these senses as alternatives to lost vestibular inputs; and (4) cognitive and behavioral problems make compliance to a vestibular exercise program difficult. Finally, intracranial injury can damage neural structures important to the compensatory process, resulting in persisting symptoms and a protracted recovery.

A comprehensive treatment plan which incorporates vestibular rehabilitation exercises, modified to adjust for the above limitations, is an effective way to gain functional independence and minimize persisting and disabling symptoms of vestibular system pathology in patients with TBI.

REFERENCES

1. Igarashi, M, et al: Physical exercise and balance compensation after total ablation of vestibular organs. Progress Brain Res 76:395, 1988.
2. Lacour, M, and Xerri, C: Vestibular compensation: New perspectives. In Flohr, H, and Precht, W (eds): Lesion Induced Neuronal Plasticity in Sensorimotor Systems. Springer-Verlag, New York, 1981.
3. Berman, J, and Fredrickson, J: Vertigo after head injury—A five year follow-up. J Otolaryngol 7:237, 1978.
4. Barber, HO: Head injury: Audiological and vestibular findings. Ann Otol Rhinol Laryngol 78:239, 1969.
5. Pearson, BW, and Barber, HO: Head injury: Some otoneurologic sequelae. Arch Otolargyngol 97:81, 1973.
6. Griffith, MV: The incidence of auditory and vestibular concussion following minor head injury. J Laryngol Otol 93:253, 1979.
7. Gibson, W: Vertigo associated with trauma. In Dix, R, and Hood, JD (eds): Vertigo. Wiley, New York, 1984.
8. Healy, GB: Hearing loss and vertigo secondary to head injury. N Engl J Med 306:1029, 1982.
9. Toglia, JU, et al: Vestibular and audiologic aspects of whiplash injury and head trauma. J Forensic Sci 14:219, 1969.
10. Baloh, RW: Dizziness, Hearing Loss and Tinnitus: The Essential of Neurotology. FA Davis, Philadelphia, 1984.
11. Black, FO: Vertigo: Current therapy. Otolaryngol Head Neck Surg 4:59, 1990.
12. Nelson, JR: Neurootologic aspects of head injury. In Thompson, RA, and Green, JR (eds): Advances in Neurology, vol. 2. Raven, New York, 1979.
13. Karnik, PP, et al: Otoneurologic problems in head injuries and their management. Int Surg 60:466, 1975.
14. Schuknecht, HF: Mechanism of inner ear injury from blows to the head. Ann Otorhinolaryngol 78:253, 1969.
15. Lindsay, JR, and Heminway, WG: Postural vertigo due to unilateral sudden partial loss of vestibular function. Ann Otol 65:692, 1956.
16. Herdman, SJ: Treatment of vestibular disorders in traumatically brain-injured patients. J Head Trauma Rehabil 5:63, 1990.
17. Jacobs, GB, et al: Post traumatic vertigo: Report of three cases. J Neurosurg 51:860, 1979.
18. Glasscock, ME, et al: Persistent traumatic perilymph fistulas. Laryngoscope 97:860, 1987.
19. Lehrer, JF, et al: Peripymphatic fistula—A definitive and curable cause of vertigo following head trauma. West J Med 141:57, 1984.
20. Grimm, RJ, and Black, FO: Perilymph fistula syndrome: Defined in mild head trauma. Acta Otol (suppl)464:1, 1989.
21. Shumway-Cook, A, and Horak, F: Vestibular rehabilitation: An exercise approach to managing symptoms of vestibular dysfunction. Semin Hearing 10:196, 1989.
22. Shumway-Cook, A, and Horak, F: Rehabilitation strategies for patients with vestibular deficits. Neurol Clin 8:441, 1990.
23. Ylikoski, J, et al: Dizziness after head trauma: Clinical and morphologic findings. Am J Otol 3:343, 1982.
24. Herdman, SJ: Assessment and treatment of balance disorders in the vestibular deficient patient. Balance, Proceedings of the APTA Forum. APTA, Alexandria, 1989.
25. Norre, ME, and De Weerdt, W: Positional (provoked) vertigo treated by postural training. Vestibular habituation training. Agressologie 22:37, 1981.
26. Epley, J: Benign paroxysmal positional vertigo: Diagnosis and non-surgical treatment. In Arenberg, IK (ed): Dizziness and Balance Disorders. New York, Kugler, 1993.
27. Semont, A, et al: Curing the BPPV with a Liberatory Maneuver. Adv Otorhinolaryngol 42:290, 1988.
28. Brandt, T, et al: Therapy for benign paroxysmal positioning vertigo, revisited. Neurology 44:796, 1994.
29. Louis, M: Visual field and perceptual deficits in brain damaged patient. Crit Care Update 8:32, 1981.
30. Stanworth, A: Defects if ocular movement and fusion after head injury. Br J Ophthamol 58:266, 1974.
31. Zee, DS: Vertigo. In Current Therapy in Neurological Disease. Decker, Philadelphia, 1985.
32. Shumway-Cook, A, and Myers, L: Management of Vestibular System Pathology in the Patient with Cervical Dysfunction. Presentation at the Washington State Orthopedic Special Interest Meeting, Fall, 1991.
33. McCollum, G, and Leen, TK: Form and exploration of mechanical stability limits in erect stance. J Motor Behav 21:225, 1989.
34. Shumway-Cook, A, and Woollacott, M: Motor Control: Theory and Practical Applications. Williams & Wilkens, Baltimore, 1995.
35. Shumway-Cook, A, and McCollum, G: Assessment and treatment of balance deficits in the neurologic patient. In Montgomery, P, and Connoly, B (eds): Motor Control: Theoretical Framework and Practical Application to Physical Therapy. Chattanooga Corp, Chattanooga, 1991.
36. Shumway-Cook, A, and Olmscheid, R: A systems analysis of postural dyscontrol in traumatically brain-injured patients. J Head Trauma Rehab 5:51, 1990.
37. Berg, K: Measuring balance in the elderly: Validation of an instrument. (Dissertation). McGill University, Montreal, 1993.
38. Shumway-Cook, A, et al: Predicting fall risk in community dwelling older adults. Phys Ther 8:812, 1997.

39. Brandstater, M, et al: Hemiplegic gait: analysis of temporal variables. Arch Phys Med Rehabil 65:583, 1983.
40. Lerner-Frankiel, MB, et al: Functional community ambulation: What are your criteria? Clin Management 6:12, 1990.
41. Lundin-Olsson, L, et al: "Stops walking when talking" as a predictor of falls in elderly people. Lancet 349:617, 1997.
42. Shumway-Cook, A, et al: The effects of two types of cognitive task on postural control in elderly fallers and non fallers. J Gerontol 52:M232, 1997.
43. Kerns, K, and Mateer, CA: Walking and chewing gum: The impact of attentional capacity on everyday activities. In Sbordone, RJ, and Long, CJ (eds): Ecological Validity of Neuropsychological Testing. GR Press, Delray Beach, FL, 1996.
44. Geurts, AC, et al: Dual task assessment of reorganization of postural control in persons with lower limb amputation. Arch Phys Med Rehab 72:1059, 1991.
45. Nashner, LM: Adaptation of human movement to altered environments. Trends Neurosci 10:358, 1982.
46. Shumway-Cook, A, and Horak, F: Assessing the influence of sensory interaction on balance. Phys Ther 66:1548, 1986.
47. Shumway-Cook, A: Unpublished observations, 1997.
48. Horak, F: Clinical measurement of postural control in adults. Phys Ther 67:1881, 1987.
49. Shumway-Cook, A, et al: Postural sway biofeedback: Its effect on reestablishing stance stability in hemiplegic patients. Arch Phys Med Rehab 69:395, 1988.
50. Bles, W, et al: Compensation for labyrinthine defects by use of a tilting room. Acta Otolaryngol (Stockh) 95:576, 1983.
51. Pfaltz, CR, and Kamath, R: Central compensation of vestibular dysfunction: (I) Peripheral lesions. Adv Otorhinolaryngol 30:335, 1983.
52. Peterka, R, et al: Age-related changes in human postural control: Sensory organization tests. J Vestib Res 1:73, 1990.

CHAPTER 21

Cervical Vertigo

Richard A. Clendaniel, PT, PhD

Cervical vertigo is a controversial subject at best. This term tends to encompass a variety of entities, some of which are theoretically more likely than others, including cervical ataxia, cervical dizziness, and cervical nystagmus. Because vertigo is defined as the illusion of movement (rotation, tilt, or linear displacement) and is therefore restrictive, the term cervical dizziness will be used in the remainder of this chapter to refer to symptoms of dizziness (including vertigo, dysequilibrium, and light-headedness) arising from the cervical spine. Several different processes may cause cervical dizziness. These pathophysiological mechanisms include irritation of the sympathetic vertebral plexus, vertebrobasilar insufficiency (VBI), and altered proprioceptive afferent signals from the upper cervical spine. This latter potential cause of dizziness is of particular interest owing to the large number of patients with either whiplash injuries or neck pain that are seen by physical therapists. This particular cause of dizziness is also perhaps the most controversial. One of the major problems in identifying patients with cervical dizziness is the lack of a concrete test that is sensitive and specific to this entity. From a therapeutic standpoint, the controversy surrounding cervical dizziness may be academic. If an individual presents with cervical symptoms as well as dizziness, the holistic approach would be to treat the cervical problem as well as the dizziness. The aim of this chapter is to review the anatomic and physiological bases for cervical dizziness, the scientific findings that lend support or detract from the cervical contribution to dizziness, and discuss possible treatment strategies for this condition.

POSTERIOR CERVICAL SYMPATHETIC SYNDROME

Barré[1] suggested that cervical problems could irritate the sympathetic vertebral plexus, leading to constriction of the labyrinthine artery and decreased perfusion of the labyrinth, which would induce vertigo. There is little objective data, however, to support this hypothesis. In addition, the intracranial circulation is controlled independent of the cervical sympathetic system. As such, it is difficult to see how a cervical injury could lead to restricted blood flow to the inner ear.

VERTEBROBASILAR INSUFFICIENCY

Another possible cause of dizziness arising from the cervical spine is occlusion of the vertebral arteries owing to osteoarthritic spurs[2] or occipitoatlantal instability.[3] The vertebral arteries can be compressed during cervical rotation or extension, as occurs during reaching for an object on an overhead shelf, turning around while backing up a car, or during cervical spine manipulations. In normal individuals, the carotid arteries provide sufficient collateral circulation to prevent symptoms.[4] In individuals with atherosclerotic vascular disease, the cerebrovascular circulation may be compromised to the extent that compression of the vertebral arteries could lead to VBI. In a study of 65 patients diagnosed with VBI, Williams and Wilson[5] found that vertigo was the initial symptom in 48 percent of the cases. Vertigo owing to VBI is generally abrupt in onset, of short duration (several minutes), and may be associated with nausea and vomiting.[6] The vertigo is generally associated with symptoms related to ischemia of the other areas supplied by the posterior circulation. These symptoms typically include visual hallucinations, drop attacks or weakness, visceral sensations, visual field defects, diplopia, and headaches.[5] The vertigo may be an isolated initial symptom, or may be intermixed with more typical symptoms of VBI.[7] The absence of associated symptoms in cases of episodic vertigo of greater than 6 months duration would suggest a cause of the symptoms other than VBI.

Testing for VBI during the physical examination is often performed with the vertebral artery compression test (cervical extension and rotation), typically performed in supine. This test is generally performed as part of the cervical screening examination. It should be noted that this test position is identical to the final position in the Dix-Hallpike test, which is used to assess for benign paroxysmal positioning vertigo (BPPV).[8] Brief (less than 1 minute) episodes of vertigo with combined vertical and torsional nystagmus associated with moving into this position are most likely due to BPPV rather than VBI. One method to differentiate between VBI and BPPV is to have the patient sit, forward flex at the hips, and at the same time extend and rotate their neck. This sequence of movements will place the cervical spine in a position identical to that obtained in the Dix-Hallpike test and the vertebral artery compression test; however, the patient's head will remain vertical. Maintaining the vertical orientation of the patient's head will prevent the occurrence of the signs and symptoms of BPPV (which is provoked by changes in head position relative to gravity). Therefore, any symptoms associated with this position change may be attributed to vertebral artery compression and VBI.

ALTERED PROPRIOCEPTIVE SIGNALS

The mechanism by which cervical pain or dysfunction could lead to symptoms of dizziness has not been identified. One hypothesis is that inflammation or irritation of the cervical roots or facet joints would lead to a mismatch among vestibular, visual, and cervical inputs. This multisensory mismatch would lead to the symptoms attributed to cervical dizziness, and these symptoms would be most apparent during head

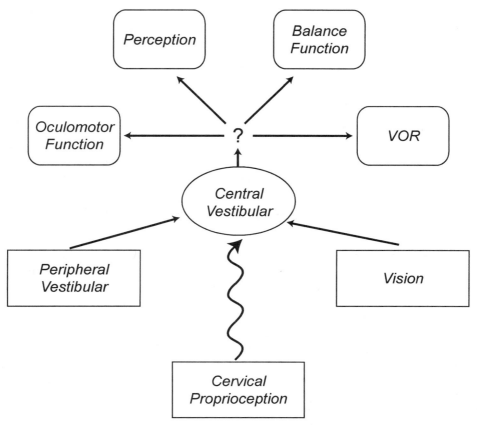

FIGURE 21–1. Schematic of the multisensory mismatch hypothesis. Peripheral inputs (vestibular, cervical, and visual) converge on central vestibular structures and affect oculomotor function, balance function, VOR, and perceptions of dizziness. Cervical dysfunction (represented by the *curved line*) would lead to a mismatch among vestibular, visual, and cervical inputs. This multisensory mismatch would lead to the symptoms attributed to cervical dizziness.

movements (Fig. 21–1). In theory, once the central nervous system (CNS) has adapted to the altered somatosensory inputs (just as the system is capable of adapting to altered vestibular inputs), the symptoms of cervical dizziness would abate even though the underlying dysfunction remained. The following sections will review the literature that addresses the role of altered cervical proprioceptive signals in the generation of signs and symptoms of dizziness.

Anatomy and Physiology

There is a convergence of cervical proprioceptive and vestibular information throughout the spinal cord, brainstem, cerebral cortex, and cerebellum.[9] A detailed review of the anatomic evidence is beyond the scope of this chapter; however, a brief review of the pertinent physiological evidence that suggests that cervical inputs may play a role in dizziness is warranted. Cervical proprioceptive signals important for postural neck reflexes arise from the joint and tendon receptors located in the deep structures of the upper cervical spine.[10] McCouch et al[10] demonstrated that the tonic neck reflexes in cats were mediated through the joint receptors rather than the cervical musculature. The role of the deep paravertebral muscle spindles in this region is not clear and may be species dependent.[11–16] In addition to its influence on postural neck reflexes, upper cervical spine proprioception is thought to be responsible for the generation of the cervical-ocular reflex (COR).[17] Rubin et al[18] recorded neurons in the vestibular nucleus that responded to both vestibular stimulation (whole body rotation) and movements of the trunk on a fixed head. Further support for the hypothesis that cervical proprioception can influence vestibular function comes from the work of Hikosaka and Maeda.[19] These investigators reported that, in the cat, vestibular excitation of the abducens nerve was inhibited by contralateral and facilitated by ipsilateral electrical stimulation of the cervical dorsal roots or facet joints. In addition, they reported that these effects were seen with stimulations at C2 and C3 and were not observed with stimulations at C5 or lower. These studies indicate that cervical proprioception may play a role in postural control and have an effect on vestibular function. It is important to remember that these studies were done on anesthetized or decerebrate animals, and that responses in awake, normally functioning animals may be entirely different. In light of the physiological findings and the anatomic convergence of cervical and vestibular inputs, the following sections will explore whether cervical proprioceptive signals can contribute to symptoms of vertigo or dysequilibrium and influence vestibular system function or postural stability.

Findings Following Cervical Spine Lesions

A number of studies have investigated oculomotor and balance changes following either experimentally induced lesions in the upper cervical spine or following cervical whiplash injuries. Based on these studies in animals and humans, it appears that there is little effect on the oculomotor and vestibular system, but that cervical injuries may lead to disturbances in balance function.

OCULOMOTOR FINDINGS

Cervical proprioceptive ablation has been performed by both sectioning of the dorsal roots and by injection of local anesthetics in the neck. Igarashi et al[20] reported on the oculomotor effects seen after both local anesthetic injections and unilateral transection of the C1 and C2 dorsal roots in squirrel monkeys. Lidocaine (1cc of 1 percent solution) without epinephrine was injected into the deep neck regions unilaterally in the experimental animals, and into either the superficial posterior neck region or abdominal wall in control subjects. The animals were placed in the dark and the eye movements were recorded. There was no evidence of spontaneous nystagmus in either the experimental or control groups postinjection. Optokinetic nystagmus was measured pre- and postinjection in 12 animals using a rotating optokinetic stimulus, which accelerated at 1° per second², from 0° to 200° per second. The investigators reported a bidirectional decline in both the slow phase eye velocity and the velocity of the fast phase component of the optokinetic nystagmus in the experimental subjects. The control groups also demonstrated that slow phase eye velocity decreases postinjection. The authors stated that there was a statistically significant difference in the slow phase eye velocity changes between the experimental and control groups, and infer from this finding that cervical proprioception contributes to oculomotor behavior. Two counter-arguments to their conclusion can be made. (1) The decline in the fast phase velocity in the experimental group and the slow phase changes seen in both control groups would argue that the local anesthetic has a systemic and diffuse effect, rather than a specific effect on the vestibular or optokinetic system through cervical proprioceptive path-ways. (2) The authors reported a statistically significant difference using a p value of .066, which is above the generally accepted probability level for statistical significance.

Similar measures were recorded in five monkeys following left C1 and C2 dorsal root section. The authors reported no spontaneous nystagmus and asymmetrical opto-kinetic responses as compared to preoperative responses. Slow phase eye velocity was diminished during clockwise optokinetic stimulation (p values ranging from .03 to .09). The postrotatory nystagmus (rotation velocity 200° per second) was measured in four monkeys preoperatively and following left C1 and C2 dorsal root sections. The first two postoperative days the monkeys demonstrated a decrease in the maximum slow phase eye velocity following counterclockwise rotations. The authors state that this was a statistically significant decrease, and that the effect was likely due to the loss of proprioceptive input from the cervical spine to vestibular nuclei. However, they again use a p value of .06 as their level of significance. This response difference was short lived, as by the fifth day following the dorsal root section, the slow phase re-sponses were greater than the control values and there was no apparent asymmetry in the responses. In addition to the questionable statistical significance, the responses to the optokinetic stimuli and the rotational stimulus are in opposite directions. The clockwise optokinetic stimulation induces nystagmus with slow phases to the right and fast phases to the left (left-beating nystagmus). In humans, this stimulation also in-duces a sense of rotation in a counterclockwise direction. The postrotatory nystagmus following counterclockwise rotation would be right beating (slow phases to the left and fast phases to the right); this would be accompanied by a sense of clockwise rota-tion in humans. Although the authors suggest that these findings support the role of cervical proprioception in normal oculomotor and vestibulo-ocular function, their in-terpretations should be taken cautiously in light of the actual data.

Several other studies have assessed oculomotor and vestibular function in hu-mans following flexion-extension injuries to the cervical spine. Oosterveld et al[21] con-ducted electronystagmographic (ENG) studies in 262 patients with symptoms of cervi-cal or cervical and upper extremity pain following acceleration injuries to the cervical spine. Eighty-five percent of these individuals had symptoms of light-headedness or a floating sensation. The authors report that none of the patients had rotational vertigo. Spontaneous nystagmus was reported in 63 percent of the patients; 110 of these 165 pa-tients (67 percent) also had positional nystagmus. Central oculomotor findings, includ-ing direction changing nystagmus, saccadic smooth pursuit, and impaired visual sup-pression of the vestibulo-ocular reflex (VOR), were found frequently. The incidence of individual central signs ranged from 26 to 43 percent. The authors also report that cer-vical nystagmus was present in 168 individuals. The authors suggest that this nystag-mus indicates a lesion in the cervical proprioceptive system; however, the observed cervical nystagmus may simply be the normal manifestation of the COR. The central oculomotor findings reported in this study support the authors' contention that cervi-cal whiplash injuries represent diffuse rather than well-localized lesions of the CNS. Caloric tests were not performed routinely in this study. Therefore, if one attributes the "vestibular signs" (spontaneous and positional nystagmus) to the cervical injury, then one has to assume that the peripheral vestibular system is normal. This is of course a questionable assumption in light of the central oculomotor findings.

Toglia[22] reported the ENG and rotational chair results in 309 patients, who had primary symptoms of dizziness following a flexion-extension acceleration injury to the cervical spine. Of these patients, 57 percent had abnormal caloric test results (40 percent had a significant canal paresis, 22.5 percent had a significant directional preponderance) and 51 percent had abnormal rotational tests. These data support the idea that peripheral vestibular system pathology is frequently present in individuals following whiplash injuries. In theory, one could make the argument that the caloric weaknesses and rotational asymmetries were due, not to peripheral vestibular dysfunction, but to impaired cervical input to the vestibular nuclei. An asymmetry of at least 25 percent was required before the caloric or rotational results were considered abnormal. Given this criterion level and the low gain of the COR as compared to the VOR, it seems unlikely that disrupted cervical inputs would lead to the observed caloric and rotational results.

Based on the anatomic convergence of vestibular, cervical proprioceptive, and visual signals from the acessory optic tract on type II neurons in the vestibular nuclei,[23,24] Karlberg and Magnusson[25] proposed that asymmetric cervical proprioception may affect optokinetic after nystagmus (OKAN). The authors measured OKAN in normal, healthy individuals with the head in neutral, passively rotated 70° to either side, and actively rotated 60° to 70° to either side. The authors found that OKAN initial velocity, duration, and cumulative eye position were significantly decreased when the optokinetic stimulus was rotated in the direction of passive head rotation when compared to the head in neutral. When the optokinetic stimulus was in the direction opposite the head rotation, there was no decrease in the OKAN response. A similar decrease in OKAN duration and cumulative eye position occurred during active head rotation. The authors suggest that this cervical influence on OKAN may play a role in the provocation of symptoms of dizziness in individuals with cervical pain and dysfunction. Although these studies were conducted in normal humans, the results may support the findings Igarashi et al[20] reported following unilateral C1 and C2 dorsal root section. Recall that they reported a decrease in the slow phase velocity of postrotatory nystagmus, when the slow phase was directed toward the side of the dorsal root section. Karlberg and Magnusson[25] reported a decrease in slow phase velocity when the optokinetic nystagmus was in the same direction as the head rotation. If one assumes that head rotation to the right induces an asymmetric input from the cervical proprioceptors (greater on the left than the right owing to stretching of the muscle spindles), then the results of the two studies are qualitatively similar. In both cases the slow phase eye velocities were decreased toward the side of decreased cervical proprioceptive input. Whether this asymmetric OKAN test can be used to identify individuals with cervical vertigo remains to be seen.

The smooth-pursuit neck torsion test (SPNT) is another test that has been proposed to identify cases of cervical dizziness. This test evaluates the smooth-pursuit eye movement system, conducted with the neck in neutral and rotated 45° to the left and to the right. Smooth-pursuit eye movements are recorded in each position. The gain (the ratio of eye velocity to target velocity) of the response is determined for each neck position, and the difference between the smooth-pursuit gain in neutral and the average gain in the rotated positions is calculated (the SPNT difference). To determine the sensitivity and specificity of this test, Tjell and Rosenhall[26] compared the performance of individuals with diagnoses of whiplash-associated disorders (with and without associated dizziness), central vertigo, Ménière's disease, and normal individuals. The authors reported a significant difference between individuals without whiplash and those with whiplash on the SPNT difference. Using two standard deviations from the mean of the healthy controls as the limit for normal, the authors report that the SPNT difference has a sensitivity of 90 percent in the whiplash with dizziness group. Fourteen of the 25 subjects with whiplash and no symptoms of dizziness had SPNT difference scores greater than the two standard deviations from normal (sensitivity of 56 percent). The authors make the statement that the specificity of the test was 91 percent. However, the authors did not report the raw data, so it is unclear how they arrived at this value. Given the "false-positive" rate of 56 percent in the whiplash group without dizziness, it seems unlikely that the SPNT would have a specificity value of 91 percent. The authors conclude that the SPNT test is therefore useful in diagnosing cervical dizziness. One should exercise care in interpreting the usefulness of this test, however, because the authors did not report the sensitivity values for the two groups with peripheral and central causes of vertigo. Given the small difference between the SPNT difference scores in the two groups of patients with whiplash injuries, the test may not differentiate between cervical dizziness and cervical pain. However, the results of this study do support the hypothesis that cervical inputs influence the oculomotor system.

Injection of local anesthetics in the posterior upper cervical musculature in animals and man reveal different oculomotor responses. De Jong et al[27] reported that injection of a local anesthetic in the cat, monkey, and rabbit induced nystagmus. The induced nystagmus in the cat and rabbit lasted from several minutes to an hour or more. The nystagmus in the monkey only lasted for several minutes and was suppressed by vision. In rabbits with bilateral labyrinthectomies, injection of the local anesthetic did not induce nystagmus, indicating that this nystagmus is generated through the vestibular system.[28] In monkeys, there was no effect of the local anesthetic on optokinetic nystagmus, OKAN, or caloric nystagmus. A local anesthetic was injected into two humans, and no nystagmus was seen in either individual. Therefore, the nature of the cervical-induced nystagmus appears to be species specific.

In summary, although there is a known cervical input to the vestibular nuclei and a convergence of cervical, visual, and vestibular inputs in the CNS, it does not appear that cervical lesions have a profound effect on the oculomotor or vestibular systems. In addition, the studies to date have not been able to differentiate between individuals with cervical pain and individuals with cervical dizziness.

BALANCE FINDINGS

In contrast to the inconclusive results of various oculomotor tests in individuals with suspected cervical dizziness, the balance tests may be more beneficial in the diagnosis of this disorder. De Jong et al[27] described ataxia across species following injections of a local anesthetic in the cervical region. Cats developed ataxia and hypotonia ipsilateral to the injection and had a tendency to fall to that side. Rabbits also displayed a complex behavior following unilateral injection. The rabbits first fell and rolled to the side of the injection, developed lateropulsion, and then demonstrated ipsilateral hypotonia. Similarly, when unilateral cervical root sections were performed in rabbits that had previously had a unilateral labyrinthectomy, the rabbits fell to the side of the labyrinthectomy and rolled along the long axis of their body. The direction of the rolling depended on the side of the labyrinthectomy and was independent of the side of the cervical root section. Although the nystagmus induced by the local anesthetic in monkeys was small compared to the cat, the ataxia was greater. The monkeys displayed a head and trunk tilt of approximately 10° toward the side of the lesion and marked ataxia of the ipsilateral limbs. Injection of a local anesthetic in the human resulted in a sense of light-headedness, and a sense of lateropulsion. There was a deviation of stance toward the side of the injection and ipsilateral past pointing. In supine, the injection produced a sense that the bed was rolling over toward the side of the injection. Although the injection of the local anesthetic was no doubt an unusually potent stimulus, it points out both postural and perceptual findings that one might expect to see in cases of altered cervical proprioceptive inputs.

Standing balance in patients with chronic cervical pain and associated symptoms of vertigo or imbalance were compared to age-matched, normal healthy controls, and patients with chronic cervical pain and no associated vertigo or imbalance. Postural sway was measured with dynamic posturography (Equitest, Neurocom International Inc, Clackamas, OR).[29] The subjects were tested with eyes open on both stable and sway-referenced platform conditions (sensory organization tests 1 and 4). The subjects performed the tests with their necks in neutral, flexion, extension, lateral flexion to the right and left, as well as rotation to the right and left. The subjects with cervical pain also performed the tests with their necks in the most painful position. When the subjects performed the tests on a stable platform, there was no difference among groups or test positions. However, when the test was performed on a sway-referenced platform, the authors found differences between groups and with different neck positions. All three subject groups generally demonstrated increased sway when their necks were held out of the anatomically neutral position. The patients with cervical pain and dizziness had significantly increased sway when their necks were in neutral as compared to the healthy controls. The subjects with cervical pain and dizziness had increased sway as compared to the subjects with cervical pain and no dizziness when their necks were held in the most painful positions. The authors conclude that dynamic posturography may be an appropriate method of determining the presence of cervical dizziness. The authors did not determine the specificity and sensitivity of this test, and this needs to be examined before the test can be clinically useful.

Karlberg et al[30,31] described changes in postural control in individuals with suspected cervical dizziness and in individuals with cervical and radiating upper extremity pain. No mention was made as to whether the individuals with the upper quarter pain had complaints of dizziness or imbalance. Postural control in these studies was assessed using a force platform and measuring the motion of the center of pressure. The authors induced body sway with vibrators attached to the gastrocnemius muscles or the posterior cervical musculature. When compared to age- and sex-matched controls, the individuals with upper quarter pain had increased velocity of sway and increased variance of sway with eyes closed when either site was vibrated.[31] In a subsequent study, postural dynamics (measures of swiftness, stiffness, and damping determined from an inverted pendulum model of stance control) were determined for three groups of individuals.[30] Using the vibration-induced body sway described previously, the authors measured the postural control parameters in individuals with suspected cervical dizziness, individuals with a recent bout of vestibular neuritis, and in normal, healthy individuals. The individuals with a suspected cervical cause to their dizziness demonstrated lower values of stiffness than either the normal or vestibular neuritis groups. In addition, the individuals with the cervical dizziness had higher values for damping than the normal individuals. Using Fisher linear discriminant analysis and the swiftness, stiffness, and damping values, the authors were able to distinguish those with cervical vertigo from both the normal individuals and the subjects with vestibular neuritis. They were also able to differentiate the individuals with vestibular neuritis from the normal individuals. The results of these two studies give further support to the hypothesis that cervical disorders lead to disturbances in postural control. The authors report that a naïve tester using this method could correctly classify 78 percent of the individuals with cervical dizziness, so this may be a test for cervical dizziness. However, as the authors note, the specificity of this test has not yet been determined.

Based on the results of the lesion induced ataxia in humans and the changes seen in stance control in individuals with cervical pain, it appears that cervical proprioception has a role in balance control. The mechanism of the postural disturbance is questionable. Individuals with cervical spine disease or cervical disc disease may have compression of the spinal cord and the spinal tracts relaying the proprioceptive information from the lower extremities, which could cause the observed postural disturbances. However, many of the individuals with cervical pain or dizziness have no findings of spinal cord compression on radiologic or clinical examination.[32] Another possible mechanism of the altered postural control is inaccurate proprioceptive input from sensitized proprioceptors in either the joint capsules or the cervical musculature. This could create a sensory mismatch between the vestibular and proprioceptive inputs, which could lead to symptoms of dizziness and altered postural control.[33] These symptoms would be greatest during head movements, where vestibular and cervical proprioceptive inputs would be changing. It remains to be seen whether any of these tests can be used to identify individuals with cervical dizziness.

EXAMINATION AND TREATMENT

With the lack of a definitive test for cervical dizziness, the diagnosis is based on the individual's signs, symptoms, and the absence of otologic or neurologic causes for the clinical findings. An individual with suspected cervical dizziness typically presents with dysequilibrium or light-headedness, cervical pain, ataxia or unsteadiness, and limited cervical motion. Head movements typically aggravate the symptoms. Other disease processes, such as cerebellar and spinal ataxia, bilateral vestibular loss, BPPV, and chronic unilateral vestibular loss, can also present with similar signs and symptoms. These otologic and neurologic causes of dizziness may also present with restricted cervical motion and neck pain owing to muscular guarding of the neck to limit head movements. Consequently, the presence of dysequilibrium or light-headedness, cervical pain, ataxia or unsteadiness, and limited cervical motion is not consistently indicative of a cervical cause of the symptoms. If the symptoms are due to an otologic or neurologic cause, this should become apparent with a comprehensive clinical examination, vestibular function tests, or radiologic evaluation. If there are no apparent neurologic or otologic causes for the symptoms, one should conduct a more detailed evaluation of the upper quarter. This should include assessment of active and passive cervical range of motion, neurological examination of the upper extremities (strength, sensation, and reflexes), palpation of the cervical spine musculature, and segmental mobility testing of the cervical spine.

Treatment in cases of supposed cervical dizziness is directed toward the clinical findings and the patient's symptoms. Treatment of the cervical spine should address restricted mobility (owing to joint restrictions or muscle tightness), increased muscle tone, trigger points, and poor cervical posture. Detailed descriptions of the treatment approaches for upper quarter dysfunction are beyond the scope of this chapter, but the therapeutic treatments may include cervical spine mobilization, range of motion exercises, cervical strengthening exercises, soft tissue mobilization, and thermal agents. Owing to the apparent role of the upper cervical spine in the generation of cervical dizziness, treatment may need to be focused on this area. There are numerous techniques available to increase joint mobility in the upper cervical spine. In the author's experience, the techniques described below have been well tolerated by patients, are relatively easy to perform, and appear to be effective in increasing cervical mobility. The first technique is atlanto-occipital distraction (Fig. 21–2). In this technique, the patient lies supine, and the patient's head is supported by the therapist. The therapist positions his hands, such that the superior nuchal line of the patient's skull is resting on the therapist's fingertips. The therapist can just let the patient's head rest on his fingertips, or the therapist can apply gentle traction to the upper cervical spine by flexing the metacarpal phalangeal joints.

The second technique is designed to increase rotation between C1 and C2 (Fig. 21–3). Again, the patient lies supine. The therapist will "lock" the patient's lower cervical spine by passively flexing the patient's neck. This can be combined with lateral flexion (not shown). The therapist then passively rotates the patient's head in the direction of restricted mobility. At end range, the patient attempts to gently rotate her neck in the opposite direction. This motion is blocked by the therapist's hand. After 10 seconds, the patient relaxes, and the therapist will gently rotate the patient's neck in the

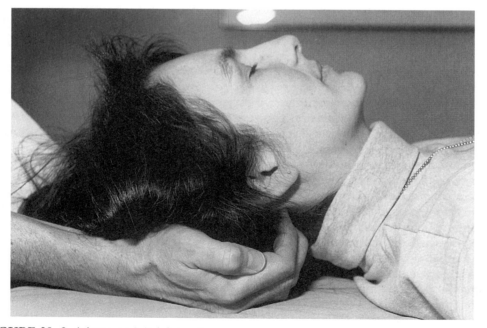

FIGURE 21–2. Atlanto-occipital distraction.

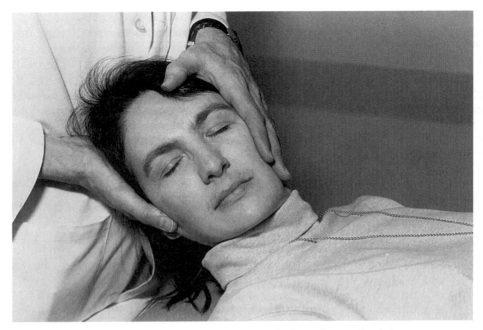

FIGURE 21–3. Mobilization of C1-C2 to increase cervical rotation to the right.

direction of the restricted motion. This treatment technique is analogous to the contract–relax stretching techniques often used with limb musculature. The force generated by the patient during the active, resisted rotation in this technique is minimal. Telling the patient to look in the direction of the rotation is often sufficient to generate the appropriate level of force. As with most mobilization techniques, it is important to follow up with active exercises to maintain the increased range. Any findings of imbalance or motion sensitivity can be treated with head movement exercises, positioning or habituation exercises, and balance exercises described elsewhere in this book (see Chapter 17).

There is evidence that treatment of cervical dysfunctions can lead to decreased symptoms of dizziness and improvements in postural stability. Karlberg et al[34] reported on the improvements in cervical pain and mobility as well as postural control in a controlled study of individuals undergoing physical therapy for cervical pain and dizziness. In this study, the type of treatment for the cervical dysfunction was not controlled owing to the variety of symptoms and physical findings. Prior to treatment, the patients displayed significantly higher body sway velocities than did healthy controls when the gastrocnemius muscles or posterior cervical musculature were vibrated. Following treatment, which was restricted to treatment of the cervical dysfunction, there was a marked improvement in the vibration-induced sway velocity. The authors reported that posttreatment the sway velocity during vibration of the gastrocnemius muscles returned to normal levels. They noted, however, that the patients continued to display increased sway velocities when tested with vibration applied to the posterior cervical musculature. The implication from this study and other anecdotal reports in the literature is that treatment of identified cervical dysfunction associated with symptoms of dizziness may lead to resolution of the dizziness as well as the cervical signs and symptoms.

CONCLUSION

The existence of a cervical cause of dizziness continues to be a topic of debate. Although individuals with cervical symptoms may have complaints of imbalance and light-headedness, there is no clear clinical test that can be used to unequivocally identify the cervical spine as the cause of the patient's symptoms. There is some anatomic and physiological evidence to suggest that the cervical spine could influence balance and perceptions of stability, but how this could actually lead to symptoms of dizziness remains unclear. As stated in the introductory comments, the debate over a cervical cause of dizziness may be academic from a physical therapy standpoint. If patients present with cervical dysfunction and imbalance, then we should treat both conditions.

CASE STUDY

HISTORY

J.B. is a 63-year-old gentleman referred by his family physician to a neurologist in the Vestibular Clinic. J.B. was evaluated by the neurologist and referred to physical therapy for treatment of possible cervical dizziness. He was initially seen in physical therapy on 11/18/96. J.B. states that he has been bothered by episodic bouts of dizziness, which started approximately 1 year ago. He states that the afternoon prior to the onset of his symptoms he had been lifting sheets of plywood out of his pick-up truck. The next morning he awoke with mild discomfort and stiffness in his neck and a strong sense of imbalance, with a tendency to lose his balance to the left. He denied having vertigo or aural symptoms associated with the onset of his symptoms. He states that since the initial onset he has been bothered by a chronic sense of light-headedness and dysequilibrium. He states that his symptoms are exacerbated by head motion, exertion, and after sitting in one position for a prolonged period of time (e.g., after driving or reading). Associated with the increased symptoms of dysequilibrium are cervical and shoulder symptoms. He describes these symptoms as mild to moderate pain and stiffness in the cervical spine and upper trapezii muscles. He does note some difficulty walking in the dark and on uneven surfaces. He denies having oscillopsia, positioning vertigo, migraine headaches, increased symptoms in busy visual environments, extremity numbness or weakness, and incoordination. J.B. states that he has had an MRI and carotid ultrasounds in the past, which were normal. ENG-Caloric test showed no evidence of unilateral hypofunction or oculomotor abnormalities. Audiograms showed bilateral, mild high-frequency sensorineural hearing loss. His medical history is unremarkable. He is taking no medications. He is a retired engineer.

CLINICAL EXAMINATION

Oculomotor Exam

J.B.'s oculomotor exam was normal. There was no spontaneous or gaze-evoked nystagmus in room light or behind Frenzel lenses. Extraocular movements were normal. His saccadic and smooth-pursuit eye movements were normal. VOR cancellation and VOR gains to both slow and rapid head rotations were normal. Behind Frenzel lenses, there was no head shaking induced nystagmus. Dix-Hallpike tests were negative bilaterally. There was no tragal compression-, valsalva-, or hyperventilation-induced nystagmus or vertigo. There was a one-line difference between static and dynamic visual acuity.

Balance Exam

J.B.'s Romberg test with eyes open was normal. With eyes closed, he performed the test for 30 seconds, but exhibited excessive sway. Romberg testing on 4-inch thick foam with eyes open was normal. With eyes closed, this test was again characterized by increased sway. Sharpened Romberg test with eyes open was normal. Sharpened Romberg test with eyes closed was positive as he could perform the test for a maximum of 20 seconds. Free gait showed normal velocity and no ataxia, but J.B. exhibited minimal head or trunk rotation. When asked to rotate his head while walking he developed a mild amount of ataxia (4 deviations from a 12-inch wide 10-yard-long path) and noted provocation of his symptoms of dysequilibrium and cervical discomfort.

Upper Quarter Exam

J.B.'s posture was characterized by a forward head. Cervical flexion and extension were mildly limited, but there was no pain or symptom provocation at end range. Cervical rotation was 75° to the right and 60° to the left. J.B. noted a provocation of his cervical symptoms and dysequilibrium at the limits of his cervical rotation to the left. Palpation of the cervical spine revealed increased muscle tone and tenderness in the left suboccipital musculature, the left upper trapezius muscle, and a trigger point in the left sternocleidomastoid muscle. Segmental evaluation revealed restricted rotation to the left at C1–C2. No other segmental restrictions were noted. Manual muscle testing of the upper extremities revealed normal, symmetrical strength. Light touch was normal in the upper extremities. Deep tendon reflexes were also normal.

IMPRESSIONS

There was no evidence of unilateral or bilateral vestibular hypofunction on examination. In addition, there were no signs or history suggestive of BPPV. His history of exertion-induced symptoms may be suggestive of a perilymph fistula. However, there were no physical findings consistent with a fistula; specifically, there was no tragal compression- or valsalva-induced nystagmus or vertigo. His balance exam shows a mild disturbance in static postural stability (increased sway in the Romberg tests with eyes closed and the positive Sharpened Romberg test with eyes closed). He demonstrates the ability to use vestibular cues to maintain upright stance. He demonstrates mild dynamic postural instability with head rotation while ambulating. The findings on J.B.'s upper quarter exam are consistent with a musculoskeletal dysfunction in the upper cervical spine. Although "cervical dizziness" is a controversial entity, this gentleman presents with cervical signs and symptoms that may be related to his symptoms of imbalance (specifically the temporal correlation between the dysequilibrium and cervical symptoms).

TREATMENT (11/18/96)

Because it was felt that J.B.'s symptoms were cervical in nature, the initial treatment was focused on his cervical problems. Treatment consisted of soft tissue mobilization of the suboccipital musculature, the left upper trapezius muscle, and the left sternocleidomastoid muscle. This was followed by mobilization of C1–C2 using a muscle energy technique (contract-relax), and active resisted isometric cervical rotation to the left at J.B.'s end range. Following treatment, J.B.'s rotation was symmetrical and symptom free. He was instructed in a home program to "correct" the forward head posture (dorsal glide of the head performed in prone), active resisted cervical rotation also performed in prone, and self-massage of the suboccipital musculature.

RETURN CLINIC VISIT (12/1/96)

J.B. returned to clinic noting a mild decrease in his symptoms of dysequilibrium and cervical discomfort. On examination, he had a normal Romberg test with eyes closed on both a firm surface and the 4-inch thick foam. His sharpened Romberg test with eyes closed and his ambulation with head rotation were unchanged. Cervical range of motion showed 70° of rotation to the left and 75° to the right. Palpation demonstrated increased muscle tone in the left suboccipital musculature and the left sternocleidomastoid muscle, as well as a mild limitation in rotation left at C1–C2. Treatment consisted of soft tissue mobilization of the suboccipital musculature and the left sternocleidomastoid muscle, spray and stretch to the left sternocleidomastoid muscle, and mobilization of C1–C2. Post-treatment, J.B. had symmetric and pain free cervical rotation. He was instructed to continue with his home exercise program.

RETURN CLINIC VISIT (12/8/96)

J.B. returned to clinic for reassessment and further treatment. He had no symptoms of dysequilibrium or cervical discomfort in the preceding week. His balance exam revealed normal static balance (sharpened Romberg with eyes closed) and no head rotation induced symptoms or ataxia while walking. He continued to demonstrate a 5° restriction in cervical rotation to the left. He was treated with joint mobilization of C1–C2: distraction, muscle energy techniques, and grade 3 oscillations to increase rotation to the left. He was instructed to continue with his home exercise program for an additional 4 to 6 weeks. Because he had been symptom free for an entire week, we felt that further outpatient physical therapy was not indicated at the time. He was instructed to call in 1 month to inform us of his progress or earlier if he became symptomatic.

TELEPHONE CALL (2/2/97)

J.B. called to say he is doing well (no dysequilibrium and no cervical symptoms). He stopped performing the home exercises 3 weeks ago, and he has noted no ill effects from stopping the exercises. He will return to clinic as needed.

REFERENCES

1. Barré, MJA: Sur un syndrome sympathique cervical posterieur et sa cause frequente: L'arthrite cervicale. Rev Neurol 45:1246, 1926.
2. Hardin, CA, et al: Vertebral artery insufficiency produced by cervical osteoarthritis spurs. Neurology 10:855, 1960.
3. Coria, F: Occipitoatlantal instability and vertebrobasilar ischemia: Case report. Neurology 32:305, 1982.
4. Fields, WS: Arteriography in the differential diagnosis of vertigo. Arch Otolaryngol 85:111, 1967.
5. Williams, D, and Wilson, TG: The diagnosis of the major and minor syndromes of basilar insufficiency. Brain 85:741, 1962.
6. Fisher, CM: Vertigo in cerebrovascular disease. Arch Otolaryngol 85:855, 1967.
7. Grad, A, and Baloh, RW: Vertigo of vascular origin: Clinical and ENG features in 84 cases. Arch Neurol 46:281, 1989.
8. Dix, M, and Hallpike, C: The pathology, symptomatology and diagnosis of certain common disorders of the vestibular systems. Ann Otol Rhinol Laryngol 61:987, 1952.
9. Mergner, T, et al: Comparison of the modes of interaction of labyrinthine and neck afferents in the suprasylvian cortex and vestibular nuclei in the cat. In Fuchs, AF, and Becker, W (eds): Progress in Oculomotor Research. Elsevier/North-Holland, Amsterdam, 1981, p 343.
10. McCouch, GP, et al: Location of receptors for tonic neck reflexes. J Neurophysiol 14:191, 1951.
11. Bakker, DA, and Richmond, FJR: Muscle spindle complexes in muscles around upper cervical vertebrae in the cat. J Neurophysiol 48:62, 1982.
12. Richmond, FJR, and Abrahams, VC: Morphology and distribution of muscle spindles in dorsal muscles of the cat neck. J Neurophysiol 38:1322, 1975.
13. Richmond, FJR, and Abrahams, VC: Physiological properties of muscle spindles in dorsal neck muscles of the cat. J Neurophysiol 42:601, 1979.
14. Richmond, FJR, and Abrahams, VC: What are the proprioceptors of the neck? In Granit, R, and Pompeiano, O (eds): Reflex Control of Posture. Elsevier/North-Holland, Amsterdam, 1979, p 245.
15. Richmond, FJR, et al: Motor and sensory fibers of neck muscle nerves in the cat. Can J Physiol Pharmacol 54:294, 1976.
16. Richmond, FJR, and Bakker, DA: Anatomical organization and sensory receptor content of soft tissues surrounding the upper cervical vertebrae in the cat. J Neurophysiol 48:49, 1982.
17. Barnes, GR, and Forbat, LN: Cervical and vestibular afferent control of oculomotor response in man. Acta Otolaryngol 88:79, 1979.
18. Rubin, AM, et al: Vestibular-neck integration in the vestibular nuclei. Brain Res 96:99, 1975.
19. Hikosaka, O, and Maeda, M: Cervical effects on abducens motoneurons and their interaction with vestibulo-ocular reflex. Exp Brain Res 18:512, 1973.
20. Igarashi, M, et al: Nystagmus after experimental cervical lesions. Laryngoscope 82:1609, 1972.
21. Oosterveld, WJ, et al: Electronystagmographic findings following cervical whiplash injuries. Acta Otolaryngol 111:201, 1991.
22. Toglia, JU: Acute flexion-extension injury of the neck. Neurology 26:808, 1976.
23. Fredrickson, JM, et al: Convergence and interaction of vestibular and deep somatic afferents upon neurons in the vestibular nuclei of the cat. Acta Otolaryngol (Stockh) 61:168, 1966.
24. Waespe, W, and Henn, V: Neuronal activity in the vestibular nuclei of the alert monkey during vestibular and optokinetic stimulation. Exp Brain Res 27:523, 1977.
25. Karlberg, M, and Magnusson, M: Asymmetric optokinetic after-nystagmus induced by active or passive sustained head rotations. Acta Otolaryngol 116:647, 1996.

26. Tjell, C, and Rosenhall, U: Smooth pursuit neck torsion test: A specific test for cervical dizziness. Am J Otol 19:76, 1998.
27. de Jong, PTVM, et al: Ataxia and nystagmus induced by injection of local anesthetics in the neck. Ann Neurol 1:240, 1977.
28. Biemond, A, and de Jong, JMBV: On cervical nystagmus and related disorders. Brain 92:437, 1969.
29. Alund, M, et al: Dynamic posturography among patients with common neck disorders. A study of 15 cases with suspected cervical vertigo. J Vestib Res 3:383, 1993.
30. Karlberg, M, et al: Dizziness of suspected cervical origin distinguished by posturographic assessment of human postural dynamics. J Vestib Res 6:37, 1996.
31. Karlberg, M, et al: Impaired postural control in patients with cervico-brachial pain. Acta Otolaryngol Suppl (Stockh) 520(Pt 2):440, 1995.
32. de Jong, JMBV, and Bles, W: Cervical dizziness and ataxia. In Bles, W, and Brandt, T (eds): Disorders of Posture and Gait. Elsevier, Amsterdam, 1986, p 185.
33. Brandt, T: Vertigo and dizziness. In Asbury, AK, et al (eds): Diseases of the Nervous System. Saunders, Philadelphia, 1986, p 561.
34. Karlberg, M, et al: Postural and symptomatic improvement after physiotherapy in patients with dizziness of suspected cervical origin. Arch Phys Med Rehab 77:874, 1996.

CHAPTER 22

Management of the Elderly Person with Vestibular Dysfunction

Susan L. Whitney, PT, ATC, PhD

The complaint of dizziness is one of the most common reasons that older adults visit the doctor's office.[1] The incidence of dizziness increases with age and accounts for 1.3 percent of all visits to internists in people age 45 to 64 years, 2.9 percent in people over 65, and 3.8 percent in people over 75. Although dizziness can be caused by many different medical conditions, it is estimated that as much as 45 percent are due to vestibular disorders.[2] The vestibular insult or injury may be the same as a younger individual's, but the functional sequelae may be very different because of the person's comorbid health status. Older adults with vestibular disorders, therefore, often present with very different problems than their younger counterparts. This chapter will provide the reader with information about the normal changes in the vestibular, visual, and somatosensory systems owing to aging as well as the pathological changes that can occur in each system. Practical suggestions are made as to how older adults may be treated differently because of their age.

VESTIBULAR FUNCTION

To understand the effect of aging on the mechanisms and potential for recovery in vestibular disease, it is important to understand the normal anatomy and physiology of the vestibular system (see Chapters 1–4). Several concepts are particularly important and will be emphasized here.

Semicircular Canal Function

The input from the receptors in the semicircular canals produce compensatory oculomotor responses (vestibulo-ocular reflex [VOR]) and compensatory postural responses (vestibulospinal reflex [VSR]). In the ideal situation, the eye movement produced by the head movement is equal (but opposite) to the head movement and the VOR is said to have a gain (eye velocity/head velocity) equal to 1. With aging, there is a decrease in the number of both hair cells and vestibular neurons.[3-5] Functionally, VOR gain decreases, although the changes appear to be frequency- and velocity-dependent.[6,7] Baloh et al[8] found that older subjects had lower visual-VOR gain as velocity increased compared with younger subjects. Although they examined this only at low frequency rotation, there appears to be a 35 percent decrease in visual-VOR gain in subjects age less than 75 years old compared with subjects age 19 to 39. If the visual-VOR gain decreases with age, especially at higher velocities, it would result in greater retinal slip and therefore poorer visual acuity during head movement. The changes in vestibular function have been compared to a progressive bilateral vestibular deficit[7-9] and may contribute to the complaints of disequilibrium (an "off-balance" sensation) and to the gait ataxia, without any true vertigo, of many older "dizzy" patients. Paige[10] suggests that this gradual, mild bilateral vestibular loss results in a mismatch in the visual and vestibular mechanisms. Interestingly, Nadol and Schuknecht[9] reported that degenerative changes can occur in only one labyrinth, producing sudden, severe vertigo or resulting in chronic vertigo and disequilibrium. Another change related to aging is a decreased ability to adapt the gain of the vestibular system.[7] This would affect the ability of the system to adjust to loss of function or other stresses to the system.

Pre-existing vestibular disorders can cause balance problems that manifest slightly differently in older individuals. There is the possibility that an older adult may have developed subclinical vestibular dysfunction when younger. Then, with the decrease in the number of hair cells and vestibular neurons with increasing age, and with the decrease in the vestibular and other systems' ability to compensate, the patient experiences symptoms of vestibular dysfunction. Thus the problems are due to decompensation, rather than a new vestibular disorder.

Bilateral vestibular disorders are more common in older adults than in younger adults. The most common cause of bilateral vestibular loss is antibiotic therapy following a major infection (see Chapters 5 and 18). The presence of visual and somatosensory changes with aging complicates the recovery from a bilateral vestibular loss. These patients are more likely to require the use of a walker or cane and will always have difficulty walking in the dark. One practical suggestion is that they increase the lighting, especially nightlights, in the house and that they carry a flashlight at night so they never have to walk in total darkness.

Utricular and Saccular Function

The presence of calcium carbonate crystals (otoconia) on the maculae of the utricle and saccule make these structures sensitive to the pull of gravity and to linear acceleration. These crystals are held in place by a gluelike substance and in all people there is a normal degeneration and regeneration of the crystals.[11] In addition, degenerative changes in the otoconia of the utricle and saccule increase with aging.[11] This may contribute to the relatively high incidence of benign paroxysmal positional vertigo (BPPV) in the elderly. The incidence of idiopathic BPPV has been reported as peaking in the sixth and seventh decades of life.[12] Baloh et al[8] report that of 116 patients aged 70 or more seen for complaints of "dizziness," 25 percent had BPPV.

Even if a patient does not present with a diagnosis of BPPV or with complaints consistent with BPPV, it is recommended that the older adult always be assessed for BPPV during the clinical examination because of its prevalence. When performing assessment or treatment for BPPV, however, it is important to consider the possibility that the patient may have cervical spine and cardiopulmonary disorders as well. Cervical spine range of motion should be assessed prior to position testing. Great care should be exercised when extending and rotating the older adult's head because of possible structural changes owing to arthritis or other cervical pathologies. Also, the patient should be screened carefully for vertebral basilar compromise. If the patient presents with a long history of cervical pathology (e.g., rheumatoid arthritis or Paget's disease), a tilt table is useful during the testing and repositioning maneuvers.

It is important to move more slowly with the repositioning maneuvers in adults over age 80 years and with the adult who has multiple medical problems.[13] The ultimate success rate in older adults is similar to that of younger persons but may require more than one visit. We think this is because it is difficult to obtain sufficient neck extension for an effective treatment. Care should also be taken with individuals who have metastatic cancer or who have had a cerebrovascular accident. We often perform the repositioning maneuver with two clinicians present to assist the patient with position changes. We also routinely monitor blood pressure in those people over 75 years old as a precaution.

Vestibular Function Tests

It is difficult to determine if dizziness is truly due to a vestibular deficit without sophisticated testing (see Chapter 6). The results of these tests in older persons must be interpreted carefully and should be based on age-related normal values.[14] For example, people in their 90s may have documented bilateral vestibular loss on caloric testing but do not actually have a bilateral vestibular loss.

VISUAL DEFICITS

Visual acuity, the ability to accommodate, and smooth pursuit normally decline with increasing age.[15,16] These normal changes associated with aging can make adaptation after a vestibular insult more difficult.

An inability to adapt to the dark has been shown in the literature to be one of the reasons why older adults may fall.[17] Combining the dark adaptation disorder with vestibular dysfunction can make it dangerous for older adults with vestibular disorders to move from areas with ample light to darkened areas. This change in light has been shown to cause temporary blindness in older adults for over a minute.[17]

In addition to dark adaptation, visual acuity and contrast sensitivity has been related to falls in older adults[18–20] and may contribute to imbalance after a vestibular disorder. Older adults may have other eye disorders including cataracts, glaucoma, and macular degeneration that impair vision.[21] Cataracts typically cloud the lens and may cause blurred vision. Those patients who have developed macular degeneration have near and distant vision affected without adversely affecting peripheral vision.[21] Individuals with glaucoma will have difficulty with their peripheral vision.[21] Depth perception disorders, such as cataracts in one eye, and double vision make maintaining upright stance more difficult for the patient. A home inspection would be very helpful for the person with glaucoma or other visual disorder to insure that their home is free of hazards. A home safety checklist that has been developed by the U.S. National Safety Council is an excellent way to determine hazards in the home[22] (Box 22–1). Any of these visual disorders can potentially increase the risk of falls and complicate the patient's rehabilitation course. A home visit to reduce hazards is very helpful for people who have visual impairments.[21]

BOX 22–1 Home Safety Checklist For Detection of Fall Hazards

Housekeeping

1.	Do you clean up spills as soon as they occur?	yes	no
2.	Do you keep floors and stairways clean and free of clutter?	yes	no
3.	Do you put away books, magazines, sewing supplies, and other objects as soon as you're through with them and never leave them on floors or stairways?	yes	no
4.	Do you store frequently used items on shelves that are within easy reach?	yes	no

Floors

5.	Do you keep everyone from walking on freshly washed floors before they're dry?	yes	no
6.	If you wax floors, do you apply 2 thin coats and buff each thoroughly or else use self-polishing, nonskid wax?	yes	no
7.	Do all small rugs have nonskid backings?	yes	no
8.	Have you eliminated small rugs at the tops and bottoms of stairways?	yes	no
9.	Are all carpet edges tacked down?	yes	no
10.	Are rugs and carpets free of curled edges, worn spots, and rips?	yes	no
11.	Have you chosen rugs and carpets with short, dense pile?	yes	no
12.	Are rugs and carpets installed over good-quality, medium-thick pads?	yes	no

Bathroom

13.	Do you use rubber mat or nonslip decals in the tub or shower?	yes	no
14.	Do you have a grab bar securely anchored over the tub or on the shower wall?	yes	no
15.	Do you have a nonskid rug on the bathroom floor?	yes	no
16.	Do you keep soap in an easy-to-reach receptacle?	yes	no

Traffic Lanes

17.	Can you walk across every room in your home, and from one room to another, without detouring around furniture?	yes	no
18.	Is the traffic lane from your bedroom to the bathroom free of obstacles?	yes	no
19.	Are telephone and appliance cords kept away from areas where people walk?	yes	no

(Continued)

(BOX 22–1   Continued)

Lighting
    20. Do you have light switches near every doorway?   yes   no
    21. Do you have enough good lighting to eliminate shadowy areas?   yes   no
    22. Do you have a lamp or light switch within easy reach from your
        bed?   yes   no
    23. Do you have nightlights in your bathroom and in the hallway
        leading from your bedroom to the bathroom?   yes   no
    24. Are all stairways well lighted?   yes   no
    25. Do you have light switches at both the tops and bottoms of
        stairways?   yes   no

Stairways
    26. Do securely fastened handrails extend the full length of the stairs
        on each side of stairways?   yes   no
    27. Do rails stand out from the walls so you can get a good grip?   yes   no
    28. Are rails distinctly shaped so you're alerted when you reach the
        end of a stairway?   yes   no
    29. Are all stairways in good condition, with no broken, sagging, or
        sloping steps?   yes   no
    30. Are all stairway carpeting and metal edges securely fastened and
        in good condition?   yes   no
    31. Have you replaced any single-level steps with gradually rising
        ramps or made sure such steps are well lighted?   yes   no

Ladders and Stepstools
    32. Do you have a sturdy stepstool that you use to reach high cupboard
        and closet shelves?   yes   no
    33. Are ladders and stepstools in good condition?   yes   no
    34. Do you always use a stepstool or ladder that's tall enough for the
        job?   yes   no
    35. Do you always set up your ladder or stepstool on a firm, level base
        that's free of clutter?   yes   no
    36. Before you climb a ladder or stepstool, do you always make sure
        it's fully open and that the stepladder spreaders are locked?   yes   no
    37. When you use a ladder or stepstool, do you face the steps and keep
        your body between the side rails?   yes   no
    38. Do you avoid standing on top of a stepstool or climbing beyond the
        second step from the top on a stepladder?   yes   no

Outdoor Areas
    39. Are walks and driveways in your yard and other areas free of
        breaks?   yes   no
    40. Are lawns and gardens free of holes?   yes   no
    41. Do you put away garden tools and hoses when they're not in use?   yes   no
    42. Are outdoor areas kept free of rocks, loose boards, and other
        tripping hazards?   yes   no
    43. Do you keep outdoor walkways, steps, and porches free of wet
        leaves and snow?   yes   no
    44. Do you sprinkle icy outdoor areas with de-icers as soon as possible
        after a snowfall or freeze?   yes   no
    45. Do you have mats at doorways for people to wipe their feet on?   yes   no
    46. Do you know the safest way of walking when you can't avoid
        walking on a slippery surface?   yes   no

(Continued)

(*BOX 22–1 Continued*)

47. Do your shoes have soles and heels that provide good traction? — yes no
48. Do you wear house slippers that fit well and don't fall off? — yes no
49. Do you avoid walking in stocking feet? — yes no
50. Do you wear low-heeled oxfords, loafers, or good-quality sneakers when you work in your house or yard? — yes no
51. Do you replace boots or galoshes when their soles or heels are worn too smooth to keep you from slipping on wet or icy surfaces? — yes no

Personal Precautions

52. Are you always alert for unexpected hazards, such as out-of-place furniture? — yes no
53. If young grandchildren visit, are you alert for children playing on the floor and toys left in your path? — yes no
54. If you have pets, are you alert for sudden movements across your path and pets getting underfoot? — yes no
55. When you carry bulky packages, do you make sure they don't obstruct your vision? — yes no
56. Do you divide large loads into smaller loads whenever possible? — yes no
57. When you reach or bend, do you hold onto a firm support and avoid throwing your head back or turning it too far? — yes no
58. Do you always use a ladder or stepstool to reach high places and never stand on a chair? — yes no
59. Do you always move deliberately and avoid rushing to answer the phone or doorbell? — yes no
60. Do you take time to get your balance when you change position from lying down to sitting and from sitting to standing? — yes no
61. Do you hold onto grab bars when you change position in the tub or shower? — yes no
62. Do you keep yourself in good condition with moderate exercise, good diet, adequate rest, and regular medical checkups? — yes no
63. If you wear glasses, is your prescription up to date? — yes no
64. Do you know how to reduce injury in a fall? — yes no
65. If you live alone, do you have daily contact with a friend or neighbor? — yes no

After identifying a fall hazard, the hazard should be eliminated or reduced. One point is allowed for each *No* answer. Score 1 to 7, excellent; 8 to 14, good; 15 and higher, hazardous.

This checklist was developed by the U.S. National Safety Council in cooperation with AARP, Itasca, IL, 1982. (Used with permission.)

SOMATOSENSORY CHANGES

Somatosensory changes occur with increasing age. Vibration sense, a decrease in the ability to detect passive motion in the foot, and an increase in lower extremity reaction times are typically seen in older adults.[23,24] Pathological changes in somatosensation include abnormal distal sensation and neuropathies.[25,26] Older adults have more difficulty sensing vibration in the distal extremities, as well as having less sensitivity with detecting the smaller sized monofilaments. Diabetes is one of the most common conditions in older adults that causes changes in distal somatosensation and vision.[27]

MUSCULOSKELETAL DEFICITS

Another potential difficulty in rehabilitating the older population with a vestibular disorder involves the musculoskeletal system. An assessment of grip strength is one of the most effective ways to get an overall idea of strength in older adults.[28] Older adults may have weakness or even muscle paralysis of various etiologies. Older adults who have preexisting conditions, such as polio or cerebral palsy and who develop late-onset vestibular disease, are more difficult to treat. Weakness is very common in the lower extremities in older adults, especially in the ankles. Careful attention to ankle strength is very important in the patient's rehabilitation. When considering the inverted pendulum model of postural control, the ankles play a critical role in the maintenance of postural control.[29] Foot and ankle muscles appear to be very weak in many older patients and strength training may be indicated.

POSTURAL HYPOTENSION

Patients who show vestibular symptoms often will complain of either dizziness and/or imbalance. The dizziness needs to be differentiated from light-headedness owing to postural hypotension associated with changes in position. Postural hypotension and vestibular-induced dizziness can be easily confused if a careful examination is not provided. Typically patients with postural hypotension become light-headed or dizzy when standing up and the symptoms last for seconds. There is also a 20-mm Hg drop in systolic pressure from supine to standing if taken immediately after rising. The patient is asked to lie in supine for up to 5 minutes, then is asked to stand with the blood pressure cuff secured to an extremity. A drop of 20 or more mm Hg is indicative of postural hypotension. Many common drugs taken by the older adult can produce postural hypotension, including diuretics. Postural hypotension alone can put a person at risk for falling because of the significant dizziness that the patient experiences when changing positions quickly.

CEREBELLAR ATROPHY

Older adults may have disturbances in coordination and tend to move slowly. Patients with cerebellar disease appear to improve with balance therapy.[30] It is not uncommon to see cerebellar atrophy as a sign of abnormal aging in the older adult. Patients with cerebellar atrophy often do not complain of dizziness, vertigo, or hearing loss. Their chief complaint often is that their balance is getting worse over a period of years. Working on the person's rhythm of gait is very helpful for these patients as their step lengths can be variable, making them unstable while ambulating.

FEAR OF FALLING

Another common problem experienced by older individuals who have vestibular disorders is fear of falling. They often experience the fear of falling, and as a result, decrease their activity level.[31–33] This fear of falling is extremely disabling to older adults and actually may prevent optimal functioning. Tinetti et al[31] suggest that therapists work with patients to decrease their fear of falling, which will also enhance their function. When asking your patient about a fall, you and the patient should be using the same definition of a fall. When taking the patient's history, one should determine if the patient has many "near falls," where they come close to hitting the ground but actually do not hit the ground. Falls with no known cause are of concern to the therapist and must be investigated further to determine why the patient fell.

ATTENTION

The role of attention in postural control in the elderly is an important one.[34–37] Shumway-Cook et al[34] have studied postural control in older adults while standing and have found that older adults allocate their resources differently than the younger adults. When they compared the young healthy and older healthy adults, the older adult's balance was more affected than the young adult's while they were concurrently performing a balance task and a simple cognitive task. Those older people who had a history of falling had significant changes in their balance as measured by center of pressure. Ludin-Olssen et al[35] determined in the nursing home setting that older adults who walked with assistive devices while they talked were more likely to fall than those who did not talk as they walked.[35] The concept of attentional resources is interesting, and one that can be incorporated into practice. Older patients who have great difficulty walking in the clinic are now told to try not to walk and talk at the same time. They are instructed to "stop walking while talking," which is the title of the Ludin-Olssen article![35]

DEPRESSION

Older adults who have vestibular disorders may be experiencing clinical depression. A simple screening exam can be performed using the Geriatric Depression Screening Scale.[38] This scale consists of 30 yes-or-no items that ask the patient to answer how they felt over the past week. The test is simple to use and can aid the therapist in making the decision for a mental health referral. Both cognition and depression will affect the ability of the patient to follow through with an exercise program. The older adult who is depressed or who has little support at home may need to be seen more frequently in the clinic and will need closer monitoring by the therapist. The patient who displays an indifferent or negative attitude towards therapeutic intervention should not be easily dismissed as "lacking motivation." Coexisting depression may be the cause of the indifference.

RISK OF FALLING IN OLDER ADULTS WITH VESTIBULAR DISORDERS

The actual risk of falling in older adults who present to a vestibular clinic is unknown. In a sample of 247 persons who presented to a vestibular clinic with a mean age of 62, 36.8 percent reported having one or more falls in the last 6 months.[39]

There are standardized tools that one can use to determine risk of falling in older adults. Specific tools that can be used to assess balance include the Berg Balance Scale (BBS)[40–47] and functional reach.[48–53] The Berg Balance Scale (BBS) has been used extensively to assess balance in older adults who have Parkinson's disease, stroke, and who are frail (Box 22–2). This 14-item exam assesses the patient's balance in increasingly difficult positions and has a maximum score of 56. As the scores decrease from 56 to 36, there is an

---

BOX 22–2   Berg Balance Scale*

1. SITTING TO STANDING

Instruction: Please stand up. Try not to use your hands for support.
Grading: Please mark the lowest category which applies.

(4)	(3)	(2)	(1)	(0)
able to stand no hands and stabilize independently	able to stand independently using hands	able to stand using hands after several tries	needs minimal assist to stand or to stabilize	needs moderate or maximal assist to stabilize

2. STANDING UNSUPPORTED

Instruction: Stand for two minutes without holding.
Grading: Please mark the lowest category which applies.

(4)	(3)	(2)	(1)	(0)
able to stand safely 2 min.	able to stand 2 min with supervision	able to stand unsupported	needs several tries to stand 30 sec	unable to stand 30 sec unassisted

IF SUBJECT ABLE TO STAND 2 MIN SAFELY, SCORE FULL MARKS FOR SITTING UNSUPPORTED. PROCEED TO POSITION CHANGE STANDING TO SITTING.

3. SITTING UNSUPPORTED FEET ON FLOOR

Instruction: Sit with arms folded for two minutes.
Grading: Please mark the lowest category which applies.

(4)	(3)	(2)	(1)	(0)
able to sit safely and securely 2 minutes	able to sit 2 minutes under supervision	able to sit 30 seconds	able to sit 10 seconds	unable to sit without support 10 seconds

4. STANDING TO SITTING

Instruction: Please sit down.
Grading: Please mark to lowest category which applies.

(4)	(3)	(2)	(1)	(0)
sits safely with minimal use of hands	controls descent by using hands	uses back of legs against chair to control descent	sits independently using uncontrolled descent	needs assistance to sit

(Continued)

(BOX 22–2 Continued)

5. TRANSFERS

Instruction: Please move from chair to bed and back again. One way toward a seat with armrests and one way toward a seat without armrests.
Grading: Please mark the lowest category which applies.

(4)	(3)	(2)	(1)	(0)
able to transfer safely with minor use of hands	able to transfer safely definite need of hands	able to transfer with verbal cuing and/or definite need of hands	needs one person to assist	needs two people to assist or supervise to be safe

6. STANDING UNSUPPORTED WITH EYES CLOSED

Instruction: Close your eyes and stand still for 10 seconds.
Grading: Please mark the lowest category which applies.

(4)	(3)	(2)	(1)	(0)
able to stand 10 sec safely	able to stand 10 sec with supervision	able to stand 3 seconds	unable to keep eyes closed 3 sec but stays steady	needs help to keep from falling

7. STANDING UNSUPPORTED WITH FEET TOGETHER

Instruction: Place your feet together and stand without holding.
Grading: Please mark the lowest category which applies.

(4)	(3)	(2)	(1)	(0)
able to place feet together independently and stand 1 min safely	able to place feet together indep. & stand for 1 min with supervision	able to place feet together independently but unable to hold for 30 sec	needs help to attain position but able to stand 15 sec feet together	needs help to attain position and unable to hold for 15 sec

THE FOLLOWING ITEMS ARE TO BE PERFORMED WHILE STANDING UNSUPPORTED.

8. REACHING FORWARD WITH OUTSTRETCHED ARM

Instructions: Lift arm to 90 degrees. Stretch out your fingers and reach forward as far as you can. (Examiner places a ruler at end of finger tips when arm is at 90 degrees. Fingers should not touch the ruler while reaching forward. The recorded measure is the distance forward that the fingers reach while the subject is in the most forward lean position.)
Grading: Please mark the lowest category which applies.

(4)	(3)	(2)	(1)	(0)
can reach forward confidently >10 inches	can reach forward >5 inches safely	can reach forward >2 inches safely	reaches forward but needs supervision	needs help to keep from falling

(Continued)

(BOX 22–2 Continued)

9. PICK UP OBJECT FROM THE FLOOR

Instructions: Pick up the shoe/slipper which is placed in front of your feet.
Grading: Please mark the lowest category which applies.

(4)	(3)	(2)	(1)	(0)
able to pick up slipper safely and easily	able to pick up slipper but needs supervision	unable to pick up but reaches 1–2 inches from slipper & keeps balance indep	unable to pick up and needs supervision while trying	unable to try/needs assist to keep from falling

10. TURNING TO LOOK BEHIND OVER LEFT AND RIGHT SHOULDERS

Instruction: Turn to look behind you over toward left shoulder. Repeat to the right.
Grading: Please mark the lowest category which applies.

(4)	(3)	(2)	(1)	(0)
looks behind from both sides and weight shifts well	looks behind one side only other side shows less weight shift	turns sideways only but maintains balance	needs supervision when turning	needs assist to keep from falling

11. TURN 360 DEGREES

Instruction: Turn completely around in a full circle. Pause, then turn a full circle in the other direction.
Grading: Please mark the lowest category which applies.

(4)	(3)	(2)	(1)	(0)
able to turn 360 safely in <4 sec each side	able to turn 360 safely one side only <4 sec	able to turn 360 safely but slowly	needs close supervision or verbal cuing	needs assistance while turning

DYNAMIC WEIGHT SHIFTING WHILE STANDING UNSUPPORTED.

12. COUNT NUMBER OF TIMES STEP TOUCH MEASURED STOOL

Instruction: Place each foot alternately on the stool. Continue until each foot has touched the stool four times.
Grading: Please mark the lowest category which applies.

(4)	(3)	(2)	(1)	(0)
able to stand independently and safely and complete 8 steps in 20 sec	able to stand independently and complete 8 steps >20 sec	able to complete 4 steps without aid with supervision	able to complete >2 steps needs minimal assist	needs assistance to keep from falling/unable to try

(Continued)

(BOX 22–2   Continued)

---

13. STAND UNSUPPORTED ONE FOOT IN FRONT OF THE OTHER FOOT

Instruction: Place one foot as close as possible in front of the other foot.
Grading: Please mark the lowest category which applies.

(4)	(3)	(2)	(1)	(0)
able to place feet tandem and holds 30 sec	able to place one foot ahead and holds 30 sec	takes small step; independently; holds 30 sec	needs help to step in place; holds 15 sec	loses balance while stepping or standing

14. STAND ON ONE LEG

Instruction: Please stand on one leg as long as you can without holding on to anything (knee does not have to be bent).
Grading: Please mark the lowest category which applies.

(4)	(3)	(2)	(1)	(0)
able to lift leg independently; able to hold for >10 sec	able to lift leg independently; or needs assist holds 5–10 sec	able to lift leg independently; holds 3 sec	tries to lift leg; unable to hold 3 sec; remains standing independently	unable to; tries or needs assist to prevent falling

TOTAL SCORE _____

MAXIMUM SCORE _____

---

increasing risk of falling.[47] Shumway-Cook et al[47] recently determined that scores of 36 and lower on the test relate to 100 percent risk of falls in community living older adults.

Another tool that is helpful for assessing risk of falls is functional reach.[48] The test was developed using older male veterans. The test is a difference score in the patient's willingness to reach forward without taking a step. Requirements to perform the test include that the patient be able to stand for 30 seconds without support in flat or no shoes and that at least 90° of shoulder flexion is present. Patients are typically instructed to raise their arm, make a fist, and then reach forward along the yardstick as far as they can without touching the wall or the yardstick. They are permitted to use any strategy that they want to complete the trials. Duncan et al[49] have determined that scores of 6 inches and less show a significant increase in the risk of falling in older adults. Individuals who reach between 6 and 10 inches are at moderate risk for falling.[49] Functional reach is related to height; those who are tall will have longer functional reach scores than those who are short. Functional reach scores have also been shown to change over the course of rehabilitation.[52] Functional reach is sometimes administered to the patient who has dizziness.[50] The functional reach test is helpful for those older adults who complain of balance problems.

QUESTIONNAIRES FOR BALANCE ASSESSMENT

The Activities-Specific Balance Scale (ABC) is a 16-item questionnaire that can be completed by the patient or administered by the caregiver (Box 22–3).[54,55] The patient's perceived confidence in performing 16 activities that are performed in and outside the house are rated by the patient from a range of 0 (no confidence) to 100 (100 percent

---

BOX 22–3 The Activities-Specific Balance Confidence (ABC) Scale[55]

For *each* of the following activities, please indicate your level of self-confidence by choosing a corresponding number from the following rating scale:

0%	10	20	30	40	50	60	70	80	90	100%
no confidence										completely confident

"How confident are you that you will *not* lose your balance or become unsteady when you. . .

1. . . . walk around the house? _____%
2. . . . walk up or down stairs? _____%
3. . . . bend over and pick up a slipper from the front of a closet floor? _____%
4. . . . reach for a small can off a shelf at eye level? _____%
5. . . . stand on your tip toes and reach for something above your head? _____%
6. . . . stand on a chair and reach for something? _____%
7. . . . sweep the floor? _____%
8. . . . walk outside the house to a car parked in the driveway? _____%
9. . . . get into or out of a car? _____%
10. . . . walk across a parking lot to the mall? _____%
11. . . . walk up or down a ramp? _____%
12. . . . walk in a crowded mall where people rapidly walk past you? _____%
13. . . . are bumped into by people as you walk through the mall? _____%
14. . . . step onto or off of an escalator while you are holding onto a railing? _____%
15. . . . step onto or off an escalator while holding onto parcels such that you cannot hold onto the railing? _____%
16. . . . walk outside on icy sidewalks? _____%

Instructions to Participants
For each of the following, please indicate your level of confidence in doing the activity without losing your balance or becoming unsteady by choosing one of the percentage points on the scale from 0% to 100%. If you do not currently do the activity in question, try and imagine how confident you would be if you had to do the activity. If you normally use a walking aid to do the activity or hold onto someone, rate your confidence as if you were using these supports. If you have any questions about answering any of these items, please ask the administrator.

Instructions for Scoring
The ABC is an 11-point scale and ratings should consist of whole numbers (0 to 100) for each item. Total the ratings (possible range = 0 to 1600) and divide by 16 to get each subject's ABC score. If a subject qualifies his/her response to items #2, #9, #11, #14 or #15 (different ratings for "up" vs "down" or "onto" vs "off"), solicit separate ratings and use the *lowest* confidence of the two (as this will limit the entire activity, for instance likelihood of using the stairs).

confident). Scores that are closer to 100 are a better score on this scale. The ABC and the Dizziness Handicap Inventory (DHI) have been shown to have a moderately negative correlation ($r = -.64$) indicating that it is a valid tool for use with persons with vestibular dysfunction.[56]

The ABC has been compared to the Modified Falls Efficacy Scale.[33] Both the Modified Falls Efficacy Scale and the ABC are sensitive tools that can be used in community-based older adults, and both discriminate those individuals who are high functioning from those who are low functioning. Scores in our clinic below 60 on the ABC are of concern. Older adults should be able to perform most of these activities with great confidence.

The Modified Fast Evaluation of Mobility, Balance, and Fear Baseline questionnaire is extremely helpful in determining risk factors for falling (Box 22–4).[57,58] The therapist fills out "yes" or "no" to the risk factors as they interview the patient or after they have obtained information from the patient's medical chart. This questionnaire has a comprehensive list of falls risk items and helps to guide intervention based on the answers to the questions.

BOX 22–4 Modified Fast Evaluation of Mobility, Balance, and Fear Baseline Questionnaire[58]

Name _____ Age____/____/____ Gender____ Height____ Weight____
Blood Pressure _____ Lives at Home, Alone _____ Lives with Somebody _____
Lives in an Institution _____

RISK FACTORS

	YES	NO
1. Needs aid for two (or more) basic activities of daily living (washing, cooking, dressing, walking, continence, feeding)	____	____
2. Needs aid for two (or more) instrumental activities of daily living (money management, shopping, telephone, medications)	____	____
3. Has had a fracture or articular problems at hips, knees, ankles, feet	____	____
4. Has visible articular sequela in the mentioned joints	____	____
5. Uses a walking device (e.g., cane, walker)	____	____
6. Limits physical activity to basic activities of daily living at home	____	____
7. Self-defines as anxious	____	____
8. Complains of vertigo	____	____
9. Complains of imbalance	____	____
10. Makes complaints suggesting an existing postural hypotension	____	____
11. Fell one or two times in the current year	____	____
12. Fell more than twice in the current year	____	____
13. Required nursing after the fall	____	____
14. Had a fracture after the fall	____	____
15. Is afraid of falling in general	____	____
16. Is afraid of falling indoors (e.g., bathtub, kitchen)	____	____
17. Is afraid of falling outdoors (e.g., bus, stairs, street)	____	____
18. Avoids going outside for fear of falling	____	____
19. Presents three or more somatic pathologies that require regular medical supervision	____	____
20. The pathologies require home-based medical-social supervision	____	____

(Continued)

(BOX 22–4   Continued)

21. Shows a specific pathology likely to induce falls: ____ ____
    - neurological (e.g., cancer, peripheral neuropathy, multiple sclerosis, lupus)
    - cardiovascular (e.g., postural hypotension)
    - musculoskeletal (e.g., total joint replacements, arthritis)
    - sensory (e.g., visual impairment)
    - other (amputation, Parkinson's disease, Alzheimer's disease)
22. Takes medications that are potentially dangerous in regard to falls: ____ ____
    - hypotensives
    - neuroleptics
    - hypnotics/anxiolytics
    - antiarrythmics
    - antiparkinsonians
    - analgesics/anti-inflammatory drugs
    - various vasoregulators

                                        Risk Factors (=total of "yes" answers): _____

TASK COMPLETION

Scores are determined for fear, pain, mobility difficulties, and lack of strength for each of the following:

                                                                                    TASK SCORE
                                                                                      (3, 2, 1)

1. Sitting on a chair, with folded arms, raises both legs horizontally   ____
2. Sitting on a chair with armrests, stands up without aid, without using banister   ____
3. Sitting on a chair, stands up without aid, walks five steps, turns around, goes back and sits down   ____
4. One-footed standing (left foot): stands on left foot without aid during 5 seconds minimum   ____
5. Repeat with one-footed standing (right foot)   ____
6. Romberg Test: stands with heels together, eyes closed, remains steady for 10 seconds   ____
7. Squatting down: without aid, squats down until buttocks reach knee level, then stands up   ____
8. Picking up a pencil from the ground without aid or support   ____
9. Standing jumping without losing balance, over a distance equal to one's own foot   ____
10. Stepping over an obstacle (foam or cardboard, 10-cm wide x 15-cm high) without touching it; the foot to arrive past the obstacle at a distance equal to its own size (left)   ____
11. Repeat with overstepping to the right   ____
12. Shoving forward to trunk; subject to remain steady following a nudge between shoulder blades (examiner's arms stretched out, nudge realized by a sudden bending of hand on trunk)   ____
13. Repeat with shoving backward (nudge on the sternum)   ____
14. Climbing stairs without losing balance, without aid or using banister (five steps minimum)   ____
15. Repeat with descending stairs (five steps minimum)   ____
16. Transfer from standing-kneeling (both knees on the ground); stable, no assistance for rising   ____

(Continued)

(BOX 22–4 *Continued*)

17. Managing the "eyes-closed forward fall"; the subject lets
    himself/herself fall, eyes closed, onto the examiner standing
    50 cm from him/her
18. Repeat with eyes-closed backward fall   ____

FEMBAF TOTAL TASK COMPLETION SCORE: ____

FEMBAF TOTAL SUBJECTIVE COMPLAINT SCORES:

fear ____   pain ____   mobility difficulties ____   lack of strength ____

3 = successfully completed without imbalance
2 = task initiated but unsteady or partially completed
1 = unable to perform or initiate task

Reprinted from DiFabio, RP, and Seavy, R. Use of the "Fast evaluation of mobility, balance, and
fear" in elderly community dwellers: Validity and reliability. Phys Ther 77:904, 1977. With
permission of the American Physical Therapy Association.

DIZZINESS ASSESSMENT

The DHI is extremely helpful in determining what type of intervention will most
benefit the patient with vestibular dysfunction.[59] This tool helps to determine the self-
perceived handicap of the individual completing the form. The patient answers 25
questions related to dizziness and/or handicap. There are three subdivisions of the test
and subscores can be calculated. The test has been divided into an emotional, physical
and functional subset. Information from this tool can significantly direct the treatment
of the patient. If the patient checks only the physical symptoms, one needs to look at
assessing positions and specific movements that predispose or increase their dizziness
and/or falls. Often older adults, who have lost mobility as a result of dizziness, check a
significant number of the emotional questions. One then needs to determine the actual
activity level of the older adult. Use of the SF-36 form can be helpful in assessing the
activity level of the patient, yet the DHI is more responsive to change after a 6- to 8-
week course of vestibular rehabilitation than the SF-36.[60,61]

TYPICAL BALANCE TESTS

If the patient is complaining of balance problems, single-leg stance (SLS), the
Romberg, and Tandem Romberg are also performed. Bohannon et al[62] have studied
older adults and have found that their SLS times significantly decrease in this group.[62]
SLS, Romberg, and Tandem Romberg help the therapist determine what kind of functional movements might be difficult for the patient.[62–66] Generally if the patient is unable to stand in SLS, they usually have great difficulty going up and down stairs without holding on to the railing. They may also have strength deficits if they are unable to

stay in SLS. The strength deficits can be determined through further testing. The patient who has difficulty with the Romberg test and Tandem Romberg often is challenged while walking through tight spaces. Standing with feet close together may be very destabilizing to the patient. Some older adults may live in homes with narrow hallways or small rooms with little clearance, and the therapist needs to consider their environment as the treatment program is designed.

HOME ASSESSMENT

Preparing your patient to function independently in the home is very important. Occasionally a home visit is necessary for older persons with vestibular dysfunction if you are concerned about their safety. Determining how many stairs the patient must ascend or descend in a home assessment is critical. Some extrinsic environmental hazards that have been identified include items such as poor lighting, uneven or slippery surfaces, loose rugs, steep stairs, objects in the pathway, long bathrobes, inappropriate furniture, and lack of handrails, especially in the bathroom.[68] Modification of the home environment so that the patient does not have to reach excessively either up or down to perform activities of daily living is helpful. Primary care physicians, especially in managed care situations, should be made aware that these services are available to their patients.

Many of the older adults seen in our clinic with complaints of dizziness and balance dysfunction do not specifically have a diagnosis. A total vestibular workup and a neurology assessment are helpful and can be performed so that the physical therapist knows what they are treating.

LENGTH OF TREATMENT

The older adult frequently needs to be treated for a longer period of time. The longer length of treatment is related to the number of risk factors present, and their fear. They may be seen in a more traditional mode of 1 to 3 times per week because of their multiple medical problems and the risk of falling when unsupervised at home. Many older patients have difficulty being transported to physical therapy. This fact can complicate rehabilitation; the older adults' cancellation rate is often higher. If their transportation system breaks down or if the weather is bad, many older adults will be forced to cancel their appointment; referral to a local agency for the aging may be indicated to assist the patient in obtaining dependable transportation.

WHAT TO DO ONCE THE RISK FACTOR
HAS BEEN IDENTIFIED

After the older person with vestibular dysfunction has been assessed, it is important to determine what problems identified in the evaluation need to be addressed, with referral being one alternative. Patients who have visual problems should be referred to an appropriate physician for further eye testing. People with undiagnosed vestibular disorders should be referred to a neurologist or otolaryngologist. If a neuropathy is suspected, a referral to a neurologist, physical therapist that specializes in EMG, or a physiatrist is recommended.

The physical or occupational therapist can also provide an environmental assessment with specific recommendations, determine if the patient needs an assistive device, and teach the patient about safety and proper clothes that they could wear to decrease their risk of falling. In addition, shoe type and wear can be determined and recommendations can be made to the patient. The older adult may have chosen to wear inappropriate shoes and they can sometimes be counseled to change.

During the environmental assessment, lighting in the patient's home may be identified as a major risk factor. Many older adults use low-wattage light bulbs or keep the lights off most of the day in order to save money. Use of nightlights is strongly suggested, especially in the bathroom. Additionally, the layout of some patient's homes may cause significant changes in contrast of light levels, which has been identified earlier as contributing to falls.[19,20] Proper lighting is something that needs to be addressed with the patient and their family.

Motor weakness is most often assessed by performing a manual muscle test or through the use of a dynamometer. Strength deficits can be addressed as patients have the potential to improve their strength, although it may take up to 6 weeks to start to see improvement.[69–71] Range of motion is a major factor that can be improved through rehabilitation. Patients can be significantly at risk for falls if they lack adequate distal range of motion in their feet. Having normal plantarflexion and dorsiflexion are extremely helpful in preventing falls and normal gait as the feet are the only things that are touching the ground while walking. Assessing flexibility of the toes and foot musculature may be of added benefit since having strong dynamic stabilizers distally may make the patient more stable. If the patient has an extremely immobile foot, performing normal balance reactions will be difficult.

CASE STUDIES

CASE #1

Mrs. H is a 91–year-old woman referred to physical therapy with a diagnosis of bilateral BPPV. She has been seen by a neurotologist that wanted her seen jointly by himself and the physical therapist for repositioning.

The patient was well-oriented and extremely pleasant older woman. Her chief complaint was that she became very dizzy 3 weeks ago when she looked up at her clock at home and also when she sat up or went from sitting to lying down. Her daughter was very concerned and worried about her mother and stated several times during the examination that she felt that her mother should move into her home. Mrs. H lived alone in a small one-bedroom apartment. She normally took the van that leaves daily from her apartment complex to the grocery store and she loves to shop! Mrs. H cleans her own apartment but has someone come in once a month to do the heavy cleaning. She arrived to the outpatient clinic carrying a straight cane while seated in a wheelchair. Patient reported that she does not use a cane in her apartment and that she has used a cane for the past 4 years. She holds onto furniture as she ambulates around the apartment and rarely uses a wheelchair except for long distances when a wheelchair is available. When she shops, she reports using the shopping cart like a wheeled walker.

Mrs. H was taking no medications except vitamins but did have a 39-year history of Paget's disease. Her laboratory findings were: calorics, severely reduced responses bilaterally with absent ice water responses; oculomotor screening, normal; rotational chair, abnormal with moderately decreased gain and a mild directional preponderance; and positional testing, normal. She was not ataxic and did not have oscillopsia.

Patient's timed "Up & Go" score was 30 seconds. She moved slowly while carrying her straight cane. Patient had a very kyphotic posture. She had decreased neck and shoulder range of motion and her overall strength was F+ to G−.

The patient had already been diagnosed with bilateral BPPV. She was more symptomatic in the left Hallpike-Dix position compared to the right Hallpike-Dix so the left ear was treated first. There were four people present for the repositioning including the physician because of the patient's age and her Paget's disease. Paget's disease produces excess bone and this excess bone production can result in narrowing of the vertebral foramen. It was decided to use a high-low table with two moveable parts. Her trunk and head were lowered as a unit and at the same time we elevated her feet to put her in the Trendelenburg position. The patient was initially brought down to the left and then was log-rolled from her left side to her right side. Movements were coordinated between the persons helping to perform the maneuver. Her head was slowly brought up as her feet were returned to the horizontal position. This positioning avoided excessive neck extension and excessive torque to her back during the modified canalith repositioning maneuver. Infrared goggles were in place through out the procedure. The patient had classic torsional and upbeating nystagmus that fatigued within 20 seconds. The second time that she was repositioned during the same session she had no symptoms.

She was told to stay upright and to not reach down towards the floor for 24 hours. The patient was instructed to sleep in a recliner. She did not have one in her apartment so her daughter decided to take her home to her house for the evening.

Patient was scheduled to return in 1 week for repositioning of the other ear. She could not make it back in any sooner because of her daughter's schedule. When the patient returned, there was no evidence of BPPV in either ear. She had been instructed to perform Brandt-Daroff habituation exercises 2 days after the repositioning. Patient reported that she had no symptoms. She could look up to her clock at home and lie down without symptoms. She had returned to her normal shopping excursions and said that she felt great.

Her daughter was very concerned about how active her mother was and wanted her to stop many of her activities. The daughter was strongly encouraged to allow her mother to stay active and to enjoy her trips out of her apartment.

During her last visit, Mrs. H was instructed in lower extremity strengthening exercises so that she could maintain her strength distally. Patient was discharged after being seen for two physical therapy visits. She no longer had any dizziness and she was satisfied with her gait.

CASE #2

Mrs. M is a 68-year-old woman seen in physical therapy with a presenting diagnosis of multi-sensory deficit. Mrs. M was well oriented and very cooperative. She stated that she had been having difficulty walking and that she had fallen twice within the last few weeks. Patient was seen by an otolaryngologist because of her falling. Quick head movements and bending made her unstable.

Her past medical history includes a silent heart attack, hypertension, cirrhosis of the liver without a history of alcoholism, mastoiditis, obesity, claustrophobia, uterine cancer, tinnitus, and stomach ulcers. In addition, the patient took medication for her knee arthritis. Past surgical history included a hysterectomy and two surgeries for cancer.

Mrs. M was on the following medications: potassium chloride, famotidine, aspirin, a multivitamin (Centrum Silver), and furosemide.

Vestibular testing results revealed that she had a normal oculomotor battery, normal static positional testing, severely reduced vestibular responses bilaterally with present ice water calorics, and reduced gain on rotational chair testing. Patient had had two previous episodes where she had been on IV antibiotics. She had osteomyelitis of her toe 10 years ago, and 2 years ago she was again treated with IV antibiotics. Furosemide is a drug that can be ototoxic so the patient was counseled to consult with her physician about whether there was another medication that could control her lower extremity swelling without the same side effects.

The patient states that she occasionally gets dizzy with changing positions. Her DHI score was 12/100. She stated that the onset of her gait instability was gradual and that it was getting worse.

Patient lives alone in a condominium that is on one floor with an elevator in the building. She formerly worked as a superintendent of schools in her area. Mrs. M was widowed at an early age and raised two children alone.

Walking with head turns and quick head movements increased her symptoms. Her ABC score was 51 percent. She did not use an assistive device.

She had fallen twice in the last few weeks. She tripped over a box the first time and the second time she got tangled in a chair cover and lost her balance. Patient states that she also has had many near falls. She stated that she almost fell the morning of the evaluation while sitting down on the commode. Mrs. M reports difficulty getting up from the floor.

Patient's strength and range of motion were generally within normal limits for her age. She had diminished vibration sense but had intact proprioception distally at her ankles. She became short of breath with exertion during functional activities and gait.

Mrs. M's timed "Up & Go" score was 12.5 seconds. Her repeated five times sit to stand test score was 16.2 seconds. Her Sensory Organization Test composite score on the EquiTest (Neurocom International, Inc.) was 77. Her Berg Balance Score was 55/56 and her Dynamic Gait Index score was 19/24. The patient was able to stand in SLS for 15 seconds on the right and 10 seconds on the left.

Overall it appeared that the patient's balance was fairly good during testing except for during dynamic gait activities. She also reported falling two times in the last 4 weeks, which put her at high risk for another fall.

Goals for Mrs. M included to: improve her DGI from 19/24 to 22/24, improve her EquiTest composite score from 77 to 85, decrease her DHI score from 12/100 to 5/100, and improve her ABC from 51 to 70 percent.

The plan was to see the patient for 3 to 4 visits over the next 2 to 3 months to improve her dynamic balance, increase her stamina, and decrease her fear of falling. She agreed to the above goals. The plan was to discuss a pool exercise program with her to attempt to have her increase her strength and mobility in a non–weight-bearing exercise program that she might enjoy to avoid any increase in knee pain associated with her increase in activity level.

Mrs. M had been prescribed the following exercises: walking with head turns to the right and left, stepping up to a stool but not onto it and down, bending down toward the floor from the sitting position, a walking program, and walking with 180° turns. She was instructed to do the exercises two times a day.

The patient was seen four times in physical therapy. During her second visit, she reported that her physician had changed her diuretic. She had not fallen since her last visit to physical therapy. During her second physical therapy visit, it took her 20 seconds to rise from the chair 5 times, which was worse than her first visit. Her ABC score had increased by 11 percent to 65 percent and her DHI score increased from 12 to 22. Her DGI score had increased from 19 to 21/24. Her composite sensory organization test on the EquiTest was 82, which was an increase of 5. Patient was prescribed standing plantarflexion next to the kitchen sink, the trace the alphabet exercise with her foot, walking and turning 180°, walking with head turns, and walking and making 360° turns. She was told to try to do the exercises two times a day.

During her third physical therapy visit, the patient stated that she had been having difficulty finding time to do the exercises. She could do the alphabet exercise without holding on to the kitchen sink. Walking and looking up was a problem for her but walking backward was easier. Mrs. M was complaining of swelling in her feet. She was instructed to keep them elevated but was also shown how to perform ankle pumps and ankle isometrics. SLS times had improved to 21 seconds on the left and 20 seconds on the right. Her five times sit to stand test was 17.3 seconds and her composite sensory organization test was 77/100. Her DHI remained at 22/100 and her ABC was 64 percent.

Mrs. M was provided written ankle exercises, a SLS exercise, a seated exercise where she rolled a rolling pin under her foot, standing weight-shift exercises, and walking with head movements.

During the patient's fourth and final visit, she stated that she had difficulty with the standing weight shifts and that moving back onto her heels while balancing was difficult. The alphabet exercise and walking backward were not a problem for her. SLS continued to be a challenge for her balance. Patient reported that she had not been walking as the therapist had requested. Her DGI score had increased to 23/24. Her DHI score had remained at 22/100. Her sensory organization test remained at 76 and her ABC score was 61 percent. Her five times sit to stand had improved to 12 seconds and her timed "Up & Go" test was now 11 seconds. SLS times had improved to 28 seconds on the left and 30 seconds on the right.

Her home exercises for the fourth physical therapy visit consisted of standing in SLS and moving her head slightly to the right and left, walking on her toes in plantarflexion and standing in SLS on a pillow. In addition, she was given instructions for rejoining her cardiac exercise group.

Mrs. M was discharged at the end of her fourth clinic visit. She had made great strides with her walking and was no longer falling. The four visits were spaced out at 3-week intervals over a 3-month period. She had met one of her goals and had partially met 3 of the other 4 goals that were initially developed in her plan of care. She was satisfied with her progress and was instructed to join the cardiac exercise group that she had belonged to after she had her silent heart attack; she hated to exercise alone. One of her neighbors from her condominium was also attending the cardiac group program so she was encouraged to join her neighbor to improve her compliance. She preferred to read and perform less physically demanding activities. The physical therapist saw Mrs. M's daughter-in-law 6 weeks after discharge and she reported that Mrs. M still had not rejoined the exercise group but that she had not been falling. Her daughter-in-law was encouraged to "remind" Mrs. M to restart the cardiac exercise program because of her shortness of breath.

SUMMARY

Older adults with vestibular disorders have some unique differences compared to younger adults. The normal physiological changes associated with aging in the vestibular apparatus, the eye, and in somatosensation can complicate the rehabilitation of the older adult with a vestibular disorder. Older adults can improve with vestibular rehabilitation but may need special care. Comorbid medical problems that may be seen in older adults with vestibular disorders require the physical therapist to think carefully before initiating an intervention program. Patient safety and encouraging compliance with the intervention are essential. By carefully identifying the patient's functional limitations, a therapeutic program can be devised to restore the older adult's function safely.

REFERENCES

1. Kroenke, K, and Mangelsdorff, AD: Common symptoms in ambulatory care: Incidence, evaluation therapy and outcome. Am J Med 86:262, 1989.
2. Collard, M, and Chevalier, Y: Vertigo. Current Opinions in Neurology 7:88–92, 1994.
3. Bergstrom, B: Morphology of the vestibular nerve. II. The number of myelinated vestibular nerve fibers in man at various ages. Acta Otolaryngol 76:173–179, 1973.
4. Richter, E: Quantitative study of human scarpa's ganglion and vestibular sensory epithelium. Acta Otolaryngol (Stockh) 90:199–208, 1980.
5. Rosenhall, U: Degenerative patterns in the degenerating human vestibular neuro-epithelia. Acta Otolaryngol (Stockh) 76:208–220, 1973.
6. Wall, C, et al: Effects of age, sex and stimulus parameters upon vestibulo-ocular responses to sinusoidal rotation. Acta Otolaryngol (Stockh) 98:270–278, 1984.
7. Paige, GD: Vestibulo-ocular reflex (VOR) and adaptive plasticity with aging. Soc Neurosci Abstr 15, 1989.
8. Baloh, RW, et al: Quantitative vestibular function testing in elderly patients with dizziness. Ear Nose Throat 68:935–939, 1989.
9. Nadol, JB, and Schuknecht, HF: The pathology of peripheral vestibular disorders in the elderly. Ear Nose Throat 68:930–934, 1989.
10. Paige, GD: Senescence of human visual-vestibular interactions. 1. Vestibular-ocular reflex and adaptive plasticity with aging. J Vestib Res 2:133, 1992.
11. Ross, MD, et al: Observations on normal and degenerating human otoconia. Ann Otol Rhinol Laryngol 85:310, 1976.

12. Baloh, RW, et al: Benign positional vertigo: Clinical and oculographic features in 240 cases. Neurology 37:371–378, 1987.
13. Epley, JM: The canalith repositioning procedure: For treatment of benign paroxysmal positional vertigo. Otolaryngol Head Neck Surg 107:399, 1992.
14. Furman, J, and Cass, S: A practical work-up for vertigo. Contemp Intern Med 7:24, 1995.
15. Spooner, JN, et al: Effect of aging on eye tracking. Arch Neurol 37:575, 1980.
16. Sharpe, JA, and Sylvester, TO: Effect of aging on horizontal smooth pursuit. Invest Ophthalmol Vis Sci 17:465, 1978.
17. McMurdo, ME, and Gaskell, A: Dark adaptation and falls in the elderly. Gerontology 37:221, 1991.
18. Duncan, PW, et al: How do physiological components of balance affect mobility in elderly men? Arch Phys Med Rehabil 74:1343, 1993.
19. Arend, O, et al: Contrast sensitivity loss is coupled with capillary dropout in patients with diabetes. Invest Ophthalmol Visual Sci 38:1819, 1997.
20. Hirvela, H, et al: Visual acuity and contrast sensitivity in the elderly. Acta Ophthalmol Scand 73:111, 1995.
21. McNulty, L: Low vision impact on rehabilitation. Geriatr Notes 5:5, 1998.
22. U.S. National Safety Council, Home Checklist: For detection of Hazards, Itasca, IL, 1982.
23. Brockelhurst, JC, et al: Clinical correlation of sway in old age-sensory modalities. Age Aging 11:1, 1982.
24. Stelmach, GE, and Worringham, CJ: Sensorimotor deficits related to postural stability: Implications for falling in the elderly. Clin Geriatr Med 1:679, 1985.
25. Richardson, J, and Ashton-Miller, J: Peripheral neuropathy: An often-overlooked cause of falls in the elderly. Peripheral Neuropathy 6:161, 1996.
26. Richardson, J, et al: Moderate peripheral neuropathy impairs weight transfer and unipedal balance in the elderly. Arch Phys Med Rehab 77:1152, 1996.
27. Braun, E, et al: Balance abilities of older adults with and without diabetes. Issues Aging 19:19, 1996.
28. Rossiter-Fornoff, J, and the FICSIT Group: A cross-sectional validation study of the FICSIT common data base static balance measures. J Gerontol 50A:M291, 1995.
29. Horak, FB, and Nashner, L: Central programming of postural movements: Adaptation to altered support surface configurations. J Neurophysiol 55:1369, 1986.
30. Gill-Body, K, et al: Rehabilitation of balance in two patients with cerebellar dysfunction. Phys Ther 77:534, 1997.
31. Tinetti, ME, et al: Falls efficacy as a measure of fear of falling. J Gerontol Psych Sci 45:P239, 1990.
32. Tinetti, M, and Williams, C: Falls and risk of admission to a nursing home. New Engl J Med 337:1279, 1997.
33. Hill, K, et al: Fear of falling revisited. Arch Phys Med Rehab 77:1025, 1996.
34. Shumway-Cook, A, et al: The effects of two types of cognitive tasks on postural stability in older adults with and without a history of falls. J Gerontol Med Sci 52A:M232, 1997.
35. Ludin-Olsson, L, et al: "Stops walking when talking" as a predictor of falls in elderly people. Lancet 349:617, 1997.
36. Lajoie, Y, et al: Upright standing and gait: Are there changes in attentional requirements related to normal aging? Exp Aging Res 22:185, 1996.
37. Maki, B, and McIlroy, W: Influence of arousal and attention on the control of postural sway. J Vestib Res 6:53, 1996.
38. Yesavage, JA, and Brink, TL: Development and validation of a geriatric depression screening scale: A preliminary report. J Psychiatr Res 17:37, 1983.
39. Whitney, SL, et al: The association between observed gait instability and fall history in persons with vestibular dysfunction. (Submitted) J Vestib Res 1999.
40. Berg, K, and Norman, K: Functional assessment of balance and gait. Clin Geriatr Med 12:705, 1996.
41. Berg, K, et al: Measuring balance in the elderly: Preliminary development of an instrument. Physiother Canada 41:304, 1989.
42. Berg, K, et al: The balance scale: Reliability assessment with elderly residents and patients with an acute stroke. Scand J Rehab Med 27:27, 1995.
43. Berg, KO, et al: Clinical and laboratory measures of postural balance in an elderly population. Arch Phys Med Rehab 73:1073, 1992.
44. Berg, KO, et al: Measuring balance in the elderly: Validation of an instrument. Canadian J Public Health 83:S7, 1992.
45. Wood-Dauphinee, S, et al: The Balance scale: Responsiveness to clinically meaningful change. Canadian J Rehab 10:35, 1997.
46. Thorbahn, LD, and Newton, RA: Use of the Berg Balance test to predict falls in elderly patients. Phys Ther 76:576, 1996.
47. Shumway-Cook, A, et al: Predicting the probability for falls in community-dwelling older adults. Phys Ther 77:812, 1997.
48. Duncan, P, et al: Functional reach: A new clinical measure of balance. J Gerontol 45:M192, 1990.
49. Duncan, PW, et al: Functional reach: Predictive validity in a sample of elderly male veterans. J Gerontol 47: M93, 1992.

50. Mann, GC, et al: Functional reach and single leg stance in patients with peripheral vestibular disorders. J Vestib Res 6:343, 1996.
51. Studenski, S, et al: Predicting falls: The role of mobility and nonphysical factors. J Am Geriatr Soc 42:297, 1994.
52. Weiner, DK, et al: Does functional reach improve with rehabilitation. Arch Phys Med Rehab 74:796, 1993.
53. Weiner, DK, et al: Functional reach: A marker of physical frailty. J Am Geriatr Soc 40:203, 1992.
54. Myers, AM, et al: Psychological indicators of balance confidence: Relationship to actual and perceived abilities. J Gerontol 51A:M37, 1996.
55. Powell, LE, and Myers, AM: The activities-specific balance confidence (ABC) scale. J Gerontol 50A:M28, 1995.
56. Whitney, SL, et al: The activities-specific balance confidence scale and the dizziness handicap inventory: A comparison. J Vestib Res (in press).
57. Arroyo, JF, et al: Fast evaluation test for mobility, balance, and fear: A new strategy for the screening of elderly fallers. Arthritis Rheum 37:S416, 1994.
58. DiFabio, RP, and Seay, R: Use of the "Fast evaluation of mobility, balance, and fear" in elderly community dwellers: Validity and reliability. Phys Ther 77:904, 1997.
59. Jacobson, GP, and Newman, CW: The development of the dizziness handicap inventory. Arch Otolaryngol Head Neck Surg 116:424, 1990.
60. Ware, JE, and Sherbourne, CD: The MOS 36-Item short-form health survey (SF-36) I. Conceptual framework and item selection. Medical Care 30:473, 1992.
61. Enloe, LJ, and Shields, RK: Evaluation of health-related quality of life in individuals with vestibular disease using disease-specific and general outcome measures. Phys Ther 77:890, 1997.
62. Bohannon, R, et al: Decrease in timed balance test scores with aging. Phys Ther 64:1067, 1984.
63. O'Loughllin, J: Incidence of and risk factors for falls and injurious falls among the community-dwelling elderly. Am J Epidemiol 137:342, 1993.
64. Vellas, BJ, et al: One-leg balance is an important predictor of injurious falls in older persons. J Am Geriatr Soc 45:735, 1997.
65. Black, FO, et al: Normal subject postural sway during the Romberg test. Am J Otolaryngol 3:309, 1982.
66. Newton, R: Review of tests of standing balance abilities. Br Injury 3:335, 1989.
67. Anacker, SL, and Di Fabio, RP: Influence of sensory inputs on standing balance in community-dwelling elders with a recent history of falling. Phys Ther 72:575, 1992.
68. Baraff, LJ, et al: Practice guidelines for the ED management of falls in community-dwelling elderly persons. Ann Emerg Med 30:480, 1997.
69. Province, M, et al for the FICSIT Group: The effects of exercise on falls in elderly patients. JAMA 273:1341, 1995.
70. Lichtenstein, M, et al: Exercise and balance in aged women: A pilot controlled clinical trial. Arch Phys Med Rehab 2:138, 1989.
71. Lord, S, and Castell, S: Physical activity program for older persons: Effect on balance, strength, neuromuscular control, and reaction time. Arch Phys Med Rehab 6:648, 1994.

CHAPTER 23

Treatment of Patients with Nonvestibular Dizziness and Disequilibrium

Neil Shepard, PhD
Annamarie Asher, PT

There are numerous causes for patients to complain of symptoms related to vertigo, disequilibrium, light-headedness, unsteadiness, or a combination thereof. Although the majority of these complaints arise associated with direct insults limited to the peripheral vestibular apparatus, other disorders can manifest symptoms of a similar nature. Components of vestibular and balance rehabilitation programs are symptom driven; that is, the exercises are chosen to treat the patient's symptoms rather than being specific to the site of lesion or the diagnosis. Therefore, these exercises are potentially applicable to the symptoms produced by a wide variety of etiologies and lesions.[1-3] Scattered results suggest that the approach utilized with the stable peripheral vestibular insult (i.e., no complaints of spontaneously occurring symptoms), may be successfully used to treat patients with nonvestibular dizziness. There are no prospectively or retrospectively designed studies to directly address this issue. This chapter will discuss the challenges of identifying patients with vestibular compared to nonvestibular dizziness. The chapter will also describe the treatment approach used for patients with nonvestibular dizziness and present outcomes for patients seen at the Vestibular Testing Center at the University of Michigan Medical Center. It is critical for the reader to understand that, because the data reported here were not developed from a designed research study, they are useful only to suggest *trends* that would require formally designed studies to verify. No effort was made to control other medical treatments that may have been provided at the same time and which may have affected symptoms.

PATIENT IDENTIFICATION

Ruling Out a Vestibular Problem

Although specific exercise programs are based on patient symptoms in our clinic, treatment of the patient with a vestibular deficit and their families in our clinic includes an explanation of vestibular function, the patient's clinical and laboratory examination findings, and the rationale for the exercise program. It is therefore important for the therapist to consider whether or not the symptoms, which are revealed in the history and physical examination, are due to vestibular involvement or not. For the patients presented later in this chapter, electronystagmography (ENG) and rotational chair results were used to determine if an individual had peripheral vestibular involvement. In reality, if laboratory testing is normal or of marginal significance, other pieces of evidence such as hearing loss, other otological symptoms, and/or history of a vestibular crisis (prolonged and severe vertigo) at the onset of the condition are used in determining the role the peripheral vestibular system is playing in generating the patient's symptoms (see Chapters 6, 8, and 9). Current vestibular testing procedures, which rely on recordings of nystagmus and measurements of a variety of parameters on rotational chair testing, focus largely on horizontal canal function and leave much of the system untested. To complicate matters further, there are disorders such as Ménière's disease in which vestibular test results may be normal.

Nonvestibular Dizziness

Conditions other than vestibular disorders may cause symptoms of dizziness and disequilibrium. For some of these conditions it is reasonable to use balance and habituation exercises in an attempt to decrease symptoms and improve function. For others the patient should be referred to an appropriate specialist for evaluation and treatment. Vascular causes of dizziness in the elderly are common. This may be due to vertebral artery compromise, which will cause dizziness when the neck is extended while laterally flexed and rotated to the involved side. A sitting vertebral artery test is used to differentiate this type of dizziness from benign positional vertigo and should be used prior to the Dix-Hallpike maneuver in all elderly patients. If the vertebral artery test is positive, the patient should be referred to their physician for further evaluation.

The other common cause of vascular dizziness in the elderly is orthostatic intolerance, which can be present even if a drop in blood pressure is not measured in the arm. The patient complains of dizziness upon rising only and it is most severe in the morning or any time they try to rise after lying down for a prolonged period. Because we do not expect this type of dizziness to reduce by repeating the provocative maneuver, habituation exercises that involve rising quickly as the primary movement are not prescribed for our elderly patients with orthostatic intolerance. These patients may benefit from exercise programs to improve muscle tone, endurance, and overall mobility. Transient ischemic attacks may cause dizziness, which is unpredictable and not related to movement or position changes. For elderly patients experiencing these types of symptoms and with a history of vascular disease a referral to a neurologist should be made. Occasionally patients are referred to our clinic with yet undiagnosed neurological conditions (e.g., seizure disorder or Arnold-Chiari malformation). If the therapist is uncomfortable treating the patient because the cause of dizziness is not clear, he or she should determine, by chart review or by speaking with the referring physician, that vascular and neurological causes of the dizziness have been ruled out or are currently being evaluated.

Dizziness is reported in the literature as being commonly associated with panic attacks and migraine disorders (see Chapters 13 and 14). It is difficult to determine to what degree these conditions cause dizziness because it varies from patient to patient. It is possible that the dizziness is completely related to the migraine or panic disorder, or it is possible that a patient with migraine or panic disorder may have another cause for their dizziness. If symptoms are appropriate, it is reasonable to use habituation exercises in an attempt to reduce these symptoms.

Several groups of patients have been identified as those for whom the symptom complaints are similar to vestibular patients and for whom exercises from a vestibular and balance rehabilitation program may be applicable. Inclusion in the therapy program is considered appropriate if the patient's symptoms are:

- Provoked by head or visual motion.
- Constant symptoms exacerbated by head or visual motion.
- Unsteadiness in gait and/or stance.

These criteria describe a stable condition, one that does not vary in its overall character with time as would occur with patients describing symptoms that only occur in a spontaneous manner without provocation. Those patients with complaints of spontaneous events of disequilibrium, involving vertigo or not, are considered either inappropriate or of a poor prognosis contingent on the frequency or duration of the spontaneous events and presence of motion-provoked symptoms between the events.[4]

TREATMENT PROGRAM FOR PATIENTS WITH NONVESTIBULAR DIZZINESS

Patients were evaluated using the same tools and procedures that we use for vestibular patients. This included stance and walking activities, motion sensitivity testing using up to 16 rapid changes in head position, which included Dix-Hallpike maneuvers, and a clinical test for dynamic visual acuity (see Chapter 15). If significant unsteadiness was discovered, the evaluation also included lower extremity strength, range of motion (ROM), and vibratory sense in the feet and ankles. Patients were questioned as to whether or not they had visually provoked symptoms. These can be described as symptoms that occur when there is movement occurring around the patient, when the patient is moving in a visually stimulating environment (e.g., grocery or department stores), or with their own eye movements. If patients responded positively to that question they were evaluated with the vestibular adaptation exercises and $\times 1$ and $\times 2$ viewing (see Chapter 17) to determine whether or not these activities could reproduce their symptoms.

The most common problems that emerged from the evaluation of these patients were motion- and visually-provoked dizziness and unsteadiness. Patients did not demonstrate significant gaze instability or specific positional vertigo. As stated, patients were not included in this discussion if they had spontaneous spells of dizziness or unsteadiness. The treatment plan was individualized depending on which of these problems existed. Motion- and visually-provoked symptoms were treated with habituation exercises (see Chapter 17). In some cases, vestibular adaptation exercises were included but not for the purpose of improving gaze stability (see Chapter 17). The ×1 and ×2 viewing paradigm exercises were used as a habituation exercise in an attempt to reduce visually provoked dizziness with repeated exposure to the provocative stimulus and symptoms. Other head motions were chosen based on their response to motion-sensitivity testing. Many patients with visual sensitivity were also instructed to walk in visually challenging environments. They were told to seek out environments that felt challenging but did not overwhelm them with dizziness, nausea, or cause symptoms that persisted for longer than 15 minutes after they left the environment. Balance activities were prescribed based on the functional deficits found in the evaluation and a discussion of these types of activities can be found in Chapter 15.

The majority of the patients were given a home exercise program to perform twice a day for 4 to 6 weeks. If the patients demonstrated significant unsteadiness on examination or for other reasons it was felt they could not safely and accurately carry out the treatment program, they were referred to physical therapy near their home for a supervised program. The patients then visited the physical therapist 1 to 3 times per week for 4 to 8 weeks. They also practiced activities at home when the therapist felt it was safe for the patient to do so. Instructions for activities based on the initial evaluation at the authors' facility were made available to the supervising therapist. Follow-up information was obtained by reevaluation at our clinic after 4 to 6 weeks or, if that was not possible owing to the patient's difficulty in traveling to our clinic, by follow-up questionnaire.

OUTCOME MEASURES

Therapy outcome was indicated by two global measures: disability score and posttherapy symptom score. Additionally, a single specific measure of sensitivity to head movement, the Motion Sensitivity quotient (MSQ), and dynamic posturography for postural control were used.[2,5] The MSQ is a single number calculated from scores

---

BOX 23–1 Disability Score

Score	Description
0	No disability; negligible symptoms
1	No disability; bothersome symptoms
2	Mild disability; performs usual work duties, but symptoms interfere with outside activities
3	Moderate disability; symptoms disrupt performance of both usual work duties and outside activities
4	Recent severe disability; on medical leave or had to change job because of symptoms, off work for less than 12 months
5	Long-term severe disability; unable to work for over 1 year or established permanent disability with compensation payments

---

BOX 23–2   Posttherapy Symptom Score

Score	Description
0	No symptoms remaining at the end of therapy
1	Marked improvement in symptoms, mild symptoms remaining
2	Mild improvement, definite persistent symptoms remaining
3	No change in symptoms relative to pretherapy period
4	Symptoms worsened with therapy activities on a persistent basis relative to pretherapy period

---

obtained by rating the intensity and duration of symptoms following each of 16 rapid head movements. The number is given in percentage, with 0 to 10 mild; 11 to 20 moderate; and greater than 30 severe. The scale is highly nonlinear but reflects a change in the symptom intensity, duration of symptoms, or the number of rapid head movements, which provoked symptoms. Details of this measure have been previously published.[5] The specific measure of dynamic posturography will not be reported because this measure was normal on the vast majority of the patients, and very few patients had it repeated at the conclusion of their active therapy period. A disability score (Box 23–1) was assigned by the authors based on questioning the patient as to the impact of the symptoms on daily activities.

A posttherapy symptom score (Box 23–2) was assigned to each patient using the follow-up questionnaire or during the final evaluation. The score was determined in response to a series of specific questions that had the patient compare symptoms at the end of active therapy to those prior to therapy.

DIAGNOSTIC CATEGORIES AND RESULTS

Each of the patient groups to be discussed met the above-listed criteria regarding their symptom presentation. To rule out the possibility of unstable peripheral vestibular involvement, none of the patients reviewed had complaints of spontaneous events. Site-of-lesion determination was made based on a full series of studies including but not limited to, ENG, extensive ocular motor evaluation, rotational chair testing, and dynamic posturography.[6] In the patients presented here, no findings were obtained that would imply peripheral vestibular system involvement except as indicated below. Age was not a restriction.

For each of the groups, Table 23–1 summarizes the two global outcome measures of disability and symptoms, with changes in MSQ when available. A negative MSQ score indicates that the patient worsened regarding intensity, duration, or the number of the 16 head movement positions that caused their symptoms by the end of active therapy.

Mal de Debarquement

Most individuals exiting from a ship (and occasionally train travel) after a cruise of a day or longer experience a continuing sensation of rocking and/or other forms of

TABLE 23–1 Therapy Outcomes

Patient Group	Disability Score (Pretreatment)	Disability Score (Posttreatment)	Change in MSQ (%)	Posttherapy Symptom Score
Mal de debarquement ($n = 4$)	2.75 ± 0.96	1 ± 0.0	1.25 ± 2.9 ($n = 2$)	1.0 ± 0.0
Migraine ($n = 6$)	2.67 ± 1.03	2.17 ± 1.3	0.33 ± 20.01 ($n = 3$)	2.0 ($n = 3$) 1.83 ± 1.2
Disequilibrium of aging ($n = 4$)	1.5 ± 0.58	1.0 ± 0.82	3.8 ($n = 1$)	1.00 ± 0.82
All tests normal ($n = 10$)	2.8 ± 1.2	1.3 ± 1.1	7.7 ± 5.1 ($n = 3$)	1.2 ± 1.1 ($n = 9$)
Primary anxiety or panic ($n = 6$)	3.3 ± 0.5	3.67 ± 0.5	0.6 ± 0.85 ($n = 2$)	2.33 ± 1.2
Central nervous system lesions ($n = 24$)	2.67 ± 1.3	2.29 ± 1.4	2.01 ± 16.45 ($n = 16$)	2.0 ± 0.9

linear shipboard movement. These perceptions are especially prominent when the individual is sitting or standing still, and typically abate after 12 to 36 hours.[7] For a small percentage of otherwise healthy persons, the feeling of movement does not resolve after the usual time interval. This perseveration of dominantly linear movement sensations when the patient is still or involved with ambulation is currently felt to be a difficulty of the central nervous system in handling changing information arising from the otolith organs.[7,8] The implication is that this disorder does not involve identifiable malfunction of the peripheral mechanism, especially that of the semicircular canals. The natural history of this disorder is spontaneous resolution within a 6- to 12-month interval. Because the majority of these patients do not have specific head motion–provoked symptoms or balance deficits, the therapy programs provided to these patients involved walking programs with head movements in the horizontal and/or vertical planes.

The outcome measures (see Table 23–1) indicate consistent improvement in symptoms and disability pre- versus posttherapy in the four patients with follow-up out of the six who were seen in our clinic during a 4.5-year interval. Caution is needed in interpreting these data given the natural history of spontaneous improvement.

Migraine

These patients carried a primary diagnosis of migraine headaches and had only complaints of head motion- or visually-provoked symptoms of disequilibrium. For some of these patients testing results would suggest the possibility of peripheral involvement from positional nystagmus, although these findings were interpreted to be manifestations of the primary disorder of migraine headaches. None of the patients reported had abnormal caloric evaluations. In addition to customized habituation and balance therapy exercises, these patients were also being treated independently with medication therapy for the headache condition.

A modest reduction in symptom score was seen in four of the six patients with migraine, with two of the patients reporting a positive change in level of disability. The treatment for each of these patients consisted of habituation exercises together with medication for prophylactic and abortive control of the headaches. Because the treatment methods were used simultaneously the relative contribution of each to the problem is not clear. In general, the prevalence of forms of dizziness with migraine headaches would be considerably greater than the 11 patients in 4.5 years reviewed.[9,10] Yet, in our clinical experience the larger percentage have spontaneous events together with motion sensitivity or only spontaneous spells of symptoms; these patients were not included in this retrospective review.

Disequilibrium Associated with Aging

Previous published work suggests that patients over the age of 65 with dominantly peripheral vestibular system insults do equally well in a vestibular and balance rehabilitation program as the younger patients; however results may take longer to achieve.[11] Work in normal elderly subjects suggests an ability to alter their biomechanical balance abilities with exercises, and the possibility that this may result in reduced risk for falls.[12–14] The implication is that the age of the patient does not alter the plasticity of the system. The patients selected in this group were all over the age of 65, carrying the diagnosis of disequilibrium associated with aging, and had no test results interpreted as indicating primary peripheral vestibular involvement. However, other systems including proprioception/somatosensory (typically in the form of reduced vibratory sensations in the distal lower limbs), vision (cataracts most commonly), and musculoskeletal (arthritic joints) involvement was not uncommon. The other important feature common to these patients was the history of gradual onset of symptoms without reported history of a vestibular crisis style event at the onset.

The four patients for whom follow-up information is available (see Table 23–1) demonstrate only modest improvement trends compared with a group of elderly having primary peripheral system involvement reported previously.[11] The other 21 individuals in this diagnostic category had supervised therapy at local facilities because the distance from their home to our laboratory was prohibitive for regular return visits; therefore, outcome measures were not available. The tendency for less improvement in this elderly group compared with the elderly population with primarily peripheral vestibular involvement may be due to their multisensory involvement, even though pretherapy disability levels are comparable between the two groups. There was, however, only slight improvement for the outcome measures used here, and the elderly patients in this type of program often describe increased function, primarily in their ability to ambulate independently outside of their home.

All Test Findings Normal

A small percentage of patients with head- and visual motion-provoked spells of vertigo, light-headedness, and unsteadiness have entirely normal findings on all of the testing and no history suggesting other causes for their symptoms. Table 23–1 gives the therapy outcomes for a group of 10 of the 25 meeting these criteria for the review. The remainder were lost to follow-up. This group was large enough to apply simple statistics with mean change in disability level of 1.8 and a mean pretherapy disability level of 2.8. The mean posttherapy symptom score was 1.2. Seventy percent (7/10) were able to decrease their disability score by at least 1 point and 78 percent (7/9) had posttherapy symptom scores of less than 3 indicating significant reduction in symptoms. The history and clinical presentation of these patients would suggest a mild form of peripheral system involvement, unable to be verified with ENG or use of rotational chair testing.

Primary Anxiety and Panic

A large percentage of patients with intractable disequilibrium, independent of the specific nature of the symptoms, develop anxiety and panic disorders. In many cases this does appear secondary to the initial symptoms associated with a vestibular insult. There is, however, a population of patients for whom the symptoms of head movement–provoked vertigo, light-headedness, unsteadiness, or combinations are a manifestation of a primary anxiety and panic disorder.[15–18] In mild forms of secondary development of anxiety and panic symptoms, the exposure therapy that occurs with habituation exercises for head and visual motion appears effective in reducing the overall symptom complex. The group of six patients reviewed, identified over an 8-week interval, are considered to have primary anxiety or panic disorders as the source of their complaints of "dizziness" with no indications of peripheral or central vestibular system involvement. Each of the patients reviewed was undergoing simultaneous treatment for their primary disorder by a psychiatrist or behavioral therapist. The vestibular and balance rehabilitation programs were administered independent of the other treatment without an effort to coordinate the two forms of treatment. It is of interest that of the six patients, three note improvement in symptoms of head movement provoked–disequilibrium, yet none of the group had improvement in their significant predisability scores (see Table 23–1). Three of the six report worsening in disability level even though one indicated concomitant reduction in symptoms. It is speculated that this dichotomy may reflect the ability to reduce the disequilibrium symptoms associated with head movement, yet the disability in this group is probably secondary to their ongoing fear to engage in routine daily activities, or volitional restriction in driving, associated with their anxiety disorder.

Central Nervous System Lesions

The largest of the special groups considered in this review are those with indications for central nervous system (CNS) disorders. Patients demonstrated repeatable indications of central vestibulo-ocular pathway involvement. General indications of vestibulocerebellar involvement were suspected in the majority of those reviewed. In only one case was a clear brainstem infarct noted. None of these patients had findings that would suggest concomitant peripheral system involvement. In this population, the principle complaint involved unsteadiness and ataxia with gait. Head motion–provoked or exacerbated symptoms were much less frequent. Of the 78 patients that were identified as appropriate for therapy, 24 were managed directly in our facility with the remaining 54 referred out to programs closer to their homes and thus were lost to follow-up. Of the 24, indications for sites of lesion were as follows:

- Sixteen with general ocular motor indications of vestibulocerebellar involvement
- Two with MRI-identified basal ganglia involvement and suspected diagnosis of progressive supranuclear palsy
- One with definite multiple sclerosis
- One olivopontocerebellar atrophy with primary cerebellar involvement by MRI
- One pons-level brainstem stroke
- Three primary cerebellar strokes

Table 23–1 gives the outcome parameter details. The mean posttherapy symptom score was 2 with a standard deviation of 0.9, suggesting a mild to moderate reduction in symptoms; yet as seen with other groups above, disability level did not show the corresponding reduction with a mean change of 0.3. Only 29 percent (7/24) of these patients were able to decrease their disability score by 1 or more points. Furthermore, 67 percent (16/24) had posttherapy symptom scores of less than 3. In a previous review[2] the central lesion patients have not differed significantly from the performance of the peripheral lesion patients; however, in that report the small group was dominated with brainstem as opposed to cerebellar lesions.

SUMMARY

Although only sparse data were available for many of the groups considered, we see no reason why the vestibular rehabilitation assessment should be altered for the various sites of lesion or diagnoses that may, by symptom complaints, be appropriate for the use of a vestibular and balance rehabilitation program. The assessment process used focused on determination of provocative activities in the form of head and/or visual motion stimuli that would cause symptoms and determination of functional deficits of balance and gait that were present as a result of the symptoms. This process also recognized deficits of balance and gait that were the primary complaint, without the presence of transient or constant symptoms of vertigo or light-headedness. Based on current knowledge, the use of a consistent format for assessment of these patients is appropriate and not in need of change to be able to achieve improved results.

For the patients in the all-test-results-normal group, overall performance is not different from those with known stationary vestibular lesions who participate in a vestibular and balance rehabilitation program. The mal de debarquement group show a trend for improvement with therapy also, but this may be nothing more than the natural history of the disorder. Whether the therapy programs help to increase the rate at which resolution of symptoms with this disorder occurs cannot be answered with the present data or other retrospective reviews.

The relatively poorer performance for the migraine, disequilibrium associated with aging, and anxiety/panic disorder patients compared to the peripheral vestibular lesion group may well be explained by the fact that these disorders do not primarily affect the vestibular system. Therefore, it is difficult to project how changes in the typical vestibular and balance rehabilitation program would allow for improved outcomes unless those changes affected the primary underlying disorder. In patients of this type, exercises are only an adjunct to the primary treatment efforts. It is reasonable that the outcome of therapy, although showing modest improvement in isolated dimensions, is ultimately dependent on the effectiveness of the primary treatment for the underlying condition.

A different line of reasoning may apply to the CNS lesion group, where the insult in the majority of the patients directly involves the pathways within the balance system, although not the labyrinth. The assumption is that a cerebellar lesion, even when stable, interferes with compensation. Clearly, although habituation exercises may reduce some of the head- or visual motion–provoked symptoms, these symptoms are not the only cause for standing or gait imbalance, as may be the case in peripheral injuries alone. Therefore, alternative approaches that also provide for direct retraining of coordination ability with the other aspects of a vestibular and balance rehabilitation program used in the peripheral cases may improve the overall outcome. What alternative approaches may be applicable has not been demonstrated; however, activities such as rhythmic patterning with dance therapy suggests the possibility of altering motor control patterns.[19–21]

Recognition of patients for whom the symptom complaints are not the direct result of an insult to the balance system per se does not prevent use of a vestibular and balance rehabilitation program as an adjunct treatment. Habituation exercises in particular appear to be a promising approach. It does, however, require counseling of the patient for realistic goals and appropriate emphasis on what should be the primary treatment modality. For those where the natural history is for spontaneous resolution, one must be cautious about assuming the effects of a therapy program.

Further efforts are needed to develop alternative treatment methods for those patients with nonperipheral vestibular system insults resulting in disequilibrium. These changes in treatment considerations could benefit the patients with multisensory deficits, such as disequilibrium associated with aging patients or head trauma patients (see Chapters 20 and 22).

REFERENCES

1. Horak, FB, et al: Effects of vestibular rehabilitation on dizziness and imbalance. Otolaryngol Head Neck Surg 106:175, 1992.
2. Shepard, NT, et al: Vestibular and balance rehabilitation therapy. Ann Otol Rhinol Laryngol 102:198, 1993.
3. Borello-France, DF, et al: Assessment of vestibular hypofunction. In Herdman, SJ (ed): Vestibular Rehabilitation. FA Davis, Philadelphia, 1994, p 247.
4. Shepard, NT, and Telian, SA: Programmatic vestibular rehabilitation. Otolaryngol Head Neck Surg 112:173, 1995.
5. Smith-Wheelock, M, et al: Physical therapy program for vestibular rehabilitation. Am J Otol 12:218, 1991.
6. Shepard, NT, and Telian, SA: Practical Management of the Balance Disorder Patient. Singular Publishing Group, San Diego, 1996.
7. Gordon, CR, et al: Clinical features of mal de debarquement: Adaptation and habituation to sea conditions. J Vestib Res 5:363, 1995.
8. Hain, TC, et al: Localizing value of optokinetic afternystagmus. Ann Otol Rhinol Laryngol 103:806, 1994.
9. Furman, JM, and Cass, SP: Balance Disorders: A Case-Study Approach. FA Davis, Philadelphia, 1996, p 108.
10. Cass, SP, et al: Migraine-related vestibulopathy. Ann Otol Rhinol Laryngol 106:182, 1997.
11. Smith-Wheelock, M, et al: Balance retraining therapy in the elderly. In Kashima, H, et al (eds): Clinical Geriatric Otolaryngology. BC Decker, Philadelphia, 1992, p 71.
12. Ledin, T, et al: Effects of balance training in elderly evaluated by clinical tests and dynamic posturography. J Vestib Res 1:129, 1991.
13. Hu, MH, and Woollacott, MH: Multisensory training of standing balance in older adults: I. Postural stability and one-leg stance balance. J Gerontol Med Sci 49:M52, 1994.
14. Hu, MH, and Woollacott, MH: Multisensory training of standing balance in older adults: II. Kinematic and electromyographic postural responses. J Gerontol Med Sci 49:M62, 1994.
15. Jacob, R: Panic disorder and the vestibular system. Psychiatr Clin North Am 11:361, 1988.
16. Furman, JM, et al: Vestibular function in patients with agoraphobia or height phobia. J Vestib Res 6:S30, 1996.
17. Furman, JM, and Cass, SP: Balance Disorders: A Case-Study Approach. FA Davis, Philadelphia, 1996, p 97.
18. Jacob, R, et al: Psychiatric aspects of vestibular disorders. In Baloh, RW, and Halmagyi, GM (eds): Disorders of the Vestibular System. Oxford University Press, New York, 1996, p 509.
19. Wolf, M: Music & TBI: A new approach to therapy. Advance for Occupational Therapists, February, 1990.
20. Altenmüller, E, et al: Music learning produces changes in brain activation patterns: A longitudinal DC-EEG Study. IJAM 5:28, 1997.
21. Thaut, MH, et al: Music versus metronome timekeeper in a rhythmic motor task. Int J Appl Music 5:4, 1997.
22. Herdman, SJ: Vestibular Rehabilitation. FA Davis, Philadelphia, 1994.

CHAPTER 24

Evaluation and Treatment of Vestibular and Postural Control Deficits in Children

Rose Marie Rine, PT, PhD

The vestibular system develops relatively early in gestation.[1-5] Investigations of the development and appropriate testing of this system have demonstrated that it is a dual function system. The functional vestibular system is comprised of vestibulo-ocular (VO) and vestibulospinal (Vsp) systems, each represented by distinct tasks and testing methods. Labyrinthine reflexes, which are mediated by the Vsp system, contribute to the postural tone necessary for the emergence of early motor milestones (e.g., rolling, sitting, standing).[6] The role of the VO system in visual stabilization, acuity, and the development of visual spatial and perception abilities has been well documented.[7-9] One can therefore logically deduce that individuals with deficits of the vestibular system since birth or very early in life will present with difficulties in either motor or visuospatial abilities, or both.[6,8,10]

The incidence of peripheral vestibular disorders in children, is similar to those in adults (e.g., Ménière's disease, perilymphatic fistula, etc.).[11-18] Furthermore, like adults with central nervous system (CNS) impairment, children with traumatic brain injury or other CNS insult may have central vestibular deficits. However, investigations of vestibular dysfunction in children with these diagnoses are scarce.[19-24] The functional integrity of the vestibular system is rarely tested in young children, and thus any impairment is undetected and untreated. This fact may be due, in part, to the child's inability to describe symptoms or even know that what they are experiencing is not "normal."[4,11] One of the major difficulties in the identification of vestibular dysfunction in children has been the unavailability or omission of traditional or recently developed tests of vestibular function for this population. This chapter will provide a review of the incidence of vestibular deficits in young children, the development of postural control abilities, and appropriate testing and intervention for this population.

INCIDENCE OF VESTIBULAR DEFICITS IN CHILDREN

There are numerous reports regarding vestibular dysfunction of various etiologies in young children.[11–17,19–24] Tsuzuku and Kaga[25] and others[21,22,26–28] have reported learning disabilities and delayed development of walking and balance abilities in children with vestibular system anomalies. Motor and balance deficits in young children with either sensorineural hearing impairment (SNHI) or evidence of vestibular hypofunction have also been reported (Figure 24–1 and Figure 24–2).[22,29–33] In spite of these reports, children with SNHI or complaints of dizziness are rarely tested for vestibular function. Casselbrandt et al[13] reported anomalies of postural control in children with otitis media that were reversed following insertion of tympanostomy tubes. However, vestibular function tests were not reported. Schaaff[28] noted that the incidence of vestibular disorders was high in developmentally delayed preschoolers with a history of otitis media. Furthermore, Eviatar and Eviatar[34] used per-rotary and cold caloric stimulation to examine vestibular function in full-term and premature infants. Their results indicated that in premature, low-birth-weight infants there is a maturational delay in vestibular system function evidenced by a reduced percent of positive nystagmus until 12 months of age. These investigators concluded that deviation of responses from the mean and standard deviation of the normative sample can be considered abnormal af-

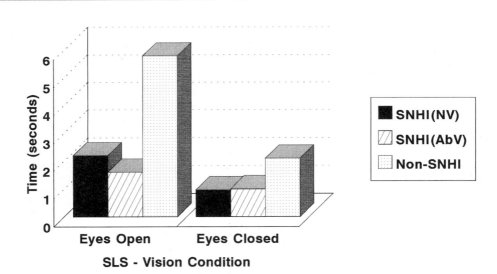

Single-leg Stance by Group

SNHI(NV) = SNHI with normal PRNT results
SNHI(AbV) = SNHI with Abnormal PRNT results
Non-SNHI = children without HI

FIGURE 24–1. Plot of mean single-leg stance times of children with and without sensorineural hearing impairment (SNHI). Children with SNHI and abnormal PRNT results score lower than those with SNHI and normal PRNT results. (From Rine, RM, et al: Balance and motor skills in young children with sensorineural hearing impairment: A preliminary study. Pediatr Phys Ther 8:55–61, 1996, with permission.)

Deviation of Mean Age Equivalent Scores From Actual Age (AE-Dev) Within the SNHI Group - by PRNT Results

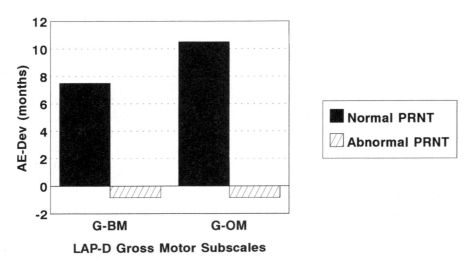

AE-Dev = Age equivalent score - chronological age
G-BM = Learning Accomplishment Profile Body Movement Scale
G-OM = Learning Accomplishment Profile Object Movement Scale

FIGURE 24–2. Plot demonstrating the difference of the mean deviation of age-equivalent scores achieved on the Learning Accomplishment Profile from chronological age between children with SNHI and normal PRNT results and those with SNHI and abnormal PRNT results. Those with abnormal PRNT achieved scores below age level. (From Rine, RM, et al: Balance and motor skills in young children with sensorineural hearing impairment: A preliminary study. Pediatr Phys Ther 8:55–61, 1996, with permission.)

ter the age of 12 months. Additionally, in spite of the documented functional relationship of the visual and vestibular systems, and the effect vestibular deficiency may have on gaze stability and oculomotor control,[8] children diagnosed with visuomotor deficits, using educational or developmental testing, are rarely tested for concurrent vestibular function or gaze stabilization deficits. However, interpretation of test results may be compounded by changes owing to adaptation or plasticity.

Investigations of plasticity and recovery of function support the idea that age at the time of injury or testing affects the neural and behavioral recovery.[35] In adults with unilateral lesions of the peripheral vestibular apparatus, recovery of function is well documented in the peripheral apparatus on vestibular tests. The fact that this recovery occurs despite no regeneration or recovery of the peripheral apparatus indicates that central neural substrate changes are responsible for the recovery. Based on evidence that the neural changes and functional recovery occurring in individuals with CNS damage depends on age at the time of the injury,[35] one can assume that the neural substrate changes seen in young children with vestibular deficits will be different from those of adults. Furthermore, these changes may mask the deficits typically noted with traditional testing methods. Rine et al[33] reported that the vestibular deficit noted during functional tasks and post-rotary nystagmus test results (on Southern California

Test of Postrotary Nystagmus or PRNT) are not identified by rotary chair testing (per-rotary nystagmus) in children diagnosed with SNHI since birth. The children with SNHI presented with delayed maturation of vestibular and vision ratios on posturography testing, hypoactive responses on PRNT, and balance abilities below age level (Figure 24–3). However, per-rotary nystagmus measures were within normal limits for the majority of the children tested. Further evidence of the dependence of recovery on age at the time of testing was reported by Horak et al[36] who found that adults with bilateral vestibular deficits since birth did not demonstrate the lack of leg muscle responses to perturbations evident in adults who had adult onset bilateral vestibular loss. However, activation of trunk muscles was delayed and smaller in amplitude in the early onset group as compared to either those without a deficit, or those with adult onset deficit (Figure 24–3). These results suggest that somatosensory inputs from the cervical and upper trunk areas compensated for the vestibular loss in the early onset but not the adult onset group. The variation of clinical symptoms seen with a peripheral vestibular deficit sustained early in life, versus in adulthood, may also be evident in children with central vestibular deficits.

Although vestibular and postural control deficits have been documented in adults with CNS involvement, similar investigations of children are scarce.[19–24] Like adults, children with traumatic brain injury or other CNS conditions should present with vestibular deficits. However, due to maturation issues involved in the development of

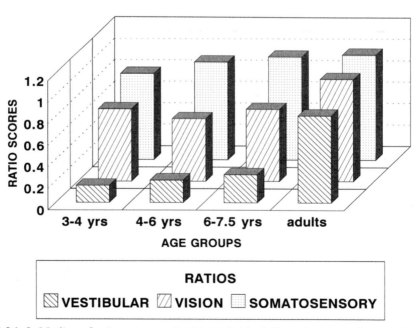

FIGURE 24–3. Median of ratio scores attained by individuals if varying age without deficits. (From Rine, RM, et al: Measurement of sensory system effectiveness and maturational changes in postural control in young children. Pediatr Phys Ther 10:16–22, 1998, with permission.)

postural control, and particularly the development of functional effectiveness of the vestibular system in postural control, the consequences to motor recovery may differ. Varied mechanisms of compensation and adaptation may mask vestibular deficits. Liao et al[23] reported poor static postural control under various sensory environments in children with spastic cerebral palsy. Although the muscle tone impairment involved is greatly responsible for these results, the fact that postural sway was significantly different between children with and without cerebral palsy only on the swayed surface (SS), eyes closed-swayed surface (ECSS), and swayed vision-swayed surface conditions (SVSS), and thus similar in all other conditions, suggests somatosensory preference, and vestibular impairment or neglect. The children with cerebral palsy did maintain balance like typically developing children with eyes closed, eyes open, and when the visual surround was sway referenced. If hypertonus alone could explain the balance deficits, abnormal sway measures should be evident on all conditions. Nashner et al[37] and others[20,22,24] reported similar results, as well as a reversal of muscle activation patterns. However, in none of these studies was vestibular function formally tested. The identification of a vestibular deficit is important to the development of appropriate intervention and for prognostic purposes. Further research is needed in this area, particularly because early identification and intervention during critical periods may affect recovery.

In summary, children, like adults, can and do have central and peripheral vestibular deficits. Reportedly, a delay in acquisition of motor skills and learning disabilities are evident in children with vestibular dysfunction.[21,22,26–28,33] To understand the implication of vestibular deficits early in life, as well as to enable the selection and interpretation of testing and the development of appropriate intervention for children, a review of the development of postural and oculomotor control as they relate to vestibular function is warranted.

DEVELOPMENT OF POSTURAL AND OCULOMOTOR CONTROL AS THEY RELATE TO VESTIBULAR SYSTEM FUNCTION

Numerous reports on the development of postural control support the idea that postural response synergies and the ability to use each of the sensory components for postural control are evident in young children learning to sit and walk. However, the muscle responses, weighting of different sensory information, and integrative abilities of postural control are not like those of adults until adolescence.[38–43] Forssberg and Nashner[38] and others[38–42] reported that, although the automatic responses to perturbation seen in adults were present and functional in young children, response latencies (e.g., short-, medium-, and long-latency) were significantly longer and matured at different rates. Haas et al[39] claimed that the change in short-latency responses to adult-like levels by 5 years of age reflected improved nerve conduction velocity. The long-latency response, reportedly an indicator of Vsp function,[39,44] was not reduced to adult-like levels until 15 years of age. The authors attributed this reduction in latency to acceleration of central polysynaptic transmission and myelinization. In addition, Woollacott and Shumway-Cook[41] noted increased variability of postural responses in 4- to 6-year-old children, and reported that the attenuation of response seen in seven year olds and adults was not observed in younger children. Additional studies demonstrated that the development of sensory integrative capacity and experience within a posture affect maturation of these muscle responses.[38,42,45]

Woollacott et al[42] reported that children without experience in sitting or standing did not demonstrate postural responses in these postures. In addition, although muscle responses occurred in response to perturbation in all experienced subjects (either sitting or standing), the temporal organization of postural responses of the youngest experienced sitters (8 to 10 months old) and standers (14 months old) differed from those of adults and older children. Instead of the typical distal to proximal sequence of muscle activation, proximal muscles (neck) initiated the response. Results of investigations by Forssberg and Nashner[38] revealed that children 3 through 10 years of age could maintain balance on all posturography test conditions. However, children less than 7.5 years of age performed like vestibular-deficient adults on the ECSS and SVSS conditions. Furthermore, Foudriat et al[45] reported that children 3 through 6 years of age had better stability on the swayed vision (SV) test, as compared to that attained on the SS test condition. Several conclusions may be gleaned from these reports: (1) experience within a posture is critical for the development of postural control abilities; (2) between 3 and 6 years of age, somatosensory function in postural control emerges, but in children less than 7.5 years, the visual and vestibular systems function in postural control is immature; (3) maturation of postural responses occurs in a stage-like pattern; and (4) the time period between the ages of 4 and 6 years is a transition period in which mature patterns are emerging. Investigators have suggested that these changes are due to maturation of individual sensory systems and the sensory integrative mechanisms contributing to postural control.[43,46-48] The integrative mechanisms involve the ability to coordinate and integrate multimodal sensory information to accurately detect vertical orientation.

Reportedly, although vision is dominant in the early stages of learning to balance in a posture, shorter latency proprioceptive responses are intact and more effectively used if visual information is removed.[42,46,47] Riach and Hayes[47] reported that the Romberg Quotients (RQ), the amount of sway with eyes closed expressed as a percentage of sway with eyes open, was below 100 in children less than 10 years of age. In adults, RQ is greater than 100. These results suggest that in young children, visual information dominates postural control but serves a destabilizing role. Riach and Starkes[46] reported that, like adults, children are able to reduce sway with visual fixation. However, younger children (3- to 5-year-olds) had an increased number of saccades during attempted visual fixation as compared to older children and adults. These investigators proposed that the increased saccades may be due to either an inability to visually fixate as well as adults, or an attempt to improve stability by increasing saccades. However, that conclusion is refuted by reports that the basic ability to stabilize visual flow with head and eye movements is acquired by 3 months of age.[8] VonHofsten and Rosander[8] noted that although a substantial lag in eye movement was evident in 1 month old infants, the lag was diminished by 3 months. This correction was attributed to maturity of both the visual and vestibular systems. Although infants can stabilize the visual environment, they may not be able to coordinate and integrate this information with other sensory system information regarding vertical orientation.

Hirabayashi and Iwasaki[43] and Rine et al[48] reported that although the effectiveness of somatosensory information was adult-like by 3 to 4 years of age, immaturity of visual and vestibular system function in postural control persisted through the age of 15. These investigators used the sensory organization test component of posturography to obtain stability scores under the varying conditions. To control for the maturational changes evident on all test conditions, ratio scores were calculated to provide a measure of sensory system effectiveness in postural control (see below).[43,48] The somatosensory ratio score (stability score on the SV condition/stability score on the eyes open [EO] condition) was similar to adults by 6 years of age. Although adult-like values on the visual function ratio (stability score on the SS condition/stability score on the EO condition) were achieved by 15 years of age, this was not true of vestibular function ratios (stability score on the ECSV condition/stability score on the EO condition).[43] However, all children over 4 years of age were able to maintain upright stance without stepping or assistance on all conditions (Figure 24–3).[43,48] This finding implies that, although at this age all sensory systems are functional in postural control, their effectiveness in postural control matures in a stage like fashion.

In summary, maturation of the functional contribution or effectiveness of the vestibular and visual systems continues through 15 years of age with the following noted: (1) although visual system effectiveness in postural control is less mature than that of the somatosensory system prior to age 7.5 years, it is the dominant source of information for postural control in standing; (2) VO mechanisms are intact and mature by 1 year of age; (3) the Vsp mechanism, or the effectiveness of the vestibular system in postural control, continues to develop beyond 15 years of age; and (4) the sensory integrative capacity required for postural control evolves between 7 and 15 years of age. The findings that development of postural control is affected by the integrity of all systems involved as well as practice and experience in a posture, suggest that deficits in any one system, in central processing capabilities, or in the ability to experience various upright postures, will impede development. Furthermore, findings that vestibular system functional contribution to oculomotor control matures by 1 year, but that its effectiveness in postural control is not adult-like until adolescence, indicates that the two vestibular motor systems mature at different rates and function separately. Therefore, a comprehensive assessment of vestibular function in children should include tests of both VO and Vsp function, which have been normed for this age group. This type of comprehensive vestibular assessment is important for: (1) the identification of deficits; and (2) the development of appropriate early interventions for children with motor, oculomotor, or postural control deficits, secondary to vestibular dysfunction.

EVALUATION

A comprehensive examination of vestibular function includes functional and diagnostic tests of VO and Vsp function.[8] Because diagnostic procedures are costly and may be uncomfortable, screening for appropriate referrals for in-depth testing is warranted for children with SNHI, recurrent inner ear infections, or symptoms indicative of vestibular dysfunction (Box 24–1). The screening, which can be provided by therapists, includes examination of motor and balance development, postural control abilities, perceptual and oculomotor control, and VO and Vsp function.[6,49] The purpose of these tests are threefold: (1) to establish that a functional balance deficit exists; (2) to isolate the contributions of the various components of the postural control system, and thus determine which component(s) is (are) problematic; and thus (3) to provide a basis for referral for further diagnostic testing and the development of remedial programs. Children who attain scores below age-appropriate levels and show a positive screening of Vsp or VO dysfunction should be referred for more comprehensive testing.

BOX 24–1   Symptoms of Vestibular Dysfunction in Children

Peripheral disorders

1. Persistent, obvious nystagmus (longer than 1 second) on head movement in the light or dark
2. Visual instability on head movement, complaints of blurring or double vision
3. Below age level balance abilities (e.g., tandem, single leg stance)
4. Complaints of spinning sensation or dizziness
5. Below age level vestibular ratios on posturography testing, unable to maintain upright on conditions 5 and 6
6. May or may not present increased latency on DPT[a] testing
7. Hypo- or hyperactive responses on PRNT[b]
8. May or may not have hearing loss or tinnitus
9. May be fearful of movement activities, or crave it
10. Complaint of incoordination

Central Disorders

1. Delay or below age level performance on gross motor tasks
2. Delay or below age level performance on visual motor, visual perception tests
3. Persistence of tonic reflexes
4. May present with increased latency and amplitude of responses on posturography DPT testing
5. Visual instability, particularly with head movement
6. Normal, hypo-, or hyperactive responses on PRNT, although majority either hypo- or hyperactive
7. Below age level performance on dynamic posturography SOT[c] with stepping or loss of balance on conditions 4 through 6
8. Below age level vision and vestibular rations on posturography SOT
9. Possible sensory integrative dysfunction

[a]Dynamic perturbation test component of posturography test
[b]Post-rotary nystagmus test
[c]Sensory organization test component of posturography test

Functionally, balance represents postural control or Vsp abilities, and aberrant persistence of labyrinthine reflexes interferes with balance ability. Clinical functional measures of balance that have been normed and standardized for use with children include the Functional Reach Test,[50] the balance subtest of the Peabody Developmental Motor Scales (PDMS)[51] and the balance subtest of the Bruininks-Oseretsky Test of Motor Proficiency (BOTMP).[52] Care should be taken in the selection of tests; not all are appropriate for all ages (Table 24–1). In addition to testing balance, the PDMS and BOTMP include visuomotor, perceptual-motor, and eye-hand coordination subtests, which enable age-appropriate functional testing of the VO system. Tasks include target skills, tracing, bilateral coordination, and pencil and paper tasks. The BOTMP and PDMS are valuable in documenting general gross and fine motor developmental status and providing more specific measures of balance and visual motor development. The prone extension test component of the Sensory Integration and Praxis Tests (SIPT)[53] also provides a test of Vsp function (Figure 24–4). Other test components of the SIPT are used primarily to assess children with learning disabilities, and focus on form and space perception, praxis, and tactile discrimination. For younger children, the Test of

Sensory Functions in Infants[54] and the DeGangi-Berk Test of Sensory Integration[40] can be used to test ocular motor control and developmental reflex integration (e.g., tonic labyrinthine, symmetric and asymmetric tonic neck reflexes; Figure 24–5). These tests of sensory integration are appropriate for children with only mild motor delays, and are reportedly valid for identifying vestibular dysfunction.[3] The use of these tests and interventions for motor planning, dyspraxia, and sensory integration are more appropriately and completely reviewed elsewhere[3] and will not be further addressed here. Children with deficits on any of the complete tests noted above, or more specifically, on the balance, reflexive, or visual motor subtests, should be examined further for sensory (vision, somatosensory, and vestibular) and postural control system effectiveness, including screening of neurological and musculoskeletal systems.

The musculoskeletal system must be examined to determine if restrictions in range of motion, pain, reduced strength, or limited endurance are present. Each of these may affect postural alignment or the availability of movement strategies to maintain equilibrium, and thus increase sway. Therefore, observation of abnormally increased sway may be due to weakness, joint instability, or CNS impairment. Use of these measures of musculoskeletal system integrity may assist in differential diagnosis of a normal CNS response to an abnormal musculoskeletal system, or an abnormal CNS response with normal musculoskeletal system activity. Subtests of the PDMS, BOTMP and the sensory integration tests can provide screening of neurological status (e.g., Romberg testing with eyes open and closed, finger to nose with eyes open and closed, developmental tonic reflex integration). Further neurological screening should include testing of deep tendon responses, cranial nerve testing, status of equilibrium reactions, and screening of the sensory systems involved in postural control.[49]

Sensory screening should include an examination of the visual, somatosensory, and vestibular systems. Somatosensory screening involves testing the integrity of the tactile and proprioceptive senses, to include testing of touch sensitivity, localization and discrimination (e.g., graphesthesia), and proprioception or position sense in the lower extremities. Visual screening should include observation of visual tracking and visual field capabilities, as well as an examination of the integrity of VO responses (see Table 24–1). VO mechanisms can be examined by noting the presence of abnormal responses, such as gaze-evoked or positional nystagmus, visual stabilization during head rotation or vestibular autorotation testing (VAT).[55] For children who cannot read, charts are available with symbols (Figure 24–6). Additional screening tests of the VO system include the head shake and post rotary nystagmus tests.[56,57] The Southern California Post Rotary Nystagmus Test (PRNT)[56] has been normed for children through 9 years of age and shown to yield reliable measures, that correlate with rotary chair test results in the identification of hypofunction.[58,59] If a balance or visuomotor deficit is evident, concomitant with evidence of VO or Vsp deficit as tested above, further diagnostic testing of vestibular function is warranted.

To isolate and test VO function, caloric and rotary chair testing are used. Normative values are available for children as young as 1 year.[7,34,59] To test Vsp function, dynamic posturography testing is used.[44,60] Dynamic posturography testing involves both a sensory organization test (SOT) and dynamic perturbation test (DPT), which complement and expand the information provided by traditional clinical testing, and yield objective, reliable[61,62] and valid[63,64] functional measure of postural control.[18] Measures obtained with these tests have been shown to identify patients with vestibular dysfunction,[63,64] and are sensitive to changes in functional abilities.[18,65] Although the

TABLE 24–1 Assessment of Vestibular Dysfunction in Children

Assessment Tool	Test Type	Vestibular System	Age Group	Items/Behaviors Tested
Peabody Developmental Motor Scales[51]	Motor development Balance ability/development Visual perception Balance, locomotor, nonlocomotor, visuomotor, and reflex subtests	Vsp[a] VO[b]	Birth through 83 months	Developmental reflexes Balance beam, EO and EC Single leg stance EO & EC Hop; tandem stand/walk Visual track and perception Target activities
Bruininks-Oseretsky Test of Motor Proficiency[52]	Balance and gross motor ability Balance, visual motor, eye-hand and bilateral coordination subtests	Vsp Vsp VO	4 through 14 years	Balance on beam in tandem and single leg stance Single leg EO and EC Target and tracing tasks Romberg test, finger to nose, bilateral coordination tasks
DeGangi-Berk Test of Sensory Integration[55]	Sensory integration and motor planning Postural control, bilateral motor and reflex integration subtests	Vsp, VO	3 through 5 years	Pivot prone and supine flexion Postural tone Diadokokinesis Tapping, jumping and bilateral tasks ATNR and STNR testing
Test of Sensory Function in Infants[54]	Sensory processing and reactivity in infants	VO, Vsp	4 through 18 months	Responses to tactile, vestibular and visual, ocular motor control

Test		System	Age	Measures
The Sensory Integration and Praxis Tests[53]	Sensory integration and motor planning abilities Visual perception	Vsp, VO	4 through 8 years	Form and space perception Praxis Tactile discrimination Vestibular integration
Southern California Post Rotary Nystagmus Test[57]	Vestibular ocular system test	VO	5 through 11 years	Nystagmus duration after rotation
Functional Reach[50]	Balance ability in standing	Vsp	5 through 15 years	Forward reaching, standing
Pediatric Clinical Test of Sensory Interaction for Balance[64,70]	Balance under varying sensory conditions			
Dynamic Posturography Testing[43,48]	Functional test of balance Effectiveness of vestibular, visual and somatosensory systems	Vsp	4 through 9 years	Measures of sway in double leg stance with EO and EC, while standing on foam or floor, or with conflict dome
Timed Up and Go test[71]	Functional stand and walk test	Vsp Vsp	Normative data 3 years through adult on SOT; DPT component, 1.5 years through adult 3 years through adult	SOT—computerized measures of sway DPT—measures EMG responses to perturbation, standing Time to rise from chair, walk 3 meters and return to sitting
Vestibular Auto-Rotation Test[56]	Visual Stability (VO function)	VO		Maintain visual stabilization with head or object movement

[a]Vestibulospinal system
[b]Vestibulo-ocular system

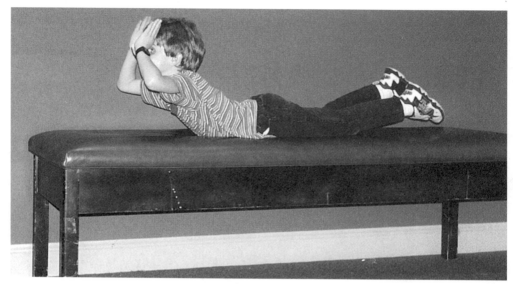

FIGURE 24–4. The prone extension test[53] examines the child's ability to assume and maintain a pivot prone position. Inability to do so is indicative of persistence of the tonic labyrinthine reflex.

sensory and motor tests noted above enable the clinician to isolate the integrity of the different components of postural control, they do not measure the functional use and effectiveness of the sensory modalities, or the integrative capabilities necessary for postural control, which the SOT provides. In addition, sensory system ratios calculated from results obtained from the SOT may be used to monitor dominance or maturation of sensory system effectiveness in postural control. Somatosensory, visual, and vestibular ratios are calculated from stability scores of the SOT as follows: somatosensory ratio = (SV score) ÷ (EO score); vision ratio = (SS score) ÷ (EO score); and vestibular ratio = (ECSS score) ÷ (EO score).[48] Recently, normative values of all SOT scores and ratio measures have been reported for children 3 through 15 years of age (see Figure 24–3).[43,48] A clinical, less sophisticated form of the sensory organization test, which requires inexpensive materials and is portable, has been developed.[66] Westcott et al[67] developed a pediatric version of this test, the Pediatric Clinical Test of Sensory Interaction for Balance (P-CTSIB), and reported fair to good reliability when combined sensory conditions scores were used. Using the P-CTSIB, the examiner documents duration of balance (up to 30 seconds), and body sway under the six SOT conditions using a dome and medium-density foam.

The DPT component of posturography includes EMG recording of selected, individual leg muscle responses to a 4° toes-up perturbation. The latency and amplitude measures obtained enable determination of the integrity of spinal and CNS function in postural control. Specifically, the short latency response of soleus is representative of spinal and peripheral level mechanisms. Measures of the response of anterior tibialis provide an indirect measure of Vsp function.[44,68] Maturation changes in these neuromotor components of postural control can, therefore, be measured and monitored. Although Muller et al[40] and Dichigans et al[44] have reported that responses are apparent with minimal maturation changes noted in the very early stages of learning to stand

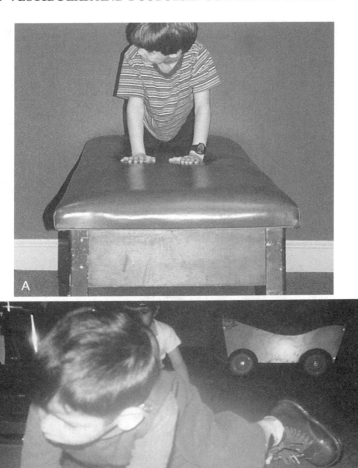

FIGURE 24–5. One method of testing if the asymmetrical tonic neck reflex is interfering with function is to request that the child maintain quadruped with elbows extended as he/she looks to the left or right: (*A*) the child without deficit is able to do so without difficulty, (*B*) the arms collapse as the child attempts to look to his right.

and walk, normative data are not yet available for children. In a recent review, Harcourt[63] reported that posturography testing may not be as sensitive as caloric testing in the identification of individuals with peripheral vestibulopathy. Yet, posturography does provide additional information and is most valuable for identifying patients with central abnormalities.

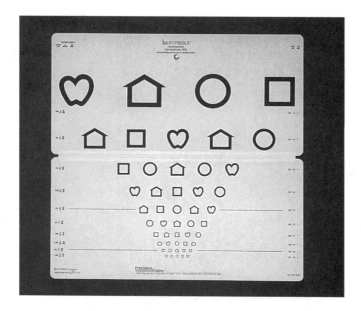

FIGURE 24–6. For children who do not know letters, vision charts with symbols can be used. (Obtained from Lighthouse Low Vision Products, 36-02 Northern Blvd., Long Island City, NY 11101.)

TREATMENT

Peripheral Disorders

Like adults with peripheral dysfunction, once a diagnosis is complete, medical management and rehabilitation should begin. Treatment may include medication, surgery, or vestibular adaptation, and vision and balance training activities (see Chapters 10, 11, and 17). The balance and adaptation training activities must be modified to the child's level of cognitive maturation and interest level, with particular consideration to the care giver. Unlike the adult who will be responsible for his or her own exercise regimen, the child depends on parents and therapists to carry out the program and assure compliance. To maximize the child's participation and cooperation, the use of toys, games, and other items to facilitate visual tracking, or the use of swings to provide the movement during visual stabilization activities, is important. Instead of letters, which are not motivating or fun, line pictures, moving ball or animal with symbols or letters, or even simple computer or video games may be used. If the child can interact, attempt to grasp or point to specific letters or symbols, while sitting, swinging, and so on, therapy becomes a game, is fun, and may minimize resistance and maximize effort and cooperation. This cooperation and effort are critical to the effectiveness of the exercise regimen. Typically, after acute symptoms have subsided, and appropriate medical treatment is rendered (e.g., surgery to repair fistula), children are eager to resume play and other age-appropriate activities. Monitoring progress is critical, and short-term training should be carried out at home with care givers (e.g., visual tracking exercises, visual stabilization regimen, balance and movement activities to resume age-appropriate levels of activity).

Central Vestibular and Postural Control Deficits

As noted previously, few studies have been conducted to examine vestibular function in children with CNS disorders. However, reports do note postural control and sensory organization deficits in children with learning disability or cerebral palsy.[22,26,69,70] In addition, investigators report that vestibular stimulation does improve motor and visual abilities in low-birth-weight premature infants and children with CNS deficit or autism.[22,71–73] Specific clinical signs and symptoms of central deficits have been delineated elsewhere in this volume. Reportedly, postural control deficits are the most consistent finding. Therefore, children with deficits of balance, postural control ability, and visual motor function should be evaluated for VO and Vsp function, and differential diagnosis of the multiple factors involved should be completed. Treatment can then be developed to either facilitate the use and integration of systems intact but not used, or to facilitate compensatory mechanisms. For example, a child with hypertonus, developmental delay, and evidence of VO and Vsp dysfunction should participate in programs that include facilitation and improvement of visual stabilization ability, movement tolerance, and balancing during visual stabilization. Balance training under varying sensory environments should be encouraged by using intact systems, and facilitating integration of information. Unlike treatment for peripheral disorders, in which the focus is on forced use of remaining vestibular mechanisms, treatment for central disorders (e.g., the peripheral vestibular apparatus is intact) should focus not only on use of vestibular information, but on all aspects and mechanisms involved in postural control. Specific treatment foci should be developed on an individual basis, because each patient demonstrates unique strengths and weaknesses (e.g., appropriate or abnormal muscle tone, sensory integrative deficit). Although there is evidence to support the efficacy of intervention in adults, the same cannot be said for the pediatric population.

CASE STUDIES

CASE 1

A 7.5-year-old girl is admitted to the hospital with complaints of dizziness, nystagmus, spinning sensation, and inability to sit or stand. She was diagnosed with vestibular neuritis, hospitalized, and treated for 3 days. At discharge, she was referred to physical therapy for evaluation and treatment of symptoms. Evaluation revealed the following:

- Equilibrium reactions: Intact; Patient was able to single leg stance with EO 2 seconds, and with EC 1 second, either leg; she was unable to walk on a 3.5-inch balance beam in forward or sideways directions; she was able to stand in tandem 3 seconds, but not walk in tandem without side stepping.
- Neurological screening: Deep tendon reflexes were intact; finger-to-nose testing was negative; rapid, alternating upper and lower extremity movements were also intact.
- Vision and VO testing: On visual tracking test, optokinetic and gaze-evoked nystagmus were noted; a tendency to maintain the head tilted to the right was observed; patient favored the left eye by semiclosure of the right during dynamic visual acuity testing, which was normal except for this "squint."
- Posturography testing: Loss of balance occurred on the ECSS and SVSS conditions; vision ratio was within normal limits, but the vestibular ratio was well below normative age values (more than 2 standard deviations below mean).

A parent was trained in visual stabilization techniques using flash cards the child enjoyed and was familiar with (e.g., single word on a card). The two activities were to be practiced daily, 2 minutes each: (1) Read card as head or card is moved: (a) child is to read card as it is moved to right and left at 1 Hz; (b) with card stabilized at midline, child is to read card as head is turned to the left and right at 1 Hz (once able to do this without difficulties, increase speed of head/card movement to 2 Hz); (2) read 4 "word cards" taped on wall at eye level of child, 6 feet from child: (a) practice reading cards as head is rotated right and left (perform binocularly and monocularly). Additional activities/instructions for the parent included: (1) encourage play as before and practice balancing by walking between tape lines 4 inches apart on floor, gradually reducing to 3 inches; progress to walking heel-to-toe on line or foot prints (practice 2 minutes daily); (2) encourage hopping games five times weekly (e.g., hop scotch, jump rope swung slowly back and forth by Mom and child to jump over it). Owing to difficulties in transportation, weekly monitoring of progress and adjustment of exercises was done via phone contact. In 2 months, all symptoms were relieved. The child was able to tandem stand and walk 5 feet. No difficulties were noted with reading or visual fixation with either card or head movement.

CASE 2

A 7-year-old boy was referred for assessment due to recent complaints of dizziness, vertigo and vision difficulties. The child was born premature with a low birth weight (1.5 pounds). Sensorineural hearing impairment was diagnosed at 18 months of age. However, with use of hearing aids, audiologic testing was within normal limits, and the child did comprehend spoken language and spoke clearly. He also had a history of frequent ear infections with drainage tubes inserted twice (bilaterally). Due to vision and reading difficulties, this child had been recently placed in a special education program for learning disability. He was referred for testing to establish vestibular functional status, and to determine if further testing or treatment was warranted. Parent reported that until recently, typical activities included playing T-ball and basketball with peers (intramural sports). Review of records indicated treatment with gentamicin and amoxicillin during the past few years.

- Vision and VO testing: Patient and parent reported dizziness with moving visual stimuli (e.g., looking up at sky and watching clouds, watching television, changing visual direction in classroom), and that at times his "eyes do funny things." When asked to demonstrate this, the child replicated nystagmus. Difficulties with smooth pursuit were noted, with corrective saccades and attempts to turn the head to maintain fixation on a moving target. Dynamic visual acuity was normal. Although nystagmus was not exaggerated on head shake test, the child reported dizziness. Hyperactive response was observed on the PRNT, with nystagmus duration of 35 seconds and complaints of severe vertigo following rotation in either direction.
- Motor and balance ability: Patient was able to single leg stance EO 6 seconds, and EC 3 seconds. He was able to walk a 3.5-inch balance beam, but not balance standing across beam in double or single leg stance. On the BOTMP, he

achieved an age equivalent score of 4 years 11 months and 7 years 8 months on the Balance and Visual-Motor Coordination subtests, respectively.

- Neurological screening: The following were within normal limits: deep tendon reflexes, rapid alternating movements, integration of labyrinthine reflexes (e.g., able to assume and hold pivot prone) and finger-to-nose test.
- Posturography (SOT): Patient relied on stepping strategy to maintain upright on the ECSS and SVSS conditions, and posturing was noted on the SS condition. He achieved a vision ratio of .29 (more than two standard deviations below norm for age) and vestibular ratios of .45 (2 standard deviations below norm for age).

The patient was referred for further medical diagnostic testing for possible fistula, which was substantiated. Surgical correction was performed. Physical therapy following surgery focused on visual stabilization and balance retraining. Within 2 months, all vertigo and dizziness were eliminated. Reading ability improved so that the child was removed from learning disability program and placed in a gifted program. Within 6 months, the child resumed all activities, including playing basketball with peers.

CASE 3

This 9-year-old girl with a diagnosis of spastic hemiplegia since birth presented with gait and balance deviations, and delayed gross motor functioning. IQ testing was within normal limits, and thus she was placed in a fully integrated classroom with itinerant physical and occupational therapy, each provided twice weekly.

- Neurodevelopmental status: Hypertonicity was evident in the right upper and lower extremity. Balance testing revealed deficits: unable to balance in single leg stance on right with EO or EC; equilibrium reactions intact but delayed (e.g., reliance on tilting reactions in quadruped and kneeling, and on protective extension stepping/staggering in upright); balance in all positions was challenged by head rotations. Persistence of developmental reflexes was noted: ATNR and STNR evidenced with increased arm extension in direction of head turning, and inability to lean forward in quadruped, with less than 120° of flexion at the hips if head was extended to look forward; tonic labyrinthine was evident with inability to assume pivot prone extension position.
- Gait and motor ability: Gait deviations included: toe-heel contact on the right, knee flexion during midstance on right, lack of arm swing, and wide base of support. Patient was unable to run. A 1-inch leg length discrepancy was noted with the right leg being shorter. Gross motor functional level was 30 months.
- Vestibular testing: Patient could not tolerate movement in a net swing (e.g., fearful and complaints of dizziness). Hyperactive nystagmus response was noted on the PRNT (duration of 90 seconds in either direction), and the patient reported that she felt "upside down" for the duration of the nystagmus following the rotation. On the P-CTSIB she was able to balance in double leg stance with EO or EC with minimal sway, but staggered when asked to stand on foam with EO or EC. She could not balance with the dome on her head standing on

the floor or dense foam (indicative of failure on SOT conditions 4 through 6). No gaze-evoked nystagmus was evident.
- Vision testing: Visual tracking was intact in all directions with no nystagmus. A difference of two lines was noted on dynamic visual acuity testing (head stationary versus rotating side to side).

Due to the lack of dizziness or complaints of vertigo, a central vestibular deficit was identified and no further diagnostic testing was performed. Physical therapy treatment continued as before with the addition of facilitation of integration of tonic reflexes by use of vestibular stimulation on a scooter board, and vestibular stimulation in a net swing with and without visual fixation. Velocity and directions of movement were gradually increased, to tolerance. Balance training activities were added to include balancing in kneeling and upright on compliant surfaces (high-density foam), the use of Romper Stompers in upright, and swinging baseball bat at ball on a "Tee" (rotation with visual fixation on ball). A 3/4-inch full sole lift was placed on the right shoe.

Initially, the child was unable to locate items on a visually complex poster when swinging in swing less than 1 Hz. Within 3 months, she was able to locate very small (.5- to 1-inch diameter) items on complex poster while swinging in net swing in both the forward-backward and side-side directions while prone. Within 6 months, she was able to complete this activity in sitting. Balance improved tremendously, with the patient being able to walk on dense foam with EO and EC within 9 months. Gait improved with heel-toe contact within 6 months. Gross motor performance increased 24 months in 9 months time (per age equivalent score on the Peabody Developmental Motor Scales). At the end of 15 months, she could roller skate and participate in all physical activities with peers. Gait deviations were essentially undetectable to the untrained eye. She was discharged from physical therapy services at school.

SUMMARY

Similar to adults, children do present with postural control and vestibular deficits, and the development of appropriate intervention is dependent upon an accurate, comprehensive evaluation. Recent research has resulted in the availability of normative data that enables in depth analysis of postural control and vestibular system function in young children. Therefore, a comprehensive assessment of these systems should be included as part of the evaluation of children presenting with evidence of balance or postural control deficits, complaints of dizziness, or a history of inner ear disease or injury. Owing to the effect of age at the time of onset on compensatory mechanisms, and maturation of sensory and integration systems, care must be given to the interpretation of test results. Based on the appropriate interpretation of the evaluation results an intervention program should begin, which may include activities to facilitate habituation, sensory integration or organization, balance and/or vestibular training, and visual stabilization exercises. Age and maturation must also be considered in the selection and design of intervention strategies to address the specific problem identified.

The intervention activities to be implemented with children must be age appropriate with regard to comprehension and interest levels. In addition, education and training of caregivers and/or parents is critical to the success of the program. Despite the paucity of research regarding treatment of this population, the case studies presented here and reports in the literature do provide evidence to support the importance of identification of, and intervention for, vestibular and postural control deficits in children.

REFERENCES

1. Kodama, A, and Sando, I: Postnatal development of the vestibular aqueduct and endolymphatic sac. Ann Otolaryngol Rhinol Laryngol 91:3, 1982.
2. Nadol, JB, and Hsu, W: Histopathologic correlation of spiral ganglion cell count and new bone formation in the cochlea following meningogenic labyrinthitis and deafness. Ann Otol Rhinol Laryngol 100:712, 1991.
3. Ayres, J: Sensory Integration and Learning Disorders. Western Psychological Services, Los Angeles, 1983.
4. Fried, MP: The evaluation of dizziness in children. Laryngoscope 90:1548, 1980.
5. Muller, K, et al: Maturation of set-modulation of lower extremity EMG responses to postural perturbations. Neuropediatrics 23:82, 1992.
6. Montgomery, P: Assessment of vestibular function in children. Phys Occupational Ther Pediatr 5:33, 1985.
7. Cioni, G, et al: Development of the dynamic characteristics of the horizontal vestibulo-ocular reflex in infancy. Neuropediatrics 15:125, 1984.
8. Von Hofsten, C, and Rosander, K: The development of gaze control and predictive tracking in young infants. Vision Res 36:81, 1996.
9. Busis, SN: Vertigo in children. Pediatr Otolaryngol Pediatr Ann 478, Aug. 1976.
10. Clark, JE, and Watkins, DL: Static balance in young children. Child Dev 55:854, 1984.
11. Balkany, TJ, and Finkel, RS: The dizzy child. Ear Hearing 7:138, 1986.
12. Bower, B: Fits and other frightening or funny turns in young children. Practitioner 225:225, 1981.
13. Casselbrant, ML, et al: Effect of otitis media on the vestibular system in children. Ann Otol Rhinol Laryngol 104:620, 1995.
14. Das, VK: Pendred's syndrome with episodic vertigo, tinnitus and vomiting and bithermal caloric responses. J Laryngol Otol 101:721, 1987.
15. Enbom, H, et al: Postural compensation in children with congenital or early acquired bilateral vestibular loss. Ann Otol Rhinol Laryngol 100:472, 1991.
16. Finkelhor, BK, and Harker, LA: Benign paroxysmal vertigo in childhood. Laryngoscope 97:1161, 1987.
17. Shirabe, S: Vestibular neuritis in childhood. Acta Otolaryngol 458:120, 1988.
18. Healy, GB, et al: Ataxia and hearing loss secondary to perilymphatic fistula. Pediatrics 61:238, 1978.
19. Barron, S, and Irvine, J: Effects of neonatal cocaine exposure on two measures of balance and coordination. Neurotoxicol Teratol 16:89, 1994.
20. Brogen, E, et al: Postural control in children with spastic diplegia: muscle activity during perturbations in sitting. Devel Med Child Neurol 38:379, 1996.
21. Bundy, AC, et al: Concurrent validity of equilibrium tests in boys with learning disabilities with and without vestibular dysfunction. Am J Occup Ther 41:28, 1987.
22. Horak, FB, et al: Vestibular function and motor proficiency of children with impaired hearing or with learning disability and motor impairments. Devel Med Child Neurol 30:64, 1988.
23. Liao, HF, et al: The relation between standing balance and walking function in children with spastic diplegic cerebral palsy. Devel Med Child Neurol 39:106, 1997.
24. Reid, DT, et al: An investigation of postural sway in sitting of normal children and children with neurological disorders. Phys Occupational Ther Pediatr 11:19, 1991.
25. Tsuzuku, T, and Kaga, K: Delayed motor function and results of vestibular function tests in children with inner ear anomalies. Int J Pediatr Otorhinolaryngol 23:261, 1992.
26. Deitz, JC, et al: Performance of children with learning disabilities and motor delays on the Pediatric Clinical Test of Sensory Interaction for Balance (P-CTSIB). Phys Occupational Ther Pediatr 16:1, 1996.
27. Morrison, D, and Sublett, J: Reliability of the Southern California Postrotary Nystagmus test with learning-disabled children. Am J Occup Ther 37:694, 1983.
28. Schaaf, RC: The frequency of vestibular disorders in developmentally delayed preschoolers with otitis media. Am J Occup Ther 39:247, 1985.
29. Rapin, I: Hypoactive labyrinths and motor development. Clin Pediatr 13:922, 1974.
30. Kaga, K, et al: Development of righting reflexes, gross motor functions and balance in infants with labyrinth hypoactivity with or without mental retardation. Adv Otorhinolaryngol 41:151, 1988.
31. Sandberg, LE, and Terkildsen, K: Caloric tests in deaf children. Arch Otolaryngol 81:350, 1965.
32. Rine, RM, et al: Balance and motor skills in young children with sensorineural hearing impairment: A preliminary study. Pediatr Phys Ther 8:55, 1996.

33. Rine, RM, et al: Relationship of vestibular function, motor and postural control ability in children with hearing impairment—A preliminary study. Pediatr Phys Ther 9:194, 1997.
34. Eviatar, L, and Eviatar, A: The normal nystagmic response of infants to caloric and perrotatory stimulation. Laryngoscope 89:1036, 1979.
35. Villablanca, JR, et al: Neurological and behavioral effects of a unilateral frontal cortical lesion in fetal kittens II. Visual system tests, and proposing an "optimal developmental period" for lesion effects. Behav Brain Res 57:79, 1993.
36. Horak, FB, et al: Vestibular and somatosensory contributions to responses to head and body displacements in stance. Exp Brain Res 100:93, 1994.
37. Nashner, LM, et al: Stance posture control in select groups of children with cerebral palsy: Deficits in sensory organization and muscular coordination. Exp Brain Res 49:393, 1983.
38. Forssberg, H, and Nashner, LM: Ontogenetic development of postural control in man: Adaptation to altered support and visual condition during stance. J Neurosci 2:545, 1982.
39. Haas, G, et al: Development of postural control in children: Short-, medium-, and long-latency EMG responses of leg muscles after perturbation of stance. Exp Brain Res 64:127, 1986.
40. Berk, RA, and DeGangi, GA: DeGangi-Berk Test of Sensory Integration. Western Psychological Services, Los Angeles, 1983.
41. Woollacott, MH, and Shumway-Cook, A: Changes in postural control across the life span—A systems approach. Phys Ther 70:799, 1990.
42. Woollacott, MH, et al: Neuromuscular control of posture in the infant and child: Is vision dominant? J Motor Behav 19:167, 1987.
43. Hirabayashi, S, and Iwasaki, Y: Developmental perspective of sensory organization on postural control. Brain Devel 17:111, 1995.
44. Dichigans, J, and Deiner, HC: The use of short- and long-latency reflex testing in leg muscles of neurological patients. In Struppler, A, and Weindl, A (eds): Clinical Aspects of Sensory Motor Integration. Berlin, Springer-Verlag, 1987.
45. Foudriat, BA, et al: Sensory organization of balance responses in children 3–6 years of age: A normative study with diagnostic implications. Int J Pediatr Otorhinolaryngol 27:225, 1993.
46. Riach, CL, and Starkes, JL: Visual fixation and postural sway. J Motor Beh 21:265, 1989.
47. Riach, CL, and Hayes, KC: Maturation of postural sway in young children. Devel Med Child Neurol 29:650, 1987.
48. Rine, RM, et al: Measurement of sensory system effectiveness and maturational changes in postural control in young children. Pediatr Phys Ther 10:16, 1998.
49. Westcott, SL, et al: Evaluation of postural stability in children: Current theories and assessment tools. Phys Ther 77:629, 1997.
50. Donahue, B, et al: The use of functional reach as a measurement of balance in boys and girls without disabilities ages 5 to 15 years. Pediatr Phys Ther 6:189, 1994.
51. Folio, MR, and Fewell, R: Peabody Developmental Motor Scales. Riverside Publishing, Chicago, 1983.
52. Bruininks, RH: Bruininks-Oseretsky Test of Motor Proficiency: Examiner's Manual. American Guidance Service, Circle Pines, MN, 1978.
53. Ayres, AJ: Sensory Integration and Praxis Tests. Western Psychological Services, Los Angeles, 1989.
54. DeGangi, GA, and Greenspan, SI: Test of Sensory Function in Infants. Western Psychological Services, Los Angeles, 1989.
55. Saadat, D, et al: High frequency horizontal vestibulo-ocular reflex testing in children. Research Forum. American Academy of Otolaryngology Head and Neck Surgery, 1994.
56. Ayres, AJ: Southern California Postrotary Nystagmus Test. Western Psychological Services, Los Angeles, 1989.
57. Nashner, LM, and Peters, JF: Dynamic posturography in the diagnosis and management of dizziness and balance disorders. Neurol Clin 8:331, 1990.
58. Keating, NR: A comparison of duration of nystagmus as measured by the Southern California Postrotary Nystagmus Test and electronystagmography. Am J Occup Ther 33:92, 1979.
59. Wiener-Vacher, SR, et al: Canal and otolith vestibulo-ocular reflexes to vertical and off vertical axis rotations in children learning to walk. Acta Otolaryngol 116:657, 1996.
60. Diener, HC, et al: Variability of postural "reflexes" in humans. Exp Brain Res 52:423, 1983.
61. Rine, RM, et al: Reliability of EMG measures obtained during dynamic balance testing. Conference Proceedings, APTA Combined Sections Meeting 1998.
62. Rine, RM, et al: Reliability of postural sway, strategy scores and muscle responses during quiet stance. Phys Ther s43, 1997.
63. Harcourt, JP: Posturography—Applications and limitations in the management of the dizzy patient. Clin Otolaryngol 20:299, 1995.
64. Furman, JMR, et al: Assessment: Posturography. Neurology 43:1261, 1993.
65. Shepard, NT: The clinical use of dynamic posturography in the elderly. Ear Nose Throat 68:940, 1989.
66. Shumway-Cook, A, and Horak, FB: Assessing the influence of sensory interaction on balance. Phys Ther 66:1548, 1986.

67. Westcott, SL, et al: Test-retest reliability of the Pediatric Clinical Test of Sensory Interaction for Balance (P-CTSIB). Phys Occup Ther Pediatr 14:1, 1994.
68. Allum, JHJ, et al: Differential control of leg and trunk muscle activity by vestibulo-spinal and proprioceptive signals during human balance corrections. Acta Otolaryngol 115:124, 1995.
69. Isaacson, JE, et al: Learning disability in children with postmeningitic cochlear implants. Arch Otolaryngol Head Neck Surg 122:929, 1996.
70. Lowes, PL: An evaluation of the standing balance of children with cerebral palsy and the tools for assessment. Medical College of Pennsylvania and Hahnemann University, 1996.
71. Gregg, CL, et al: The relative efficacy of vestibular-proprioceptive stimulation and the upright position in enhancing visual pursuit in neonates. Child Devel 309, 1997.
72. Slavik, BA, et al: Vestibular stimulation and eye contact in autistic children. Neuropediatrics 15:33, 1984.
73. Wincent, MM, and Engel, JM: Vestibular-proprioceptive abilities in children experiencing recurrent headaches. Phys Occup Ther Pediatr 14:63, 1994.

CHAPTER 25

Physical Therapy Diagnosis for Vestibular Disorders

Susan J. Herdman, PT, PhD

Diagnosis can be defined as "the art of distinguishing one disease from another."[1] In medicine, the identification of a particular disease leads to specific medical and/or surgical treatment. A physical therapy (PT) diagnosis differs from a medical diagnosis in that, rather than attempting to identify a particular disease, a constellation of symptoms and signs toward which physical (and occupational) therapy will be directed is identified. Once the PT diagnosis is achieved, the general exercise approach can be identified (Table 25–1). Certainly there will be times when the medical diagnosis and the PT diagnosis are the same, for example, benign paroxysmal positional vertigo (BPPV). However, there will be times when the diagnoses will differ. For example, vestibular neuronitis would be a medical diagnosis. As therapists, however, we do not treat the inflammatory process of vestibular neuronitis. A more appropriate PT diagnosis would be vestibular hypofunction.

The diagnostic schematic presented here is a "work in progress." It is offered as a framework for arriving at a physical diagnosis for patients with vestibular problems. Each of the PT diagnoses presented should demonstrate commonalities across all persons with that diagnosis. There are two phases to making the PT diagnosis. The first is in the history of the patient's complaints; the second consists of some simple clinical tests of the vestibulo-ocular system.

HISTORY

Of special importance in the patient's history are the nature of the patient's symptoms and the temporal quality of those symptoms. The *nature* of the symptom refers to whether the patient is complaining of *vertigo* (an illusion of movement, typically vertigo or spinning) or of *disequilibrium* (the sense of being off-balance). The *temporal* quality of the symptoms refers to whether the symptoms are episodic or continuous in na-

TABLE 25–1 Diagnosis-Driven Treatment

Diagnosis	Treatment Options
BPPV	Canalith repositioning, liberatory, Brandt-Daroff
Unilateral vestibular hypofunction	Adaptation, substitution (habituation)
Motion sensitivity	Habituation
Bilateral vestibular loss	Substitution, adaptation
Central vestibular	Habituation

ture. If the symptoms are episodic, it is important to establish the duration of the episode. For example, episodes of vertigo lasting seconds or less than 1 minute suggest BPPV.

CLINICAL EXAMINATION

The first of simple clinical tests of the vestibulo-ocular system is positional testing. A positive response to positional testing would consist of vertigo *and* nystagmus being provoked when the patient's head is in specific positions. The duration and direction of the nystagmus is used to diagnose positional vertigo that is peripheral (e.g., BPPV; see Chapter 19) or central in origin.

The second clinical test is the assessment of the gain of the vestibulo-ocular reflex (VOR) using rapid (high-acceleration) head movements (head-thrust test; see Chapters 6 and 15). The presence of the corrective saccade (positive head-thrust test) indicates the low gain of the vestibular system. If the person makes a corrective saccade following a head thrust to the right, the vestibular loss is on the right. If the person makes corrective saccades with head thrusts to the right and to the left, it indicates a bilateral vestibular loss. The sensitivity of the head-thrust test for identifying patients with unilateral vestibular loss is actually fairly low (35%) but its specificity is very high (95%).[2] That is, many patients with unilateral vestibular loss will not have a positive head-thrust test, but if the patient does have a positive test, it is likely that the patient has a vestibular deficit. Our results with patients with bilateral vestibular loss suggest that there may be a higher sensitivity of the head-thrust test for this patient group. Another simple clinical test that can be used to assess vestibular function is the measure of visual acuity during horizontal head movement (dynamic visual acuity [DVA]) (see Chapter 15). The sensitivity of the clinical DVA test for vestibular deficits is approximately 85% and its specificity is 55%.[3]

DIAGNOSTIC FLOWCHART

The first question asked is whether or not the patient has complaints of vertigo (Figure 25–1). If the patient has a history of vertigo (spinning), the next step is to determine the duration of the vertigo. Spells of vertigo lasting for brief periods of time (< 1 minute) suggest BPPV, the most common cause of vertigo owing to a peripheral vestibular problem (see Chapter 19 for the diagnostic flowchart for BPPV). It is important to

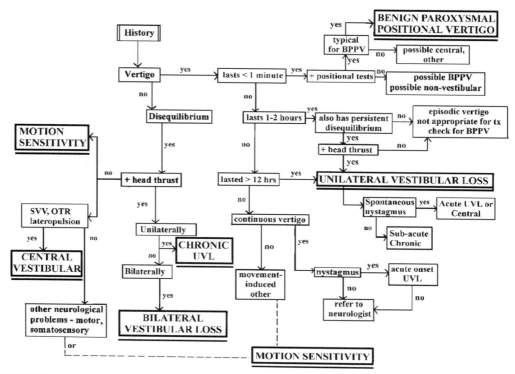

FIGURE 25–1. This flow diagram begins with the *history* (upper left). The patients should be asked if they have experienced *vertigo* (a sense of spinning). If the answer is "yes," the next series of questions deals with the temporal nature of that vertigo. (Column to the right: <1 minute, 1–2 hours, >12 hours, continuous). The temporal quality of the vertigo then leads to diagnoses of BPPV, episodic vertigo, unilateral vestibular loss, continuous vertigo, and motion sensitivity. Note that some of these diagnoses are appropriate for PT treatment, while others are not. If, on history, the patient states that he or she has not experienced vertigo but rather has complaints of *disequilibrium*, the path leads to diagnoses that must be distinguished based on clinical examination. Note how the presence or absence of corrective saccades to rapid head thrusts is used to identify unilateral and bilateral vestibular loss. UVL = unilateral vestibular loss, SVV = subjective visual vertical, OTR = ocular tilt reaction.

distinguish whether the nystagmus is typical for BPPV (combined torsional and vertical or horizontal), is typical for a central lesion (pure vertical), or if the history suggests another problem like a perilymphatic fistula. Note that positional testing may not provoke vertigo and nystagmus. However, this does not mean that the patient does not have BPPV. The appearance of vertigo and nystagmus during testing is notoriously inconsistent. A diagnosis of BPPV may be reached, at least tentatively, by history alone. Also note that the possibility of a diagnosis of BPPV is raised regardless of the patient's description of the duration of the spell of vertigo. Patients are often poor historians and may believe the vertigo lasted for extended periods of time because they continue to feel poorly even after the actual spinning has stopped. In fact, all patients should be tested for BPPV, including those without complaints of true vertigo. BPPV is very common and has been identified in patients who also have unilateral or bilateral vestibular loss (see Chapters 17 and 18).

Vertigo that lasts for several hours is most likely to be from Ménière's disease (see Chapter 5) or may be a migraine-related event (see Chapter 13). These types of *episodic vertigo* are not appropriate for treatment using vestibular rehabilitation, and must be managed medically. The exception would be the patient who has persistent complaints of imbalance between these episodes of vertigo who might have developed *unilateral vestibular hypofunction* with repeated episodes of Ménière's disease. The head-thrust test may help to identify this problem, although formal vestibular function tests may be necessary.

Vertigo lasting 12 hours to days typically signifies the sudden onset of *unilateral vestibular hypofunction* (see Chapter 5). Spontaneous nystagmus in the light would be observed during the acute period following onset. This spontaneous nystagmus should resolve within 1 to 2 weeks. Failure of spontaneous nystagmus to resolve strongly suggests central involvement of the structures responsible for compensation. Thus, the presence of spontaneous nystagmus in the light should be correlated with time from onset to determine if there is central involvement.

Continuous vertigo has several possible explanations. First, the patient may be in the acute phase following onset of unilateral dysfunction. This can be easily verified by determining when the vertigo started. Second, the patient may not be actually experiencing vertigo continuously or may be misusing the word vertigo. For example, the patient may be experiencing movement-provoked symptoms or *motion sensitivity*. This implies that movement of the individual or, more often, movement of the environment, produces symptoms that may include lightheadedness, nausea, and even an illusion of movement. Although this can occur following unilateral or bilateral vestibular loss, it can also occur in patients with other, non-vestibular problems such as migraine. Finally, complaints of continuous vertigo of long duration suggest problems for which the patient should be referred to a neurologist.

The patient may deny a history of vertigo but may complain of *disequilibrium*. There are many underlying etiologies for the complaint of disequilibrium, both vestibular and non-vestibular. The head-thrust test can be used to identify whether the patient has *chronic unilateral vestibular hypofunction* (positive to one side only) or *bilateral vestibular loss* (positive with head thrusts in both directions). Patients with apparently normal VOR to rapid head thrusts may still have a vestibular deficit so further testing (DVA, vestibular function tests) may be needed to reach this diagnosis.

The complaint of disequilibrium may also be an aspect of motion sensitivity. If patients with disequilibrium specifically have complaints of *lateropulsion* (and abnormal subjective visual vertical and an ocular tilt reaction) they probably have a *central vestibular* problem above the level of the vestibular nuclei (see Chapter 12). Finally, disequilibrium may be related to other neuromuscular problems

IDENTIFICATION OF MODIFIERS

Once a PT diagnosis has been achieved, it is necessary to perform other assessments to identify other problems that will modify the exercise program for each individual patient. These modifiers include disorders affecting other systems, subjective complaints, psychological factors, and the patient's premorbid activity level (Box 25–1). Finally, there are specific assessments that must be performed to establish the patient's baseline performance so that changes in status can be assessed following treatment (Table 25–2).

BOX 25–1 Modifiers of Treatment

Other system involvement
  Visual—Cataracts, macular degeneration, field
  Somatosensory—Peripheral neuropathy
  Musculoskeletal—Cervical, back, arthritis, strength, range of motion
  Central nervous system—Stroke (e.g., brainstem), cerebellar disease
Psychological
  Anxiety, depression
  Perception of disability
  Somatoform, conversion
  Severity of subjective complaints
  Secondary gain issues
Activity Level
  Basic ADL—bath, dress, meals, clean
  Fall history—circumstance, frequency, injury
  Driving—day, night
  Work—harder to perform, changed jobs, not working

SUMMARY

The use of this paradigm should enable the therapist to arrive at a diagnosis in which all patients have a common group of symptoms and signs and that will indicate the appropriate treatments for that patient. The complete examination, including assessment of those factors that will result in modifications in how those exercises are applied, should enable the therapist to develop a problem list, goals, and treatment plan for the patient.

TABLE 25–2 Functional Assessment of Vestibular Dysfunction

Problem	Tests
Subjective complaints	Visual analog scales
	Symptom scale
	DHI
Visual acuity during head movement	Clinical Dynamic Visual Acuity Test
	Computerized dynamic visual acuity test
Balance in stance	Romberg
	Sharpened Romberg
	Single leg stance
	Fukuda's stepping test
Balance while ambulating	Qualitative gait description
	Dynamic Gait Index
	Gait deviations
	Gait with head turn

REFERENCES

1. Dorland's Illustrated Medical Dictionary, ed 24. WB Saunders Company. London, 1965, p 411.
2. Harvey, SA, et al: Relationship of the head impulse test and head-shake nystagmus in reference to caloric testing. Am J Otol 18:207, 1997.
3. Venuto, PJ, et al: Interrater reliability of the clinical dynamic visual acuity test. Scientific Meeting and Exposition of the American Physical Therapy Association, 78:S21, 1998.

Index

An "f" following a page number indicates a figure; a "t" indicates a table.